Urinary Diversion

Second Edition

Urinary Diversion

Second Edition

Edited by

Karl J Kreder MD FACS

Professor and Clinical Vice Chair, Director of Urodynamics and Reconstructive Urology, Department of Urology
University of Iowa Hospitals and Clinics, Iowa City, IA, USA

Anthony R Stone MD

Professor and Vice Chair, Director of Urology, Department of Urology
University of California, Davis, Sacramento CA, USA

Taylor & Francis
Taylor & Francis Group
LONDON AND NEW YORK
A MARTIN DUNITZ BOOK

First published in the United Kingdom in 2005
by Taylor & Francis, an imprint of the Taylor & Francis Group, 2 Park Square,
Milton Park, Abingdon, Oxfordshire OX14 4RN

Tel.: +44 (0) 20 7017 6000
Fax.: +44 (0) 20 7017 6699
E-mail: info@dunitz.co.uk
Website: http://www.dunitz.co.uk

A CIP record for this book is available from the British Library.

Library of Congress Cataloging-in-Publication Data

Data available on application

ISBN 1 84184 353 9

Distributed in North and South America by

Taylor & Francis
2000 NW Corporate Blvd
Boca Raton, FL 33431, USA

Within Continental USA
Tel.: 800 272 7737; Fax.: 800 374 3401
Outside Continental USA
Tel.: 561 994 0555; Fax.: 561 361 6018
E-mail: orders@crcpress.com

Distributed in the rest of the world by
Thomson Publishing Services
Cheriton House
North Way
Andover, Hampshire SP10 5BE, UK
Tel.: +44 (0)1264 332424
E-mail: salesorder.tandf@thomsonpublishingservices.co.uk

Composition by J&L Composition, Filey, North Yorkshire

Printed and bound in Italy by Printer Trento S.r.l.

Contents

SECTION VI: PREVENTION OF REFLUX

SECTION VI: CONDUIT URINARY DIVERSION

Contributors

Joseph B Abdelmalak MD
Glickman Urologic Institute
Cleveland Clinic Foundation
Cleveland, OH, USA

Hassan Abol-Enein MD PhD
Professor of Urology
Urology and Nephrology Center
Mansoura, Egypt

Daniela Andrich MD MRCS
Institute of Urology
London, UK

Ramesh Babu MS MCH FRCS (Paeds)
Specialist Registrar in Paediatric Urology
Department of Paediatric Urology
Wessex Regional Centre for Paediatric Surgery
Southampton University Hospitals NHS Trust
Southampton, UK

Abdellatif Benchekroun MD
Professor
Department of Urology
Hospital Avicenne
Rabat R.P., Morocco

Fiona C Burkhard MD
Department of Urology
University of Berne
Inselspital-Anna Siler-Haus
Berne, Switzerland

Maurice Camey
Professor of Urology (retired)
Paris, France

Lesley K Carr MD FRCS(C)
Medical Director, Women's Pelvic Health Centre
Division of Urology
Sunnybrook and Women's College Health Science Centre
Toronto, Ontario, Canada

Pasquale Casale MD
Assistant Professor of Urology
University of Pennsylvania
Children's Hospital of Philadelphia
Division of Pediatric Urology
Philadelphia, PA, USA

Christopher Chapple BSc MD FRCS(Urol)
Consultant Urological Surgeon
Department of Urology
Royal Hallamshire Hospital
Sheffield, UK

Lise L Christensen MD
Institute of Experimental Clinical Research and Department of Urology
Skejby Hospital
University Hospital in Aarhus
Aarhus, Denmark

Morten Colding-Jørgensen MD MSc
Department of Medical Physiology
The Panum Institute
University of Copenhagen
Copenhagen, Denmark

Christopher S Cooper MD
Associate Professor
Director, Pediatric Urology
The University of Iowa
Iowa City, IA, USA

Joseph A Costa MD
Assistant Professor of Surgery
University of Florida College of Medicine
Head, Section of reconstructive Surgery and Neuourology
University of Florida shands Jacksonville
Jacksonville, FL, USA

Thomas Davidsson MD PhD
Associate Professor
Department of Urology
University Hospital Lund
Lund, Sweden

Jens Christian Djurhuus MD
Professor of Clinical Surgery
Institute of Experimental Clinical Research
University of Aarhus
DK-8200 Aarhus North
Denmark

Ahmed S El-Azab MD
Clinical Research Fellow
Section of Female Urology and Voiding Dysfunction
Glickman Urologic Institute
Cleveland Clinic Foundation
Cleveland, OH, USA

Margit Fisch MD
Professor of urology
Center of Urology and Pediatric Urology Hamburg
Allgemeines Krankenhaus Harburg
Hamburg, Germany

John A Freeman MD
Medical Director
Nevada Urology Associates
Reno, NV, USA

Jorgen Frokiaer MD
Consultant in Clinical Physiology
Institute of Experimental Clinical Research
Department of Clinical Physiology/Nuclear Medicine
Skejby Hospital
University Hospital in Aarhus
Aarhus, Denmark

Elmer W Gerharz MD
Associate Professor of Urology
Department of Urology
Julius Maximilians-University Medical School
Würzburg, Germany

Mohamed A Ghoneim MD PhD
Urology and Nephrology Center
Mansoura University
El Mansoura, Egypt

Inderbir S Gill MD MCh
Glickman Urologic Institute
Cleveland Clinic Foundation
Cleveland, OH, USA

Arthur C Grabowski MD
Sunnybrook & Women's College
Health Science Center
Toronto, Ontario, Canada

Tamsin Greenwell MD FRCS (Urol)
Consultant Urological Surgeon
Institute of Urology
London, UK

Michael Guralnick MD FRCSC
Assistant Professor
Department of Urology
Medical College of Wisconsin
Milwaukee, WI, USA

Rudolf Hohenfeller MD
Head Professor of Urology
University of Mainz
Department of Urology
Mainz, Germany

Mark Horowitz MD
Assistant Professor, Pediatric Urology
Director, Pediatric Voiding Dysfunction Center &
Urodynamics Laboratory
Weill Medical College of Cornell University
New York Presbyterian Hospital
New York, NY, USA

Regina Hovey MD
UCI Medical Center
University of California
Irvine, CA, USA

Christopher Iselin MD
Clinique D'Urologie
Geneva, Switzerland

Troels Munch Jørgensen MD
Department of Urology
Section of Pediatric Urology
Aarhus University Hospital
Aarhus, Denmark

Badrinath Konety MD MBA
Assistant Professor of Urology and Epidemiology
Department of Urology
University of Iowa
Iowa City, IA, USA

Martin A Koyle MD
Professor or Surgery and Paediatrics
Chairman, Department of Paediatric Urology
University of Colorado Health Sciences Center and
The Children's Hospital
Denver, CO, USA

Karl J Kreder MD FACS
Professor and Clinical Vice Chair
Director of Urodynamics and Reconstructive Urology
Department of Urology
University of Iowa Hospitals and Clinics
Iowa City, IA, USA

Eric A Kurzrock MD
Assistant Professor of Pediatrics and Urology
Chief of Pediatric Urology
University of California Davis Children's Hospital
Department of Urology
Sacramento, CA, USA

Jerilyn M Latini MD
Fellow, Female and Reconstructive Urology
Department of Urology
University of Iowa
Iowa City, IA, USA

Alain LeDuc MD
Professor of Urology
Service D'Urologie
Hopital Saint-Loise
Paris, France

Cheryl T Lee MD
Assistant Professor of Urology
Comprehensive Cancer Center
University of Michigan
MI, USA

Birger Lindegård MD PhD
Associate Professor
Department of Nephrology
Lund University Hospital
Lund, Sweden

Padraig SJ Malone MCh FRCSI FRCS
Consultant Paediatric Urologist
Department of Paediatric Urology
Wessex Regional Centre for Paediatric Surgery
Southampton University Hospitals NHS Trust
Southampton, UK

Wiking Månsson MD PhD
Consultant Urologist
Associate Professor
Department of Urology
Lund University Hospital
Lund, Sweden

Stephen D Mark MD
Urologist
Christchurch Hospital
Department of Urology
Christchurch, New Zealand

W Scott McDougal MD
Chief of Urology
Department of Urology
Massachussets General Hospital and
Walter S Kerr Jr Professor of Urology
The Harvard Medical School
Boston, MA, USA

Andrew C McGregor MD
Urology Resident
University of Kentucky
School of Medicine
Lexington, KY, USA

Steven R Mindrup MD
Resident in Urology
Department of Urology
University of Iowa
Iowa City, IA, USA

Michael E Mitchell MD
Professor, University of Washington
Chief, Division of Pediatric Urology
Children's Hospital and Regional Medical Center
Seattle, WA, USA

James E Montie MD
Chairman, Department of Urology
Valassis Professor of Urologic Oncology
University of Michigan
Department of Urology
Taubman Center
Ann Arbor, MI, USA

Anthony Mundy MS MRCP FRCS
Institute of Urology
London, UK

Thiagarajan Nambirajan MS DNB MCh (Urol) FRCSUrol
Specialist Registrar in Urology
Regional Urology Service
Belfast City Hospital
Belfast, Northern Ireland

Mike Minh Nguyen MD
Resident Physician
Department of Urology
University of California
Davis School of Medicine
Sacramento, CA, USA

Karl Obrant MD PhD
Professor
Department of Orthopedics
University Hospital MAS
Malmö, Sweden

Andrew C Peterson MD
Chief
Reconstructive Urology
Female Urology and Urodynamics
Department of Surgery
Urology Service
Madigan Army Medical Center
Fort Lewis, WA, USA

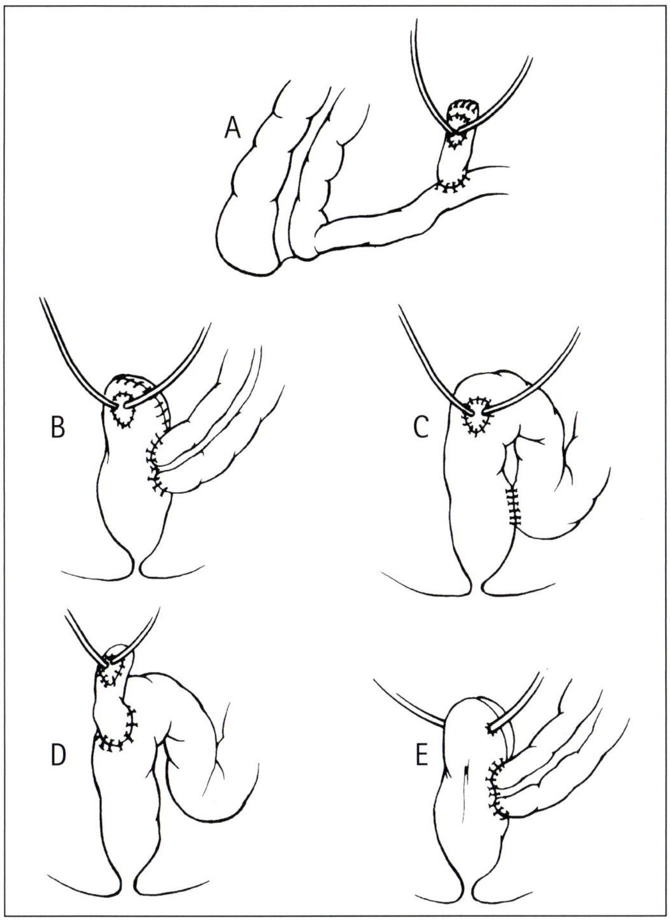

Figure 1.5 Implantation of ureters into a partially excluded intestinal segment. (a) Nagano's anastomosis of trigone to an isolated portion of ileum (1901); (b) Müller's anastomosis of trigone to isolated lower sigmoid colon (1903); (c) Borelius and Berglund's anastomosis of trigone to dome of sigmoid loop (1905); (d) Uretero-ileosigmoidostomy of Berg (1907); (e) Descomps' direct anastomosis of ureters to upper rectal pouch (1909). (After Hinman and Weyrauch.[1])

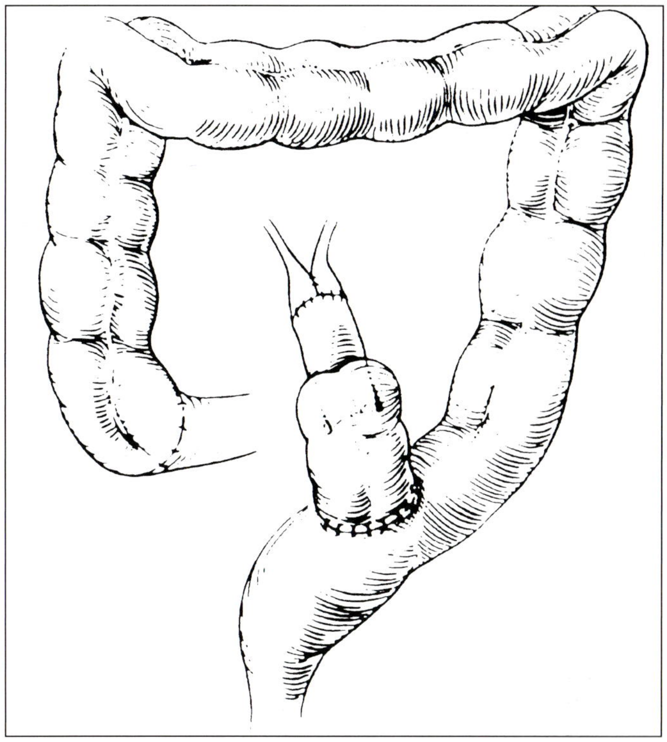

Figure 1.6 Hendren's uretero-ileocecosigmoidostomy (1983). (With permission from Rink RC et al. In: Bladder Reconstruction and Continent Urinary Diversion. Chicago: Yearbook Medical Publishers, 1987.[37])

North Carolina, 'as a means to avoid the risk of late malignancy seen after conventional ureterosigmoidostomy when the ureters are anastomosed directly to the sigmoid with the bowel in continuity'.[37,38]

Augmented valved rectum

Although the simplicity of urinary continence achieved with ureterosigmoidostomies and rectal bladders are attractive, each suffers from unique complications making the procedures undesirable. In the case of ureterosigmoidostomy, a significant number of patients suffer from metabolic disturbances, pyelonephritis, and are also at risk for development of malignancy at the ureterointestinal anastomotic site. Conversely, patients with rectal bladders and an abdominal colostomy have the disadvantage of having to wear an abdominal appliance to collect the feces, and those with a perineal colostomy are often incontinent of stool.

In 1975, Knox and Jago reported the value of intussusception of the colorectal junction in piglets.[39] In 1988, Kock and associates from Sweden and Egypt rediscovered and refined this technique, first in experimental animals and later, clinically preventing the regurgitation of urine throughout the colon. This reduced the metabolic imbalance observed in ureterosigmoidostomy patients.[40,41] They devised a novel procedure in which the rectum was augmented by anastomosing an ileal patch to the anterior rectal wall (see Chapter 30). Reflux of the rectal contents towards the colon was prevented by creating a colorectal intussusception valve. Stool was temporarily diverted using a transverse colostomy, then closed 2 months later. The ureters were implanted in an antireflux fashion within the intussuscepted colorectal segment. Alternatively, in the case of larger aperistaltic ureters that would not fit into a sigmoid intussusception, the ureters were implanted into an afferent limb of an intussuscepted ileal nipple, which was then anastomosed into the rectum directly. Kock initially reported a mean rectal reservoir capacity of 800 ml with low pressure, daytime continence and no nocturnal enuresis with no emptying up to two times per night.[41] Ghoneim has now successfully performed this procedure in over 501 patients in Egypt. However, he stresses the importance of longitudinal review to assess the long-term effect on renal function, and the incidence of tumor development at the anastomotic site.[42]

Appliance-dependent urinary diversion

Gastric conduit

On 30 June, 1956, Edwin Sinaiko of Chicago was the first to use a segment of the antrum of the stomach to create a gastric conduit in a 38-year-old woman with metastatic bladder cancer and uremia secondary to bilateral ureteral obstruction.[43] He attempted this procedure after performing a significant number of gastric conduits in experimental animals.[44,45] These experiments revealed that when stomach is used as:[43]

> an artificial bladder, hyperchloremic acidosis and azotemia do not occur. There is no hypokalemia because very little potassium is lost. A partially continent bladder substitute and a continent urinary bladder would be physiologically feasible. The contact of urine with gastric mucosa, especially antrum, did not stimulate through the gastrin mechanism acid secretion in the main stomach. There was no obvious damage to the ureters and kidneys from possible regurgitation of acid from the stomach. In this substitute bladder, the gastric acidity and lysozyme provides a bacteriostatic and bacteriocidal protective medium which is desirable in preventing serious retrograde infection in the kidneys. Stomach tissue beyond the needs of the animal is available for use as an artificial urinary bladder. The length of the ureters is more than enough to reach the pouch easily … Loss of HCl in the gastric juice secreted by the pouch did not produce hypochloremia.

The stoma of the first gastric conduit was managed with a permanent catheter placed into the pouch. The woman's renal function and intravenous pyelogram returned to normal, and she gained 3.6 kg (8 lbs). She survived for 18 months, dying of carcinomatosis; however, she was noted to have normal renal function and no symptomatic urinary infections.[46] Sinaiko subsequently improved his technique by creating a second gastric fundus along the greater curvature, basing the vasculature on the left gastroepiploic artery. The left and right ureters were brought intraperitoneally through the mesentery of the left and right colons, respectively. The stoma was placed within the existing paramedian incision at the level of the umbilicus.[46] In 1978, Leong of Hong Kong reported the successful creation of a gastric conduit in 21 patients.[47] Having had significant experience with gastric neobladders and gastrocystoplasties, Leong used the whole gastric pyloric antrum based on the left gastroepiploic artery, and brought it through an opening in the transverse mesocolon, placing the stoma in the right iliac fossa.

Jejunal conduit

In 1935, Seiffert performed jejunal conduits in two patients, with one patient surviving 3 years, and the other dying early of renal failure.[3,48] The jejunal conduit became popular in the 1960s, paralleling the use of radiotherapy for pelvic malignancies. Both jejunal and transverse colon conduits were used, since these segments of bowel were less likely to have been damaged during radiotherapy. However, many patients with jejunal conduits experienced significant electrolyte disturbances (i.e. hypochloremic hyponatremic acidosis), hence the technique is rarely used today.[49,50]

Ileal conduit

In 1911, Zaayer reported the results of ileal conduits in two patients.[51] The first case was 'successful' although the patient died 11 days postoperatively due to extensive cervical malignancy. The second case, performed in a patient with carcinoma of the bladder, died 6 days postoperatively of peritonitis. In 1927, Bollman and Mann performed ileal conduits in experimental animals,[1] however, they died of electrolyte imbalances, felt to be secondary to bowel segments which were too long.

Eugene M Bricker, a general surgeon from Barnes Hospital in St Louis, is responsible for the refinement and repopularization of the ileal conduit technique (Figure 1.7).[52] Bricker had previously abandoned the creation of a continent urinary diversion using the ileocecal segment due to persistent postoperative incontinence (Figure 1.8). He subsequently admitted that he copied the technique to create an ileal conduit from Dr Heinz Haffner at the St Louis City Hospital, who, then 'unable to use the cecum as a reservoir was forced to use an isolated segment

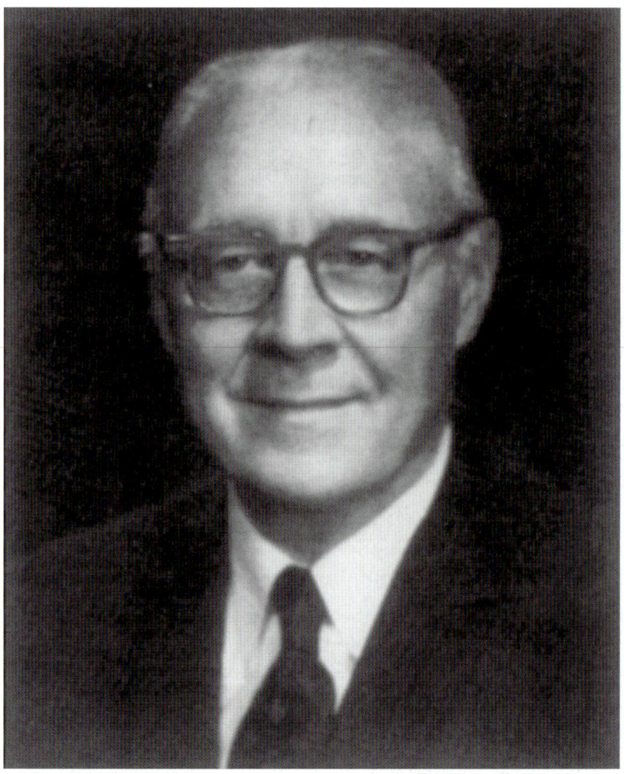

Figure 1.7 Eugene M Bricker, general surgeon who contributed much to urinary diversion techniques.

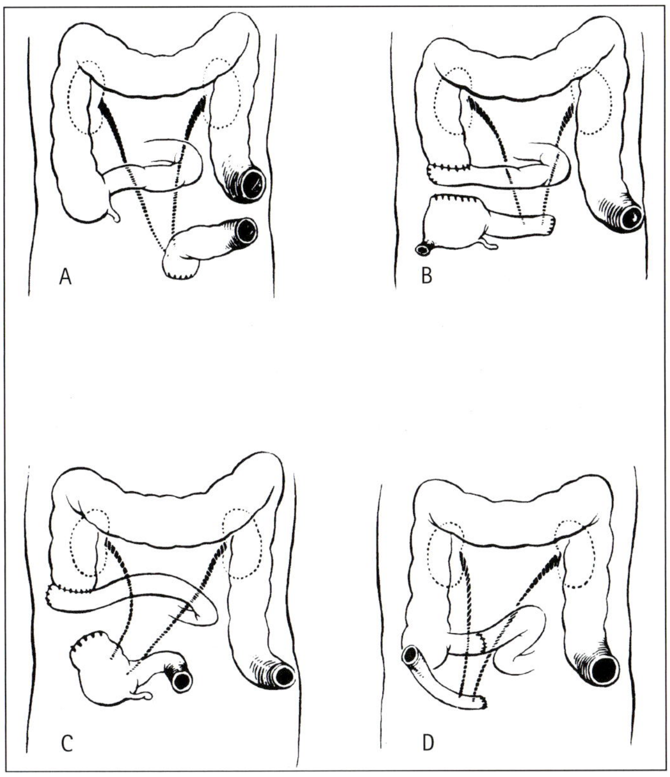

Figure 1.8 Bricker's contributions included: (a) sigmoid colon conduit; (b,c) two techniques of ileocecal conduits which were originally meant to be continent diversions; and (d) ileal conduit. (With permission from Bricker EM. Surg Clin North Am 1950; 30: 1511–21.[52])

of the ileum alone'.[52] He reported the results of ileal conduits in four women undergoing pelvic exenteration over a 2-month period, using a simple mucosa-to-mucosa ureteroileal anastomosis as described by Justin J Cordonnier (also a general surgeon at the Barnes Hospital in St Louis) a year earlier for ureterosigmoidostomy.[14] In reference to an antireflux uretero-intestinal technique, Bricker wrote in 1950: 'We believe that the day of "dunking" and "tunneling" ureters is past. There should be no fundamental difference between anastomosing the ureter with the intestine and anastomosing the bowel itself.'[52] The stoma of the conduit was simple; the ileal mucosa sutured to the skin without the creation of a bud. He used the Rutzen bag (an improved ostomy appliance which Bricker became familiar with during the care of trauma patients during the Second World War) to collect the urine exiting from the ileal conduit stoma. At the conclusion of his classic report on the ileal conduit, Bricker stated:

> We ourselves are pleased with the procedure because we feel that it is the acme of simplicity and because we believe that the various factors previously mentioned are going to prove its superiority over other methods of dealing with the ureters after pelvic evisceration. At the present time we are ready to drop the project of trying to develop a continent intra-abdominal urinary pouch in favor of this method which provides for prompt elimination of the urine without stagnation into an extra-abdominal urinary reservoir which is convenient, sanitary and under the control of the patient.

Wallace of London and Turnbull, a general surgeon at the Cleveland Clinic, modified the ileal conduit in the 1960s and 1970s. In 1966, Wallace described a technique of ureteroileal anastomosis which aimed 'to provide a method of diversion with a minimum of suturing, to speed the operating time', and as a result decreased the ureteroileal anastomosis stricture rate.[53] The technique entails large spatulation of the ureters which are then jointly anastomosed side to side, 'together forming a circular stoma' which is then anastomosed to the butt-end of the ileal conduit. In 1975, at the Annual Meeting of the Pelvic Surgeons, Turnbull reported and popularized the loop-end myotomy ileostomy in obese patients.[54,55] Turnbull reported excellent results in more than 500 patients, a technique which now carries his name. The Turnbull loop stoma has since been confirmed to have a decreased risk of stomal stenosis; however, it also has a higher risk of parastomal hernias.[56–58]

Simple, rapid to build and with minimal short-term complications, the ileal loop is still widely used today as a standard urinary diversion against which other forms of diversion are compared. Recently, Madersbacher et al from Bern, Switzerland have reviewed the long-term outcomes of ileal conduits.[59] They followed 131 patients for an average of 98 months finding 192 conduit-related complications in 87 (66%) of the patients. Of these, upper urinary tract changes (27%), stoma complications including stenosis and parastomal hernia (24%), bowel problems (24%) and infections (23%) are most common. Ureteroileal anastomotic complications were seen in 18 (14%), 13 of those being stenosis of the anastomosis needing surgical or endoscopic revision. Stones formed in 9% of patients, and renal function was preserved in the majority with hyperchloremic, metabolic acidosis forming in only two patients. However, 27% of patients in their group experienced renal function deterioration over 15 years of follow-up.[59]

Ileocecal conduit

In 1950, Bricker and Eiseman reported two cases in which ileocecal conduits were successfully employed (see Figure 1.8).[60] In 1947, they anastomosed the ureters of a 68-year-old man with rectal cancer to the terminal ileum of an isolated ileocecal segment and created a permanent cecostomy through which the patient used a continuous drainage catheter. A year later, they performed an ileocecal pouch in a 48-year-old woman with rectal cancer. In the second case, the ureters were anastomosed to the cecum, and a urinary stoma utilizing the terminal ileum was created in the midline of the abdomen, near a sigmoid fecal colostomy. The appendix in both pouches was left intact, and although the ileocecal valve was placed between the skin stoma and the cecal pouch in the second patient, the reservoir was totally incontinent. Presumably, because continence could not be achieved, Bricker abandoned this more complicated procedure in favor of the ileal conduit.[52]

The ileocecal conduit was reintroduced in 1975 by Zinman and Libertino of Boston.[61,62] They anastomosed the ureters to the terminal ileum and augmented the ileocecal valve by approximating the cecum around the ileum for a length of 1 cm proximal to the valve with seromuscular sutures. The entire cecal diameter was brought to the skin as a stoma. In this fashion, an augmented ileocecal valve prevented reflux.

Transverse colon conduit

Although it is speculated that the use of colon conduit was performed prior to the 1960s, no clear documentation of such cases exists. Similar to jejunal conduits, the popularity of neoadjuvant radiotherapy for the treatment of pelvic malignancies in the 1960s and 1970s created the need for a bowel segment in urinary diversion which was relatively free of radiation damage. Various reports exist utilizing transverse colon conduits from 1975 to the early 1980s.[63–67] Perhaps the earliest of these procedures was performed by Morales and Golimbu of New York, but it was Schmidt of Iowa and later San Diego who popularized the technique.[63–65] This is still a viable option for diversion in those patients with an irradiated pelvis.

Sigmoid colon conduit

In 1940, Bricker, while in Columbia, Missouri, used the sigmoid colon conduit in four patients (see Figure 1.8).[52] He placed the urinary stoma near the opened colostomy stoma of patients undergoing pelvic exenteration, leading to poor results in half the patients surviving the perioperative period. This led Bricker to other techniques of urinary diversion as previously discussed. In 1959, Turner–Warwick of London refined Bricker's technique by placing the sigmoid colostomy in the left abdomen and the sigmoid urinary conduit in the right abdomen as a one-stage procedure.[68] However, although detailed descriptions were given, no clinical experience was reported using this simplified technique. In 1965, Mogg of England popularized the use of sigmoid urinary conduits in children with abnormal urinary tracts secondary to neurogenic bladders,[69] whereby the stoma was brought to the left lower abdominal quadrant. He was unable to perform the sigmoid colon conduit in two of 50 children secondary to 'vascular anomalies of the inferior mesenteric artery'. Dramatic stabilization of the upper urinary tract was noted in this patient population. A decade later, Hendren of Boston continued to popularize the use of the sigmoid colon conduit in pediatric urology.[70] Prior to the development of the Mainz continent diversion, Altwein and Hohenfellner of Mainz, West Germany, used the sigmoid and rectosigmoid colon as their preferred method of urinary diversion.[71]

Richie and Skinner reported that ischemic bowel may be a complication of sigmoid colon conduits in patients who have undergone pelvic radiotherapy or are undergoing cystectomy.[72,73] The superior hemorrhoidal artery, a branch of the hypogastric artery, is sometimes ligated during the creation of a sigmoid conduit. In the case of a patient with an irradiated pelvis, the distal colon and rectum may have insufficient blood supply secondary to radiation damage to the smaller collateral vessels. Similarly, because the hypogastric arteries are sometimes sacrificed during a cystectomy, the blood supply to the rectum may be compromised after sigmoid conduit in this patient population. However, the sigmoid conduit is an accepted and useful option if careful patient selection and technique are employed.

Continent urinary diversion

Gastric reservoir

In 1977, Rudick and associates of New York developed a continent urinary reservoir using stomach in dogs.[74] They constructed a pouch using a large wedge of gastric fundus and implanted the ureters using a modification of the Paquin technique. A continent stoma was created using a modification of the Janeway–Depage tubovalvular gastrostomy. Although the initial capacity of the reservoir was approximately 200 ml, by 2 weeks the pouch retained over 1 l of volume, remaining completely continent in a 6-month follow-up. Nguyen and Mitchell of Seattle have had some experience with the continent gastric reservoir, in which the appendix or ureter may be used to create a continent stoma.[75]

Ileal reservoir

Continent urine reservoirs made from small bowel have evolved tremendously with time. One of the most important advances involves creation of a low pressure, continent bladder. The advantages of detubularized bowel segments in urinary reconstruction were well known in Sweden in the late 1950s when Giertz and Franksson of Stockholm noted improved continence in neobladders (see Figure 1.11d later).[76] The U-shaped ileocystoplasty reported by Goodwin and associates in 1958, demonstrated further advancement in the use of detubularized bowel segments.[77–79] In 1967, Kock (Figure 1.9) and associates of Göteborg, Sweden, developed a low-pressure ileal pouch for patients with fecal ileostomies following proctocolectomy.[80,81] Dissatisfied with the continence achieved with their preliminary technique, in 1972 they performed an intussuscepted ileal nipple valve in the fashion initially described by Watsuji in 1899 for gastrostomies.[81–83] Various modifications of the intussuscepted ileal nipple were developed due to the high initial incidence of detussusception associated with using sutures.

Kock and associates described the use of staples to secure the ileal nipple valve, with a collar of fascia or Marlex mesh placed around the base of the valve.[81] Animal studies demonstrated the ileal pouch preserved the upper urinary tracts and also resulted in few electrolyte abnormalities.[84] Kock and associates commenced their clinical experience in 1975 when a 28-

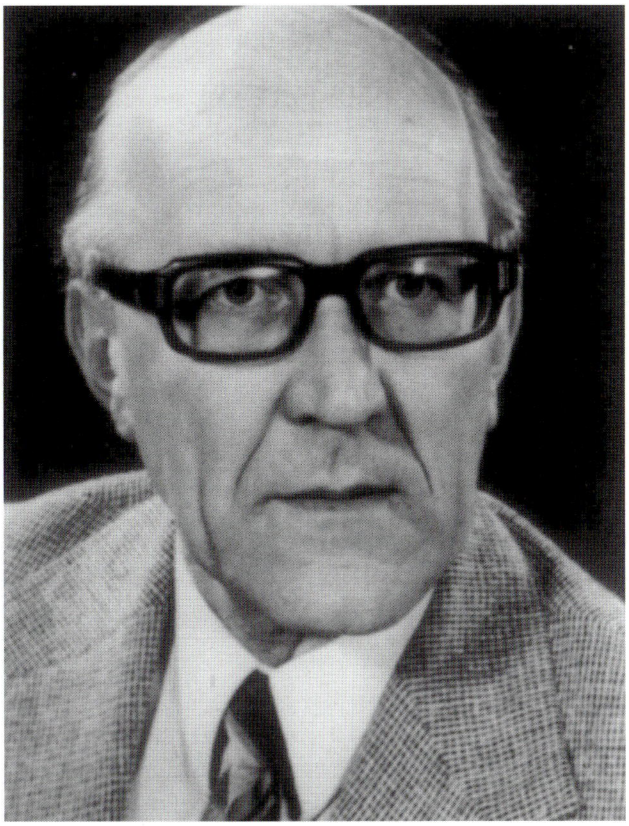

Figure 1.9 Nils Kock, prominent Swedish surgeon responsible for the refinement of the intussuscepted ileal nipple.

year-old woman, with neurogenic bladder of unclear etiology, underwent conversion of an ileal loop to the Kock reservoir, achieving perfect continence.[85] In 1976, Madigan in England, and Leisinger et al of Zurich, Switzerland, reported a small series of patients undergoing the Kock pouch for continent urinary diversion.[86–88] By 1982, Kock and associates had performed the procedure on 12 patients, seven of them requiring revisions of their efferent nipples over a mean follow-up of 32 months.[89] The technique used approximately 60–70 cm of distal ileum, with the pouch created from two central 20–22-cm segments which were completely detubularized (see Chapter 23). The afferent and efferent intussuscepted nipples used to prevent reflux and maintain continence, respectively, were formed from 15–17-cm limbs on each side of the central segments. An interesting editorial comment by Donald Skinner followed this 1982 manuscript by Kock et al:[90]

> The concept of a continent ileal conduit is attractive. Patients are asking about it ... However, it should be emphasized that on all forms of urinary diversion the early results look good, but long-term followup is not yet available and the operation is more time-consuming than other forms of diversion. Will it become an innovative but rarely used procedure like Gilchrist's operation or will it become a more acceptable alternative for urinary diversion than the standard ileal conduit?

Between August 1982 and August 1985, Skinner and associates constructed these ileal reservoirs in 250 patients.[91,92] In short-term follow-up (10–44 months), they reported a high rate of reoperation (23%), primarily for efferent nipple revision, 'to achieve continence or to eliminate a parastomal hernia and/or difficult catheterization'.[92] Although there is a significant learning curve with this procedure, a significant reoperation rate also still exists in the best hands, leading many who initially performed this procedure to perform continent ileocolonic reservoirs (GD Webster, personal communication, March 1994).

Abol-Eniem and Ghoneim developed a novel ureteroileal reimplantation technique in 1994 to avoid the pitfalls of the intussuscepted ileal vale.[93] This T-pouch was constructed from 44 cm of ileum with a second, separate proximal 8–10 cm segment of ileum for the antireflux limb. The 44-cm segment layed out in a 'V' configuration. The distal 3–4 cm of the 8-cm spearate piece is anchored into the serosal lined trough formed by the base of the two adjacent 22-cm lengths of the longer segment. The distal portion of the afferent short segment is staple reduced to a 30-Fr size and the detubularized pouch is re-approximated over it to form a flap valve. Skinner and his group incorporated this technique to provide an antirefluxing valve to orthotopic ileal neobladders in 1998 with no added complications.[94] This procedure can be used to provide continent catheterizable reservoirs as well by creating a 'Double T-pouch continent ileal reservoir'.

Ileocecal reservoirs, continent right colon pouch

In 1908, Verhoogen of Brussels devised an operation isolating the ileocecal region as a continent reservoir, with the appendix brought to the right lower quadrant where it could be catheterized periodically (Figure 1.10a).[95,96] He performed the one-stage operation unsuccessfully in two patients with carcinoma of the bladder. In 1910, Makkas successfully completed the work of Verhoogen by performing the operation in two stages and implanting the entire trigone into the pouch (Maydl's technique) rather than individual ureters.[97] Moreover, Makkas performed a side-to-side anastomosis of the ileum to the mid-transverse colon rather than the hepatic flexure as Verhoogen had done. In 1912, Lengemann further modified the technique by isolating an additional 30 cm of ileum to which he implanted the trigone extraperitoneally at a second operation.[98] He performed this technique in 12 patients, with nine patients dying perioperatively.

In 1946, Gallo of Argentina reported the results of a previous autopsy (1940) on a patient who had lived 13 years following implantation of both ureters into an isolated ileocecal reservoir with appendectomy. The patient had an intact upper urinary tract noted at death.[99] Also in 1946, Ramirez Gutiérrez of Bogota, Colombia, described the technique for a two-stage ileocecal continent pouch in the fashion of Verhoogen.[100] In the first stage, an ileocecal reservoir was created with the

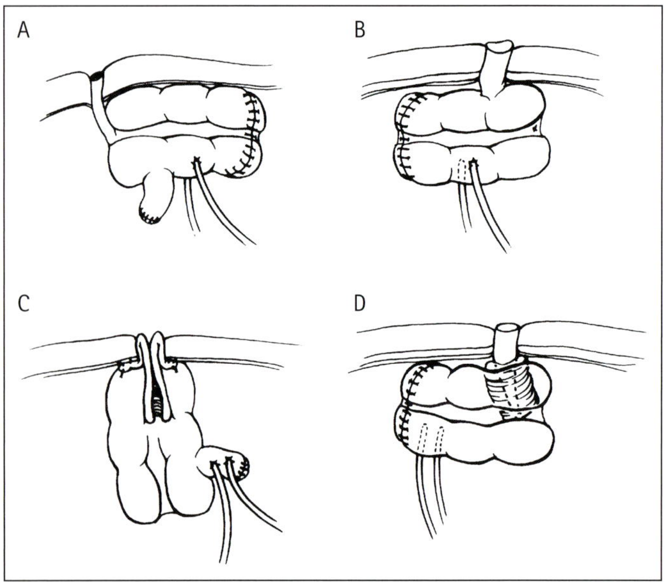

Figure 1.10 Ileocecal reservoirs. (a) Verhoogen's ileocecal continent reservoir with appendicostomy (1908); (b) Gilchrist and associates' continent ileocecal reservoir (1949); (c) Ashken's continent ileocecal reservoir (1974); (d) Zingg and Tscholl's continent ileocecal reservoir (1977).

appendix as the catheterizable stoma. In the second stage, 1–2 months later after 'sterilizing' the cecal reservoir by multiple antiseptic irrigations, the ureters were implanted into the cecal reservoir. Inspired by this work from South America, Gilchrist, Merricks, Hamlin and Rieger of Chicago reported a successful continent ileocecal reservoir in 1950 (Figure 1.10b).[101] They initially performed the surgery in several dogs, first creating the pouch with the ileum brought out to the skin and secondly implanting the ureters into the cecum. They then performed the surgery on a 63-year-old man who had had five prior operations for leiomyosarcoma of the perirectal tissues over the previous 2 years, including an abdominoperineal resection. On 13 October, 1949, the ileocecal pouch was created after appendectomy, with a catheter brought through the 23-cm segment of ileum, with intermittent catheterizations through this stoma 1 week postoperatively. Each ureter was implanted into the cecum by a modified Coffey I anastomosis. On the sixteenth postoperative day it was no longer possible to catheterize the pouch secondary to an ileal kink approximately 12.7 cm from the skin. The ileum was revised to a straight 10-cm segment from the skin (at McBurney's point) to the ileocecal valve, which was readily catheterized. One month later, a pelvic exenteration was performed, and cystoscopy of the pouch revealed healthy mucosa and ureteral orifices (following indigo carmine intravenous injection) with an estimated capacity of 220 ml. Continence was dependent on the competence of the ileocecal valve; the patient remained continent if catheterization was performed frequently enough. In self critique, the authors felt that a larger segment of right colon would have resulted in improved continence and a shorter initial segment of ileum used would facilitate catheterization. In 1951, this group reported the capacity of the pouch in this patient had increased and that catheterization was performed every 4 hours.[102] They reported an additional three patients in whom a continent ileocecal reservoir was performed, with only one of the three surviving the perioperative course. The survivor had metastatic prostate cancer (stage D1) and underwent orchiectomy 2 months following the creation of the reservoir. He required catheterization every 5–6 hours to prevent leakage with a pouch capacity of 300 ml.

In 1952, Romero Lobo and Santander of Venezuela successfully performed a continent ileocecal reservoir, as described by Gilchrist and associates, on a 15-year-old girl with a rectovaginal fistula, with excellent early continence.[103] In 1973, a long-term follow-up report on 40 patients who had undergone this procedure between 1949 and 1963 revealed a 94% complete continence rate, with the patients performing catheterizations every 4–6 hours during the day and once at night.[104] In these patients, a modified Coffey II technique was used for the ureterocecal anastomosis, with reflux noted in only 7% of their patients. Pouch stones occurred in three patients in whom nonabsorbable sutures were used in closing the outer layers of the reservoir. However, later reports suggested that in the hands of other surgeons, the urinary continence rates were difficult to reproduce when relying on the ileocecal valve as the sole mechanism of continence; therefore, the technique fell out of favor.[90,105]

It was not until 1974 that Ashken of Norwich, England, revived some interest in the continent ileocecal reservoir.[106] He isolated the right colon along with 15 cm of distal ileum and anastomosed the ureters to the terminal ileum using the split-cuff nipple technique of Ricard. An additional 20 cm of ileum was isolated on its vascular pedicle, intussuscepted and sutured to the open end of the cecum (Figure 1.10c). This ileal nipple (Kock technique) was then brought to the skin as the continent stoma. Three of seven patients subsequently underwent detussusception of the catheterizable ileal nipple. A modification, in which the ileal spout valve was brought through the true ileocecal sphincter similarly failed, as did an ileal spout system fashioned as a flutter valve sewn into the open end of the cecum.[107,108] Benchekroun of Rabat, Morocco, reported in 1977 a modification of the first Ashken technique.[109] Instead of intussuscepting the ileum anastomosed to the open cecum, he 'invaginated' this segment so that the mucosal surfaces were opposed, therefore having the serosal surfaces forming the luminal and external surfaces of the nipple. However, evagination continued to occur in 17% of a series of 160 patients.[110]

In 1977, a continent cecal reservoir using silk-sutured intussusception of a 12-cm segment of terminal ileum through the ileocecal valve to form a nipple into isolated cecum was reported by Zingg and Tscholl of Berne, Switzerland (Figure 1.10d).[111] Two of three surviving patients were continent at short-term follow-up. In 1977, Mansson and associates of Lund, Sweden, developed a series of continent ileocecal reservoir techniques in which an intussuscepted ileocecal valve was used as the continence mechanism.[112–114] Their technique utilized a detubularized right colonic segment, staples for maintenance of the intussuscepted ileal nipple valve and anchoring of the nipple base to the anterior rectus sheath.[115] In 1986, Webster and Bertram of Durham, North Carolina, described a stapling technique and the use of a Marlex strip (after Kock) to stabilize the intussusception of the ileocecal valve.[116] In attempting to avoid the use of staples, in 1985, King and coworkers of Durham, North Carolina, reported stabilization of the intussusception by suturing the intussuscepted nipple to the reservoir wall, using muscle-to-muscle anastomosis with absorbable sutures.[117]

In 1985, Thüroff and associates of Mainz, West Germany, described an ileocecal reservoir performed since 1983 which uniquely detubularized and combined both the ileal and cecal bowel segments (see Chapter 16).[118,119] Although they used staples and mesh to stabilize a catheterizable segment of intussuscepted ileum (not ileocecal valve), in theory it was less likely to detussuscept, since compared to previous pouches, a larger capacity, low-pressure reservoir had been created. In the initial reservoir technique, referred to as the 'mixed augmentation ileum 'nzecum' (Mainz) pouch, the native ileocecal valve was defunctionalized during the detubularization process, and the ureters were implanted in an antireflux fashion directly into the cecum. In 1988, after noting that detussusception of the ileal nipple was still a problem, Thüroff and associates modified their technique by staple fixation of the ileal nipple not only to the bowel wall, but also to a maintained ileocecal valve.[120]

In 1985, Rowland and coworkers of Indianapolis, reported that since 1982, rather than an intussuscepted ileocecal valve, a plicated terminal ileum was used to create the continent catheterizable stoma of an ileocecal continent reservoir (see Chapter 25).[121] In their initial version, later referred to as the 'Indiana continent urinary reservoir', they performed no detubularization of the right colon. They soon realized the need for detubularization after noting 'bolus contractions' of the right colon causing incontinence in their patients. They used approximately 20 cm of right colon with a 15-cm segment of terminal ileum, along with an additional 15 cm of ileal patch anastomosed to the opened upper cecal segment in order to create a low-pressure system. They plicated the catheterizable terminal ileum to a 12-Fr caliber using two layers of silk sutures. In 1987, Rowland and associates reported a series of 29 patients, of whom 24 had abdominal stomas, two women had vaginal stomas, and three men had neobladders.[122] The detubularization of the cecum was performed using an ileal patch in 15, sigmoid patch in two, and Heineke–Mikulicz reconfiguration in two. The ureteral reimplantations were performed using the Leadbetter technique. Using this plicated ileal segment, over 90 and 70% of the patients maintained daytime and nighttime continence, respectively. Since 1985, the Indiana group has adopted (i) transverse folding or Heineke–Mikulicz technique to detubularize the right colon, (ii) stapled rather than sutured ileal tapering[123] and (iii) examination of the competency of the ileocecal valve with the reservoir open after tapering the ileum, with further plicating silk sutures in Lembert fashion.[124]

In 1988, Bejani and Politano not only introduced stapled tapering of the ileum, but also a purse-string plication of the ileum at the junction of the ileocecal valve for added continence resulting in perfect early continence in 10 patients.[123] Moreover, in their reservoir, the right colon and half of the transverse colon were used as the detubularized reservoirs described in 1987 by Lockhart of Miami and refined by Lockhart and associates of Tampa, Florida.[125,126]

In 1989, Koff and associates of Columbus, Ohio, based on laboratory animal experience, described an ingenious, albeit more time-consuming, technique to create a continent catheterizable ileal stoma in an ileocecal reservoir.[127–129] Their reservoir used the entire right colon and 20 cm of distal ileum. A 4-cm mesenteric window was made at the distal ileum (next to the ileocecal valve) and the right colon detubularized in the Heineke–Mikulicz fashion. The ileum was divided into two segments of equal length, and the proximal end of the free ileal segment incised 4 cm along its antimesenteric border. This is then anastomosed to the site of the cecum near the ileocecal valve. The distal (already opened) end of the free ileal segment was wrapped around the distal ileum (next the ileocecal valve) where the mesenteric window had been created, and sutured in place. In this fashion, Koff and associates created a 'more physiologic' reservoir, which allows increased resistance of the outlet during filling of the pouch. This 'ileal servomechanism' allowed urine to enter the ileal segment surrounding the imbricated distal ileum; therefore as the reservoir fills added resistance is provided aiding in continence. This was verified by urodynamic studies in seven of their patients.[128]

Transverse colon reservoir

In 1989, Bihrle and associates of Indianapolis reported an experimental animal model of a continent transverse colon reservoir.[130] Using a detubularized segment of transverse colon, they implanted the ureters utilizing the Leadbetter antireflux technique, and anastomosed a tunneled and tubularized gastric segment based on the right gastroepiploic artery into the reservoir, thus creating a new continence mechanism. They developed the technique primarily for patients who had had prior pelvic irradiation and desired a continent urinary diversion. Excellent results were reported in four patients with greater than 1-year follow-up; the only major complication was stomatitis which was readily controlled by an H_2-blocker.[131]

Orthotopic bladder replacement

The first report of a successful neobladder was published in 1988 by Guido Tizzoni and Alfonso Poggi of Bologna, who performed a two-stage technique using small bowel in a dog. In the first stage they isolated 7-cm segment of lavaged small bowel which they united in a loop. One month later they anastomosed the ureters to the segment and the segment to the neck of the bladder. The dog was continent and tolerated three pregnancies successfully. The animal died 30 months later with normal renal anatomy (Figure 1.11a).[1,132,133]

In 1912, Georges Lemoine of Brussels performed a cystectomy and implantation of the ureters into the rectum as a treatment for a man with cancer.[3,134] However, because of recurrent pyelonephritis, he subsequently displaced the rectum forward and anastomosed it to the urethra, with the sigmoid colon brought down to the anal canal. Although the patient died of sepsis on the eighteenth postoperative day, Lemoine may be credited as performing the first human orthotopic bladder substitution.

Gastric neobladder

In 1972, Leong and Ong of Hong Kong were the first to report the successful use of gastric antrum to create a neobladder in 10 of 26 dogs after total cystectomy.[135] They stated that a similar operation had been performed on three human patients, the first being performed in 1969. In a later report, Leong reported the results of a gastric neobladder using the pyloric antrum in eight men and one woman in whom a radical cystectomy had been performed between 1969 and 1975 (Figure 1.12).[136] The segment of antrum was brought to the pelvis based on the left gastroepiploic artery with the omentum remaining intact. Continuity of the bowel was performed utilizing a Billroth I gastroduodenostomy, the gastro-urethral anastomosis was performed using 3-0 catgut suture, and ureteral implantation performed using the Leadbetter submucosal tuneling technique. Two patients died immediately postoperatively (due to an anesthetic complication in one and an undiagnosed pheochromocytoma in the other). Three patients died several months later secondary to carcinoma, intestinal obstruction and persistent gastrourethral urinary leakage. Of those who survived, excellent urinary streams, minimal residuals, and initial bladder capacities of 100–150 ml with subsequent bladder capacities of 300 ml at 18 months follow-up were reported. No statement on urinary continence was made.

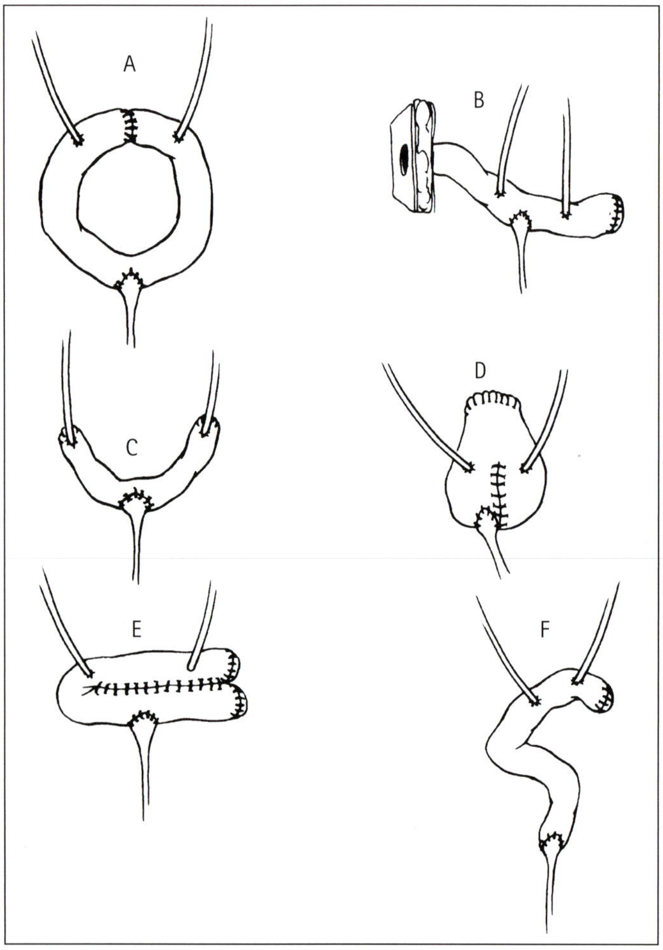

Figure 1.11 Ileal neobladders. (a) Tizzoni and Poggi (1888); (b) Couvelaire (1951); (c) Pyrah and Raper (1955); (d) Giertz and Franksson (1957); (e) Mellinger and Suder (1958); (f) Gandin (1960).

Ileal neobladders

In 1951, 40 years following Lemoine's rectal neobladder, Couvelaire of St Louis Hospital, Paris, reported the first clinical use of ileum for complete bladder substitution following cystectomy for cancer in a 45-year-old man (Figure 1.11b).[137] He performed the surgery in two stages. First, he closed one end of the bowel loop, performed the ileo–prostatic urethral anastomosis on the antimesenteric border, and brought the other end of the loop to the skin as a safety valve. In the second stage, he closed the end stoma. The patient was able to void without using a catheter. In 1955 Pyrah and Raper from Leeds, England, reported their results in three patients using a U-loop shaped segment of ileum (Figure 1.11c).[138] Two of the three patients survived, and both were completely continent during the day. In 1957, Giertz and Franksson of Stockholm reported 19 patients in whom an ileal orthotopic bladder was successfully completed (Figure 1.11d).[76] Their initial case consisted of a simple anastomosis between the distal end of the isolated loop of ileum to the urethra. In the remaining 18 cases they detubularized the segment of bowel by folding a 15-cm loop of ileum upon itself, and anastomosing the two limbs together to make a

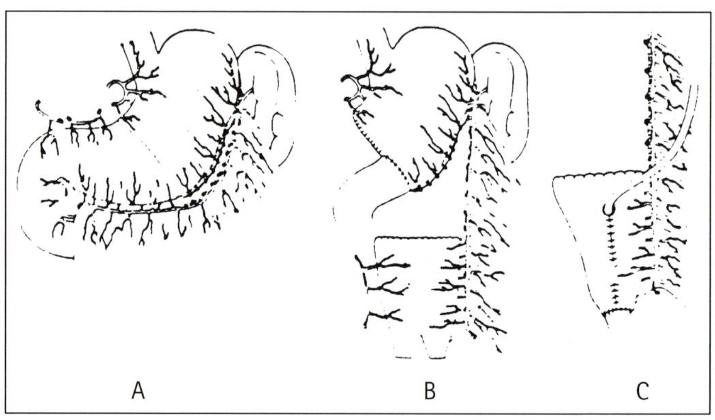

Figure 1.12 Leong and Ong's gastric neobladder (1969).

single cup-shaped cavity. Interestingly, 2 of the 18 were women and 14 of the 19 patients survived the peri-operative period. Although their patients voided by Valsalva, had no significant residual urine or reflux, and were continent during the day, over half the patients suffered from nocturnal incontinence. Indeed, Giertz and Franksson should be credited as being the first to use detubularized segments of bowel for neobladders. In 1958, Mellinger and Suder of Cincinnati reported a C-shaped ileal loop with closed ends (Figure 1.11e) and in 1960, Gandin, from Calfornia, described using a straight loop of ileum with the ureters separately attached to one end and the urethra to the opposite end of the bowel segment (Figure 1.11f).[139,140]

Camey of Paris is thought by many to have been responsible for the popularization of total bladder replacement using ileum. He performed the so-called Camey I ileal neobladder in 1959, a technique fashioned after that reported by Pyrah and Raper 4 years earlier.[138,141,142] This technique utilized an intact 35-cm segment of bowel with the center of its antimesenteric border anastomosed to the urethra following cystectomy. He later described the Camey II, wherein he detubularized a 65-cm segment of ileum in the manner of Mellinger and Suder (see Chapter 14).[139,143]

In 1987, Hautmann and associates of Ulm, West Germany, described the creation of the 'ileal neobladder' in 11 men following cystectomy.[144] They used a 60–70-cm segment of distal ileum which was detubularized in a W or M shape, anastomosed to the urethra, and the ureters sewn into the reservoir as tunneled implants in the Le Duc–Camey fashion (see Chapter 33).[145] In 1987, Tscholl and coworkers of Switzerland, reported their experience of seven patients using the S pouch, which was originally described for anorectal reconstruction.[146] The procedure utilized a 55-cm length of ileum, arranged into three segments of 13-cm subsegments in the form of the letter S. The cephalad 19-cm segment was used to create the antireflux nipple for ureteral implantation. Melchior et al of Kassel, West Germany, in 1988 described a segment of 40 cm of ileum opened on its antimesenteric border, except for the proximal 8-cm segment, which was intussuscepted to create an antirefluxing afferent nipple into which both ureters were reimplanted.[147] The open ileal segment was then situated in a U shape, anastomosed to the urethral remnant and closed as a cylindrical detubularized reservoir. Also in 1988, Studer and associates of Berne, Switzerland, reported a 50–60-cm ileal segment of bowel opened along its antimesenteric border and folded twice according to 'Goodwin's cup-patch technique' in order to create a neobladder (see Chapter 14).[148,149] They used three forms of antireflux mechanisms, with the proximal 10–25-cm segment of ileum which included creation of an intussuscepted ileal valve, split-cuff nipple, or a 20-cm tubular isoperistaltic afferent limb which had minimal antireflux properties.

In 1987, Ghoneim, Kock and associates of Mansoura, Egypt, and Göteborg, Sweden, reported excellent results in 16 men undergoing cystoprostatectomy, in whom a modified version of the Kock ileal continent diversion was performed. A 60-cm segment of ileum was used as an orthotopic reservoir by excluding the 17-cm efferent nipple (see Chapter 14).[150] Skinner and associates of Los Angeles have since popularized this technique of ileal neobladder, reporting in 1991 a large series of 126 patients with excellent results.[151] In 1996, the same group from Los Angeles updated their large series by reporting now on 295 patients undergoing this operation, again with outstanding results.[152] Many other ileal configurations such as the T-pouch mentioned earlier have been reported and are too numerous to be mentioned.

Ileocecal neobladders

In 1965, Hradec of Prague and Gil-Vernet of Barcelona individually reported their experiences in performing ileocecal neobladders.[153,154] Hradec performed ileocecal neobladders in 10 patients. He anastomosed the left ureter to the proximal end of the ileal segment, the right ureter to the upper right colon, and the urethra to the cecum (Figure 1.13a).[153] In contrast, Gil-Vernet implanted the ureters into the ileum allowing native ileocecal valve to prevent reflux and then anastomosed the urethra to the side of the upper right colon (Figure 1.13b).[154]

In 1975, Khafagy and associates of Cairo, reported 10 patients undergoing ileocecal orthotopic bladder replacement following radical cystectomy for carcinoma of the bilharzial bladder.[155] They described anastomosing the lower part of the cecum to the prostatic urethra or bladder neck, while the ureters were

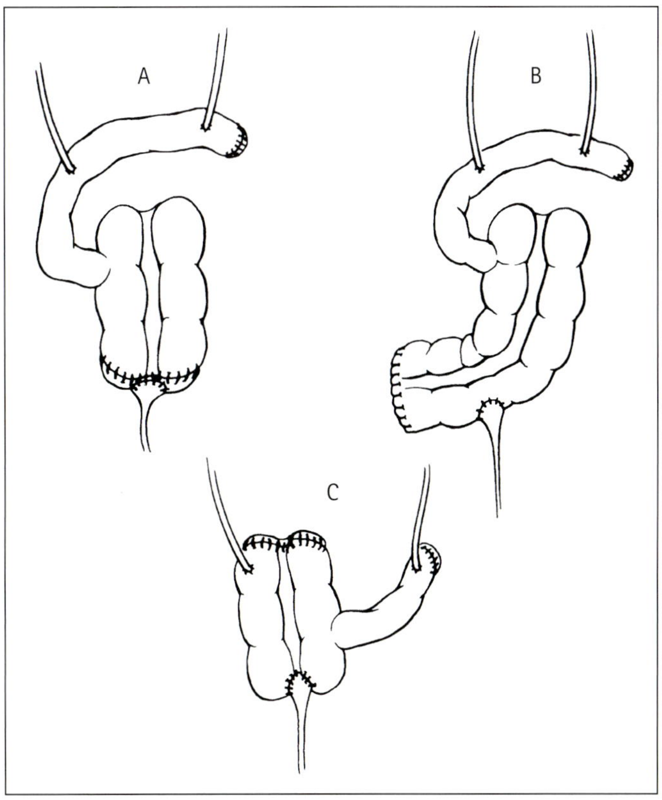

Figure 1.13 Ileocecal neobladders. (a, b) Gil-Vernet (1965); (c) Hradec (1965).

implanted in the ileum (again allowing the native ileocecal valve to reduce reflux). By 1987, they had performed this procedure on 130 patients (22 female) with a mortality rate of 15% with five patients developing fistulas.[156] They recommended maintaining the bladder neck whenever possible for improved continence. Although overall continence was reported to be acceptable (82% daytime and 24% nocturnal continence), they did not differentiate male and female urinary control rates. Alcini and coworkers of Rome, in 1988, reported 26 patients undergoing a similar technique for ileocecal neobladder with 100% daytime continence and 100% nocturnal enuresis.[157]

In 1986, Zinman and Libertino of Burlington, Massachusetts, described a modified version of the ileocecal neobladder technique developed by Gil-Vernet.[158] First, during cystectomy, the prostatic urethra was excised by enucleating the prostate, leaving the prostatic capsule behind. Secondly, the ileocecal valve was plicated after seromuscular longitudinal incisions were made and the redundant cecum was wrapped around the terminal ileum. Finally, the ureters were anastomosed to the proximal end of the ileum using the Wallace technique and the upper end of the right colon was anastomosed to the prostatic capsule. They performed this technique on 14 men. Three patients (21%) were totally incontinent and an additional four patients (29%) had nocturnal enuresis. All of the above-mentioned ileocecal neobladders were constructed in a tubularized fashion.

In 1986, Light and Englemann of Houston, Texas, reported the construction of detubularized ileocecal neobladders in two men (see Chapter 16).[159] Detubularization consisted of antimesenteric incisions of both the ileum and cecum, leaving 5 cm of the proximal ileum tubularized for anastomosis to the remnant urethra. The ureters were reimplanted using the Goodwin–Gallo technique. One patient required an artificial urinary sphincter for neurogenic reasons, while the other patient was continent during the day but required an adult diaper overnight.

Both the Mainz and Indiana continent urinary reservoirs have been modified for use as neobladders instead of continent diversions (see Chapters 16 and 25).[160,161] The Mainz neobladder was constructed by Thüroff et al from 10–15 cm of proximal right colon and 25 cm of terminal ileum and remodeled in an N configuration.[160] Instead of forming an efferent intussuscepted ileal-ileocecal valve, the appendiceal stump is anastomosed directly to the urethra. In 1987, Rowland and coworkers reported use of the Indiana neobladder in two boys with exstrophy and one man, anastomosing the intact efferent tapered ileal segment to the urethra.[161] This form of urinary diversion is not commonly used today because of significant mucus production from the colonic mucosa.

Right colon neobladders

Goldwasser of Israel is to be credited for the use of a segment of detubularized right colon without any ileal segment tail (see Chapter 17). In 1986, while at the Mayo Clinic, he and associates first described this technique in a series of seven men.[162] The entire right colon, including the proximal transverse colon, was used, and the entire segment, except the most dependent 5 cm of cecum, was detubularized in a Heineke–Mikulicz reconfiguration. Goldwasser and associates have performed this technique in over 40 men, with two-thirds of the patients continent at night 'if they wake every 2–3 hours to void'.[163,164]

Sigmoid colon neobladders

In 1956, Palken, of Seattle, Washington, successfully used a tubularized 20.3-cm segment of sigmoid colon as a bladder substitute in a 57-year-old man.[165] Prior to performing what was the first recorded human sigmoid neobladder, Palken completed the procedure in dogs in a similar fashion to that described in animals by Bisgard of Nebraska and Rubin of Baltimore, Maryland (Figure 1.14a).[166,167] In Stockholm, Giertz and Franksson (1957) reported that in addition to their larger series of ileal neobladders, they had performed sigmoid neobladders in four patients, three being detubularized bowel segments.[76] They discovered that their patients with detubularized ileal segments had a less morbid course than patients in whom segments of sigmoid were used; in fact, only two of four of their sigmoid patients survived the post-operative course.

In 1959, Bourque of Montreal favored the use of sigmoid neobladder and reported excellent results in 25 cases of U-loop anastomosis.[168] Gil-Vernet of Barcelona refined the use of the tubular sigmoid colon as a neobladder following radical cystoprostatectomy (Figure 1.14b). He and Gosalvez first reported their results in 1957 and by 1962 had a series of 41 patients.[169,170] Their patients with tubularized sigmoid suffered significant daytime frequency and nocturnal enuresis.[170] In 1965, Hradec of Prague reported 68 patients who had undergone tubularized sigmoid neobladders with reasonable continence results.[153] In 1991, Reddy of Minnesota routinely used a detubularized sigmoid neobladder following radical cystoprostatectomy, being careful not to ligate the hypogastric artery in the left side of the bladder pedicles, which would compromise

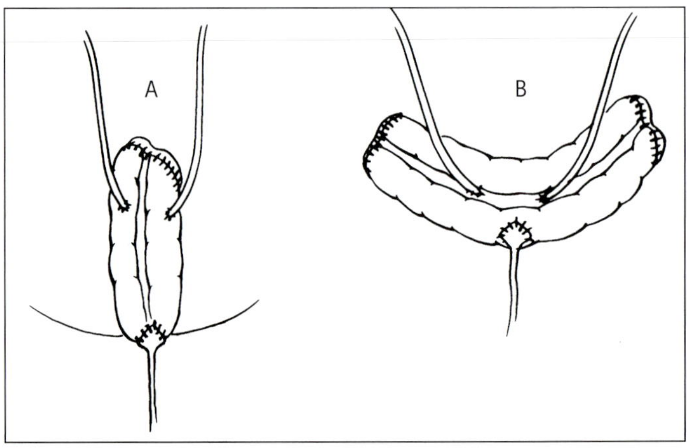

Figure 1.14 Sigmoid neobladders. (a) Method of Bisgard, Rubin and Palken (1943, 1948 and 1956, respectively); (b) Method of Gil-Vernet and Bourque (1957 and 1959, respectively).

the rectal vasculature (see Chapter 18).[171,172] He reported excellent daytime continence; however, 30% of the patients suffered nocturnal enuresis. Currently, the use of the tubularized large bowel is discouraged because of high pressure and low storage volumes.

Outcomes of orthotopic bladder reconstruction

The long-term outcomes of orthotopic, continent urinary diversion are well reported. Studer of Switzerland and Hautmann of Germany both report good outcomes with these types of diversions with excellent patient satisfaction, physiologic function of the bladder and preservation of the upper urinary tracts with no adverse effects on cancer cure rates.[173–176]

With continued evolution of techniques and surgical care, creation of the orthotopic neobladders can now be performed safely and rapidly in even patients with significant comorbidities. Parekh et al from Vanderbilt University showed no difference in short-term morbidity between 117 patients undergoing orthotopic reconstruction and 81 patients with ileal loop diversion.[177] The same group in 2002 showed that orthotopic neobladder reconstruction was a safe alternative to ileal loop diversion in patients with high perioperative risk and comorbidities with no increase in perioperative morbidity or mortality.[178] This indicates that in experienced hands, while orthotopic reconstruction of many types may result in longer operative times than the ileal loop diversion, this does not necessarily translate to higher morbidity, longer hospitalization or worsened outcomes.

Laparoscopic urinary diversion

Recently, laparoscopic surgical techniques have become commonplace in general, urologic, gynecologic and other surgical specialties. Laparoscopic techniques have advanced dramatically over the past 10 years with laparosopic renal surgery being performed routinely. Laparoscopic prostatectomy is being performed in many surgical centers with some centers performing laparoscopic cystectomy and urinary diversion. Interest for laparoscopic urinary diversion has grown recently with the first urinary loop diversion being performed by Kozminiski and Partamian in 1992.[179]

As the technology grew and continued to improve, researchers turned attention toward intracorporal reconstruction with continent diversions. In 2000, Inderbir Gill and his group at the Cleveland Clinic, Cleveland, Ohio, performed the first completely laparoscopic cystectomy with ileal loop urinary diversion on two patients.[180] They continued to modify the procedure performing the challenging surgery through a transperitoneal route using six laparoscopic ports (two 5-mm ports, two 10-mm ports and two 12-mm ports). The Studer pouch was constructed with 65 cm of small bowel as described elsewhere with good results.[181]

Some modifications to the technique were necessary in order to allow completely intracorporal, laparoscopic construction. The posterior plate was constructed by cutting the bowel with endoshears and the harmonic scalpel. The posterior urethral anastomotic sutures were placed into the posterior wall of the pouch and urethra, the anterior closure being started at the urethra and continued to the proximal end of the pouch. All suturing and knot tying was performed intracorporally using free-hand laparoscopic techniques only.

Hand-assisted laparoscopy was first performed in the early 1990s by inserting the finger or hand through a small very tight incision.[182,183] Leakage of carbon dioxide and spraying of blood limited its usefulness. In 1996 the first hand-assisted laparoscopy port was approved by the Food and Drug Administration for use in the USA and since has been used extensively in many surgical specialties.[184] Peterson et al of Madigan Army Medical Center in Washington State reported the first case of hand-assisted, laparoscopic cystoprostatectomy with urinary diversion in a human.[185] The bladder was removed through the hand port. After the cancer surgery was completed, the hand port served as a mini-laparotomy incision and an ileal loop performed extracorporally. The patient did well with rapid return to normal activities 4 weeks after surgery.

The appendix and reconstructive urology

In more recent years, the use of the appendix has become popular, particularly in the construction of a catheterizable neourethra as part of a continent urinary reservoir. Most refer to this technique as the Mitrofanoff principle after the Russian surgeon who, in 1980, reported the use of the appendix in order to create a continent vesicostomy.[186] In actuality, however, the appendix had been used many years earlier in reconstructive urology. It was used in 1908 by Verhoogen of Brussels and in 1927 the appendix was used in Argentina as a continent catheterizable stoma for right colon reservoirs.[95,99] From 1910 to 1914, three reports by Eaton, Kennedy and Babcock described the direct anastomosis of a ureter into the appendix.[3,187,188] In Mitrofanoff's initial report, a series of 16 children underwent implantation of the catheterizable appendix into the native bladder. Since that time he has also used the native ureter for similar implantation. Duckett and Snyder of Philadelphia are primarily responsible for the popularization of this technique which they summarized as:[189]

> A narrow conduit (appendix or ureter) brought to the skin, a large, leak-proof urine storage reservoir (bladder, augmented bladder, or colon segment), an antirefluxing connection to the reservoir to provide continence, and an easy self-catheterizing maneuver to drain the system.

References

1. Hinman F, Weyrauch HM. A critical study of the different principles of surgery which have been used in ureterointestinal implantation. Trans Am Assoc Genitourin Surg 1936; 29: 15–156.

2. Goodwin WE. Experiences with intestine as a substitute for the urinary tract. In: King LR, Stone AR, Webster GD (eds). Bladder Reconstruction and Continent Urinary Diversion. Chicago: Year Book Medical Publishers, 1991; 1–24.
3. Murphy LJT. Ureteric repairs and replacement, urinary diversion, artificial bladders and allied subjects. In: The History of Urology. Springfield, Illinois: Charles C Thomas, 1972; 288–332.
4. Thorne ID, Resnick MI. The use of bowel in urologic surgery: an historical perspective. Urol Clin North Am 1986; 13: 179–91.
5. Simon J. Extropia vesicae (absence of the anterior walls of the bladder and pubic abdominal parietes); operation for directing the orifices of the ureters into the rectum; temporary success; subsequent death; autopsy. Lancet, 1852; ii: 568–9.
6. Lloyd. Extropia vesicae (absence of the anterior walls of the bladder) operation; subsequent death. Lancet, 1851; ii: 370–2.
7. Smith T. An account of an unsuccessful attempt to treat extroversion of the bladder by a new operation. St Barth Hosp Rep 1879; 15: 29–35.
8. Maydl K. Ueber die Radikaltherapie der Ectopia Vesicae Urinariae. Wien Med Wochenschr 1894; 44: 25.
9. Ricard. As stated by Heitz-Boyer M and Hovelacque A. Création d'une nouvelle vessie et d'un nouvel urètre. J Urol (Paris) 1912; 1: 237–58.
10. Coffey RC. Physiologic implantation of the severed ureter or common bile duct into the intestine. JAMA 1911; 56: 397–403.
11. Coffey RC. Transplantation of the ureters into large intestine in the absence of a functioning urinary bladder. Surg Gynecol Obstet 1921; 32: 383–91.
12. Nesbit RM. Uretero-sigmoid anastomosis by direct elliptical anastomosis. J Urol 1949; 61: 728.
13. Cordonnier JJ. Ureterosigmoid anastomosis. Surg Gynec Obstet 1949; 88: 441–6.
14. Cordonnier JJ. Ureterosigmoid anastomosis. J Urol 1950; 63: 276–85.
15. Leadbetter WF. Consideration of problems incident to performance of ureteroenterostomy: report of a technique. J Urol 1950; 65: 818–30.
16. Woodruff LM, Cooper JF, Leadbetter WF. Ureteroenterostomy: experimental studies. J Urol 1952; 71: 873–9.
17. Weyrauch HM, Young BW. Evaluation of common methods of uretero-intestinal anastomosis: an experimental study. J Urol 1952; 67: 880–91.
18. Leadbetter WF, Clarke BG. Five years' experience with ureteroenterostomy by the 'combined' technique. J Urol 1954; 73: 999–1008.
19. Clarke BG, Leadbetter WF. Ureterosigmoidostomy: collective review of results in 2897 reported cases. J Urol 1955; 73: 67–82.
20. Goodwin WE, Harris AP, Kaufman JJ, Beal JM. Open transcolonic ureterointestinal anastomosis: a new approach. Surg Gynecol Obstet 1953; 97: 295–300.
21. Le Duc A, Camey M. Un Procédé d'implantation uretero-ileal anti-reflux dans l'enterocystoplastie. J Urol (Paris) 1979; 85: 449.
22. Le Duc A, Camey M, Teillac P. An original antireflux ureteroileal implantation technique: long-term follow-up. J Urol 1987; 137: 1156–8.
23. Kristjansson A, Grubb A, Månsson W. Renal tubular dysfunction after urinary diversion. Scand J Urol 1995; 29: 407–12.
24. Giordano D. Sulla questione se si possano trapiantare gli ureteri nel retto: note critico-sperimentale. Clin Chir (Milan) 1894; 2: 80.
25. Mauclaire P. De quelques essais de chirurgie expérimentale applicables au traitement (a) de l'exstrophie de la vessie, (b) des abouchements anormaux du rectum, (c) des anus contre nature complexes. Assoc Franc Chir 1895; 9: 546.
26. Schloffer H. Ziele bei der Behandlung der Blasenektopie. Zbl Chir 1916; 43: 749.
27. Boyce WH, Vest SA. A new concept concerning treatment of exstrophy of the bladder. J Urol 1952; 67: 503–17.
28. Boyce WH, Kroovand RL. The Boyce–Vest operation for extrophy of the bladder. Urol Clin North Am 1986; 13: 307–19.
29. Gersuny R. Cited by Foges. Officielles protokol der Gesellschaft der Aerzte in Wien. Wien Klin Wochenschr 1898; 11: 989–90.
30. Lotheissen G. Uber Uretertransplantationen. Wien Klin Wochenschr 1899; 12: 883.
31. Heitz-Boyer M, Hovelacque A. Création d'une nouvelle vessie et d'un nouvel urètre. J Urol (Paris), 1912; 1: 237–58.
32. Lowsley OS, Johnson TH, Rueda AE. A new operation for diversion of the urine with voluntary control of feces and urine. J Int Coll Surg 1953; 20: 457–64.
33. Levitsky V. Transplantation of the ureters into isolated ampulla of rectum after total cystectomy. Am J Surg 1953; 85: 91–7.
34. Johnson TH. Further experiences with a new operation for urinary diversion. J Urol 1956; 76: 380–6.
35. Ghoneim MA, Shoukry I. The rectal bladder with perineal colostomy for urinary diversion. Urology 1974; 4: 511–19.
36. Hendren WH. Ureterocolic diversion of urine: management of some difficult problems. J Urol 1983; 129: 719–29.
37. Rink RC, Retik AB. Ureteroileocecalsigmoidostomy and avoidance of carcinoma of the colon. In: King LR, Stone AR, Webster GD (eds). Bladder Reconstruction and Continent Urinary Diversion. Chicago: Year Book Medical Publishers, 1987; 172–8.
38. Kim KS, Susskind MR, King LR. Ileocecal ureterosigmoidostomy: an alternative to conventional ureterosigmoidostomy. J Urol 1988; 140: 1494–8.
39. Knox AJ, Jago RH. The value of intestinal valves in urinary diversion: an experimental study. Br J Urol 1975; 47: 391–7.
40. Kock NG, Berglund B, Ghoneim MA et al. Urinary diversion to the augmented and valved rectum. Scand J Urol Nephrol 1988; 22: 227–33.
41. Kock NG, Ghoneim MA, Lycke KG, Mahran MR. Urinary diversion to the augmented and valved rectum: preliminary results with a novel surgical procedure. J Urol 1988; 140: 1375–9.
42. Ghoneim MA. Urinary diversion to the modified rectal bladder (the augmented and valved rectum): an anal sphincter-controlled bladder substitute. In: King LR, Stone AR, Webster GD (eds). Bladder Reconstruction and Continent Urinary Diversion. Chicago: Year Book Medical Publishers, 1991; 228–44.
43. Sinaiko ES. Artificial bladder in man from segment of stomach. Surg Forum 1957; 8: 635–9.
44. Sinaiko ES, Walker L, Necheles H. Artificial bladder from stomach pouch. Am J Physiol 1954; 179: 3.

45. Sinaiko ES. Artificial bladder from segment of stomach and study of effect of urine on gastric secretion. Surg Gynecol Obstet 1956; 102: 433.
46. Sinaiko ES. Artificial bladder from a gastric pouch. Surg Gynecol Obstet 1960; 111: 155–62.
47. Leong CH. Use of the stomach for bladder replacement and urinary diversion. Ann R Coll Surg Engl 1978; 60: 283–9.
48. Seiffert L. Die Darm-siphon-blase. Arch Klin Chir 1935; 183: 569–74.
49. Morales PA, Whitehead ED. High jejunal conduit for supravesical urinary diversion: report of 25 cases. Urology 1973; 1: 426–31.
50. Golimbu M, Morales P. Jejunal conduits: technique and complications J Urol 1975; 113: 787–95.
51. Zaayer. Discussion. Intra-abdominale plastieken. Ned Tijdschr Geneesk 1911; 65: 836.
52. Bricker EM. Bladder substitution after pelvic evisceration. Surg Clin North Am 1950; 30: 1511–21.
53. Wallace DM. Ureteric diversion using a conduit: a simplified technique. Br J Urol 1966; 38: 522–7.
54. Turnbull RB Jr, Weakley FL. Atlas of Intestinal Stomas. St Louis: CV Mosby, 1967.
55. Turnbull RB Jr, Hewitt CR. Loop-end myotomy ileostomy in the obese patient. Urol Clin North Am 1978; 5: 423–9.
56. Skinner DG. The craft of urologic surgery. Urol Clin North Am 1978; 5: 423.
57. Bloom DA, Lieskovsky G, Rainwater G et al. The Turnbull loop stoma. J Urol 1983; 129: 715–18.
58. Emmott D, Noble MJ, Mebust WK. A comparison of end versus loop stomas for ileal conduit urinary diversion. J Urol 1985; 133: 588–90.
59. Madersbacher S, Schmidt J, Eberle JM et al. Long term outcome of ileal conduit diversion. J Urol 2003; 169: 985–90.
60. Bricker EM, Eiseman B. Bladder reconstruction from cecum and ascending colon following resection of pelvic viscera. Ann Surg 1950; 132: 77–84.
61. Zinman L, Libertino JA. Ileocecal conduit for temporary and permanent urinary diversion. J Urol 1975; 113: 317–23.
62. Libertino JA, Zinman L. Ileocecal conduit for temporary and permanent urinary diversion. Urol Clin North Am 1986; 13: 241–50.
63. Morales P, Golimbu M. Colonic urinary diversion: 10 years of experience. J Urol 1975; 113: 302–7.
64. Schmidt JD, Hawtrey CE, Buchsbaum HJ. Transverse colon conduit: a preferred method of urinary diversion for radiation-treated pelvic malignancies. J Urol 1975; 113: 308–13.
65. Schmidt JD, Buchsbaum HJ, Nachsheim DA. Long term followup, further experience with, and modification of the transverse colon conduit in urinary tract diversion. Br J Urol 1985; 57: 284–8.
66. Leoning SA, Navarre RJ, Narayana AS, Culp DA. Transverse colon conduit urinary diversion. J Urol 1982; 127: 37–9.
67. Beckley S, Wajsman Z, Pontes JE, Murphy GP. Transverse colon conduit: a method of urinary diversion after pelvic irradiation. J Urol 1982; 128: 464–8.
68. Turner-Warwick RT. Technique for the separate diversion of urine and faeces. Lancet 1959; i: 1021–22.
69. Mogg RA. Treatment of neurogenic urinary incontinence using colon conduit. Br J Urol 1965; 37: 681–6.
70. Hendren WH. Nonrefluxing colon conduit for temporary or permanent urinary diversion in children. J Pediatr Surg 1975; 10: 381.
71. Altwein JE, Hohenfellner R. Use of the colon as a conduit for urinary diversions. Surg Gynecol Obstet 1975; 140: 33–8.
72. Richie JP. Sigmoid conduit urinary diversion. Urol Clin North Am 1986; 13: 225–32.
73. Skinner DG, Lieskovsky G, Skinner E, Boyd S. Urinary diversion. Curr Probl Surg 1987; 24: 401–71.
74. Rudick J, Schonholz S, Weber HB. The gastric bladder: a continent reservoir for urinary diversion. Surgery 1977; 82: 1–8.
75. Nguyen DH, Mitchell ME. Gastric bladder reconstruction. Urol Clin North Am 1991; 18: 649–57.
76. Giertz G, Franksson C. Construction of a substitute bladder with preservation of urethral voiding after total and subtotal cystectomy. Acta Chir Scand 1957; 113: 218–28.
77. Tasker JH. Ileo-cystoplasty: a new technique: an experimental study with report of a case. Br J Urol 1953; 25: 349–53.
78. Goodwin WE, Winter CC, Barker WF. 'Cup-patch' technique of ileocystoplasty for bladder enlargement or partial substitution. Surg Gynecol Obstet 1959; 108: 240–4.
79. Ekman H, Jacobsson B, Kock N et al. The functional behaviour of different types of intestinal urinary bladder substitutes. Congr Int Soc Urol Lond 1964; 2: 213.
80. Kock NG. Intra-abdominal 'reservoir' in patients with permanent ileostomy. Arch Surg 1969; 99: 223–31.
81. Kock NG. The development of the continent ileal reservoir (Kock pouch) and its application in patients requiring urinary diversion or bladder replacement. In: King LR, Stone AR, Webster GD (eds). Bladder Reconstruction and Continent Urinary Diversion. Chicago: Year Book Medical Publishers, 1991; 247–71.
82. Kock NG. Continent ileostomy. Prog Surg 1973; 12: 180–201.
83. Watsuji H. Eine kombinierte Anwendung des Hackers und fontanschen Verfahrens bei der Gastrostomie. Mitt Med Ges 1899; 13: 879–82.
84. Kock NG, Nilson AE, Norlen L, Sundin T, Trasti H. Changes in renal parenchyma and the upper urinary tracts following urinary diversion via a continent ileum reservoir: an experimental study in dogs. Scand J Urol Nephrol (Suppl) 1978; 49: 11–22.
85. Kock NG, Nilson AE, Norlen L, Sundin T, Trasti H. Urinary diversion via a continent ileum reservoir: clinical experience. Scand J Urol Nephrol (Suppl) 1978; 49: 23–31.
86. Madigan MR. The continent ileostomy and the isolated ileal bladder. Ann R Coll Surg Engl 1976; 58: 62–9.
87. Leisinger HJ, Sauberli H, Schauwecker H, Mayor G. Continent ileal bladder: first clinical experience. Eur Urol 1976; 2: 8–12.
88. Leisinger HJ, Schauwecker H, Sauberli H. Dynamics of the continent ileal bladder: an experimental study in dogs. Invest Urol 1977; 15: 49–54.
89. Kock NG, Nilson AE, Nilsson LO et al. Urinary diversion via a continent ileal reservoir: clinical results in 12 patients. J Urol 1982; 128: 469–75.
90. Skinner DG. In search of the ideal method of urinary diversion [Guest editorial]. J Urol 1982; 128: 476.

91. Skinner DG, Boyd SD, Leiskowsky G. Clinical experience with the Koch continent ileal reservoir for urinary diversion. J Urol 1984; 132: 1101–7.
92. Skinner DG, Lieskovsky G, Boyd SD. Continuing experience with the continent ileal reservoir (Kock pouch) as an alternative to cutaneous urinary diversion: an update after 250 cases. J Urol 1987; 137: 1140–5.
93. Abol-Eniem H, Ghoneim MA. A novel uretero-ileal reimplantation technique: A serosal lined tunnel. A preliminary report. J Urol 1994; 151: 1193.
94. Stein JP, Lieskovsky G, Ginsberg DA, Bochner BH, Skinner DG. The T pouch: an orthotopic ileal neobladder incorporating a serosal lined ileal antireflux technique. J Urol 1998; 159: 1836–42.
95. Verhoogen J. Neostomie urétero-caecale: formation d'une nouvelle pouche vesicale et d'une nouvel urètre. Assoc Franc d'Urol 1908–1909; 12: 362–5.
96. Verhoogen J, de Graeuve, A. La cystectomie totale. Folia Urol 1909; 3: 629–73.
97. Makkas M. Zur Behandlung der Blasenektopie umwandlung der ausgeschalteten Coecum zur Blase und der Appendix zur Urethra. Centralbl Chir 1910; 37: 1073–6.
98. Lengemann P. Ersatz der extirpierten Harnblase durch das Coecum. Zentralbl Chir 1913; 40: 14–15.
99. Gallo AG. A Propósito de operación de triana: nueva técnica de exclusion de la vejiga utilizando el ciego aislando como receptacullo urinario. Bol Trab Acad Argentina Cirujanos 1946; 30: 604–10.
100. Ramirez Gutiérrez A. Operación de triana neo-vejiga cecal. Rev Fac Med Bogota (Columbia) 1946; 15: 3161.
101. Gilchrist RK, Merricks JW, Hamlin HH, Rieger IT. Construction of a substitute bladder and urethra. Surg Gynecol Obstet 1950; 90: 752–60.
102. Merricks JW, Gilchrist RK, Hamlin H, Rieger IT. A substitute bladder and urethra, using cecum as bladder and ileum as urethra. J Urol 1957; 65: 581–9.
103. Romero Lobo F, Santander E. Construcción de un reservorio vestical (neo vejiga) a expensas del ciego y colon ascendente con abocamiento de los ureteres en el mismo acto quirúrgico y formación de una uretra ileal. Bol Hosp Vargas de San Cristobal (Venezuela) 1952; 1: 61–75.
104. Sullivan H, Gilchrist RK, Merricks JW. Ileocecal substitute bladder: long-term followup. J Urol 1973; 109: 43–5.
105. Harper JG, Berman MH, Hertzberg AD, Lerman F, Brendler H. Observations on the use of the cecum as a substitute urinary bladder. J Urol 1954; 71: 600–2.
106. Ashken MH. An appliance-free ileocecal urinary diversion: preliminary communication. Br J Urol 1974; 46: 631–8.
107. Ashken MH. Continent ileocaecal urinary reservoir. J Roy Soc Med 1978; 71: 357–60.
108. Ashken MH. Urinary cecal reservoir. In: King LR, Stone AR, Webster GD (eds). Bladder Reconstruction and Continent Urinary Diversion. Chicago: Year Book Medical Publishers, 1987; 238.
109. Benchekroun A. Continent caecal bladder. Eur Urol 1977; 3: 248–50.
110. Benchekroun A. The ileocecal continent bladder. In: King LR, Stone AR, Webster GD (eds). Bladder Reconstruction and Continent Urinary Diversion. Chicago: Year Book Medical Publishers, 1991; 324–36.
111. Zingg E, Tscholl R. Continent cecoileal conduit: preliminary report. J Urol 1977; 118: 724–8.
112. Mansson W, Colleen S, Sundin T. Continent cecal reservoir in urinary diversion. Br J Urol 1984; 56: 359–65.
113. Mansson W, Colleen S, Sundin T. The continent cecal reservoir in urinary diversion. World J Urol 1985; 3: 173–8.
114. Mansson W, Colleen S. Experience with a detubularized right colonic segment for bladder replacement. Scand J Urol Nephrol 1990; 24: 53.
115. Mansson W. Continuing experience with the right colon as a continent reservoir for urine. In: King LR, Stone AR, Webster GD (eds). Bladder Reconstruction and Continent Urinary Diversion. Chicago: Year Book Medical Publishers, 1991; 283–8.
116. Webster GD, Bertram RA. Continent catheterizable urinary diversion using the ileocecal segment with stapled intussusception of the ileocecal valve. J Urol 1986; 135: 465–9.
117. King LR, Robertson CN, Bertram RA. A new technique for the prevention of reflux in those undergoing bladder substitution or undiversion using bowel segments. World J Urol 1985; 3: 194–6.
118. Thüroff JW, Alken P, Riedmiller H et al. The Mainz-pouch (mixed augmentation ileum 'n zecum for bladder augmentation and continent urinary diversion. World J Urol 1985; 3: 179–84.
119. Thüroff JW, Alken P, Riedmiller H et al. The Mainz-pouch (mixed augmentation ileum and cecum) for bladder augmentation and continent urinary diversion. J Urol 1986; 136: 17–26.
120. Thüroff JW, Alken P, Riedmiller H et al. 100 cases of Mainz-pouch: continuing experience and evolution. J Urol 1988; 140: 283–8.
121. Rowland RG, Mitchell ME, Bihrle R. The cecoileal continent urinary reservoir. World J Urol 1985; 3: 185–90.
122. Rowland RG, Mitchell ME, Bihrle R et al. Indiana continent urinary reservoir. J Urol 1987; 137: 1136–8.
123. Bejany DE, Politano VA. Stapled and nonstapled tapered distal ileum for construction of a continent colonic urinary reservoir. J Urol 1988; 140: 491–4.
124. Bihrle R, Foster RS. Continent ileocecal reservoirs: the Indiana pouch. In: King LR, Stone AR, Webster GD (eds). Bladder Reconstruction and Continent Urinary Diversion. Chicago: Year Book Medical Publishers, 1991; 308–15.
125. Lockhart JL. Remodeled right colon: an alternative urinary reservoir. J Urol 1987; 138: 730–4.
126. Lockhart JL, Pow-Sang M, Persky L et al. A continent colonic urinary reservoir: the Florida pouch. J Urol 1990; 144: 864–7.
127. Koff SA, Cirulli C, Lucero SP, Hamoudi A. An operation to create a continent catheterizable urinary sphincter from a short intestinal segment. J Urol 1987; 138: 996–9.
128. Koff SA, Cirulli C, Wise HA. Clinical and urodynamic features of a new intestinal urinary sphincter for continent urinary diversion. J Urol 1992; 142: 293–6.

129. Koff SA, Wise HA. Continent urinary diversion using an ileal servomechanism sphincter. Urol Clin North Am 1992; 19: 611–16.
130. Bihrle R, Foster RS, Steidle CP et al. Creation of a transverse colon-gastric composite reservoir: a new technique. J Urol 1989; 141: 1217–20.
131. Bihrle R, Klee LW, Foster RS. Transverse colon-gastric tube composite reservoir. Probl Urol 1991; 5: 292–8.
132. Tizzoni G, Poggi A. Die wiederherstellung der Harnblase: experimentelle untersuchunger. Centrlbl Chir 1888; 15: 921–4.
133. Tizzoni G, Poggi A. Resultato ultima di un esperimento sulla recostruzione della vescica orinaria. Mem R Acad Sci (Bologna) 1890; 1: 525.
134. Lemoine G. Création d'une vessie nouvelle par un procédé personnel après cystectomie totale pour cancer. J Urol Med Chir 1913; 4: 367–72.
135. Leong CH, Ong GB. Gastrocystoplasty in dogs. Aust N Z J Surg 1972; 41: 272–9.
136. Leong CH. Use of the stomach for bladder replacement and urinary diversion. Ann R Coll Surg Engl 1978; 60: 283–9.
137. Couvelaire R. Le réservoir ileal de substitution après la cystomie totale chez l'homme. J d'Urol 1951; 57: 408–17.
138. Pyrah LN, Raper FP. Some uses of an isolated loop of ileum in genito-urinary surgery. Br J Surg 1955; 42: 337–57.
139. Mellinger GT, Suder GL. Ileal reservoir (ureteroileourethral anastomosis). JAMA 1958; 167: 2183–6.
140. Gandin MM. Uretero-ileo-urethral anastomosis: case report. J Urol 1960; 83: 279–82.
141. Camey M, Le Duc A. L'enterocystoplastie avec cystoprostatectomie totale pour cancer de la vessie. Ann d'Urol 1979; 13: 114–23.
142. Camey M. Bladder replacement by ileocystoplasty following radical cystectomy. World J Urol 1985; 3: 161.
143. Camey M, Richard F, Botto H. Ileal replacement of bladder. In: King LR, Stone AR, Webster GD (eds). Bladder Reconstruction and Continent Urinary Diversion, 2nd edn. Chicago: Mosby Year Book, 1991; 389–410.
144. Hautmann RE, Egghart G, Frohneberg D, Miller K. Die Ileumneoblase. Urologe 1987; 26: A67–73.
145. Hautmann RE, Egghart G, Frohneberg D, Miller K. The ileal neobladder. J Urol 1988; 139: 39–42.
146. Tscholl R, Leisinger HJ, Hauri D. The ileal S-pouch for bladder replacement after cystectomy: preliminary report of 7 cases. J Urol 1987; 138: 344–7.
147. Melchior H, Spehr C, Knopf-Wagemann I et al. The continent ileal bladder for urinary tract reconstruction after cystectomy: a survey of 44 patients. J Urol 1988; 139: 714–18.
148. Studer UE, Ackermann D, Casanova GA, Zingg EJ. A newer form of bladder substitute based on historical perspectives. Semin Urol 1989; 6: 57.
149. Studer UE, Ackerman D, Casanova GA, Zingg EJ. Three years experience with an ileal low pressure bladder substitute. Br J Urol 1989; 63: 43–52.
150. Ghoneim MA, Kock NG, Lycke G, Shebab El-din A. An appliance-free sphincter-controlled bladder substitute: the urethral Kock pouch. J Urol 1987; 138: 1150–4.
151. Skinner DG, Boyd SD, Liekovsky G, Bennet C, Hopwood B. Lower urinary tract reconstruction following cystectomy: experience and results in 126 patients using the Kock ileal reservoir with bilateral ureteroileal urethrostomy. J Urol 1991; 146: 756–60.
152. Elmajian DA, Stein JP, Esrig D et al. The Kock ileal neobladder: updated experience in 295 male patients. J Urol 1998; 156: 920–5.
153. Hradec EA. Bladder substitution: indications and results in 114 operations. J Urol 1965; 94: 406–17.
154. Gil-Vernet JM. The ileocolic segment in urologic surgery. J Urol 1965; 94: 418–26.
155. Khafagy M, El-Bolkainy MN, Barsoum RS, El-Tatawy S. The ileocecal bladder: a new method for urinary diversion after radical cystectomy (a preliminary report). J Urol 1975; 113: 314–16.
156. Khafagy MM, el-Kalawy M, Ibrahim A et al. Radical cystectomy and ileocecal bladder reconstruction for carcinoma of the urinary bladder. Br J Urol 1987; 160: 60–3.
157. Alcini E, d'Addessi A, Giustacchini M et al. Bladder reconstruction after cystectomy: use of ileocecal segment in 3-loop ileal reservoir. Urology 1988; 531: 10–13.
158. Zinmann L, Libertino JA. Right colocystoplasty for bladder replacement. Urol Clin North Am 1986; 13: 321–9.
159. Light JK, Engelmann UH. Le Bag: total replacement of the bladder using an ileocolonic pouch. J Urol 1986; 136: 27–31.
160. Thüroff JW, Alken P, Riedmiller H et al. 100 cases of Mainz-pouch: continuing experience and evolution. J Urol 1988; 140: 283–8.
161. Rowland RG, Mitchell ME, Bihrle R et al. Indiana continent urinary reservoir. J Urol 1987; 137: 1136–8.
162. Goldwasser B, Barrett DM, Benson AC. Bladder replacement with use of a detubularized right colonic segment: preliminary report of a new technique. Mayo Clin Proc 1986; 61: 615–21.
163. Goldwasser B, Mansson W, Davidsson T et al. Cystourethrometric findings in patients with detubularized right colonic segment for bladder replacement. J Urol 1992; 145: 538–41.
164. Goldwasser B, Ramon J. Total bladder replacement using detubularized right colon. In: Webster G, Kirby R, King L, Goldwasser B (eds). Reconstructive Urology. Boston: Blackwell Scientific Publications, 1991; 477–86.
165. Palken M. Urinary bladder substitution. Northwest Med 1956; 55: 1347.
166. Bisgard JD. Substitution of the urinary bladder with a segment of sigmoid: an experimental study. Ann Surg 1943; 117: 106–9.
167. Rubin SW. The formation of an artificial urinary bladder with perfect continence: an experimental study. J Urol 1948; 60: 874–906.
168. Bourque JP. The indications and techniques of bowel substitution after total cystectomy. Br J Urol 1959; 31: 448–60.
169. Gil-Vernet JM, Gosalvez R. Ileocystoplastie ou colocystoplastie. J Urol Med Chir 1957; 63: 466–82.
170. Gil-Vernet JM, Escarpenter G, Perez-Trujillo Vic JB. A functioning artificial bladder: results of 41 consecutive cases. J Urol 1962; 87: 825–36.

171. Reddy PK. Detubularized sigmoid reservoir for bladder replacement after cystoprostatectomy. Urology 1987; 29: 625–8.
172. Reddy PK, Lange PH, Fraley EE. Total bladder replacement using detubularized sigmoid colon: technique and results. J Urol 1991; 145: 51.
173. Lee KS, Montie JE, Dunn RL, Lee CT. Hatumann and Studer orthotopic neobladders: a contemporary experience. J Urol 2003; 169: 2188–91.
174. Hautmann RE, Petriconi RD, Gottfried HW. The ileal neobladder: complications and functional results in 363 patients after 11 years of followup. J Urol 1999; 161: 422–8.
175. Thoeny HC, Sonnenschein MJ, Madersbacher S, Vock P, Studer UE. Is ileal orthotopic bladder substitution with and afferent tubular segment detrimental to the upper urinary tract in the long term? J Urol 2002; 168: 2090–4.
176. Hautmann RE, Simon J. Ileal neobladder and local recurrence of bladder cancer: patterns of failure and impact on function in men. J Urol 1999; 162: 1963–6.
177. Parekh DJ, Gilbert WB, Koch MO, Smith JA Jr. Continent urinary reconstruction versus ileal conduit: a contemporary single-institution comparison of perioperative morbidity and mortality. Urology 2000; 55: 852–5.
178. Parekh DJ, Clark T, O'Connor J et al. Orthotopic neobladder following cystectomy in patients with high perioperative risks and co-morbid medical conditions. J Urol 2002; 168: 2454–6.
179. Kozminski M, Partamian KO. Case report of laparoscopic ileal loop conduit. J Endourol 1992; 6: 147.
180. Gill IS, Fergany A, Klein EA et al. Laparoscopic radical cystoprostatectomy with ileal conduit performed completely intracorporeally: the inital 2 cases. Urology 2000; 56: 26–9.
181. Gill IS, Kaouk JH, Meraney AM et al. Laparoscopic radical cystectomy and continent orthotopic ileal neobladder performed completely intracorporeally: the initial experience. J Urol 2002; 168: 13–18.
182. Tschada RK, Rassweler JJ, Schmeller N. Laparoscopic tumor nephrectomy – the German experiences. J Urol 1995; 153 (Suppl): 479A.
183. Winefield HN, Chen RN, Donovan JF. Laparoscopic trick of the trade: how to overcome lack of tactile feedback. J Endourol 1996; 10: S189.
184. Nakada SY, Moon TD, Gist M et al. Use of the pneumo sleeve as an adjunct in laparoscopic nephrectomy. Urology 1996; 49: 612.
185. Peterson AC, Lance RA, Ahuja SK. Laparoscopic hand assisted radical cystectomy with ileal conduit urinary diversion. J Urol 2002; 168: 2103–5.
186. Mitrofanoff P Cystostomie continente trans-appendiculaire dans le traitement des vessies neurologiques. Chir Pediatr 1980; 21: 297–305.
187. Kennedy B. Uretero-appendiceal anastomosis for transplantation of the ureter shorted by disease or accident. Surg Gynecol Obstet 1912; 15: 464–6.
188. Babcock W. A note as to the recognition of the ureter: report of a case of anastomosis of the ureter into the appendix. Surg Gynecol Obstet 1914; 18: 119–20.
189. Duckett JW, Snyder HM. Use of the Mitrofanoff principle in urinary reconstruction. World J Urol 1985; 3: 191–3.

2 Anatomy of the stomach, small and large bowel as it applies to urinary tract reconstruction

Jacob Ramon

Introduction

For more than a century the gastrointestinal tract has been employed in numerous creative and sophisticated procedures to correct abnormalities of the genitourinary tract. A myriad of procedures incorporating stomach, jejunum, ileum, different parts of the colon and a combination of the above bowel segments have been used in diverting, reconstructing and remodeling different portions of the urinary tract. A thorough knowledge of the surgical anatomy of these structures is necessary in order to properly isolate, mobilize and fashion them according to the requirements of the reconstructive procedures being performed.

This chapter reviews the anatomy of the gastrointestinal tract[1,2] and provides an overview of the anatomical considerations in the use of bowel segments in urinary reconstructive surgery.

Stomach

The stomach is the most dilated part of the alimentary canal. Its mean capacity varies with age, being about 30 ml at birth, increasing gradually to about 1000 ml at puberty, and commonly reaching about 1500 ml in the adult. Normally, the stomach lies in the epigastric, umbilical and left hypochondriac regions of the abdomen, but its position may vary markedly, either as a physiologic anatomic difference or as a result of disease. Its shape and size are extremely variable and are modified by many factors, including the state of gastric physiologic activity, the amount and character of the gastric contents, individual eating habits, changes in the position of the surrounding viscera, changes in the tension of adjacent supporting ligaments and the presence of gastric disorders.

The proximal portion of the stomach, which includes the cardia, fundus and the body of the stomach, is designed for storage and digestion. Its distal part, which includes the antrum and pylorus, is adapted to the role of mixing and evacuation.

When the stomach is empty and its walls contracted, its surfaces are almost superior and inferior, but when it is distended they become anterior and posterior, respectively. The lesser curvature, extending between the cardiac and pyloric orifices, forms the right (or posterosuperior) border of the stomach. The greater curvature is directed anteroinferiorly, and is four or five times as long as the lesser curvature.

The stomach has a blood supply so extensive and interconnected that three of its four major nutrient arteries can be ablated without incurring necrosis or even significant dysfunction. A submucosal plexus of arterioles provides for rapid healing of wounds and a low incidence of anastomotic disruption after operative manipulation. The major arterial supply to the stomach is shown in Figure 2.1. The lesser curvature of the stomach is supplied primarily by the left gastric artery, which arises from the celiac axis. This vessel connects with the right

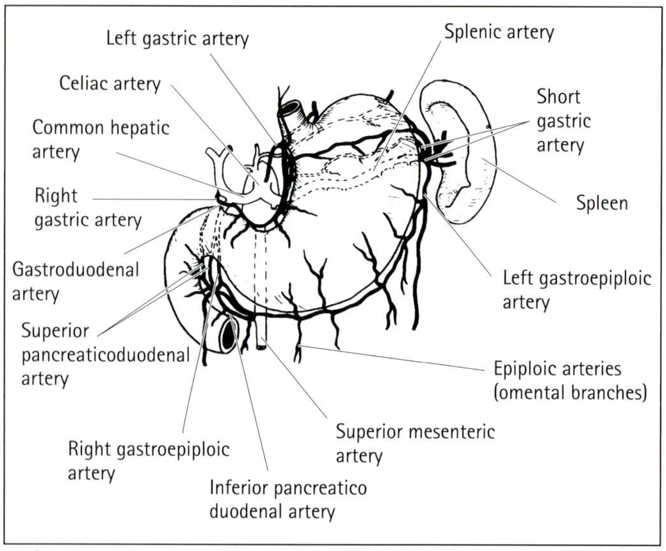

Figure 2.1 Arteries of the stomach.

gastric artery, a branch of the common hepatic artery that provides branches to the pylorus and the first part of the duodenum. Right and left gastroepiploic arteries arise from the gastroduodenal and splenic arteries, respectively. They form an arcade along the greater curvature, the right providing blood to the antrum and the left supplying the body and the lower portion of the fundus. The mid-portion of the greater curvature corresponds to a point at which the gastric branches of the vascular arcade change direction. The short gastric arteries arising from the splenic and left gastroepiploic arteries provide blood to the fundus and to the most proximal portion of the body of the stomach.

The gastric veins commence as straight vessels between the glands of the mucosa and these drain into submucosal veins which then drain into larger veins. The larger veins accompany the main arteries and ultimately drain into the splenic and superior mesenteric veins, but some pass directly to the portal vein. The lymphatic drainage of the stomach follows the distribution of the blood supply.

The greater omentum hangs from the greater curvature of the stomach. Between the greater curvature and the transverse colon are the two descending anterior layers of the greater omentum, known as the gastrocolic ligament. This ligament contains between its two layers, close to the curvature of the stomach, the left and right gastroepiploic vessels.

Utilizing the gastroepiploic vessels, a pedicle of stomach may be mobilized to the pelvis for gastrocystoplasty. There are two forms of gastrocystoplasty: one uses the antrum and the other a wedge resection of the greater curvature. The antral gastrocystoplasty uses the antrum with a blood supply consisting of the left gastroepiploic artery. In mobilizing the right side of the greater curvature to facilitate antral resection, it should be borne in mind that there is a frequent relationship of the middle colic artery and its branches to the subpyloric area of the stomach. If ligated, the loss of these vessels may cause gangrene of the mid-transverse colon. Occasionally, the left gastroepiploic artery will be atretic at some point in its course and will not provide an adequate blood supply. The right gastroepiploic artery is found to be much more constant in its course and caliber. The wedge gastrocystoplasty uses a large wedge-shaped segment of the body of the stomach which is removed with its blood supply. (The right gastroepiploic artery is preferred.) The gastric flap is brought retroperitoneally into the pelvis through windows made in the base of the transverse mesocolon, and in the mesentary of the distal ileum (Figure 2.2).[3] Alternatively, the pedicle can be placed in the right gutter after reflecting the cecum, ascending colon, and hepatic flexure, medially.

Small bowel

The small bowel extends from the pylorus to the cecum. The length of the small intestine depends entirely upon the state of bowel activity at the time of measurement. Estimates provide

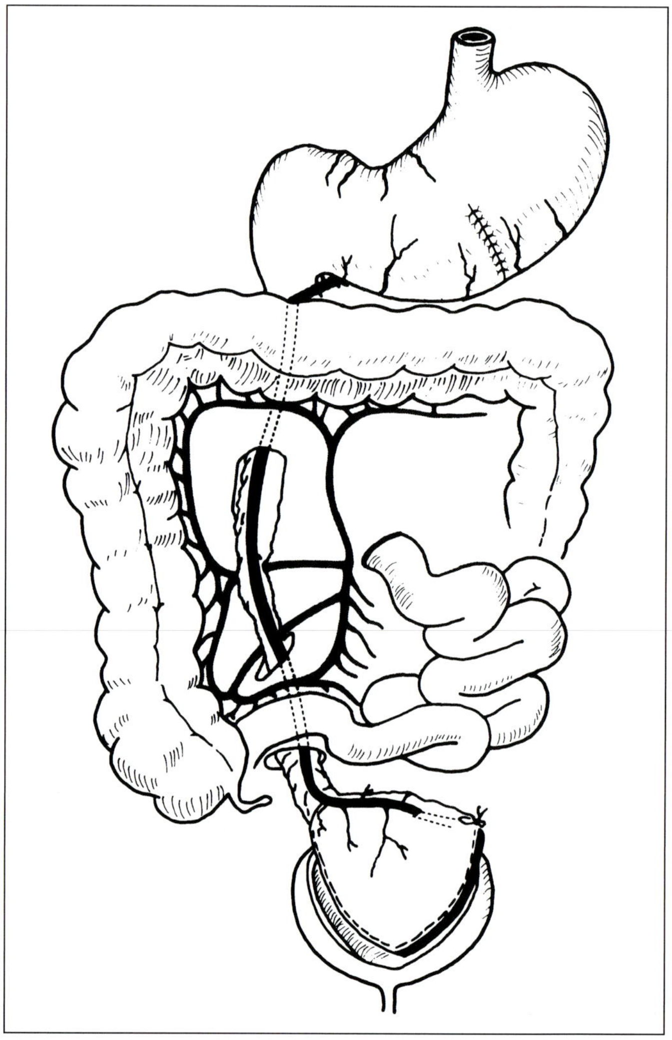

Figure 2.2 Gastrocystoplasty. The retroperitoneal path of a wedge-shaped gastric flap, based on the right epiploic artery.

Anatomical considerations

The colon requires mobilization from its fixed position for urinary reconstruction. The mesentery to the ileocecal and the ascending colon generally provides sufficient length for segments of this portion of bowel to be drawn into the pelvis for bladder augmentation or replacement. On occasion, it is necessary to sever the right colic artery at its origin in order to mobilize the distal portion the ascending colon towards the pelvis. The transverse colon is mobilized by detaching the gastrocolic omentum along the avascular plane of its attachment to the colon. Its mesentery is generally not long and allows only adequate mobility for the performance of a transverse colon conduit. The descending colon is mobilized much as the right colon by incising the avascular line lateral to the colon. Its mesentery allows for considerable mobility. The mesentery attached to the sigmoid colon permits the use of this segment in vitually all forms of reconstructive urinary diversion.

Conclusion

A variety of techniques are available to the urologist for incorporation of bowel into the urinary tract. The segments of bowel which urologists frequently deal with include the stomach, small and large bowel and rectum. As mentioned before, with thorough knowledge of the surgical anatomy and the anatomical variations of these structures, reconstruction of the urinary tract may be performed with the appropriate segment of intestine, with the least morbidity, to the urinary and gastrointestinal tracts.

References

1. Williams PL, Warwick R (eds). Gray's Anatomy, 36th edn. Edinburgh: Churchill Livingstone, 1980.
2. Lindner HH (ed). Clinical Anatomy. New York: Appleton and Lange, 1989.
3. Adams MC, Mitchel ME, Rink RC. Gastrocystoplasty: alternative solution to the problem of urological reconstruction in severely compromised patients. J Urol 1988; 140: 1152–6.
4. Skinner DG, Boyd SD, Lieskovsky G. Clinical experience with the Kock continent reservoir for urinary diversion. J Urol 1984; 132: 1101–7.
5. Thüroff JW, Alken P, Riedmiller H, Jacobi GH, Hohenfellner R. 100 cases of Mainz pouch: continuing experience and evaluation. J Urol 1988; 140: 283–8.
6. Ramon J, Leandri P, Rossignol G, Botto H. Orthotopic bladder replacement using ileum: techniques and results. In: Webster G, Kirby R, King L, Goldwasser B (eds). Reconstructive Urology. Boston: Blackwell Scientific Publications, 1993: 445–7.
7. Woodhouse CRJ, Malone PR, Cumming J, Reilly TM. The Mitrofanoff principle for continent urinary diversion. Br J Urol 1989; 63: 53–57.

3 Metabolic implications and electrolyte disturbances

Cigdem Tanrikut and W Scott McDougal

Introduction

Since intestine was neither meant to serve as a conduit nor as a means of storage for urine, its use in urologic reconstructive procedures may result in numerous short- and long-term complications. Metabolic complications include electrolyte abnormalities, nutritional disturbances, calculus formation, alterations in hepatic metabolism; changes in glucose metabolism; abnormal drug metabolism; and bone disease and growth disturbances.

Many of these metabolic complications are influenced by the degree of solute absorption across the bowel segment. Solute absorption is impacted by: (i) the segment of bowel used; (ii) the surface area of bowel used; (iii) the time of retention of urine; (iv) the concentration of solutes in the urine; (v) renal function; and (vi) the pH and osmolality of the urine. These factors affect the amount of solute absorbed as well as the type and severity of metabolic complication.

Electrolyte abnormalities

A range of electrolyte and metabolic abnormalities may develop based on the segment of the gastrointestinal tract used during urinary reconstruction (Table 3.1). Knowledge of normal physiologic function of a particular segment of the gastrointestinal tract is helpful in predicting which abnormalities are likely to develop.

Stomach

When stomach is used in urinary diversion, a hypokalemic, hypochloremic metabolic alkalosis can occur.[1] Although this complication is rarely significant in the presence of normal renal function, it can be marked in the patient with severely limited renal function. The cause of this metabolic abnormality is related to the normal physiologic function of the stomach. A H^+/K^+ antiport in the stomach secretes a hydrogen ion into the lumen in exchange for a potassium ion. The hydrogen ion is derived from carbonic acid, which also generates a bicarbonate ion. The bicarbonate ion is released into the systemic circulation, and then excreted by the kidney into the urine. When diverted through the gastric segment, secreted hydrogen ions are partially neutralized by the excess bicarbonate ions. If renal function is severely limited, bicarbonate excretion by the kidney is compromised which can lead to development of significant metabolic alkalosis. On rare occasions, patients may develop severe manifestations of this abnormality, i.e. lethargy, seizures or death. To reduce hydrogen ion secretion, proton-pump inhibitors such as omeprazole or lansoprazole can be used with good effect.

The gastric antrum produces gastrin, a hormone that stimulates hydrogen ion secretion by the parietal cells. Gastrin release is stimulated by mechanical stretch of the stomach, nerve stimulation and local enteric reflexes. Delivery of alkaline urine to the gastric segment and mechanical stretch can stimulate local acid secretion and gastrin production. Alterations in acid production can produce ulcers and dysuria. The hematuria-dysuria syndrome may result due to excess acid secretion and is characterized by suprapubic pain, bladder spasm, hematuria, and dysuria.[2,3] Treatment includes administration of proton-pump inhibitors.

Jejunum

Electrolyte abnormalities, which are difficult to manage, occur more commonly when jejunum is employed for urinary diversion than with the use of ileum or colon. Metabolic derangements include hyponatremia, hypochloremia, hyperkalemia, azotemia, and acidosis.[4] These abnormalities occur as a consequence of

Table 3.1 Electrolyte/metabolic abnormalities that may occur following urinary reconstruction with a bowel segment and their treatment

Segment	Physiologic function	Abnormality	Treatment	Prevention
Stomach	Secretion of H^+, Cl^-, K^+	Hypochloremic, hypokalemic metabolic alkalosis	Saline administration, KCl replacement, proton-pump inhibitors	Proton-pump inhibitors, KCl supplementation
	Gastrin secretion	Metabolic alkalosis, hematuria-dysuria syndrome	Saline administration, KCl replacement, proton-pump inhibitors	Proton-pump inhibitors, KCl supplementation
Jejunum	Secretion of Na^+, Cl^- Reabsorption of K^+, H^+	Hyponatremic, hyperkalemic, hypochloremic metabolic acidosis, azotemia. Can result in jejunal conduit syndrome (i.e. lethargy, nausea, vomiting, dehydration, weakness, fever)	Saline administration, correction of acidosis with $NaHCO_3$ administration	Oral NaCl supplementation, hydration
Ileum, colon	Absorption of NH_4^+, Cl^- Inability to absorb K^+	Hyperchloremic metabolic acidosis ± hypokalemia	Correction of acidosis with $NaHCO_3$ administration with simultaneous K^+ replacement	Oral $NaHCO_3$ or bicitrates. Chlorpromazine or nicotinic acid can reduce the need for alkalinizing agents

enhanced sodium and chloride secretion with concurrent dehydration.[5] As a result of the dehydration and hypovolemia, the kidney produces renin. This increases aldosterone production which, in turn, stimulates sodium reabsorption by the kidney. In addition, renal acid excretion is hindered by hyperkalemia, leading to acidosis. A low-sodium, high-potassium, hyperosmotic urine is delivered to the jejunal segment diversion.[6] The jejunal segment reabsorbs potassium and secretes more sodium, chloride and water, perpetuating the problem. When severe, the patient may develop the jejunal conduit syndrome:[7] lethargy, nausea, vomiting, dehydration, weakness and fever. Treatment includes hydration, salt repletion and correction of the acidosis. Due to the severity of metabolic abnormalities when large segments of jejunum are employed the jejunal segment, if used, should be as short as possible. In general, other segments are a better choice for urinary diversion.

Ileum and colon

With the interposition of ileum or colon into the urinary tract, hyperchloremic metabolic acidosis ensues.[8,9] This imbalance is caused by net absorption of ammonium and chloride from the urine.[5] The ammonium ion substitutes for sodium in the Na^+/H^+ antiport.[10,11] Hypokalemia may also occur in patients with ileal and colon segments. Ileum possesses better ability to absorb potassium; therefore, hypokalemia is more common with colonic segments.[12]

The majority of patients with ileal conduits exhibit some degree of hyperchloremic metabolic acidosis,[9,13] although clinical symptoms are relatively few. Patients with orthotopic or continent urinary diversions may be more likely to exhibit the metabolic abnormalities than those with conduits due to the increased contact time of urine to mucosa.[14] Patients with compromised renal function are less able to compensate for the increased acid load and, thus, are also more likely to exhibit sequelae of the acidosis. Correction of acidosis is further impaired by pyelonephritis, urinary obstruction, or urinary stasis.

Treatment includes correction of acidosis with concomitant potassium repletion. Correction of acidosis without potassium repletion may lead to a marked hypokalemia because potassium will re-enter the cells and move out of the bloodstream as the serum pH rises.[15] Normal acid–base balance can be achieved by administration of sodium bicarbonate or sodium citrate plus citric acid. Patients on a low-sodium diet can be administered potassium and sodium citrate,[13] as long as potassium supplementation is not contraindicated. For patients on a sodium- and potassium-restricted diet, chlorpromazine[16] or nicotinic acid[17] may be useful. These medications partially inhibit intestinal chloride absorption, limiting the development of acidosis and thus reducing the need for alkalinizing agents.

Nutritional disturbances

Various nutritional deficiencies may result due to alterations in absorption following resection of segments of the gastrointestinal tract for urologic reconstructive purposes (Table 3.2). Removal of a significant portion of stomach can lead to vitamin B_{12} deficiency due to decreased secretion of intrinsic factor. Vitamin B_{12} deficiency can also be induced after resection of the distal ileum because of consequent impairment of vitamin absorption.[18] Body stores of vitamin B_{12} may last several years before a decrease in serum levels is noted.[19] Persistent vitamin B_{12} deficiency if left untreated leads to megaloblastic anemia and peripheral sensory neuropathy.

Resection of distal ileum and/or loss of the ileocecal valve can cause reduced bile salt absorption and fat malabsorption.[20] Bile salts that have been inadequately absorbed in the ileum have secretory effects on the colonic mucosa, resulting in diarrhea. This can be treated by oral administration of cholestyramine, which binds the bile salts. With loss of the ileocecal valve, transit time may be decreased and bacteria can reflux from the colon into the small bowel contributing to overgrowth-mediated fat malabsorption and resultant steatorrhea. Treatment of diarrhea induced by fat malabsorption is with low-fat diet. As a consequence of fat malabsorption, absorption of fat-soluble vitamins (vitamins A, D, E and K) may be reduced. In rare cases, these deficiencies may be clinically significant.[21] Fat malabsorption may also lead to an increased incidence of gallstone formation.[22]

Loss of colonic segments is generally well tolerated and causes few nutritional problems. Diarrhea may occur when long segments of colon are removed. When alkaline ileal contents drain into a significantly shortened segment of colon, acidosis and dehydration may result due to loss of electrolytes and fluid in the stool.

Calculus formation

Patients with intestinal urinary diversions are at higher risk for development of urinary tract calculi than the general population through a variety of mechanisms (Box 3.1). Risk of calculus formation can be minimized by encouraging adequate hydration, implementing citrate supplementation, treatment of urea-splitting bacteriuria, and routine bladder irrigation for those patients using clean intermittent self-catheterization. In addition, routine radiographic screening for stones is recommended.

BOX 3.1 POTENTIAL CAUSES OF URINARY CALCULUS FORMATION FOLLOWING URINARY DIVERSION

- Urinary stasis associated with continent urinary diversion[23,24]
- Chronic bacteriuria with urease-producing bacteria[25]
- Metabolic abnormalities[26] resulting in hypercalciuria, hypocitruria, hyposulfaturia
- Foreign bodies, e.g. staples or sutures which serve as a nidus for mineral deposition
- Hyperoxaluria due to lipid malabsorption[27]
- Abnormal mucus production by the intestinal segment

Hepatic metabolism

The venous return of all intestinal segments commonly used for urinary diversion drains directly into the portal circulation. As a result, the liver is exposed to significant alterations in blood solute concentrations. It quickly adapts to this increased load by accelerating its ability to clear the solutes presented. This adaptive capability of the liver is illustrated by its metabolism of ammonia. Ammonia is generated in the renal tubule and excreted in the urine. It may also be produced from urea by the action of urease, an enzyme produced by urea-splitting bacteria. With interposition of intestine into the urinary tract, there is a marked increase in the absorption of urinary ammonia into the portal circulation. In the liver, the ammonia is incorporated into the ornithine cycle to create urea. A normally functioning liver rapidly adapts to the increased ammonia load by increasing its capacity for ureagenesis, with the end result of imperceptible alterations in the serum concentration of ammonia.[5]

Table 3.2 Nutritional abnormalities following urologic reconstruction and their treatment

Segment resected	Physiologic function	Abnormality	Treatment
Stomach	Intrinsic factor secretion	Vitamin B_{12} deficiency	Replacement with parenteral vitamin B_{12}
Jejunum	Folic acid absorption	Folic acid deficiency	Replacement with parenteral folic acid
Ileum, colon	Absorption of bile salts	Diarrhea	Cholestyramine
	Absorption of lipids and lipid-soluble vitamins	Steatorrhea, deficiency of fat-soluble vitamins	Low-fat diet, replacement of fat-soluble vitamins
	Absorption of vitamin B_{12}	Vitamin B_{12} deficiency	Replacement with parenteral vitamin B_{12}

Decreased liver function can interfere with ammonia metabolism in the liver, even in the absence of clinical indices of hepatic dysfunction.[28] Presence of small amounts of endotoxin can also interfere with ammonia metabolism.[29] Hyperammonemia manifests itself as change in mental status.[30,31] Therefore, when hyperammonemia does occur, one should suspect underlying liver dysfunction or systemic bacteremia associated with urinary infection with urea-splitting bacteria. An underlying obstruction of the diversion must also be ruled out. Management of hyperammonemia and associated ammoniagenic coma includes drainage of the urinary intestinal diversion in order to relieve possible urinary tract obstruction, as well as to decrease urine to mucosa contact time. Systemic antibiotics should be administered to treat urease-producing bacterial infection. Protein intake is restricted and oral neomycin is given to reduce the ammonia load from the gastrointestinal tract. Lactulose may be given orally or by rectum to prevent ammonia absorption in the gut. In severe circumstances, arginine glutamate serves as a substrate to complex ammonia by forming glutamine.[32]

Glucose metabolism

The presence of an intestinal segment in urinary diversion patients can indirectly affect systemic glucose metabolism. In the case of a hyperglycemic diabetic patient in whom the proximal tubule of the kidney is overloaded and unable to completely reabsorb glucose filtered by the glomerulus, the excess glucose will 'spill' into the urine. When this urine is presented to the intestinal mucosa of the conduit, the excess glucose could potentially be transported into the mucosal cells and ultimately be reintroduced into the bloodstream, resulting in further exacerbation of the patient's hyperglycemia.[33]

One study compared glucose absorption from urine in diabetic and non-diabetic patients with ileal conduits.[34] Glucose was instilled into the conduit; the non-diabetic patients demonstrated no significant glucose absorption. In contrast, one of three diabetic patients showed significant absorption. Thus, it appears that diabetic patients may have an enhanced ability to resorb glucose from urine in the lumen of the intestinal conduit.

Abnormal drug metabolism

Patients who have undergone urinary diversion using an intestinal segment may experience altered drug metabolism. Medications that are most likely to cause such a problem are those that are absorbed by the gastrointestinal tract, then excreted unchanged or as an active metabolite by the kidney into the urine. The excreted drug or metabolite in the urine is exposed to the intestinal segment, which then absorbs it, returning it to the bloodstream. This can lead to toxic serum levels and adverse effects, even death. Examples of such drugs include phenytoin,[35] some antibiotics, as well as some chemotherapeutic agents, such as methotrexate[36,37] and cisplatin. In order to reduce toxicity, one must carefully monitor drug levels at regular intervals during the course of treatment. In addition, for patients with continent urinary diversion undergoing administration of the aforementioned drugs, one should consider continuous pouch drainage to minimize contact time with the intestinal mucosa.

Bone disease and growth disturbances

It has been suggested that one of the long-term effects of intestinal urinary diversion is alteration of bone mineral content. Boyd first proposed this concept in 1931,[38] noting an association between ureterosigmoidostomy, chronic acidosis and metabolic bone disease. Explanations have attributed these skeletal effects to impaired absorption of calcium and vitamin D,[39] as well as effects of chronic acidosis.[40,41] Persistent metabolic acidosis is buffered by carbonate extracted from bone; this also results in calcium release into the bloodstream, which is then cleared by the kidney. Increased absorption of phosphate and sulfate in the setting of chronic acidosis may induce further renal loss of calcium. It has also been reported that metabolic acidosis impairs the 1-α-hydroxylation of 25-hydroxyvitamin D_3 to 1,25-dihydroxyvitamin D_3 in the kidney.[42,43]

Previously published studies have implicated intestinal urinary diversion as a risk for impaired bone metabolism, growth, and development.[44,45] Osteomalacia in adults and rickets in children have been observed in patients with ureterosigmoidostomy, ileal ureters, and augmentation cystoplasty.[46–49] Bone density abnormalities have been demonstrated in adult intestinal urinary diversion patients who exhibit a chronic low-grade metabolic acidosis.[50] Patients may have increased risk of fracture and problems with malunion when orthopedic procedures are performed. Subtle differences in growth have been demonstrated in myelodysplastic children. Because of the large variations in development, it has been difficult to conclusively demonstrate significant differences in the growth and development of intestinal urinary diversion patients who are otherwise normal when compared with normals as established by standard growth curves.[51]

Conclusion

Metabolic and nutritional complications are common after intestinal urinary diversion. Knowledge of potential consequences and initiation of preventive measures can help to minimize these problems. In addition, careful surveillance of the diversion patient and early intervention as indicated should help minimize morbidity.

References

1. Gosalbez R Jr, Woodard JR, Broecker BH, Warshaw B. Metabolic complications of urinary diversions: an overview. J Urol 1993; 150: 710–12.
2. Nguyen DH, Bain MA, Salmonson KL et al. The syndrome of dysuria and hematuria in pediatric urinary reconstruction with stomach. J Urol 1993; 150: 707–9.
3. Plawker MW, Rabinowitz SS, Etwaru DJ, Glassberg KI. Hypergastrinemia, dysuria-hematuria and metabolic alkalosis: complications associated with gastrocystoplasty. J Urol 1995; 154: 546–9.
4. Klein EA, Montie JE, Montague DK, Kay R, Straffon RA. Jejunal conduit urinary diversion. J Urol 1986; 135: 244–6.
5. Koch MO, McDougal WS. The pathophysiology of hyperchloremic metabolic acidosis after urinary diversion through intestinal segments. Surgery 1985; 98: 561–70.
6. Golimbu M, Morales P. Jejunal conduits: technique and complications. J Urol 1975; 113: 787–95.
7. Golimbu M, Morales P. Electrolyte disturbances in jejunal urinary diversion. Urology 1973; 1: 432–8.
8. Castro JE, Ram MD. Electrolyte imbalance following ileal urinary diversion. Br J Urol 1970; 42: 29–32.
9. Mills RD, Studer UE. Metabolic consequences of continent urinary diversion. J Urol 1999; 161: 1057–66.
10. Stampfer DS, McDougal WS. Inhibition of the sodium/hydrogen antiport by ammonium ion. J Urol 1997; 157: 362–5.
11. McDougal WS, Stampfer DS, Kirley S, Bennett PM, Lin CW. Intestinal ammonium transport by ammonium and hydrogen exchange. J Am Coll Surg 1995; 181: 241–8.
12. Koch MO, Gurevitch E, Hill DE, McDougal WS. Urinary solute transport by intestinal segments: a comparative study of ileum and colon in rats. J Urol 1990; 143: 1275–9.
13. McDougal WS. Metabolic complications of urinary intestinal diversion. J Urol 1992; 147: 1199–208.
14. Boyd SD, Schiff WM, Skinner DG et al. Prospective study of metabolic abnormalities in patients with continent Koch pouch urinary diversion. Urology 1989; 33: 85–8.
15. Koff SA. Mechanism of electrolyte imbalance following urointestinal anastomoses. Urology 1975; 5: 109–14.
16. Koch MO, McDougal WS. Chlorpromazine: adjuvant therapy for the metabolic derangements created by urinary diversion through intestinal segments. J Urol 1985; 134: 165–9.
17. Koch MO, McDougal WS. Nicotinic acid: treatment for the hyperchloremic acidosis following urinary diversion through intestinal segments. J Urol 1985; 134: 162–4.
18. Racioppi M, D'Addessi A, Fanasca A et al. Vitamin B_{12} and folic acid plasma levels after ileocecal and ileal neobladder reconstruction. Urology 1997; 50: 888–92.
19. Stein R, Lotz J, Andreas J et al. Long-term metabolic effects in patients with urinary diversion. World J Urol 1998; 16: 292–7.
20. Olofsson G, Fjalling M, Kilander A, Ung KA, Jonsson O. Bile acid malabsorption after continent urinary diversion with an ileal reservoir. J Urol 1998; 160: 724–7.
21. Saltzman JR, Russell RM. Nutritional consequences of intestinal bacterial overgrowth. Compr Ther 1994; 20: 523–30.
22. Holmes DG. Long-term complications related to the modified Indiana pouch. Urology 2002; 60: 603–6.
23. Nurse DE, Mundy AR. Stone after enterocystoplasty. Br J Urol 1996; 77: 684.
24. Turk TM, Koleski FC, Albala DM. Incidence of urolithiasis in cystectomy patients after intestinal conduit or continent urinary diversion. World J Urol 1999; 17: 305–7.
25. Cohen TD, Streem SB, Lammert G. Long-term incidence and risks for recurrent stones following contemporary management of upper tract calculi in patients with a urinary diversion. J Urol 1996; 155: 62–5.
26. Terai A, Arai Y, Kawakita M, Okada Y, Yoshida O. Effect of urinary intestinal diversion on urinary risk factors for urolithiasis. J Urol 1995; 153: 37–41
27. Earnest DL, Johnson G, Williams HE, Admirand WH. Hyperoxaluria in patients with ileal resection: an abnormality in dietary oxalate absorption. Gastroenterology 1974; 66: 1114–22.
28. McDermott WV Jr. Diversion of urine to the intestines as a factor in ammoniagenic coma. N Engl J Med 1957; 256: 460.
29. McDougal WS, Heimburger S, Wilmore DW, Pruitt BA Jr. The effect of exogenous substrate on hepatic metabolism and membrane transport during endotoxemia. Surgery 1978; 83: 55–61.
30. Kaveggia FF, Thompson JS, Schafer EC, Fischer JL, Taylor RJ. Hyperammonemic encephalopathy in urinary diversion with urea-splitting urinary tract infection. Arch Int Med 1990; 150: 2389–92.
31. Edwards DH. Hyperammonemic encephalopathy related to ureterosigmoidostomy. Arch Neurol 1984; 41: 1211–12.
32. Silberman R. Ammonia intoxication following ureterosigmoidostomy in a patient with liver disease. Lancet 1958; ii: 937.
33. Onwubalili JK. Overt diabetes mellitus without glucosuria in a patient with cutaneous ureteroileostomy. BMJ 1982; 284: 1836–7.
34. Sridhar KN, Samuell CT, Woodhouse CRJ. Absorption of glucose from urinary conduits in diabetes and non diabetes. BMJ 1983; 287: 1327–9.
35. Savarirayan F, Dixey GM. Syncope following ureterosigmoidostomy. J Urol 1969; 101: 844–5.
36. Bowyer GW, Davies TW. Methotrexate toxicity associated with an ileal conduit. Br J Urol 1986; 60: 592.
37. Fossa SD, Heilo A, Bormer O. Unexpectedly high serum methotrexate levels in cystectomized bladder cancer patients with an ileal conduit treated with intermediate doses of the drug. J Urol 1990; 143: 498–501.
38. Boyd JD. Chronic acidosis secondary to ureteral transplantation. Am J Dis Child 1931; 42: 366–71.
39. Gafter U, Kraut JA, Lee DBN et al. Effect of metabolic acidosis on intestinal absorption of calcium and phosphorus. Am J Physiol 1980; 239 (Suppl): G480–G484.
40. Lemann J Jr, Litzow JR, Lennon EJ. Studies of the mechanism by which chronic metabolic acidosis augments urinary calcium excretion in man. J Clin Invest 1967; 46: 1318–28.
41. Lemann J Jr, Litzow JR, Lennon EJ. The effects of chronic acid loads in normal man: further evidence for participation of bone mineral in the defense against chronic metabolic acidosis. J Clin Invest 1966, 45: 1608–14.

42. Cunningham J, Bikle DD, Avioloi LV. Acute, but not chronic, metabolic acidosis disturbs 25-hydroxyvitamin D_3 metabolism. Kidney Int 1984; 24: 47–52.
43. Kawashima H, Kraut JA, Kurokawa K. Metabolic acidosis suppresses 25-hydroxyvitamin D_3-1α-hydroxylase in the rat kidney. J Clin Invest 1982; 70: 135–40.
44. Mundy AR, Nurse DE. Calcium balance, growth and skeletal mineralisation in patients with cystoplasties. Br J Urol 1992; 69: 257–9.
45. McDougal WS, Koch MO, Shands C 3rd, Price RR. Bony demineralization following urinary intestinal diversion. J Urol 1988; 140: 853–5.
46. Green RC, Boyd JA. Rickets secondary to chronic hyperchloremic acidosis in ureterosigmoidostomy. AMA Arch Intern Med 1959; 103: 807–13.
47. Harrison AJ. Clinical and metabolic observations on osteomalacia following ureterosigmoidostomy. Br J Urol 1958; 30: 455–61.
48. Salahudeen AK, Elliott RW, Ellis HA. Osteomalacia due to ileal replacement of ureters: report of 2 cases. J Urol 1984; 131: 335–7.
49. Specht EE. Rickets following ureterosigmoidostomy and chronic hyperchloremia. J Bone Joint Surg 1967; 49: 1422–30.
50. Stein R, Fisch M, Andreas J et al. Whole-body potassium and bone mineral density up to 30 years after urinary diversion. Br J Urol 1998; 82: 798–803.
51. Gerhaz EW, Ransley PG, Woodhouse CRJ. Growth failure revisited: a second look at the metabolic consequences of enterocystoplasty in childhood. J Urol 2001; 165 (Suppl): A433.

4 The mechanics of tubular and detubularized bowel for bladder substitution

Morten Colding-Jørgensen and Kenneth Steven

Introduction

Bladder substitution has become a standard method of urinary diversion. Substitution with closed tubular bowel segments allows normal micturition and reliable daytime continence but has the disadvantage of resulting in nighttime incontinence.[1–3] The nocturnal incontinence is caused by peristaltic contractions occurring early on during filling.[4] The reduced level of consciousness during sleep makes it impossible to increase the urethral sphincter pressure in response to these contractions. Also, the capacity of tubular bowel substitutes is inadequate to store the overnight urine production resulting in overflow incontinence even in the absence of contractions.[5] Bladder substitution using detubularized bowel has been successfully introduced to improve nighttime continence.[6–9]

We present a revision of our study[10] which gives a theoretical analysis of the mechanics of tubular and detubularized bowel bladders and compare the results with urodynamic findings and clinical observations. A comprehensive analysis of the mechanics of smooth-muscle reservoirs has been presented by Colding-Jørgensen and Steven.[11]

Theory

Reservoir geometry

The purpose of detubularization is to create a reservoir with the highest capacity for a given length of bowel. To accomplish this, the bowel segment is opened along its antimesenteric border and fashioned into the shape of a U-, S- or, W-pouch or the Kock reservoir.

To construct a cylindrical reservoir from an isolated bowel segment, part of the segment must be used to close the ends of the cylinder.[12] With the relaxed length of bowel, L_0, and radius, r_0, the reference volume, V_0, is given by:

$$V_0 = \pi(nr_0)^2\left(\frac{L_0}{n} - nr_0\right), \qquad (1)$$

where n assumes the value 1 for the tubular, and 2, 3, 4 for the U, S and W pouches, respectively.

It is not possible to fashion a bowel reservoir into the shape of a perfect cylinder, so it will assume an ovoid configuration. It can be shown[10,11] that the ovoid reservoirs may be considered as consisting of a central cylindrical part with radius nr and with curved ends which may be shaped as hemispheres. The construction of the two hemispherical ends requires a surface area of $4\pi(nr_0)^2$ of the total cylinder surface $2\pi r_0 L_0$, so the central cylindrical part will have length $L_0/(n-2nr_0)$. The two hemispherical ends contribute to the reservoir volume by $\frac{4}{3}\pi(nr_0)^3$, so the total volume is given by:

$$\begin{aligned} V_0 &= \pi(nr_0)^2\left(\frac{L_0}{n} - 2nr_0\right) + \frac{4}{3}\pi\,(nr_0)^3 \qquad (2)\\ &= \pi(nr_0)^2\left(\frac{L_0}{n} - \frac{2}{3}nr_0\right). \end{aligned}$$

For reservoirs with $L_0 > 2n^2r_0$ the volumes of the non-spherical reservoirs calculated by eqn. (2) and the corresponding ellipsoid reservoirs differ by less than 2% if the length:diameter ratio is

<12. The difference is even less for reservoirs with higher ratios. Accordingly, eqn. (2) serves as a simple and accurate approximation to calculate the volumes of both near-spherical and cylindrical reservoirs.

Figure 4.1 shows the effect of detubularization on reservoir volume. To make the results generally applicable, dimensionless units are used with bowel length expressed in fractions of bowel diameter, $d_0 = 2r_0$, and reservoir volume, V_0, in fractions of the volume, V_{tub}, of corresponding tubular bowel ($n = 1$). It is evident that detubularization, particularly with a spherical reservoir, increases reservoir volume substantially, unless very short sections of bowel are used.

Figure 4.2 shows how the reservoir volume is influenced by the number of segments the bowel section is fashioned into. To calculate the values for a bowel section of a given length and arbitrary diameter the number of segments, n, are allowed to assume non-integer values. The interrupted line shows the optimum number of segments, n_{opt}, for each particular section of bowel, L_0/d_0, that allows for the construction of a spherical reservoir. From eqn. (2) it follows that:

$$n_{opt} = \sqrt{L_0/d_0}\ .$$

For a particular bowel section, the number of segments can be found as the integer: $n < n_{opt}$. Accordingly, both the use of a higher or a lower number of segments than n_{opt} for construction will reduce the volume below that of the ideal, spherical reservoir. Furthermore, detubularization will not be worthwhile if n_{opt} is well below 2. The curve optimums are relatively flat, so deviations from the spherical shape will only give minor changes in volume.[10] All calculations are based upon the assumption that no tissue is lost during surgery.

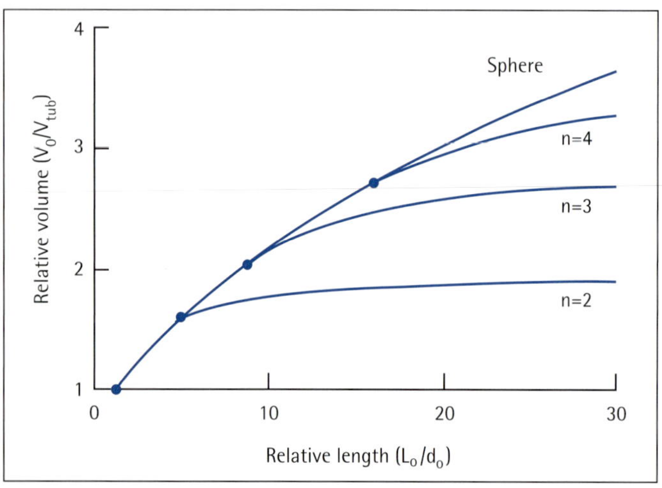

Figure 4.1 Volumes of different types of relaxed reservoirs calculated as a function of the length of bowel used for construction. Volume is expressed in fractions of the volume of tubular bowel ($n = 1$) and length, L, in fractions of bowel diameter, d. The number of segments a bowel section is fashioned into is given by n, where $n = 2$ corresponds to a U-pouch, $n = 3$ to an S-pouch and $n = 4$ to a W-pouch.

To summarize: surgery should result in the construction of an ovoid reservoir with a ratio between length and diameter well below 4 ($n_{opt} << 2$). The optimum is a spherical reservoir with ratio 1, but, as a rule of thumb, any ovoid reservoir with a length:diameter ratio between 1 and 2 will provide a perfectly good reservoir.

Pressure

The law of Laplace relates the pressure difference, P, across a thin curved membrane-to-membrane tension, T, and is usually expressed by:

$$P = \left(\frac{1}{r_1}+\frac{1}{r_2}\right) \times T, \tag{3}$$

where r_1 and r_2 are the two principal radii (the largest and the smallest) of the membrane surface. The equation is valid only if tension is the same in all directions as for fluid–fluid or fluid–air interfaces, so it does not generally apply to tissue membranes, and must be transformed to:[13]

$$P = \frac{T_1}{r_1} + \frac{T_2}{r_2}, \tag{4}$$

where T_1 is the tension (N/m) along the path with curvature r_2 and T_2 along the path with curvature r_1. For a thick wall, both the radii and tensions change through the wall, but according to the integral mean value theorem there exists a position in the wall, where eqn. (4) is satisfied. For bowel consisting of an inner mucosal layer and an outer, weak longitudinal muscular layer a value of two-thirds of the wall thickness appears to be a reasonable approximation.[10]

For the uniform spherical reservoir, $r_1 = r_2 = r_s$ and $T_1 = T_2 = T$, so:

$$P_s = 2T/r_s. \tag{5}$$

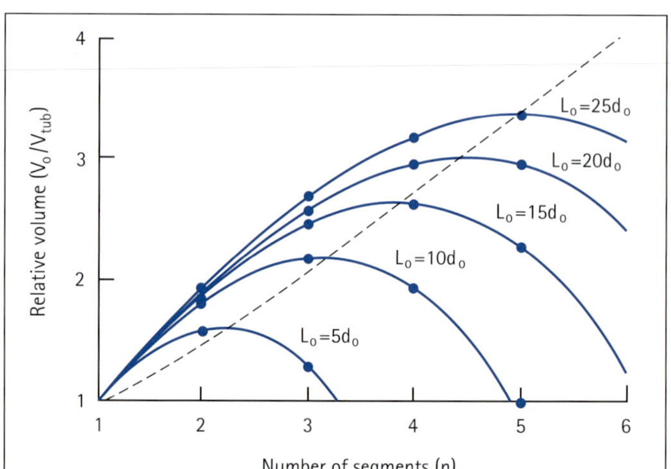

Figure 4.2 The effect on volume of the number of segments (n) a bowel section is fashioned into for the construction of a detubularized reservoir.

For a cylindrical tube with the circumferential tension T_1 the longitudinal tension T_2 is $T_1/2$, and because r_2 is infinite the pressure is $P_c = T_1/r_1$.

The non-spherical reservoir usually has an ovoid shape, and with $r_2 > r_1$ and assuming rotational symmetry around the long axis eqn. (4) reduces to:

$$P = \left(1 + Q\right) \times \frac{T_1}{r_1}, \tag{6}$$

where the form factor:

$$Q = \frac{r_1 T_1}{r_2 T_2}$$

assumes a value between 0 (cylinder) and 1 (sphere).

The form factor depends upon the exact shape of the reservoir. For most reservoirs, Q will be almost proportional to the ratio between reservoir diameter, d, and length, L (Colding-Jørgensen, unpublished data) so with $r = d/2$ and the circumferential tension, T, eqn. (6) can be approximated by:

$$P = \left(1 + \frac{d}{L}\right) \times \frac{T}{r}. \tag{7}$$

Stress–strain relation

The stress, σ, is expressed by the force per unit area of relaxed tissue. The passive, elastic stress is given by:[11,13]

$$\sigma_e = 20\,\{\exp(8\lambda_\Omega) - 1\}, \tag{8}$$

where σ_e is expressed in kPa and the surface stretch ratio $\lambda_\Omega = \Omega/\Omega_0$ where Ω is the actual and Ω_0 the relaxed surface area.

The active stress, σ_a, produced by muscular contraction depends upon the circumferential stretch ratio $\lambda_r = r/r_0$. The stress–strain relation can be approximated by a triangular relation with a maximum value at $\lambda_r = 1.11$ and a slope, $d\sigma_a/d\lambda_r$, of 1.125. The contraction strength is then defined as a fraction, ψ, of the maximum force, σ_{max}, of contraction so:

$$\sigma_a = \sigma_{max}\,\psi\,(1 - 1.125\,|\,\lambda_r - 1.11\,|), \tag{9}$$

with $\sigma_{max} = 150$ kPa for the spherical and 200 kPa for the non-spherical reservoir.[11] This applies when $\sigma_a > 0$. Under all other conditions $\sigma_a = 0$. The total stress, σ_m, is:

$$\sigma_m = \sigma_e + \sigma_a, \tag{10}$$

With the relaxed wall thickness, δ_0, the actual circumferential tension, T, is given by

$$T = \delta_0 \sigma_m / \lambda_L, \tag{11}$$

where $\lambda_L = L/L_0$ is the longitudinal stretch ratio. Substitution into eqn. (7) and with $\lambda_\Omega = \lambda_r \lambda_L$ gives

$$P = \left(1 + \frac{d}{L}\right) \times \frac{\delta_0 \sigma_m}{r_0 \lambda_\Omega}. \tag{12}$$

For the spherical reservoir $\lambda_L = \lambda_r$, so $\lambda_\Omega = \lambda_r^2$. For non-spherical reservoirs the variation in λ_L is generally small, so it is assumed that $\lambda_L = 1$ giving $\lambda_\Omega = \lambda_r$. Given σ_m, the pressure is calculated by insertion in eqn. (12).

Pressure–volume relation

For a given volume, V, the radius and hence $\lambda_r = r/r_0$ is found from

$$V = \pi r^2 (L - \tfrac{2}{3} r)$$

with $L - 2r$ for the spherical and $L = L_0$ for the non-spherical reservoir. This radius expresses some mean radius positioned within the wall. With w as the part of the wall inside this radius, the fluid volume is $V - w$. Knowing λ_r, the pressure, P, is calculated using the eqns (8) to (12).

Figure 4.3 shows the pressure–volume relations for tubular and detubularized bowel. The muscle tone is taken to be 15% of the maximum value throughout ($\psi = 0.15$). Figure 4.3a shows the relations for ileal reservoirs each constructed from a 40-cm segment of bowel with a diameter of 3.2 cm and a wall thickness of 0.2 cm in the relaxed state. The pressure–volume relation for the tubular reservoir ($n = 1$) is compared with those of the detubularized U ($n = 2$), S ($n = 3$) and spherical reservoirs. The pressures corresponding to the reference volumes (V_0) are indicated by dots. It is apparent that the tubular reservoir has substantially smaller capacity and a larger pressure at V_0 than the detubularized reservoirs. Consequently, detubularization both improves reservoir capacity for geometrical reasons (see Figure 4.1), and assures a pressure reduction by increasing reservoir radius in accordance with Laplace's law.

Figure 4.3b shows the pressure–volume relation for right colon reservoirs each constructed from either a 15- or 24-cm bowel segment. The lengths are selected so the reference volume (V_0) of the 15-cm tubular cecal reservoir matches that of the tubular ileal reservoir, and so the reference volume of the 24-cm spherical cecal reservoir matches that of the spherical ileal reservoir. In accordance with the results shown in Figure 4.1, detubularization of the 15-cm cecal segment only gives a slight gain in volume owing to the length:diameter ratio of only 2.7. In contrast, detubularizing the 24-cm cecal segment with a length:diameter ratio of 4.4 produces a substantial volume gain.

The pressure–volume relations may change during filling owing to the viscoelasticity of the bowel wall.[14] These changes have not been taken into account.

Contractions

Reservoir contractions increase wall tension. The magnitude of the resulting pressure rise depends upon the curvature of the reservoir wall and can be approximated by eqn. (12). Peristaltic

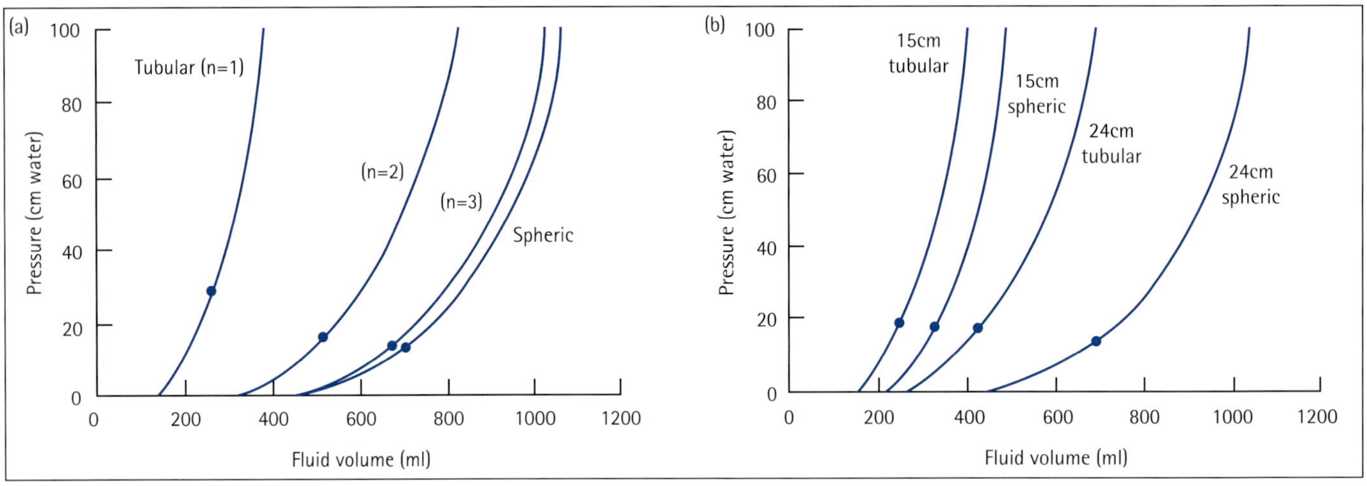

Figure 4.3 The pressure–volume relation of different types of ileal and right colon reservoirs. Resting muscle tone is taken to be 15% of the maximum value throughout. (a) Tubular (n = 1) and different types of detubularized ileal reservoir each constructed from 40 cm of bowel. (b) Tubular (n = 1) and spherical right colon reservoirs each constructed from either a 15- or a 24-cm section of bowel.

contractions usually only include part of the bowel, so if one part of the reservoir contracts, the remainder will be distended. With a low degree of filling the distension will be slight, and consequently the resulting pressure rise small.

Tubular versus detubularized ileal reservoir

Figure 4.4 shows the effect of partial contractions on reservoir pressure. The pressures are calculated for a tubular and a detubularized spherical reservoir each constructed from a 40-cm segment of ileum.[10] The resting tone of the reservoir wall is taken to be 15% of the maximum force of contraction. During contractions, the muscle tone is assumed to increase from 15% (ψ = 0.15) to 65% (ψ = 0.65) of the maximum value involving an area of contraction of 40, 50 or 60% of the reservoir wall, respectively.

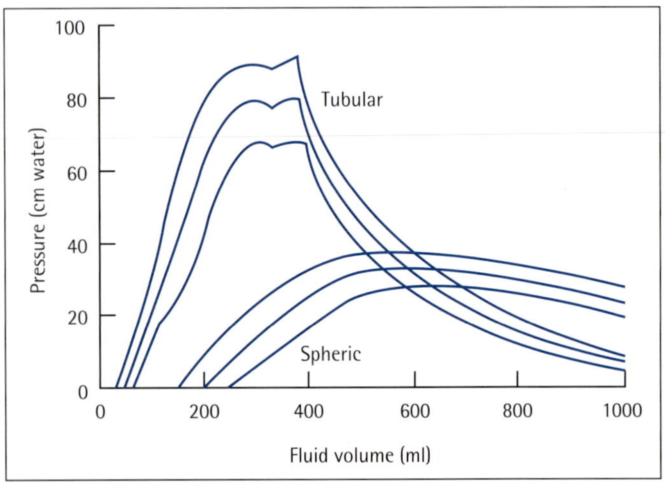

Figure 4.4 Calculated pressure rises in tubular and detubularized spheric ileal reservoirs produced by contractions including part of the reservoir wall (60, 50 or 40% from top to bottom). During contraction, muscle tone increases from 15 to 65% of the maximum force of contraction.

It is apparent that the shapes of the curves for the two types of reservoir are similar, but the volume range for the tubular is only about half while the pressure range is about twice that of the spherical reservoir. Hence detubularization delays the onset and reduces the amplitude of the pressure rise caused by partial contractions. Consequently, the detubularized reservoir accommodates a higher volume at a lower pressure than the tubular reservoir, which may account for the improved nighttime continence. Partial contractions are calculated to result in a measurable pressure rise of about 10 cmH_2O at a volume of <100 ml in the tubular against more than 200 ml in the detubularized reservoir. Accordingly, the absence of a pressure rise early on during cystometry cannot be taken as evidence against the existence of contractions. Also, abdominal straining is needed to empty particularly the detubularized reservoir which may predispose to residual urine. It is also apparent from Figure 4.4 that overdistension reduces the pressure rise produced by partial contractions which may lead to urinary retention.

Right colon reservoirs

The tubular right colon reservoirs have a larger radius and are shorter than the tubular ileal reservoirs. Figure 4.5 shows the pressure–volume relation during partial contractions for both tubular and detubularized right colon reservoirs, each constructed from a 15- or 24-cm segment with a diameter of 5.75 and a wall thickness of 0.2 cm. The area of contraction includes 50% of the wall, and during contraction the muscle tone increases from 15% (ψ = 0.15) to 65% (ψ = 0.65) of the maximum force of contraction.

The maximum pressure rises are smaller in the tubular cecal reservoirs than in the tubular ileal reservoir owing to their large radii. Conversely, the onset of the pressure rise is similar in the tubular ileal and the tubular 15-cm cecal reservoir but is delayed in the 24-cm tubular cecal reservoir owing to its higher volume.

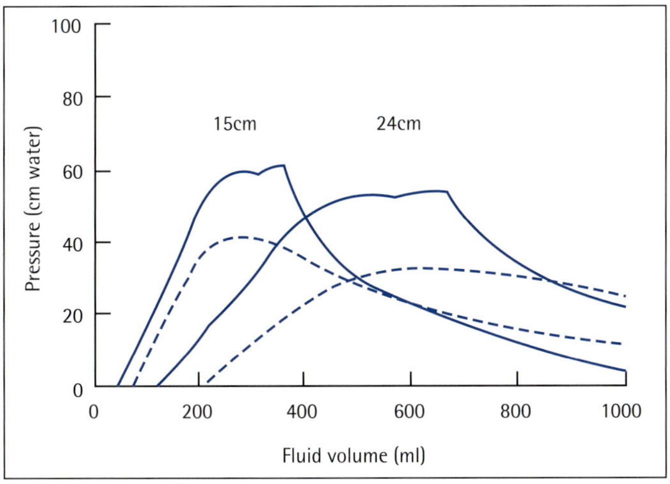

Figure 4.5 Calculated pressure rises in tubular (——) and detubularized spherical right colon reservoirs (----) produced by contractions including 50% of the bowel wall. During contraction, muscle tone increases from 15 to 65% of the maximum force of contraction.

Both the maximum and the onset of the pressure rise match in the spherical ileal and 24-cm right colon reservoirs owing to their equal volume and shape.

Patients

Urodynamics

Cystometry

Table 4.1 summarizes the results of medium-fill water cystometry. The detubularized ileal Kock reservoir has a substantially higher capacity than the tubular ileocecal bladder (595 ml against 330 ml at 3 years, $P < 0.05$). Also, in accordance with the theoretical calculations, detubularization delays the onset of the pressure rise produced by contractions (268 ml against 80 ml at 6 months, $P < 0.05$). In further agreement with the theoretical predictions, the amplitude of the pressure waves is smaller in the detubularized bladder substitutes (33 cmH_2O against 59 cmH_2O at 3 years, $P < 0.05$). Consequently the maximum pressure is about 21% less in detubularized Kock reservoirs (56 cmH_2O against 68 cmH_2O at 3 years, $P < 0.05$).

Clinical results

Continence (Table 4.2)
Daytime continence is achieved consistently in both groups but sooner in patients with a detubularized bowel bladder (96% against 69% at 6 months, $P < 0.05$). Detubularization improves nighttime continence considerably. By 2 years, 87% of the patients with the urethral Kock reservoir have obtained nighttime continence against only 17% with the tubular ileocecal bladder ($P < 0.05$). Age has an adverse effect on nighttime continence which appears to improve with the length of postoperative follow-up.

Micturition (Table 4.3)
The peak urine flow rates are similar in the two groups of patients reflecting that voiding is accomplished by straining. The voiding intervals are considerably longer in patients with detubularized bowel substitutes (4 hours against 2.5 hours at 1 year, $P < 0.05$) presumably owing to the higher bladder capacity. The disadvantage of detubularization is a higher incidence of urinary retention. None of our patients with a tubular bladder substitute has urinary retention. In contrast, by 6 months, 12% and by 1 year, 25% of the patients with the detubularized

Table 4.1 Medium-fill cystometry in patients with tubular ileocecal and detubularized ileal Kock bladder substitutes. Follow-up at 6 months and 3 years

	Reservoir type, median values (range)			
	Tubular (ileocecal)		Detubularized (Kock)	
Parameter	6 months	3 years	6 months	3 years
Patients (*n*)	15	7	60	16
Capacity (ml)	300 (175–650)	330 (175–468)	445* (208–970)	595* (401–1115)
Volume 1st contr. (ml)	80 (40–350)	88 (38–130)	268* (60–490)	314 (50–550)
Amplitude maximum contr. (cmH_2O)	54 (15–96)	59 (30–100)	35 (2–67)	33* (8–51)
Maximum pressure (cmH_2O)	77 (35–102)	68 (58–123)	55 (7–94)	56* (32–88)

* $P < 0.05$, between tubular and detubularized bladder substitutes.
Contr., contraction.

Table 4.2 Continence in patients with tubular ileocecal and detubularized ileal Kock bladder substitutues at 6 months and 2 years follow-up

	Tubular (ileocecal) reservoir		Detubularized (Kock) reservoir	
Parameter	6 months	2 years	6 months	2 years
Patients (*n*)	16	12	60	28
Daytime	69%	100%	96%*	100%
Nighttime	0%	17%	65%	87%*
Age <60 (*n*)	0% (8)	20% (5)	71% (21)*	100% (7)*
Age >60 (*n*)	0% (8)	14% (7)	62% (39)*	81% (21)*

* $P < 0.05$, between tubular and detubularized bladder substitutes.

Table 4.3 Voiding characteristics (median values and range) in patients with tubular ileocecal and detubularized ileal Kock bladder substitutes at 6 months and 1 year follow-up

	Tubular (ileocecal) reservoir		Detubularized (Kock) reservoir	
Parameter	6 months	1 year	6 months	1 year
Patients (*n*)	15	8	59	44
Peak flow rate (ml/s)	18 (8–38)	24 (9–42)	17 (5–70)	17 (4–44)
Voiding interval (hours)	2.0 (1.0–3.0)	2.5 (2.0–3.0)	3.0* (1.5–7.0)	4.0* (1.0–7.0)
Urinary retention (postvoid residual > 100 ml: SIC)	0%	0%	12%	25%

* $P < 0.05$, between tubular and detubularized bladder substitutes.
SIC, intermittent self-catheterization.

urethral Kock reservoirs have a postvoid residual urine above 100 ml and need intermittent self-catheterization. These patients present with urgency and frequency, so to appreciate this condition, determination of the postvoid residuals should be performed at regular intervals.

Discussion

The results of the theoretical analysis are borne out by our clinical observations showing that detubularization increases reservoir capacity, delays the onset and reduces the amplitude of the pressure rise produced by contractions. These findings both account for the markedly improved nighttime continence, the longer voiding intervals, and also for the predisposition to urinary retention following bladder substitution with detubularized bowel. Consequently, measurements of postvoid residuals should be performed periodically in these patients. Furthermore, it is apparent from theory that the absence of a pressure rise early on during cystometry cannot be used as evidence against the occurrence of reservoir contractions.

The theoretical results are corroborated by clinical studies showing that the capacity of the W-pouch, the ellipsoid S-pouch, and the near-spherical Kock reservoir are similar[9,15–17] and higher than that of the U-pouch.[8,18] Furthermore, the cystometric characteristics of the S-pouch and the Kock reservoir have been found to be almost the same.[17] This observation supports the conclusion founded on the theoretical analysis that the essence of detubularization is to create a high-capacity reservoir and that its exact geometric shape is of secondary importance. A length:diameter ratio between 1 and 2 will produce a perfectly good reservoir.

The improvement in nighttime continence with postoperative follow-up from 65% at 6 months to 87% at 2 years is in accordance with that reported by others.[19] Also, the finding of an adverse effect of age on nighttime continence with the detubularized Kock pouch is consistent with the results of a previous study[19] showing that 80% of patients with a W-pouch under the age of 70 years achieve nighttime continence against only 56% above this age limit.

The calculated cystometric characteristics of the tubular ileocecal bladder substitute are in accordance with our clinical observations and those of the tubular ileal bladder are consistent with previous clinical studies.[1,3,18] The pressure rise produced by contractions during filling is calculated to be smaller in the tubular cecal than in the tubular ileal reservoir, which may result in slightly improved continence. Conversely, the urodynamic characteristics of the detubularized 24-cm right colon and detubularized ileal reservoirs are calculated to match in terms of capacity, maximum pressure and onset of the pressure rise produced by partial contractions.

References

1. Camey M. Bladder replacement by ileocystoplasty following radical cystectomy. World J Urol 1985; 3: 161–6.
2. Steven K, Klarskov P, Jakobsen H, Bay-Nielsen H, Rasmussen F. Transpubic cystectomy and ileocecal bladder replacement after preoperative radiotherapy for bladder cancer. J Urol 1986; 135: 470–5.
3. Roehrborn CG, Teigland CM, Sagalowsky AI. Functional characteristics of the Camey ileal bladder. J Urol 1987; 138: 739–42.
4. Jakobsen H, Steven K, Stigsby B, Klarskov P, Hald T. Pathogenesis of nocturnal incontinence after ileocecal bladder replacement: continuous measurement of the urethral closure pressure during sleep. Br J Urol 1987; 59: 148–52.
5. McDougal WS. Bladder reconstruction following cystectomy by uretero-ileo-colourethrostomy. J Urol 1986; 135: 698–701.
6. Goldwasser B, Barrett DM, Benson RC Jr. Bladder replacement with use of a detubularized right colon segment: preliminary report of a new technique. Mayo Clin Proc 1986; 61: 615–21.
7. Ghoneim MA, Kock NG, Lycke G, El-Din ABS. An appliance-free sphincter-controller bladder substitute: the urethral Kock pouch. J Urol 1987; 138: 1150–4.
8. Melchior H, Spehr C, Knop-Wagemann I, Persson MC, Juenemann KP. The continent ileal bladder for urinary tract reconstruction after cystectomy: a survey of 44 patients. J Urol 1988; 139: 714–18.
9. Wenderoth UK, Bachor R, Egghart G et al. The ileal neobladder: experience and results of more than 100 consecutive cases. J Urol 1990; 143: 492–7.
10. Colding-Jørgensen M, Poulsen AL, Steven K. Mechanical characteristics of tubular and detubularised bowel for bladder substitution: theory, urodynamics and clinical results. Br J Urol 1993; 72: 586–93.
11. Colding-Jørgensen M, Steven K. A model of the mechanics of smooth muscle reservoirs applied to the intestinal bladder. Neurourol Urodynam 1993; 12: 59–79.
12. McDougal WS. Mechanics and neurophysiology of intestinal segments as bowel substitutes: an editorial comment. J Urol 1987; 138: 1438–9.
13. Lee M-C, Fung Y-C, Shabetal R, LeWinter MM. Biaxial mechanical properties of human pericardium and canine comparisons. Am J Physiol 1987; 249: H75–H82.
14. Colding-Jørgensen M, Nordling J, Steven K. A model for the plasticity of soft tissues. In: Mosekilde E (ed). Proceedings of the 1st Copenhagen Symposium on Computer Simulation in Biology, Ecology and Medicine. San Diego, California: Simulation Council Inc, 1993; 153–7.
15. Bachor R, Frohneberg D, Miller K, Egghart G, Hautmann R. Continence after total bladder replacement: urodynamic analysis of the ileal neobladder. Br J Urol 1990; 65: 462–6.
16. Boyd SD, Lieskovsky G, Skinner DG. Kock pouch bladder replacement. Urol Clin North Am 1991; 18: 641–8.
17. Shaaban AA, Dawaba MS, Gaballah MA, Ghoneim MA. Urethral controlled bladder substitution: a comparison between Parks S pouch and Hemi-Kock pouch. J Urol 1991; 146: 973–6.
18. Camey M, Botto H, Thebaut Y. Ileal cystoplasty. Probl Urol 1991; 5: 307–15.
19. Hautmann RE, Miller K, Steiner U, Wenderoth U. The ileal neobladder: 6 years of experience with more than 200 patients. J Urol 1993; 150: 40–5.

5 Bacteriuria in patients with reconstructed lower urinary tracts

Björn Wullt and Wiking Månsson

Introduction

The main indications for reconstruction of the lower urinary tract are bladder cancer requiring cystectomy, and benign conditions such as interstitial cystitis and neuropathic bladder disorders, where augmentation of the bladder is needed. The reconstruction involves interposition of isolated intestinal tissue in the lower urinary tract, and in most cases a neoanastomosis between the ureter and intestine. Protection of renal function is a main goal in these patient groups why the anastomosis is crucial. There may be stenosis and/or reflux. Since patients with reconstructed lower urinary tracts frequently have bacteriuria, the reflux involves a risk for pyelonephritis, with potential development of kidney scars and decrease in renal function. Therefore antireflux ureteric implantation techniques have been advocated. However, stenosis of the ureteric anastomosis or insufficiency of the antireflux mechanism may occur resulting in exposure of the upper urinary tract to contaminated urine. Therefore an understanding of the frequency and composition of bacteriuria in patients with reconstructed lower urinary tract is of major importance. It should, however, be recognized that issues as the local host response and the role of antibacterial defenses in the reconstructed lower urinary tract are not well understood.

This chapter reviews the current knowledge of microbial colonization of the reconstructed lower urinary tract, the role of possible antibacterial defense mechanisms and the implications for antireflux surgery as a protective measurement for renal function.

Frequency of bacteriuria in the reconstructed lower urinary tract

Historically, the most commonly used techniques of urinary diversion have been ureterosigmoidostomy and ileal conduit. A variety of new techniques for reconstruction of the lower urinary tract have now been introduced. Orthotopic bladder substitution and continent cutaneous urinary diversion have gained much popularity, and large clinical series have documented that results are satisfactory regarding complication rate, functional outcome and patients' quality of life. In fact, when radical cystectomy is performed, many centers use the orthotopic bladder substitute as the standard reconstruction, also in females. Enterocystoplasty is usually performed in benign disorders, where augmentation of the bladder capacity or decrease in hyperactivity is needed.

Conduit diversion

Conduit urine is bacteriuric in practically all cases, mostly with a Gram-positive mixed dermal flora (i.e. streptococci species and *Staphylococcus epidermidis*), occasionally including uropathogenic strains (Gram-negative enterobacteriaceae such as *Escherichia coli*, *Proteus*, *Pseudomonas* and *Enterococcus faecalis*).[1–5] Urine, when sampled through a double lumen catheter avoiding contamination from the skin, the stoma and the distal part of the conduit, showed less frequent growth than urine sampled from the stoma, indicating a route of infection through the mucocutaneous junction.[1,2] Obviously the urostomy appliance attached to the skin creates a moist chamber favoring bacterial growth. Residual conduit urine,[6] and reflux from the collecting device have been found to promote bacterial growth.[7]

Continent reservoir with abdominal stoma

Most patients with a continent urinary reservoir have bacteriuria,[8–11] that is a mixture of the dermal flora with intermittent growth of uropathogenic strains. Ileal reservoir patients followed for 5 months showed bacteriuria, in most cases *E. coli*, and a frequent change in species was observed. Various anaerobic strains were found occasionally in urine, but always at the stoma/peristomal area.[8] In a series of 42 patients from our department, we obtained weekly urine cultures for 3 weeks from well-functioning continent cecal reservoirs or detubularized right colonic reservoirs (unpublished results). The patients had been followed for 2–15 years and none was on antibiotics. No patient had sterile urine on all test occasions. Bacterial growth in high densities was found in 33 cases, with a single species in all cultures from 20 of the patients. In cultures with single species growth, *E. coli* was the most frequent finding. Many cultures showed growth of multiple species: the dermal flora and uropathogenic strains. The continent cutaneous reservoir is emptied by clean intermittent catherization (CIC), which probably contributes to the contamination of the reservoir urine. It is not known if incomplete emptying influences colonization rate, but it seems likely. Leakage due to imperfect closure of the nipple valve correlates with bacterial growth.[8]

Orthotopic bladder substitution

The rates of bacteriuria in neobladder patients vary considerably in clinical reports, from 3%[12,13] to 30%.[14] However, reports with strict protocols and repeated urine sampling show that 30–80% of urine samples from this patient group show bacterial growth.[15–17] In a recent study, semiquantitative aerobic and anaerobic culture techniques in repeated urine samples from patients with ileal and colonic orthotopic bladder substitutes showed abundant growth of the skin flora and anaerobic strains in urine in 34/40 of the patients tested.[18] Individual samples frequently contained more than one microbial species. Repeated urine samples from the individual patients revealed a substantial variation in bacterial growth and species recovered. Twenty-three of the patients had bacteria in all urine samples, 11 patients had bacteria in some specimens and six patients had sterile urine on all sampling occasions. Uropathogenic strains, the majority being *E. coli*, were detected in 18/40. In this study, it was shown that the correct cut-off value for significant bacteriuria was 10^4 CFU/ml and that the culture of only one or two urine samples collected over a 6-month period would not have detected uropathogenic colonization in nearly half of the patients.[18] Thus, correct sampling and culture techniques significantly influence the data collected, a fact probably explaining the variation in the reported rate of bacteriuria in this patient group.

Augmentation cystoplasty

This patient group has a 'mixed lower urinary tract' with bladder tissue and ileal or colonic tissue. Furthermore, the extent of the cystoplasty differs within this patient group, from 'clam' to cup-patch after subtotal cystectomy. The remaining bladder tissue is in some cases affected by diseases like interstitial cystitis and other conditions, constituting an important determinant of susceptibility to urinary tract infection (UTI). Bacteriuria in these patients seems to be severely influenced by the use of CIC.[19–21] In our department, 22 of 23 patients with enterocystoplasty and on CIC, had positive urine cultures at three consecutive weekly tests. The flora was fairly stable in almost all cases, with *E. coli* by far the most common organism. Of the 11 patients with ileal cystoplasty and spontaneous voiding, five had negative cultures on all three test occasions, two had persistent *E. coli* and/or enterococci, while in four the cultures revealed Gram-positive members of the dermal flora (unpublished results).

Summary

The incorporation of intestinal segment in the urinary tract seems to favor urinary growth of the skin flora, anaerobic bacteria and uropathogenic strains. The route suggested for infection is ascending; bacteria enter the urethra, or the abdominal stoma, followed by colonization of the reconstructed lower urinary tract. Bacteriuria is common in all kind of reconstructions, however, neobladders with complete emptying have been reported to be at low risk for carrying bacteriuria. CIC and residual urine seem to increase the bacterial colonization. The augmentation cystoplasty constitutes a distinct subgroup, in which the remaining part of the bladder tissue is an important determinant of UTI susceptibility.

Factors involved in the antibacterial defense

The foregoing data clearly show that the lower urinary tract, reconstructed with an interposed intestinal segment, in the large majority of cases is heavily colonized by a variety of microorganisms. However, these patients seldom experience subjective signs of local infection. This paradox potentially could be explained by the intrinsic qualities of the interposed intestinal mucosa. In contrast to the gastrointestinal tract, the normal urinary tract is sterile, due to efficient antibacterial defense. The protection against ascending infection is usually achieved by cooperation between the specific and native defenses. Specific immunity requires an antigenic exposure, homing and T and B lymphocyte activation resulting in specialized responses such as antibody production. The native defenses are present at the site of infection and represents a wider spectrum of responses including mechanical forces like the urine flow and regular bladder emptying, epithelial defensins, mucosal inflammation etc. In the reconstructed lower urinary tract these defenses are compromised or removed. However, the interposed intestinal segment has its own intrinsic bacterial tolerance mechanisms to deal with bacterial colonization and other antigens present in the gastrointestinal tract. The mechanisms, both non-immunological and immunological, together constitute the intestinal 'mucosal barrier'. This chapter discusses some of these mechanisms. For indepth information, the interested reader is referred to a recent review covering this topic.[22]

Specific immunity

The intestine is the body's largest immunological organ. Protection of its vast mucosal surface from multiple antigens – microbial, parasitic, toxic, etc. (immune exclusion) – while recognizing and allowing non-harmful antigens to present themselves at the mucosal surface without hypersensitivity reactions (oral tolerance) requires a complex, integrated immune system. Whereas oral tolerance involves many rather poorly defined mechanisms, probably including generations of specific T-suppressor cells in the small-bowel mucosa, there is now considerable understanding of immune exclusion.

Intestinal immune exclusion operates via antibodies produced by the mucosa, chiefly secretory immunoglobulin A (s-IgA), the body's predominant immunoglobulin, while s-IgM plays a lesser role. Production of s-IgA is induced when the antigen presents to the mucosa. Antigenic priming occurs in lymphoepithelial structures, that is solitary lymphoid follicles or aggregations such as in the lymphoid tissue of Peyer's patches, also termed gut-associated lymphoid tissue (GALT). The antigen is taken up by M (membrane) cells in a specialized follicle-associated epithelium. Committed B lymphocytes are thereafter released from Peyer's patches to the blood via the mesenteric lymph nodes and the thoracic duct. As mature B-cells they then 'home' to the intestinal lamina propria, using 'addressins' on the endothelium of the mucosal venules that recognize specific receptors on the B-cell, to become antibody-producing plasma cells. Such plasma cells are found near the epithelial cells of exocrine glands in all parts of the body, but especially in the intestine. The plasma cells produce IgA mainly as dimers with a small peptide-joining (J) chain, which acts as a ligand for a receptor in the membrane of the epithelial cells, the secretory compent (SC). After binding to the SC the now complete s-IgA molecule is transported across the epithelial cells and appears on the mucosa.

Local production of immunoglobulins continues in excluded intestinal segments incorporated into the urinary tract.[16,23,24] It is not yet known if the density of GALT is affected by the mucosa's contact with urine. The immunoglobulin production probably retains its local character, i.e. a response to antigens in the conduit/reservoir, as in the classic experiments when poliovirus introduced into a distal colonic segment via a double-barreled colostomy stimulated secretion of IgA in that segment but not elsewhere in the gut.[25] In a pilot study in our department, we used a per oral cholera vaccine,[26] as an antigen, introduced into colonic neobladders. Two weeks after the antigenic exposure significantly elevated serum titers were observed, which suggest that the interposed intestinal segment possesses intact immunological mechanisms (unpublished results).

The antibacterial role of the intestinal specific responses in the reconstructed lower urinary tract is not clear. However, there exists some data suggesting a protective role. Prevention of bacterial adherence to enterocytes and uroepithelial cells by reaction of immunoglobulins with bacterial ligands such as fimbriae and other surface adhesions has been demonstrated in vitro and in vivo.[27,28]

Raised levels of s-IgA in reservoir urine were found to be more potent in inhibiting bacterial adherence to uroepithelial cells than s-IgA in urine from intact systems.[24] As there appears to be a strong non-covalent interaction between s-IgA and mucus, it is probable that s-IgA is 'held' within the mucus gel and concentrated near the mucosal surface to provide the specific immune protection.[29] This potency may confer special protection in cases of reflux after urinary diversion or enterocystoplasty.

Inflammation

The normal urinary tract is sterile, due to an efficient antibacterial defense. It has been shown that mucosal inflammation (but not specific defenses) is a prerequisite for the early clearance of bacteria from the intact urinary tract.[30,31] When bacteria are established in the urinary tract, the uroepithelium is activated, and start to excrete cytokines like interleukin-6 (IL-6) and IL-8.[32] Cytokines are small proteins that function as signal mediators between cells, and they play an important role in the regulation of the host defenses against local or systemic bacterial infections.[33] Patients with asymptomatic bacteriuria (ABU) secrete no, or very low, levels of IL-6 in urine in contrast to patients with febrile UTI and pyelonephritis, who have elevated local and systemic concentrations of IL-6.[34] At disease recovery IL-6 levels are normalized.[35] IL-8 is a neutrophil chemoattractant and a powerful inducer of neutrophil chemotaxis.[36] In patients with febrile UTI or ABU urinary IL-8 levels correlate with pyuria.[37]

As described above ABU in the reconstructed lower urinary tract is frequent. In our department we recently tested urine samples, obtained weekly for 3 weeks, from patients with ileal and colonic neobladders. Pyuria was present in most urine samples, also in patients with sterile urine. Concentrations of IL-6 and IL-8 were low, or absent, in urine from colonic neobladder patients, but present in significantly higher concentrations in urine from ileal neobladders (unpublished results). These findings indicate that ABU in the neobladder patients does cause a local mucosal host response, and that this response seems to be higher in those with an ileal neobladder.

Mucus

Mucus, the viscous slippery gel covering the mucous membranes of the gastrointestinal tract, consists of a complex mixture of glycoproteins, water, various serum and cellular macromolecules, electrolytes, microorganisms and sloughed cells.[29] Its main organic constituent is mucin, which is a high molecular weight glycoprotein. The molecule has an extended rod-like configuraton with a peptide core, and oligosaccharide chains radiating like the bristles of a brush.[38] This structure accounts for the viscoelasticity of the mucin. As the carbohydrate chains are extremely hydrophilic and interdigitate with each other to produce stable non-covalent interactions, water is bound, accounting for the gel-forming property of mucin. These chains also protect the central peptide core from the destructive proteases present in enzymes and bacteria. By polymerization of the mucin monomer, highly cross-linked aggregates are formed – the mucinous gel. Mucin is produced in the goblet cells, the numbers of which increase aborally. Histologic studies of ileal and cecal reservoirs indicate that these cells are present in normal amounts also after urinary diversion (see Chapter 6). The mucus gel covers the enterocytes, in a layer of up to 400 μm, and loss from the luminal side by digestion and peristalsis is offset by a continuous baseline production of mucus which accelerates in response to stimuli like cholinergic agonists, noxious chemical agents, inflammatory mediators, bacterial toxins etc.

The ability of pathogens to adhere to the mucosal surface is important for their virulence.[39–41] Adherence of enteropathogenic *E. coli* is mediated by pili on the bacterial surface. The intestinal mucus layer seems to posses mechanisms which can prevent microbial attachment to the enterocytes.[42] The mucus film in the ileum and colon has a large and varied population of bacteria and protozoa.[29] In ileal conduits and continent cecal urinary reservoirs the mucus likewise is heavily colonized by bacteria, virtually none of them adhering to the enterocytes.[43,44] The intestinal mucus has been shown to contain specific receptors, analogous to those of the enterocytes, to which enteropathogenic *E. coli* expressing pilus adhesions can bind,[28,45] and the binding of *E. coli* to microvillous membranes of the enterocytes was found to be inhibited by purified mucin of golbet cell origin.[46,47] These observations suggest that binding of bacteria to mucus may prevent their adhesion to the enterocyte surface, probably by competitive inhibition, although non-specific interactions are also possible.[47] In reconstructed urinary tracts, the mucus thus may function as an important host defense.

Residual urine

The complete and regular emptying of the urinary bladder constitutes a potent antibacterial defense,[48] and it has been suggested that the antibacterial effect is provided through bacterial contact with the bladder mucosa. If residual urine is present bacteria escape these bactericidal mechanisms. Small amounts of residual urine support stable growth of bacteria in high densities, despite regular emptying.[49,50] In the reconstructed lower urinary tract, intestinal mucosa carries an innate tolerance for bacterial growth, and bactericidal effects through bacterial–mucosal contacts are not likely to occur. Neobladder emptying, even in the most perfect case, results in intestinal folds with small pockets of residual urine probably in amounts enough for maintenance of stable bacteriuria. These factors provide optimal conditions for bacterial growth. However, it has been shown that patients with neobladders and with very low amounts of post-void residual urine (<20 ml) have significantly lower rates of bacteriuria or have sterile urine compared with those with incomplete emptying.[18] These findings suggest that measures for optimizing neobladder emptying should reduce the bacteriuria rate, which has been suggested in clinical reports. The underlying mechanisms explaining the antibacterial defense provided by the complete, or nearly complete, neobladder emptying are unknown, and merits further studies.

Type of interposed intestine

The specific ecological properties of the ileal and colonic tissue have gained surprisingly little interest. It has been reported that mixed flora was more frequent in ileal than in colonic conduits, and that monocultures were common in urine from colonic continent reservoirs and conduits.[3,5] As the functional properties of the reconstructed lower urinary tract influence the bacteriuria rate, we investigated two strictly defined groups of ileal and colonic neobladder patients; those with complete neobladder emptying and those on CIC.[18] In the group with complete bladder emptying, urine from the ileal neobladder group invariably had bacteria, whereas all the colonic neobladder patients had sterile urine. In the CIC group the bacterial colonization, including uropathogenic growth, was similar regardless of the intestinal segment used for reconstruction. However, there was heavier growth of non-pathogenic aerobic strains in urine cultures from colonic neobladder patients, whereas anaerobic bacteria significantly predominated the cultures of ileal neobladder patients. Further, *Ureaplasma urealyticum* was found only in urine samples from the colonic neobladder group. These data do suggest that ileal and colonic tissue provide specific ecological niches that may influence the local host response differently.

Role of the prostate

Reconstruction of the lower urinary tract compromises many of the natural defenses against UTIs. In the neobladder constructed after cystoprostatectomy the absence of the prostate and its antibacterial secretions may contribute to decreased protection against ascending infection. However, in patients who have undergone radical prostatectomy, no, or a very low rate of bacteriuria, has been demonstrated.[16,18] This indicates that the increased rate of bacterial colonization in patients with reconstructed lower urinary tracts is mainly because of factors other than the missing prostatic antibacterial defenses. It also suggests that the antibacterial properties of the prostate in the intact lower urinary tract may be weaker than previously assumed.

Altered urine composition

When an intestinal segment is interposed in the urinary tract, the flux of substances across the mucosa gives the urine a composition different from that in the intact bladder. Physicochemical influences on bacterial growth in urine were studied in reconstructed urinary tracts.[51] The optimal pH for growth of pathogens in the urinary tract is 6.0–7.0. In cecal reservoir urine, the pH was slightly higher than normal and with considerably less individual variation,[51] the stability probably due to the flux of ions across the mucosa. The level and stability of pH thus could make cecal reservoir urine a more favorable medium for bacterial growth than ordinary urine. Zinc and magnesium, with known antibacterial activity, have been proposed as factors counteracting UTI,[52,53] but the concentration of these ions did not differ significantly between normal urine and cecal reservoir urine.[51] Although the 24-hour excretion of urea, another bactericidal constituent,[54] was similar in normal and reservoir urine, its concentration was lower in the reservoir, and it may be a factor promoting bacterial growth. Urine in contact with intestinal mucosa contains a surplus of substances that can act as microbial nutrients, including carbohydrates and serum proteins. The oligosaccharides of mucin, for instance, were found to be substrates for certain anaerobes, and by releasing carbohydrate from mucin they also provide for nutrition of bacteria.[29] Although the differences between reservoir urine and normal urine may imply better conditions for growth in the former, this has, however, not been shown to be the case in experimental work.[51]

Summary

The increased rate of bacteriuria in the reconstructed patients indicates a lack of 'antibacterial defenses' and suggests mucosal tolerance for bacterial growth, thus creating a basis for symptom-free carriage of bacteria. The roles of the specific and non-specific inflammatory antibacterial responses in the reconstructed lower urinary tract are mainly unknown. The absence of antibacterial prostatic secretions in neobladder patients does not seem to increase the susceptibility for bacterial colonization. Residual urine increases the rate of bacteriuria in neobladder patients.

The clinical importance of bacteriuria

The clinical relevance of bacteriuria in the reconstructed lower urinary tract is dependent on subjective signs of infection and presence of pathology of the upper urinary tract. Outflow obstruction due to stenosis of the ureterointestinal anastomosis, hydronephrosis, neobladder and kidney stones, recurrence of malignant disease or other pathologic conditions must be ruled out and treated adequately. If the patient has subjective signs of local infection, and/or engagement of the upper urinary tract, antibacterial treatment must be given. Treatment of ABU in the absence of risk factors is controversial. If the patient has a history of recurrent pyelonephritis, prophylactic antibiotic treatment is usually tried. However, the protective value of this approach has not been evaluated in clinical studies.

Prophylactic antibiotic treatment

Some centers advocate prophylactic low-dose antibiotic therapy in patients with reconstructed lower urinary tracts. Two reasons have been suggested: (i) the bacteriuria indicates an active infection and that this should be avoided, and (ii) that a future episode of pyelonephritis is caught up. Some data are available regarding the first. The systemic host response was studied in a group of patients with continent reservoirs. Serum levels of C-reactive protein (CRP) were not raised, and circulating antibodies against uropathogenic strains in the urine were not detected. Local host response parameters have shown to be increased in ileal but not in colonic neobladder patients (see above), which is indicative of an activated mucosal response towards the bacteriuria in the ileal neobladder. Patients with reconstructed lower urinary tracts and bacteriuria, even in the case of uropathogenic growth, are practically always asymptomatic – thus the clinical situation supports that the bacteriuria rather reflects a silent colonization, identical with ABU in the intact urinary tract, than an active infection with deeper penetration of the tissue. If this is the case, there is no basis for active treatment, nor for prophylactic antibiotic therapy. Furthermore, recent studies have shown that prophylactic antibiotic therapy does not influence the rate of bacteriuria,[17,18] and that growth of *E. coli* in the urine frequently recurs after treatment.

Regarding the second indication, there is no doubt that a patient with recurrent pyelonephritis has to be treated actively, and individual risk factors have to be identified. Hydronephrosis prior to the reconstruction will in some cases prevail after surgery. Frequently after reconstruction, upper urinary tracts that were normal beforehand dilate. A recent study[15] showed that bacteriuria was the main risk factor, but not hydronephrosis, for bacteriemia in patients with an ileal bladder substitute without antireflux surgery. The study, however, did not report on bacterial strains found, and there was no evaluation of the neobladder function. Even though this finding indicates benefits of active treatment of ABU in the ileal neobladder lacking reflux protection, it is important to notice that no prospective study has been done to examine if low-dose prophylactic antibiotic therapy reduces the risk for pyelonephritis.

An important issue is the influence of prophylactic antibiotic therapy on the microbial ecology. In a recent study,[18] we investigated the microbial flora in patients with ileal neobladders, treated with trimethoprim 160 mg daily as a prophylactic measure. The rate of positive urine cultures was higher, anaerobic bacteria were more frequent, and the rate of occurence of uropathogenic bacteria was lower than in ileal bladder patients not treated with antibiotics. However, about a third of the patients tested carried uropathogenic isolates, in most cases *E. faecalis*, a bacterium usually not sensitive to trimethoprim. These findings suggest that prophylactic antibiotic treatment interfers with, rather than suppresses bacterial colonization, and that the carriage of uropathogenic isolates is only moderately lowered. Future studies are needed to elucidate the long-term effects of low-dose antibiotic treatment on the microbial ecology in patients with neobladders, the selective effect regarding microbial antibiotic resistance, and the possible benefits of this treatment.

Stone formation

Routine follow-up should rule out stone formation in the reconstructed urinary tract. Special attention must be given to patients having local discomfort or recurrent bacteriuria with *Proteus* spp., and investigations such as endoscopy and radiographic examinations should be done frequently. The use of staples in the urinary tract should be avoided. Exposed staples serve as a nidus for stone formation, and a very high incidence of stones has been found in patients with Kock pouches.[55] The struvite and carbonate apatite stones always harbor *Proteus* spp. that persist until all stones and staples are removed. Even stapled closure of a conduit from the outside entails risk of stone formation.[56] Absorbable staples may not be wholly without such risk, as the absorption time is very long.

Renal function

Clinical studies investigating the fate of renal function after urinary diversion, have focused on the issue of 'low' and 'high pressure' reconstructions, and if the ureteric implantation is performed with antireflux technique or not. Generally, incontinent urinary diversions are considered low-pressure type with theoretically unhindered outflow of urine. Consequently, antireflux surgery, with its higher risks for stenosis of the neoureter anastomosis, would be superfluous in these patients. However, in the mid 1970s reports showed that the ileal conduit had a high incidence of renal function deterioration attributed mainly to reflux and bacteriuria,[57] a view that received experimental support.[58] Clinically asymptomatic or 'silent' pyelonephritis in patients with refluxing ileal conduit has been reported to be frequent.[59,60] These observations encouraged the introduction of antireflux ureteric implantation in colon conduits. However, the superiority of this approach has not been confirmed.[61] In a recent long-term follow-up of patients with ileal conduit without reflux protection, a high incidence of complications regarding kidney function was reported.[62] In a prospective randomized study, we compared renal function after ileal or colonic conduit reconstruction, with or without antirefluxing ureteric anastomosis. Total and separate renal function was determined preoperatively and at follow-up in each of the included patients. After a mean 5 years' observation, glomerular filtration rate (GFR) reduction did not differ between the groups, and this was also seen at later follow-up.[63,64] Although separate GFR did not differ between refluxing and antirefluxing anastomosis in the conduit groups, renal scarring at DMSA scan was more common in the refluxing units,[65] indicating a benefit of the antireflux surgery.

In continent urinary reconstruction, an important measure is to lower the intraluminal pressure by detubularizing the isolated intestinal segment. However, it is well known that the continent cutaneous reservoir with a reliable outlet closure mechanism may have high intraluminal pressures in the period between the regularly emptying by CIC, and therefore antireflux surgery is generally recommended in this patient group. Serum antibody titers against *E. coli*, found in the urine from patients reconstructed with continent ileal reservoirs having antireflux protection, were not significantly increased indicating that 'silent pyelonephritis' was not present.[10]

One of the main arguments against antireflux surgery in neobladder reconstruction is that high pressures are not achieved, since an overextended neobladder will result in urinary leakage, thus resulting in a 'pop-off' effect of the intraluminal pressure. However, in a recent prospective study, the 5-year risk for urosepsis was as high as 18% in patients with an ileal neobladder constructed with an ileal afferent loop and a ureterointestinal anastomosis without antireflux protection.[15] Interestingly, a similar type of neobladder[12] was not shown to produce reflux in a study using radionucleotide cystography.[66] Clinical reports from patients with neobladders and antireflux ureteric implantation have reported a very low risk for pyelonephritis, unless risk factors such as stenosis of the ureterointestinal anastomosis or failure of the antireflux protection mechanism is present.[67–70] It has been shown that reflux and histologic evidence of pyelonephritis occurred in a low pressure enterocystoplasty canine model,[71] findings which were rare in non-refluxing control kidneys. Bacteriuria, however, may be present in the upper urinary tract even in the absence of reflux.[72]

These contradictory data may be a reason for the lack of consensus on the need for antireflux surgery in neobladder construction (for a review see reference 73), and point out the importance of carrying out randomized prospective trials. Another drawback is that there is no standard for renal function assessment, making it difficult to compare different clinical series. It is important to emphasize that intravenous urography and creatinine measurements are unsatisfactory for the evaluation of renal function. In the absence of detailed information on long-term renal function or morphology, and since bacteriuria is common in the reconstructed lower urinary tract, we believe that refluxing anastomosis should not be recommended for patients judged to have long life expectancy, until studies showing satisfactory results are available.

Conclusion

Incorporation of intestinal segments into the urinary tract favors bacteriuria, including growth of uropathogenic strains. The bacterial colonization is in practically all cases asymptomatic, and studies have shown that systemic host responses are not triggered. It has been suggested that the interposed isolated intestine segment carries with it its innate tolerance, thus providing conditions favoring the asymptomatic carriage of bacteria. Several factors seem to influence the occurrence of bacteriuria: pre-existing anatomical and functional abnormalities of the urinary tract, residual urine, CIC and bacterial colonization at mucocutaneous junctions. Antibiotic treatment for asymptomatic bacteriuria is not recommended, however, patients with recurrent symptomatic infections have to be actively treated and investigated regarding risk factors, i.e. stones in the urinary tract, upper urinary tract outflow obstruction and reflux. To protect the kidneys, antireflux ureteric implantation should still be advocated, even when the urinary receptacle is of so called low-pressure type.

References

1. Bishop RF, Smith ED, Gracey M. Bacterial flora of urine from ileal conduit. J Urol 1971; 105: 452–5.
2. Morris EJ, Bracken RB, Hopfer RL, Mills K, Rodriguez DB. Urinary findings in 20 asymptomatic patients with an ileal conduit. J Enterostomal Ther 1982; 9: 24–7.
3. Hill MJ, Hudson MJ, Stewart M. The urinary bacterial flora in patients with three types of urinary tract diversion. J Med Microbiol 1983; 16: 221–6.
4. Chan RC, Reid G, Bruce AW, Costerton JW. Microbial colonization of human ileal conduits. Appl Environ Microbiol 1984; 48: 1159–65.
5. Husmann DA, McLorie GA, Churchill BM. Nonrefluxing colonic conduits: a long-term life-table analysis. J Urol 1989; 142: 1201–3.
6. Bergman B, Kaijser B, Nilson AE. Conduit urinary diversion and urinary-tract infection. II. Raised serum antibody titers against *Escherichia coli* and *Proteus mirabilis* in relation to bacteriologic findings. Scand J Urol Nephrol 1979; 13: 71–7.
7. Stewart W, Cass AS, Matsen JM. Variation in bacteriuria with intestinal loop urinary diversions. J Urol 1974; 111: 117–19.
8. Månsson W, Colleen S, Mårdh PA. The microbial flora of the continent cecal urinary reservoir, its stoma and the peristomal skin. J Urol 1986; 135: 247–50.
9. Åkerlund S, Berglund B, Kock NG, Philipson BM. Voiding pattern, urinary volume, composition and bacterial contamination in patients with urinary diversion via a continent ileal reservoir. Br J Urol 1989; 63: 619–23.
10. Åkerlund S, Campanello M, Kaijser B, Jonsson O. Bacteriuria in patients with a continent ileal reservoir for urinary diversion does not regularly require antibiotic treatment. Br J Urol 1994; 74: 177–81.
11. Arai Y, Kawakita M, Terachi T et al. Long-term followup of the Kock and Indiana pouch procedures. J Urol 1993; 150: 51–5.
12. Studer UE, Zingg EJ. Ileal orthotopic bladder substitutes. What we have learned from 12 years' experience with 200 patients. Urol Clin North Am 1997; 24: 781–93.
13. Hautmann RE, de Petriconi R, Gottfried HW et al. The ileal neobladder: complications and functional results in 363 patients after 11 years of followup. J Urol 1999; 161: 422–7; discussion 427–8.
14. Steven K, Poulsen AL. The orthotopic Kock ileal neobladder: functional results, urodynamic features, complications and survival in 166 men. J Urol 2000; 164: 288–95.
15. Wood DP Jr, Bianco FJ Jr, Pontes JE, Heath MA, DaJusta D. Incidence and significance of positive urine cultures in patients with an orthotopic neobladder. J Urol 2003; 169: 2196–9.
16. Iwakiri J, Freiha FS, Shortliffe LM. Prospective study of urinary tract infections and urinary antibodies after radical prostatectomy and cystoprostatectomy. Urol Clin North Am 2002; 29: 251–8, xii.
17. Keegan SJ, Graham C, Neal DE et al. Characterization of *Escherichia coli* strains causing urinary tract infections in patients with transposed intestinal segments. J Urol 2003; 169: 2382–7.
18. Wullt B, Holst E, Steven K et al. Microbial flora in ileal and colonic neobladders. Eur Urol 2004; 45: 223–9.
19. Fenn N, Conn IG, German KA, Stephenson TP. Complications of clam enterocystoplasty with particular reference to urinary tract infection. Br J Urol 1992; 69: 366–8.
20. Nurse DE, Mundy AR. Assessment of the malignant potential of cystoplasty. Br J Urol 1989; 64: 489–92.
21. Gonzalez R, Sidi AA, Zhang G. Urinary undiversion: indications, technique and results in 50 cases. J Urol 1986; 136: 13–16.
22. Mowat AM. Anatomical basis of tolerance and immunity to intestinal antigens. Nat Rev Immunol 2003; 3: 331–41.
23. Månsson W, Colleen S, Low K, Mårdh PA, Lundblad A. Immunoglobulins in urine from patients with ileal and colonic conduits and reservoirs. J Urol 1985; 133: 713–16.
24. Trinchieri A, Braceschi L, Tiranti D et al. Secretory immunoglobulin A and inhibitory activity of bacterial adherence to epithelial cells in urine from patients with urinary tract infections. Urol Res 1990; 18: 305–8.
25. Ogra PL, Karzon DT. Distribution of poliovirus antibody in serum, nasopharynx and alimentary tract following segmental immunization of lower alimentary tract with poliovaccine. J Immunol 1969; 102: 1423–30.
26. Jertborn M, Svennerholm AM, Holmgren J. Immunological memory after immunization with oral cholera B subunit – whole-cell vaccine in Swedish volunteers. Vaccine 1994; 12: 1078–82.
27. Fubara ES, Freter R. Protection against enteric bacterial infection by secretory IgA antibodies. J Immunol 1973; 111: 395–403.
28. Mouricout MA, Julien RA. Pilus-mediated binding of bovine enterotoxigenic *Escherichia coli* to calf small intestinal mucins. Infect Immun 1987; 55: 1216–23.
29. Neutra M, Forstner J. Gastrointestinal mucus: synthesis secretion and function. In: Johnson L (ed). Physiology of the Gastrointestinal Tract. 2 edn. New York: Raven Press, 1987: 975–1009.

30. Svanborg-Edén C, Hagberg L, Briles D, McGhee J, Michalek S. Susceptibility to *Escherichia coli* urinary tract infection and LPS responsiveness. In: Skamene E (ed). Genetic Control of Host Resistance to Infection and Malignancy. New York: Alan R Liss Inc, 1985; 385–91.
31. Svanborg Eden C, Briles D, Hagberg L, McGhee J, Michalec S. Genetic factors in host resistance to urinary tract infection. Infection 1984; 12: 118–23.
32. Agace W, Hedges S, Andersson U et al. Selective cytokine production by epithelial cells following exposure to *Escherichia coli*. Infect Immun 1993; 61: 602–9.
33. Svanborg C, Godaly G, Hedlund M. Cytokine responses during mucosal infections: role in disease pathogenesis and host defence. Curr Opin Microbiol 1999; 2: 99–105.
34. Hedges S, Stenqvist K, Lidin-Janson G et al. Comparison of urine and serum concentrations of interleukin-6 in women with acute pyelonephritis or asymptomatic bacteriuria. J Infect Dis 1992; 166: 653–6.
35. Otto G, Braconier J, Andreasson A, Svanborg C. Interleukin-6 and disease severity in patients with bacteremic nonbacteremic febrile urinary tract infection. J Infect Dis 1999; 179: 172–9.
36. Baggiolini M, Clark-Lewis I. Interleukin-8, a chemotactic and inflammatory cytokine. FEBS Lett 1992; 307: 97–101.
37. Agace W, Hedges S, Ceska M, Svanborg C. Interleukin 8 and the neutrophil response to mucosal Gram-negative infection. J Clin Invest 1993; 92: 780–5.
38. Lamont JT. Mucus: the front line of intestinal mucosal defense. Ann N Y Acad Sci 1992; 664: 190–201.
39. Svanborg-Edén C, Hanson L, Jodal U, Sohl-Åkerlund A. Variable adherence to normal urinary tract epithelial cells of *Escherichia coli* strains associated with various forms of urinary tract infection. Lancet 1976; i: 490–2.
40. Bruce AW, Chan RC, Pinkerton D, Morales A, Chadwick P. Adherence of Gram-negative uropathogens to human uroepithelial cells. J Urol 1983; 130: 293–8.
41. Savage D. Colonization by and survival of pathogenic bacteria on intestinal mucosal surfaces. In: Bitton G, Marshall K (eds). Microorganisms to Surfaces. New York: John Wiley, 1980: 175–206.
42. Blomberg L, Krivan HC, Cohen PS, Conway PL. Piglet ileal mucus contains protein and glycolipid (galactosylceramide) receptors specific for *Escherichia coli* K88 fimbriae. Infect Immun 1993; 61: 2526–31.
43. Bruce AW, Reid G, Chan RC, Costerton JW. Bacterial adherence in the human ileal conduit: a morphological and bacteriological study. J Urol 1984; 132: 184–8.
44. Carlen B, Willen R, Mansson W. Mucosal ultrastructure of continent cecal reservoir for urine and its ileal nipple valve 2–9 years after construction. J Urol 1990; 143: 372–6.
45. Laux DC, McSweegan EF, Williams TJ, Wadolkowski EA, Cohen PS. Identification and characterization of mouse small intestine mucosal receptors for *Escherichia coli* K-12(K88ab). Infect Immun 1986; 52: 18–25.
46. Drumm B, Roberton AM, Sherman PM. Inhibition of attachment of *Escherichia coli* RDEC-1 to intestinal microvillus membranes by rabbit ileal mucus and mucin in vitro. Infect Immun 1988; 56: 2437–42.
47. Mack DR, Sherman PM. Mucin isolated from rabbit colon inhibits in vitro binding of *Escherichia coli* RDEC-1. Infect Immun 1991; 59: 1015–23.
48. Cox CE, Hinman F Jr. Factors in resistance to infection in the bladder. 1. The eradication of bacteria by vesical emptying and intrinsic defense mechanisms. In: Kass EH (ed). Progress in Pyelonephritis. Philadelphia: FA Davies, 1965: 563.
49. O'Grady F, Cattel WR. Kinetics of urinary tract infection. I . Upper urinary tract. Br J Urol 1966a; 38: 156.
50. Gordon DM, Riley MA. A theoretical and experimental analysis of bacterial growth in the bladder. Mol Microbiol 1992; 6: 555–62.
51. Månsson W, Colleen S, Mårdh PA. Urine from continent caecal reservoirs. Studies on chemical composition and bacterial growth. Eur Urol 1989; 16: 18–22.
52. Colleen S, Mårdh PA, Schytz A. Magnesium and zinc in seminal fluid of healthy males and patients with non-acute prostatitis with and without gonorrhoea. Scand J Urol Nephrol 1975; 9: 192–7.
53. Fair WR, Couch J, Wehner N. Prostatic antibacterial factor. Identity and significance. Urology 1976; 7: 169–77.
54. Schlegel JU, Cuellar J, O'Dell RM. Bactericidal effect of urea. J Urol 1961; 86: 819–22.
55. Ginsberg D, Huffman JL, Lieskovsky G, Boyd S, Skinner DG. Urinary tract stones: a complication of the Kock pouch continent urinary diversion. J Urol 1991; 145: 956–9.
56. Brenner M, Johnson DE. Ileal conduit calculi from stapler anastomosis: a long-term complication? Urology 1985; 26: 537–40.
57. King L. Editorial comment. In: The Year Book of Urology. Chicago: Year Book Medical Publishers, 1974: 203.
58. Richie JP, Skinner DG, Waisman J. The effect of reflux on the development of pyelonephritis in urinary diversion: an experimental study. J Surg Res 1974; 16: 256–61.
59. Bergman B. Studies on patients with ileal conduit diversion with special regard to renal infection. Scand J Urol Nephrol Suppl 1978; 47: 1–32.
60. Schwarz GR, Jeffs RD. Ileal conduit urinary diversion in children: computer analysis of followup from 2 to 16 years. J Urol 1975; 114: 285–8.
61. Hill JT, Ransley PG. The colonic conduit: a better method of urinary diversion? Br J Urol 1983; 55: 629–31.
62. Madersbacher S, Schmidt J, Eberle JM et al. Long-term outcome of ileal conduit diversion. J Urol 2003; 169: 985–90.
63. Månsson W, Ahlgren G, White T. Glomerular filtration rate up to 10 years after urinary diversion of different types. A comparative study of ileal and colonic conduit, refluxing and antirefluxing ureteral anastomosis and continent caecal reservoir. Scand J Urol Nephrol 1989; 23: 195–200.
64. Kristjansson A, Wallin L, Månsson W. Renal function up to 16 years after conduit (refluxing or anti-reflux anastomosis) or continent urinary diversion. 1. Glomerular filtration rate and patency of uretero-intestinal anastomosis. Br J Urol 1995; 76: 539–45.
65. Kristjansson A, Bajc M, Wallin L, Willner J, Mansson W. Renal function up to 16 years after conduit (refluxing or anti-reflux anas-

tomosis) or continent urinary diversion. 2. Renal scarring and location of bacteriuria. Br J Urol 1995; 76: 546–50.
66. Waidelich R, Rink F, Kriegmair M, Tatsch K, Schmeller N. A study of reflux in patients with an ileal orthotopic bladder. Br J Urol 1998; 81: 241–6.
67. Skinner DG, Lieskovsky G, Boyd S. Continent urinary diversion. J Urol 1989; 141: 1323–7.
68. Ahlering TE, Weinberg AC, Razor B. Modified Indiana pouch. J Urol 1991; 145: 1156–8.
69. Bloch WE, Bejany DE, Penalver MA, Politano VA. Complications of the Miami pouch. J Urol 1992; 147: 1017–19.
70. Månsson W, Davidsson T, Konyves J et al. Continent urinary tract reconstruction – the Lund experience. BJU Int 2003; 92: 271–6.
71. St Clair SR, Hixson CJ, Ritchey ML. Enterocystoplasty and reflux nephropathy in the canine model. J Urol 1992; 148(2 Pt 2): 728–32.
72. Gonzalez R, Reinberg Y. Localization of bacteriuria in patients with enterocystoplasty and nonrefluxing conduits. J Urol 1987; 138(4 Pt 2): 1104–5.
73. Ghoneim MA. Ureterointestinal anastomosis in continent urinary diversion: an antirefluxing procedure – is it necessary? Tech Urol 2001; 7: 203–8.

6 Structural and functional changes of the gastrointestinal mucosa in contact with urine

Wiking Månsson, Thomas Davidsson and Roger Willén

Introduction

Exclusion of a gastrointestinal segment for incorporation in the urinary tract induces structural and functional changes both in the remaining alimentary tract and in the isolate exposed to urine. Indeed, resection and bypass have been the most widely used methods for studying the morphological and functional adaptability of the gut. For an overview of the various factors regulating growth of the gastrointestinal mucosa, readers are referred to Thompson et al.[1]

Morphological changes in the gastrointestinal mucosa exposed to urine range from varying degrees of atrophy to frank neoplasia. The development of benign and malignant tumors is more extensively discussed in Chapter 9. Other mucosal structural changes, however, may have important functional implications. Thus the production of host defense factors such as immunoglobulins and mucus may be affected, as may the absorption of different solutes in the urine. Permeability of microorganisms or toxic substances is more likely to be a risk factor when the mucosal lining is abnormal. Acute and chronic inflammation may cause symptoms from a pouch as well as affecting the strength of the wall. Mural fibrosis can reduce distensibility of the intestine, leading to secondary obstruction or decreased capacity. In this chapter we review the literature on mucosal studies and present some work by our own research group.

Normal intestinal mucosa

At light microscopy the villi of the normal small-bowel mucosa appear as finger- or leaf-like projections, 0.5–0.8 mm high in the proximal jejunum and somewhat lower in the ileum, surrounded by crypts. The villus:crypt index varies from 3:1 to 5:1. The mucosa in direct contact with the luminal contents, covering the villi and lining the crypts, is monolayered. The crypt epithelium is formed by actively proliferating undifferentiated cells which mature into absorptive cells, mucus-secreting goblet cells, enterochromaffin and other endocrine cells and also Paneth cells. The cells rest on the basement membrane measuring 4–6 μm. The Paneth cells produce lysozyme and may be important in regulating the intestinal microflora. They remain in the crypt, while the other cells migrate in the villus and are extruded from its tip. The epithelial coating of the villus thus contains mature columnar cells, enterocytes with absorptive functions, goblet cells, a few endocrine cells and specialized 'M' cells overlying the apex of Peyer's patches.

Below the epithelial layer is the lamina propria, forming the connective-tissue core of the villi and containing immunologically important structures – plasma cells, lymphocytes, macrophages – in addition to eosinophils and mast cells. The deepest layer is the muscularis mucosae, a very thin sheet of muscle cells separating the mucosa from the submucosa. The function of this layer is not clear, but it has been claimed to serve as the structural foundation of the mucosa. Large aggregates of lymphoid tissue, Peyer's patches, are located primarily in the mucosa, but extend into the submucosa.

In contrast, the colonic mucosal surface is flat, lacks villi but has microvilli on the surface. Tubular crypts extending down towards the muscularis mucosae contain columnar epithelial, endocrine and some Paneth cells and rich amounts of Peyers plaque. The connective tissue part of the mucosa is basically built up as the small intestine. The submucosa is rich in vessels, nerves and ganglia. The submucosa ends at the lamina muscularis propria with its two thick layers of muscles intercepted by nerve cell ganglia and pacemaker cells (cells of Cajal).

Electron microscopy has considerably expanded knowledge of the small intestine's absorptive cells.[2] Briefly, their luminal surface is provided with microvilli 0.5–1.5 μm high, through which ions and solutes pass and which manifoldly increase the absorptive surface. The surface coating of the microvilli, the glycocalyx, consists of glycoproteins and glycolipids. A number of 'brush-border' enzymes, non-enzymatic proteins and transport proteins involved in absorption are associated with the glycocalyx and the underlying plasma membrane. Below the microvilli is a narrow area, the terminal web, into which the filamentous core rootlets from the microvilli extend. Organelles in the cytoplasm beneath the terminal web are lysosomes, the endoplasmic reticulum (which appears as a continuous network throughout the cell), mitochondria and Golgi apparatus. The oval nucleus of the enterocyte is situated in the basal third of the cell. Except for its apical surface, the cell is surrounded by the basolateral membrane which at the cell base is in close contact with the basement membrane and the lamina propria. The membranes of adjacent cells are closely apposed to each other, but during fluid absorption the intercellular space can widen appreciably, especially along the cells' basal half. Apically, the cells are attached to each other through the junctional complex, consisting of the tight and intermediate junctions and the desmosomes. The junctions appear to play a major part in regulating the paracellular flow of water and solutes.

The density of goblet cells increases aborally. Mucin, consisting of conjugated glycoprotein, is produced and stored in these cells, from which it oozes out to form a viscous covering for the surface cells. Mucin secretion accelerates in response to many physiological and pathological stimuli. The important functions of the secreted mucin include cytoprotection in the stomach, lubrication and protection against toxins and bacteria. The composition of mucin is heterogeneous, varying between regions of the gastrointestinal tract and between individuals. Using periodic acid–Schiff (PAS) and high iron diamine-alcian blue (HID-AB) stains, mucin can be histochemically classified as neutral or acid, the latter as sialomucin or sulfomucin, containing sialic acid and sulfate, respectively. Sialomucin is dominant in the ileum and sulfomucin in the cecum and sigmoid colon. Intestinal malignancy, ulcer, cystic fibrosis and inflammatory bowel disease have been reported to cause changes in mucin composition.

Mucosal adaptation in the bypassed intestinal segment

Extensive experimental studies have been done on intestinal adaptation following transection, resection, transposition, pancreaticobiliary diversion and bypass. In the bypassed intestinal segment, either a self-emptying blind loop or a Thiry–Vella fistula, i.e. a loop with its two ends exteriorized as cutaneous stomas, there is considerable hypoplasia with reduction of mucosal weight, villus height, mucosal surface area and crypt-cell production rate.[3] Mucosal protein and DNA content are also reduced, changes described as 'disuse atrophy'.[4] Restoration of the bypassed segment to its original position promptly reverses the changes,[5] testifying to the influence of luminal chyme with its content of known nutrients, pancreaticobiliary secretions and possibly luminal growth factors. Systemic factors, perhaps humoral, however, also appear to be significant in both small and large bowel.[6,7]

Functional changes accompany these morphological developments. Thus the mucosal and brush border enzymes decrease in Thiry–Vella loops[8] and absorption of glucose and amino acids is diminished.[9–11] This hypofunction probably is an effect of the hypoplasia rather than an expression of reduced enterocyte activity per se, as the decrease correlates well with the diminution in mucosal DNA content.

Morphological changes in intestinal mucosa after exposure to urine: effect of urine or of 'disuse'?

Clinical extrapolation of the above-cited experimental findings requires caution. Clearly, however, human intestinal mucosa undergoes distinct morphological changes when exposed to urine. The dominant feature is mucosal atrophy, sometimes with complete local absence of villi. The changes seem to be much more extensive than could be expected solely from disuse of normal absorptive functions. As regards the effect of urine on the mucosa, the noxious influence may come not only from the urine per se, but also from the altered microbial ecology in such reconstructed urinary tracts, with enteropathogens such as *Escherichia coli*.

To shed some light on this question, experiments were performed in a rat model.[12] An ileocolonic segment was used for construction of an ileocolocystoplasty or an ileocolocutaneostomy (blind loop) and sham-operated animals were used for controls. The rats were killed after 8 weeks. In the sham-operated group the intestinal mucosa was intact, with microvilli, approximately 1.5 μm long in ileum, and 0.6 μm in colon (Figure 6.1). There was no fibrosis and the content of neutral mucins, sialomucins and sulfomucins in the goblet cells

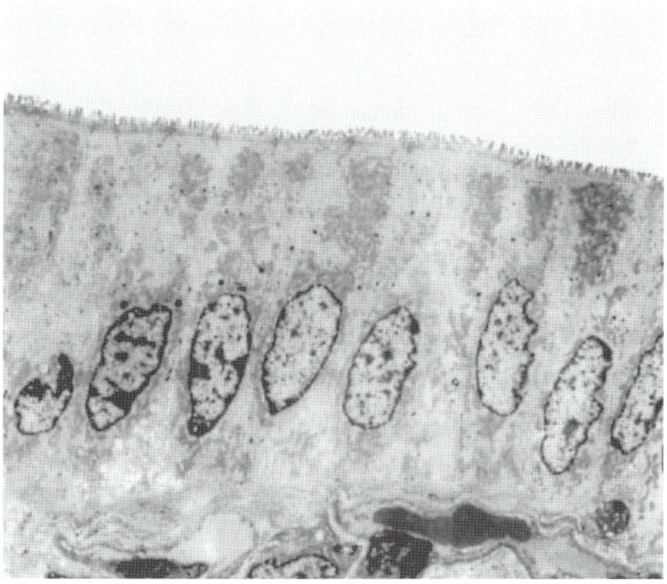

Figure 6.1 Normal rat colonic mucosa. (Original magnification ×1650.)

was normal. In the group with isolated loops, major histopathological changes were found in the ileum – pronounced atrophy of the villi and minor inflammation and fibrosis. A marked increase in the sulfated acidic mucins was noted in both enteric segments. The colonic mucosa was mainly unchanged. Ultrastructural examination showed moderately reduced height of microvilli, down to 1.1 μm in ileum and 0.5 μm in colon. In the ileum abundant ribosome-like structures were located apically in the enterocytes, just beneath the cell membrane (Figure 6.2). These structures surrounded the filamentous core rootlets, which were extremely long and prominent. In the smooth-muscle cells of the muscularis mucosae the pinocytic vesicles, i.e. inclusions of the cell membrane typical for such cells, were somewhat increased in numbers and size. In the colonic enterocytes the most obvious change was haphazard orientation of the filamentous core rootlets.

In the group of rats with ileocolocystoplasty, ileal mucosa exposed to urine differed markedly from control mucosa. Atrophy of the villi ranged from minor to moderate. The inflammatory response was accentuated and there was slight fibrosis. The amount of sulfated mucin was increased, but not the neutral or the sialomucin. No epithelial dysplasia was found. The colonic mucosa showed minimal inflammatory reaction, slight fibrosis and change in mucin content resembling that in ileum. Despite the atrophied villi, the microvillus height was essentially normal in ileum (1.4 μm), with minor edema. In the colon, too, the height of the microvilli was normal (0.6 μm), but their numbers were reduced, with some areas totally denuded and showing blebs (Figure 6.3). Such bleb formation has been described after hypoxic injury and is reversible if oxygenation is restored.[13] Ileum exposed to urine contained numerous glycocalyceal bodies (C-bodies), i.e. membrane-bound spherical vesicular

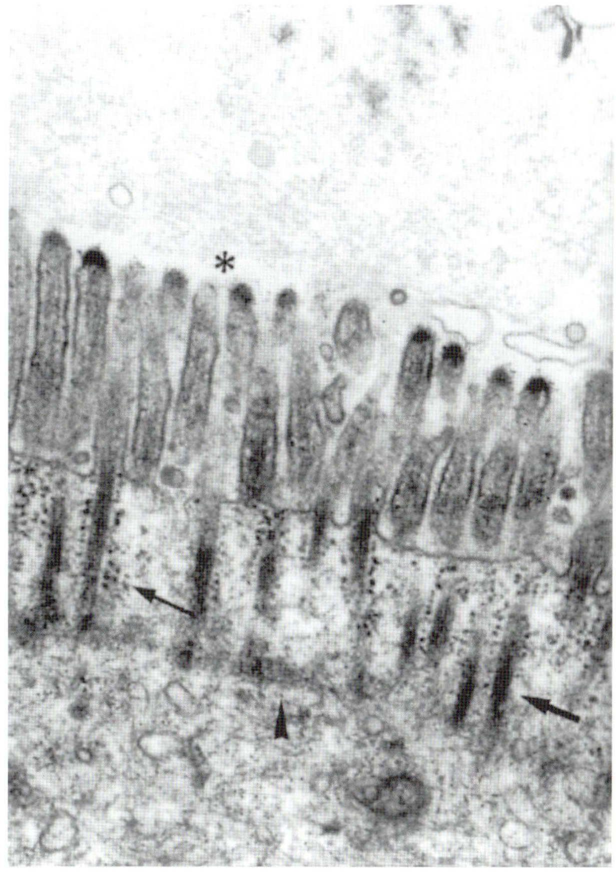

Figure 6.2 Rat ileal mucosa from exteriorized blind loop. Part of an enterocyte with glycocalyx (*), ribosome-like structures (small arrow), rootlets (large arrow) and terminal web (arrowhead). The microvilli are moderately reduced in height. (Original magnification ×28 500.)

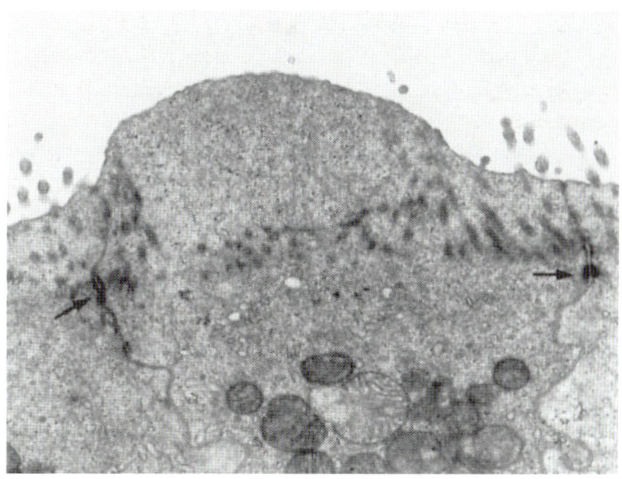

Figure 6.3 Rat colonic mucosa exposed to urine, showing a bleb with total denudation of microvilli. However, the junctional complexes (arrows) are intact. (Original magnification ×15 500.)

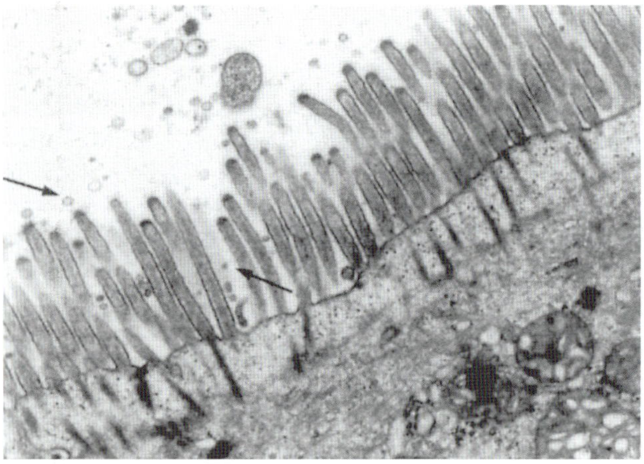

Figure 6.4 Rat ileal mucosa exposed to urine. Remarkably well-preserved microvilli with formation of glycocalyceal bodies (arrows). (Original magnification ×15 500.)

structures, in the intermicrovillus spaces (Figure 6.4). The functional implications of these bodies are not clear. They are present in normal and diseased human colon, but their presence in healthy small bowel has been disputed.[14] An interesting finding was that the intracellular organelles were more affected in the urine exposed group than in the blind loop group. Thus, the filamentous core rootlets were more prominent and randomly orientated. Enhancement of ribosomes seen apically and the mitochondrial cristae appeared dilated. Increased number of intracellular vacuoles was found.

This study thus showed that reduction of the fecal stream with its nutritional factors as well as contact with urine induces tissue damage with atrophy. Presence of urine had a more pronounced effect intracellularly than simply exclusion of an intestinal segment. It is of interest to note that the microvillus height was better preserved in ileum exposed to urine than in the ileum of the blind loop, suggesting that factors present in urine may be of importance for the metabolism of epithelial cells.

Ileal mucosa in contact with the faecal stream

Changes in the morphological structures of ileal mucosa are also seen when exposed to an abnormal fecal content as in the continent Kock ileostomy or in the ileoanal pouch. Atrophy, chronic inflammation of different degrees, fibrosis and changes in the mucin pattern have been described (Figure 6.5).[15] The reaction pattern of the ileum in contact with urine on a fecal stream seems very similar. Also in this context the risk of malignancy has been discussed. In a 30 year follow-up study of ileal pouch mucosa in patients operated for ulcerative colitis, only minor atypia and dysplasia were found and the risk of malignancy was considered low.[16] It is thus obvious that the environment to which the intestinal mucosa is exposed was of importance for the surface characteristics as well as the intracellular content of the enterocyte.

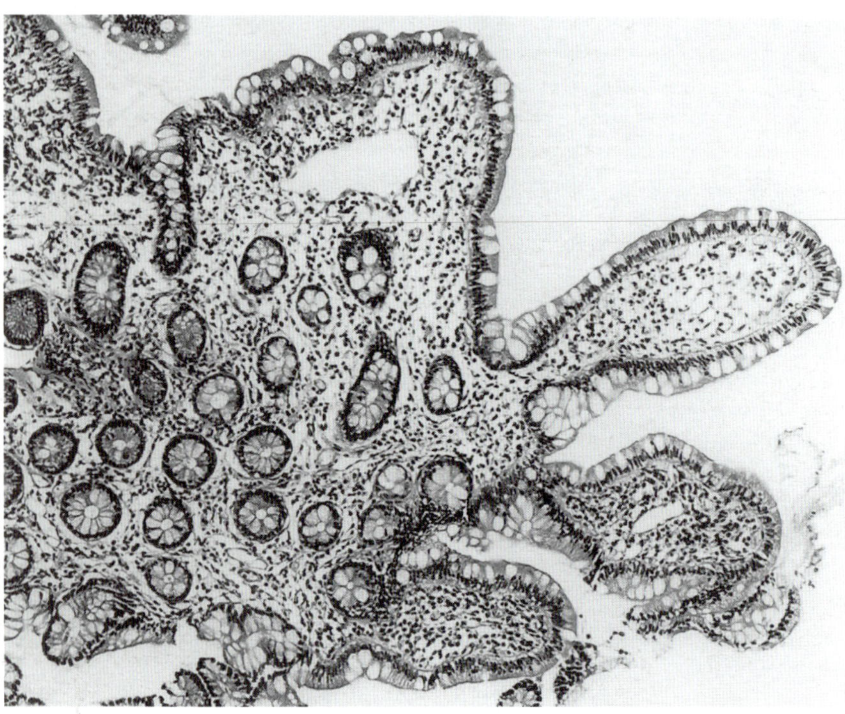

Figure 6.5 Human ileal mucosa exposed to fecal content in a continent Kock ileostomy for 18 years. Reduced and broadened villi, intact epithelium and increased amount of inflammatory cells in lamina propria. (H & E ×10.)

Gastric mucosa

Gastric segments have been used for diversion and orthotopic substitution, but mainly for gastrocystoplasty. Although the high incidence of hematuria and dysuria has hampered its use, there are some indications for this procedure. We have found no report on the response of human gastric mucosa to contact with urine. Observations on animals were somewhat contradictory. Rudick et al.[17] constructed continent urinary reservoirs from gastric fundus in dogs, and 6 months later found the macroscopic and microscopic features to be normal. This time may have been too short for changes to appear, since in the rats in the report by Castro-Diaz et al,[18] the gastric mucosa was well-preserved at 3–6 weeks after gastrocystoplasty. Further studies of gastrocystoplasty in the rat model with longer follow-up with focus on the transition zone between gastric mucosa and urothelium revealed prominent histopathological changes, with formation of papilloma, marked squamous epithelial hyperplasia and metaplastic lesions.[19,20] Frank neoplastic lesions, so also after ileocystoplasty as well as colocystoplasty, was described in one study.[21] In the latest contribution to this field, Mitchell's group also described hyperplastic changes in the junctional area, benign on histological examination, but with cell cycle and DNA ploidy abnormalities.[22] The significance of these premalignant changes is unknown, as is the true risk for humans to develop tumors at the transistion zone after such surgery. The gastric mucosa distant to this zone in the rat showed no other abnormality other than atrophy.[22]

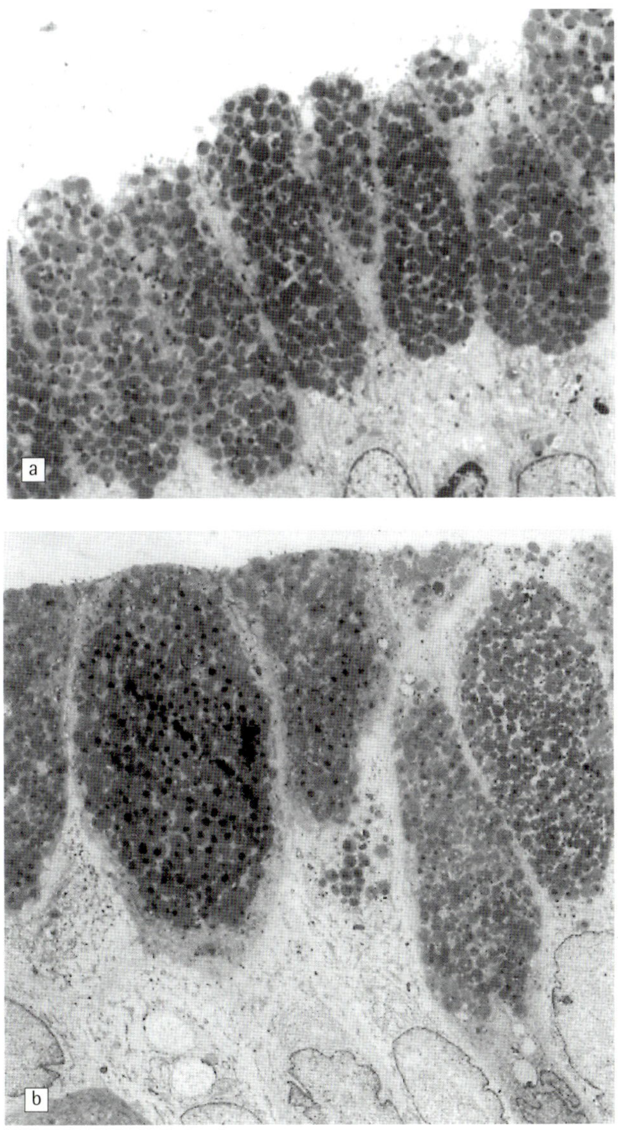

Figure 6.6 (a) Peri-operatively obtained biopsy from fundus region of the stomach with mucus-secreting epithelial cells. Original magnification ×2200. (b) Biopsy from the conduit 2 years later, showing flattened luminal surface, but preserved intracellular structures. (Original magnification ×1650.)

We studied the mucosa from the gastric fundus region in a patient before and 2 years after urinary diversion using that segment as conduit. No essential change was found at light microscopy. At electron microscopy the luminal surface of the mucus-secreting epithelial cells had a flattened appearance after contact with urine (Figure 6.6). Microvilli, intercellular spaces and cell organelles remained normal. No malignant transformation of stomach used as conduit or reservoir or for cystoplasty has been described in humans.

Jejunal mucosa

Because of the high risk of electrolyte disturbance when a jejunal segment is incorporated in the urinary tract, jejunum is rarely used in urological reconstruction. We know of no histological report describing human jejunal mucosa after exposure to urine. In studies on rats with Thiry–Vella fistulas created from jejunal or ileal segments, hypoplasia of similar degree was found in both segment types, with decrease of total mucosal thickness and villus height and reduced epithelial cell migration rate and turnover time.[9] These observations may indicate, but do not prove, similarity of response to contact with urine of jejunal and ileal mucosa.

Ileal conduit mucosa

The histological appearance of ileal urinary conduits has been described in several studies.[23–28] The main feature is mild to total atrophy of villi and microvilli. Opinions differ concerning relationship of these changes to age of the conduit, though in general their severity seems to increase with time (Figure 6.7). The total height of the lamina mucosa decreases, and substantial reduction of villus height together with crypt hyperplasia gives a considerably reduced villus:crypt index. The microvilli decrease in height and number. No correlation was detected with quantitative aspects of the microbial flora or symptomatic urinary tract infection.[26,28] Ultrastructurally, the main cellular elements of the mucosa are preserved.[28] Presence of glycocalyceal bodies, not normally found in ileum, was reported in one

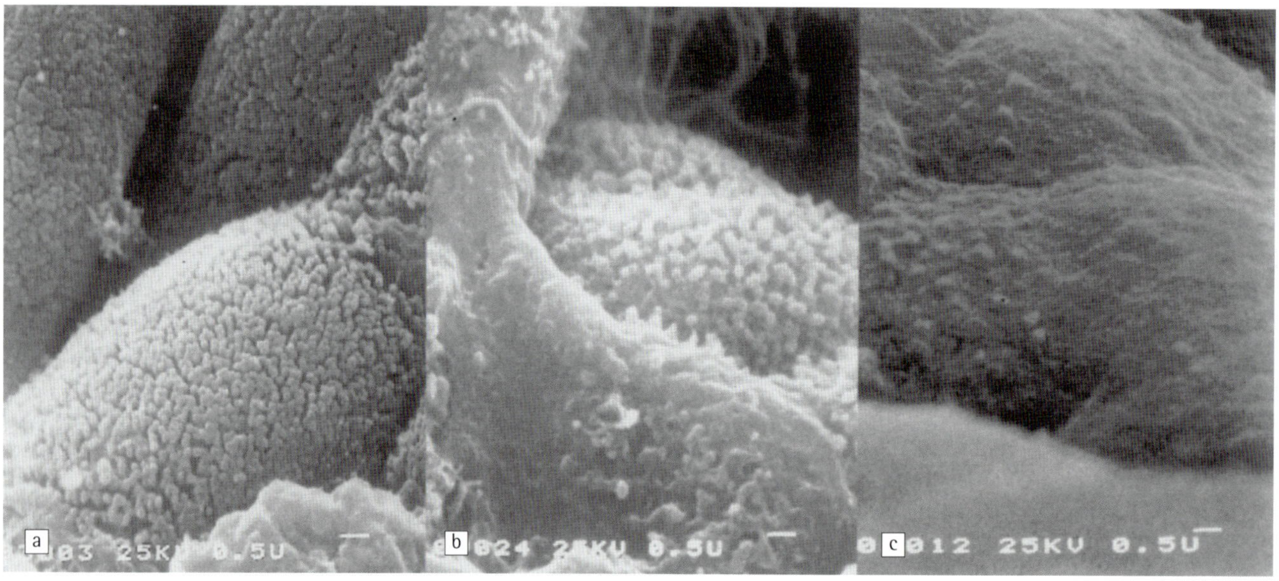

Figure 6.7 Human ileal mucosa. (a) Normal ileum with well-preserved microvilli. (b) Partial atrophy of microvilli 1 year after construction of ileal conduit. (c) After 3 years there is total atrophy of microvilli, giving a smooth cell surface. SEM bar 0.5 mm. (Courtesy of Professor P Hanke, Fulda, Germany and Urologia Internationalis.)

study,[26] but its significance is unknown. Slight to moderate chronic inflammatory reaction is often seen, with edema and inflammatory cells in the mucosa, sometimes extending into the submucosa. Goblet and enterochromaffin cells are present, and Paneth cells seem particularly resistant. Histochemical studies showed that sialomucin, the conjugated glycoprotein normally prevalent in ileum, was replaced in ileal conduits by sulfomucin,[27] which is more common in colon. Flow cytometric DNA histograms demonstrated an increased proportion of cells in the G2 phase and mitosis, indicating hyperplasia and complementing the findings of crypt hyperplasia.[27]

Ileal conduit stenosis – an enigma

Conduit stenosis seems to affect only ileum. It has not been reported in colonic conduits; thus testifying to different properties of the intestine when in contact with urine. Nor has this type of inflammation and fibrosis been described in pouches. The conduit narrowing is typically segmental, single or multiple, often appearing at the site of ureteric implantation. It usually involves short segments, but sometimes the whole conduit, and as a rule is a late sequela of urinary diversion. The clinical picture is produced by obstruction of the upper urinary tracts, causing symptomatic infection, colicky flank pain and sometimes damaging renal function. The diagnosis is usually clear when intravenous pyelography reveals dilatation of the upper urinary tract and loopogram shows segmental narrowing with proximal dilatation.[29–31] Loopоscopy completes the clinical work-up. Between 1981 and 1994 we diagnosed 12 cases of conduit stenosis appearing 7–30 years (mean 14) after construction of the ileal loop.[32] Treatment was extirpation of the conduit in five cases and partial conduit resection with ureteric reimplantation in four. Three patients with loopograms showing typical segmental stenosis were not operated on, because of high age or complicating disease. Macroscopically the walls of the excised conduits were greatly thickened (Figure 6.8) and histologically there was ulcerated mucosa, in places totally denuded, intermingled with non-ulcerated mucosa which, however, often was severely atrophic. Usually there was a strong, both acute and chronic, cell reaction, and in several cases transmural inflammation with lymphoid follicles somewhat resembling a Crohn's reaction. Severe fibrosis was found in the lamina propria (Figure 6.9). Transmission electron microscopy showed reduced microvillus height and presence of glycocalyceal bodies (Figure 6.10), as observed in non-diseased ileal conduits. The junctional complexes in non-denuded mucosal areas were tight and the subcellular structures seemed intact. The numbers of goblet cells were normal, except at sites of ulceration and severe inflammation, and Paneth and enterochromaffin cells likewise appeared normal. Immunostaining for IgA was positive in plasma cells and also in the cytoplasmic and surface compart-

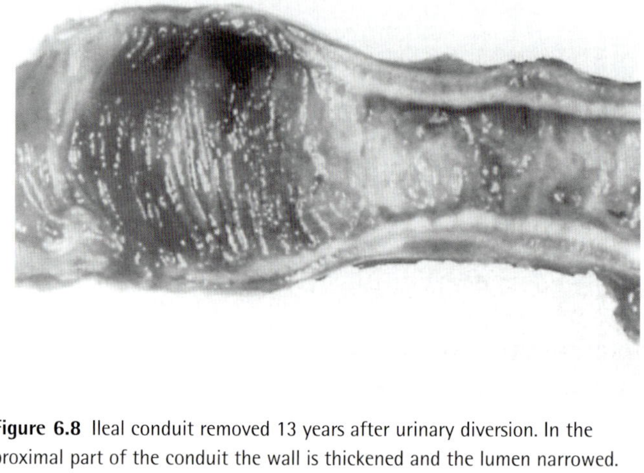

Figure 6.8 Ileal conduit removed 13 years after urinary diversion. In the proximal part of the conduit the wall is thickened and the lumen narrowed.

ments of enterocytes, indicating active production and storage of IgA, with beneficial implications for immune protection.

The main difference between normal and stenotic ileal conduits thus seemed to be the latter's severe transmural inflammation and fibrosis. Another difference, of uncertain validity, was lack of change in the mucinous pattern in our cases, i.e. sialomucin was present in the ileal conduits and not, as previously reported, replaced by sulfomucin.[27]

The cause of ileal conduit stenosis is unknown. Proposed theories include microvascular insufficiency, reaction to some noxious agent in urine, immunologic defects and mechanical causes.[29,31] Treatment is partial or, more commonly, total extirpation of the conduit, but successful balloon dilatation has been described.[33] Although local or systemic steroid treatment might be beneficial if instituted before fibrosis develops, the insidious onset of stenosis preceding obstruction largely rules out such measures. Descriptions of Crohn's disease in ileal conduits[34,35] indicate an immunologic role in such cases.

Ileal pouch mucosa

The histologic and functional features of the continent ileal pouch were extensively studied by the Gothenburg group[36–38] and essentially resembled those in ileal conduits. Thus the villi showed progressive atrophy, sometimes beginning within a few months after diversion. After 2–3 years, villus-free areas could be found mingled with islets of better preserved mucosa, especially in the caudal part of the pouch (Figure 6.11). Areas denuded of epithelium were also seen. Histomorphometrical

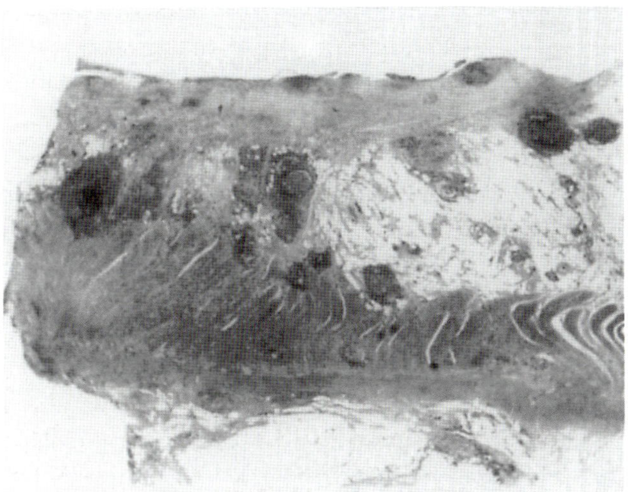

Figure 6.9 Same conduit as in Figure 6.8, showing total denudation of the mucosa, fibrosis and severe inflammatory cell reaction with lymphoid follicles throughout the wall. Severe transmural inflammation, to some extent mimicking Crohn's disease. (H & E ×8.)

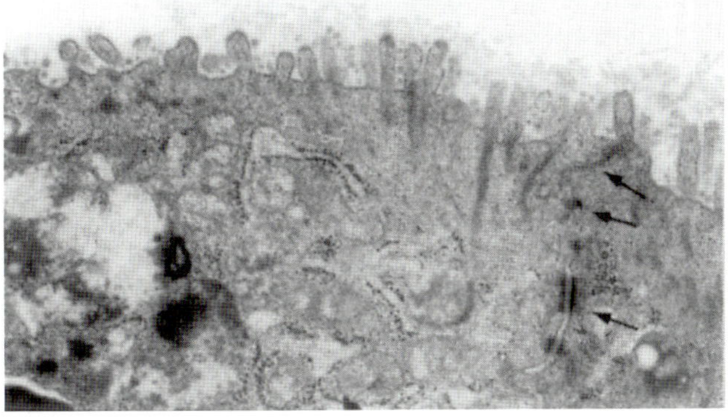

Figure 6.10 Same conduit as in Figures 6.8 and 6.9. Microvillus height only 0.5 mm, but well-preserved junctional complexes (arrows) and intracellular structures. (Original magnification ×16 100.)

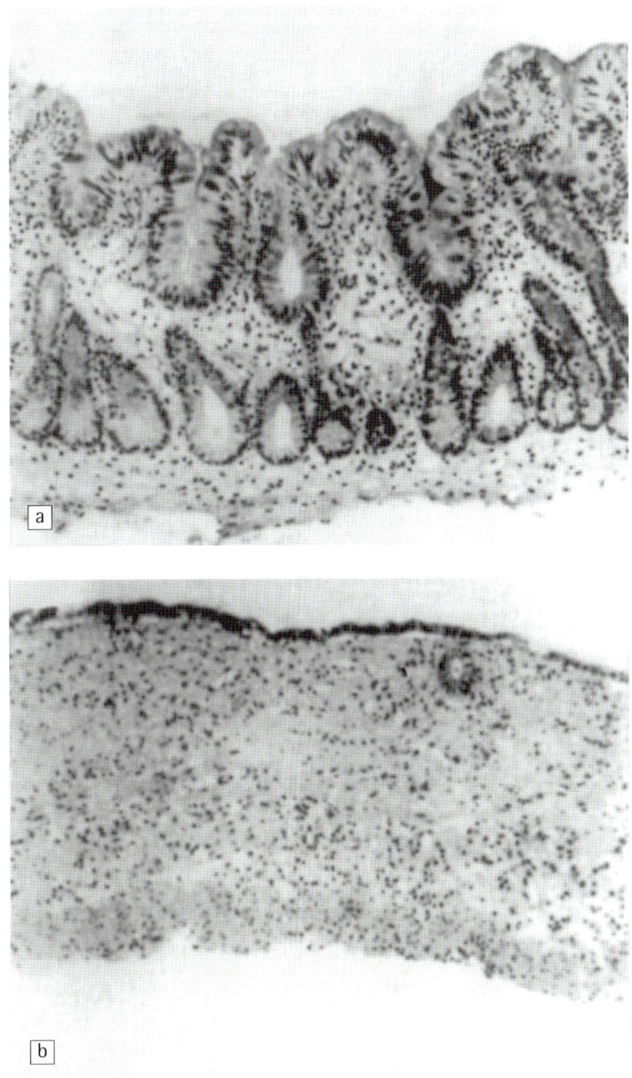

Figure 6.11 Ileal pouch 5 years after construction. In the same patient the mucosal appearance varies from areas with villi and lengthened crypts (a) to areas that are totally villus-free (b). (Reproduced from Philipson BM et al. Gut 1983; 24: 392–8[36] with permission from the BMJ Publishing Group.)

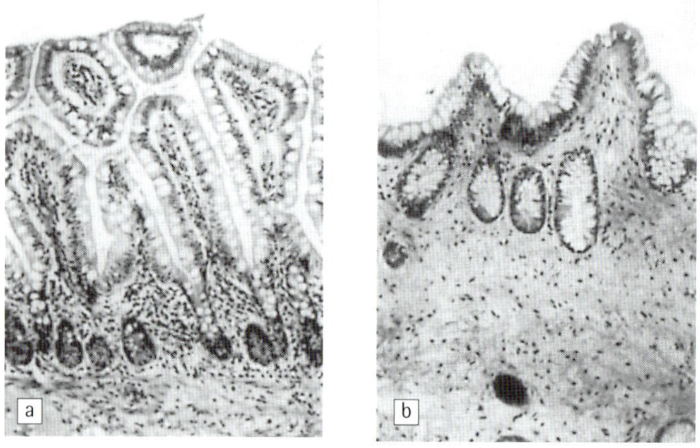

Figure 6.12 (a) Perioperatively obtained biopsy from ileum, showing normal villi and only small amounts of inflammatory cells in the stroma. (b) Biopsy of ileal nipple valve 76 months postoperatively, reveals atrophic flattened villi and severe mucosal fibrosis. (H & E x160.) (Reproduced from Månsson and Willèn. J Urol 1988; 139: 1199–201 with permission from Lippincott Williams and Wilkins.)

studies showed reduction of villus height and deepening of crypts. Numerical increase of goblet cells was found only a month postoperatively, possibly in response to the noxious stimuli of urine and its microbial content. No fibrosis was found, and only a mild inflammatory cell reaction. Other studies, however, showed various grades of thickening of the muscularis mucosae and chronic inflammation and fibrosis of the lamina propria.[39] Severe fibrosis of the efferent nipple valve[39,40] was not surprising, as the valve's construction implies mesenteric exclusion with consequent reduction of bowel-wall vascularity (Figure 6.12). As in ileal conduits, the composition of mucin changes from sialomucin to sulfomucin.[41] Transmission electron microscopy of ileal pouch wall[38] showed that in time the enterocytes assumed a cuboidal or even flattened shape, changes not recorded in studies of ileal conduits and possibly attributable to stretching of the ileal pouch wall and/or intraluminal pressure. The microvilli were markedly decreased in numbers and height. There was loss of filaments in the terminal web and distinct numerical reduction of cell organelles such as lysosomes and lysosome-related structures. One group found only few remaining microvilli after 12 months and changes of the intracellular cytoplasmic structures so pronounced that the process could be defined as a real de-differentiation of the enterocytes. Contrary, the junctional complexes were completely intact[42] (Figure 6.13).

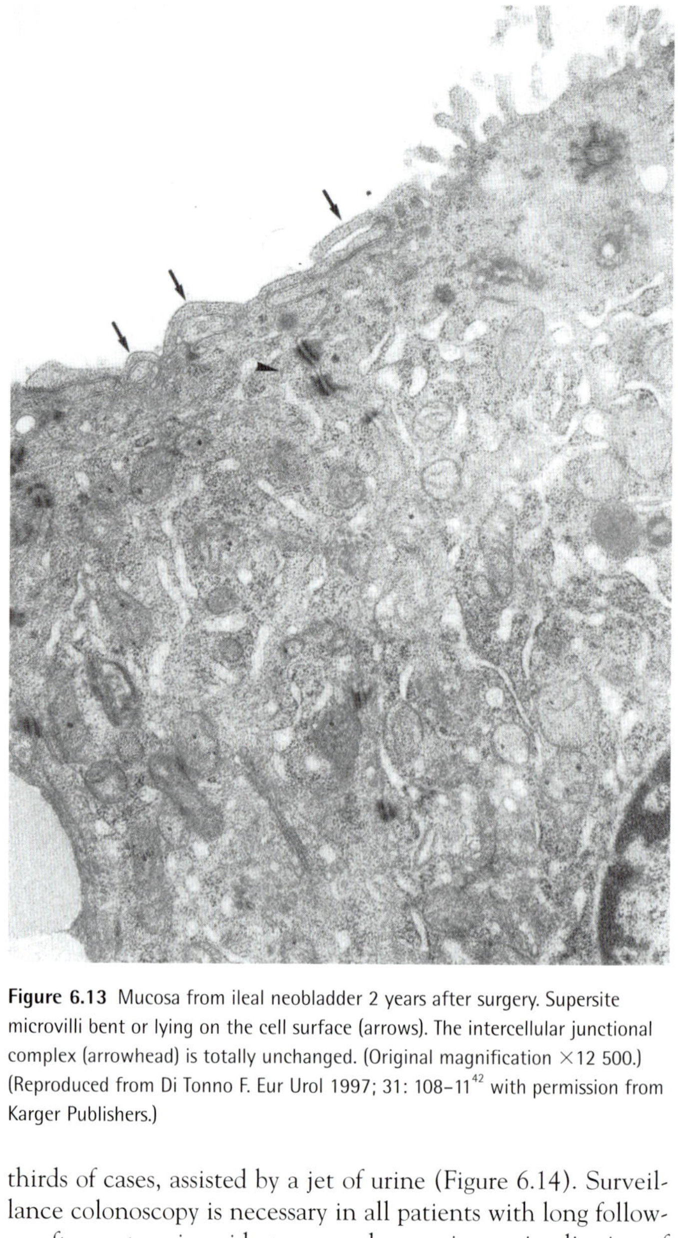

Figure 6.13 Mucosa from ileal neobladder 2 years after surgery. Supersite microvilli bent or lying on the cell surface (arrows). The intercellular junctional complex (arrowhead) is totally unchanged. (Original magnification ×12 500.) (Reproduced from Di Tonno F. Eur Urol 1997; 31: 108–11[42] with permission from Karger Publishers.)

Colonic mucosa after ureterosigmoidostomy

As a rule the colonic mucosa at surveillance colonoscopy in these cases is macroscopically normal[43] though there may be slight redness. We could identify the ureteric orifices in two-thirds of cases, assisted by a jet of urine (Figure 6.14). Surveillance colonoscopy is necessary in all patients with long follow-up after ureterosigmoidostomy, and must aim at visualization of the orifices.

Light microscopy often shows mild chronic inflammation in sites near the ureteric orifices, decreasing further away from them. Focal fibrosis of the lamina propria with a gap in the regular order of the crypts is common close to the ureteric implantation. No consistent changes were found in numbers of goblet cells or thickening of the basal lamina.[43,44] Completely normal histologic patterns have also been reported.[45]

The risk of secondary malignancy after urinary tract reconstruction has attracted considerable interest (see Chapter 9). Of 19 patients endoscopically studied at our hospital,[43] six were found to have small polyps, which in three cases proved to be dysplastic tubular adenomas. No adenocarcinoma has been reported as a colonoscopic finding in asymptomatic patients with ureterosigmoidostomy, although the literature reports around 100 cases of colonic carcinoma associated with such diversion[46]

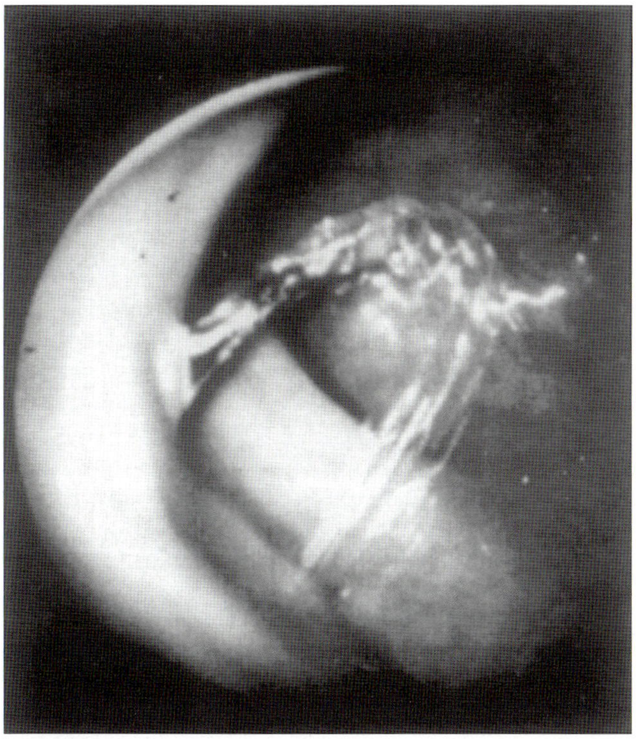

Figure 6.14 Surveillance colonoscopy shows normal colonic mucosa and jet of urine from ureteric orifice. (Reproduced from Berg et al. Endoscopy 1987; 19: 60–3.[43])

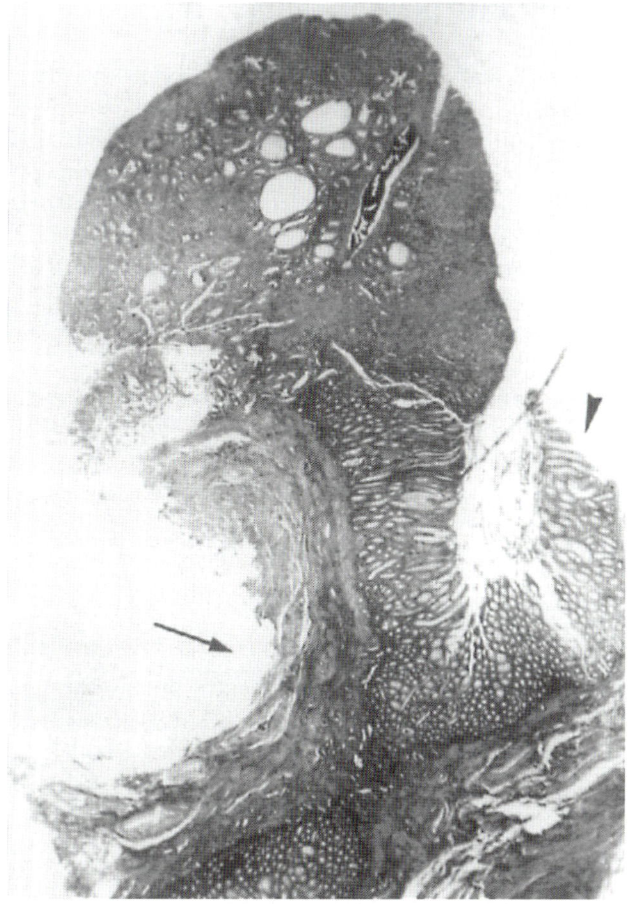

Figure 6.15 Colonic carcinoma at site of ureteric implantation in a 23-year-old woman 23 years after ureterosigmoidostomy because of bladder exstrophy. The ureteric wall appears devoid of mucosa (arrow). Close to the tumor there is normal colonic mucosa (arrowhead). (H & E ×10.)

and one case was reported from our hospital (Figure 6.15).[47] Colonic polyps, including tubular adenomas, are common in elderly persons, and colonic carcinoma as a late complication of ureterosigmoidostomy is believed to develop from such adenomas.[48] The polyps, notably, are often close to the ureterosigmoid anastomosis.[48,49] The incidence of colonic adenoma in younger patients with ureterosigmoidostomy was observed to be appreciably higher than that expected for the age, suggesting a causal relationship between the mode of urinary diversion and the development of adenoma and carcinoma.[48]

Sulfomucins are the dominant secretions in the lower two-thirds of the crypts in normal colonic mucosa, with some sialomucin in the upper third.[50] From the observed shift of sulfomucin towards sialomucin in apparently normal mucosa surrounding colonic carcinoma, Filipe and Branfoot[51] coined the term 'transitional mucosa' to express such change and interpreted it as a precursor of malignancy. The mucin pattern was stated to resemble that in human fetal gut.[51] Such abnormal patterns of mucin secretion, indicating metabolic derangement of the goblet cells, are found after ureterosigmoidostomy and various types of urinary diversion utilizing colon.[40,45,52,53] Several authors have doubted that this mucin change is a precursor of malignancy, as the same phenomenon has been observed in many benign conditions, such as solitary ulcer syndrome and other lesions with displacement of the colonic mucosa into the lumen. One explanation may be altered submucosal blood supply producing fibrosis and subsequent change of mucin pattern due to prolapsing forces at the margins of mucosal tumors. More advanced histochemical changes in larger tumors are consistent with the prolapse theory.[54]

Ultrastructural studies showed that in 'transitional mucosa' immature and intermediate cells persisted at higher levels of the crypts than in normal mucosa, suggesting that cells are prematurely shed into the crypts.[55] This may be interpreted as premalignancy, but also as a regenerative phenomenon, thereby explaining the occasional observation of 'transitional mucosa' remote from carcinoma. The presence of such mucosa in most patients with ureterosigmoidostomy or other types of colonic urinary diversion suggests that the changes should not be regarded as predictors of tumor development, but probably as effects of urine.[52,53]

In addition to changes in the composition of mucus, abnormal lectin-binding patterns are another sign of abnormal mucin secretion after ureterosigmoidostomy.[45,56] Probably, however, such changes are due to non-specific factors rather than to synthesis of a cancer-related mucosubstance indicating preneoplasia.

Colonic conduit mucosa

In patients who had undergone colonic conduit diversion 4 years previously, the conduit mucosa showed numerous inflammatory cells in the lamina propria.[43] The superficial epithelium in all these patients was higher and its goblet cells were more numerous and larger than in mucosa from patients with ureterosigmoidostomy. The number of enterochromaffin cells and small lymph follicles was normal and no atypia was seen. Similar well-preserved mucosa in colonic conduits was previously reported,[23,45,52,57] but in one series there was progressive increase of chronic inflammation during the follow-up time,[57] which was interpreted as a possible precursor of malignancy. There is, however, no proof of such a link. Severe, infiltrative chronic inflammation of a sigmoid conduit with destroyed mucosa was described in a patient with severe bleeding from the conduit.[58]

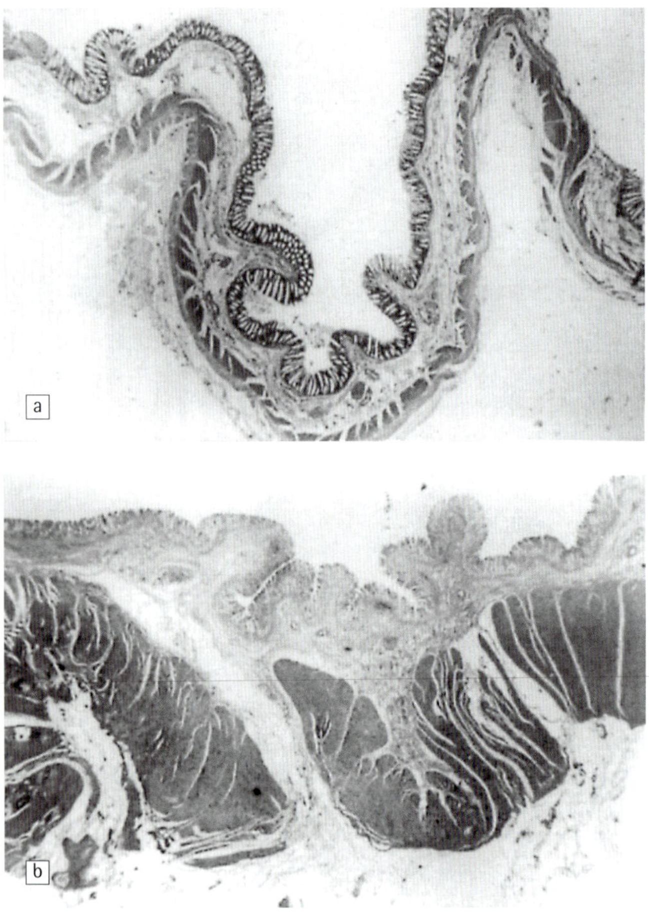

Figure 6.16 Autopsy findings in a 65-year-old woman with cecal urinary reservoir for 43 years. (a) Normal ascending colon. (b) Biopsy of cecal wall revealing well-preserved mucosa but severe hypertrophy of the muscularis propria. (H & E ×9.5.) (Courtesy of Professor F Linell, Malmö, Sweden.)

Colonic pouch mucosa

Since 1977 we have used the cecum or a right colonic segment for continent urinary reconstruction, and we have described the morphological changes after long-term exposure to urine,[40,59] i.e. mild mucosal atrophy and slight increase of inflammatory cells and collagen fibers. In a cecal reservoir with appendiceal outlet for continent cutaneous diversion, the mucosa was seen to be well preserved on light microscopy 43 years after surgery, while the muscularis propria was severely hypertrophied (Figure 6.16), suggesting high intraluminal pressure/hyperactivity.[60] Our studies showed mucin production from goblet cells to be preserved or increased, with a shift from predominant sulfomucin to sialomucin, similar to findings after ureterosigmoidostomy. This change was found soon after diversion and interpreted as a secondary, non-specific phenomenon unrelated to risk of malignant transformation. At scanning electron microscopy the mucosal surface appeared normal (Figure 6.17). Transmission electron microscopy, however, revealed that, as in ileal mucosa, ultrastructural changes were present in colonic pouch mucosa and consisted of reduced height and number of microvilli, with shortening of the filamentous core rootlets extending into the terminal web (Figure 6.18). Glycocalyceal bodies were present in most cases. Edema was a common feature and seemed to correlate with the inflammatory cell reaction. The junctional complexes were normal. Ultrastructurally, preformed anatomical structures such as neurogenic processes, the enterochromaffin cells and Paneth cells were completely preserved, as in the ileal pouches.

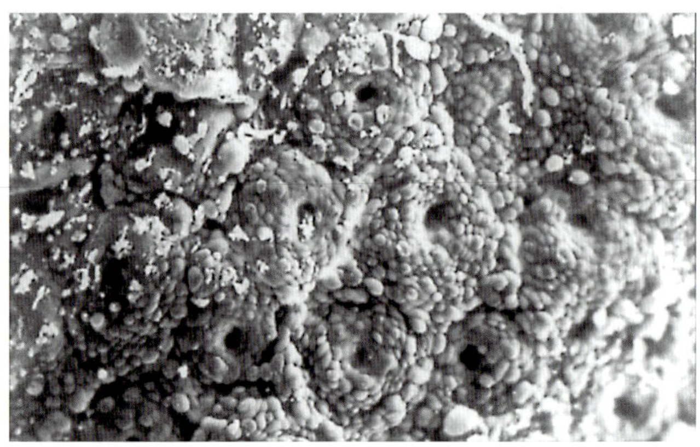

Figure 6.17 Mucosa from cecal reservoir for urine 68 months after construction. Regular mucosal surface with well-defined enterocyte borders and clearly visible crypt openings. Bar 40 mm. (Reproduced with permission from Månsson. Scand J Urol Nephrol 1984 suppl; 85: 1–37.)

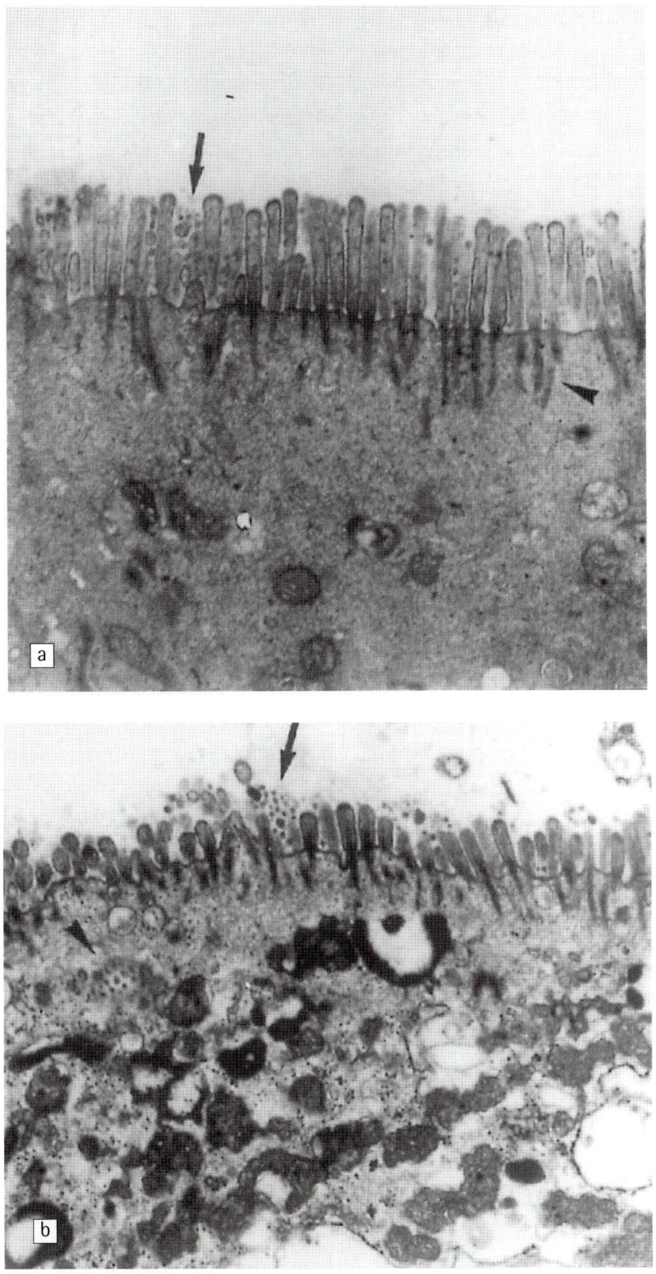

Figure 6.18 (a) Normal colon. Microvilli of normal height, with prominent filamentous core rootlets (arrowhead) and glycocalyceal bodies (arrow). (b) Biopsy specimen from cecal urinary reservoir 9 years postoperatively. Microvilli markedly reduced in numbers and height. Preserved glycocalyceal bodies (arrow) and R-body (arrowhead) containing vesicles and rod-like profiles. (Original magnification ×26 000.)

Functional changes in intestinal mucosa after exposure to urine

Parallel with structural changes, the mucosa undergoes functional modifications. The altered mucin composition of both ileum and colon soon after contact with urine begins probably as a non-specific phenomenon, perhaps mirroring the change in luminal content. Histochemical studies revealed decreased activity of brush-border enzymes such as succinic dehydrogenase (SDH), glucose-6-phosphate dehydrogenase (G-6-PD), alkaline phosphatase (ATPase) and leucine aminopeptidase (LAP) in ileal conduits and continent pouches.[36,61] These expressions of decreased functional capacity of the villous cell were confirmed by in vitro and in vivo measurements of absorption of the amino acid L-phenylalanine after continent ileal pouch urinary diversions.[36,62] The in vitro uptake correlated with morphologic findings, being lower in biopsies from avillous areas than in those from mucosa with well-preserved villous structures. The clinical study showed progressive, time-related decrease in absorption after diversion.

The morphologic features of mucosa after ileal pouch construction, coupled with these functional changes, have been regarded as advantageous adaptation to a new environment, helping to prevent absorption of harmful substances from the urine and metabolic disturbances. Experimental studies, however, clearly showed that in ileal segments chronically exposed to urine, despite morphological changes, transport of electrolytes remains similar to that in control segments, and thus the low incidence of metabolic acidosis after ileal reservoir diversion is not due to reduced absorptive capacity of the ileal mucosa.[63] Clinically, electrolyte disturbances can occur years after incorporating intestine into the urinary tract despite atrophy of the villi, testifying to the importance of mechanisms not related to morphologic changes.

Permeability

The barrier function of the normal intestinal mucosa is of utmost importance to prevent potentially noxious substances, e.g antigenic molecules, endotoxins and bacteria, from permeating.[64] A case report of a shock syndrome caused by toxin from *Staphylococcus aureus* in urine of a continent pouch highlights the hazards of a damaged barrier function.[65] The barrier function of the intestinal mucosa has been assessed mainly in vivo by studying the passage of orally given marker molecules into the blood circulation or into urine. We used in vivo technique to study permeability of ileal and colonic mucosa exposed to urine in continent reservoirs and found no or negligible permeation of ^{51}Cr-EDTA and PEG 400.[66] To circumvent the problems associated with in vivo studies we have also studied permeability of marker molecules with different molecular weights in vitro.[67] The passage of the markers through mucosa from man and rat was studied using modified Ussing diffusion chambers. In man, there were no permeability differences between colonic mucosa exposed to urine and control mucosa and in rats there was in fact less passage of the markers in ileal and colonic mucosa from cystoplasties than in control mucosa. Nor was there any differences between ileal and colonic segments in this model. These studies confirm intact barrier integrity after exposure to urine.

Conclusions

The structural changes in intestinal mucosa exposed to urine have received fairly extensive study. The dominant feature is atrophy of villi and microvilli, which, however, is less pronounced than the atrophy found after simple exclusion of an intestinal segment. On the other hand, subcellular structures are more affected. Hence the urine, with its content of solutes and microorganisms, exerts direct effects on the mucosa, but without disrupting the integrity of the cellular lining. Ileal conduit stenosis remains an enigma, and it remains to be seen if similar changes can be expected in ileal pouches.

There are comparatively few studies on possible functional changes in enterocytes in contact with urine. As anticipated, the activity of some enzymes involved in absorption was found to be diminished. Further investigation is needed, not only of functional changes in the absorptive cells, but also of the endocrine and goblet cells. The assumed protective effect of mucus, and certainly the function of the lymphoid tissue involved in immune defense in isolated intestinal segments, also require clarification. Despite the morphologic changes found, intestinal mucosa in chronic contact with urine maintains its barrier function.

Acknowledgements

Some of the studies referred to in this chapter were aided by grants from the Swedish Cancer Society, the Medical Faculty of Lund University, the Gunnar, Arvid and Elisabeth Nilsson Fund, Helsingborg, and the Dir. Albert Påhlsson Foundation, Malmö, Sweden. The excellent photographic work of Jenny Melchert and Mikael Petersson is gratefully acknowledged.

References

1. Thompson JS, Saxena SK, Sharp JG. Regulation of intestinal regeneration: new insights. Microsc Res Tech 2000; 51: 129–37.
2. Madara II, Trier IS. Functional morphology of the mucosa of the small intestine. In: Johnson LR (ed). Physiology of the Gastrointestinal Tract, 2nd edn. New York: Raven Press, 1986: 1209–49.
3. Bristol JB, Williamson RCN. Nutrition, operations and intestinal adaptation. J Parenter Enter Nutr 1988; 12: 299–309.
4. Williamson RCN, Ross JS, Malt RA. Disuse atrophy of the intestinal tract. Clin Nutr 1984; 3: 169–70.
5. Terpstra OT, Peterson, Dahl E, Williamson RCN. Colostomy closure promotes cell proliferation and dimethylhydrazine induced carcinogenesis in rat distal colon. Gastroenterology 1981; 81: 475–80
6. Albert V, Young GP, Morton CL, Robinson P, Bhatal PS. Systemic factors are trophic in bypassed rat small intestine in the absence of luminal contents. Gut 1990; 31: 311–16.
7. Delvaux G, Caes F, Willems G. Refeeding of fasting rats stimulates epithelial cell proliferation in the excluded colon. Gastroenterology 1984; 86: 802–7.
8. Bishop WP, Kim S, Yamazato M, Yoshino H, Kimura K. Mucosal morphology in isolated bowel segments: importance of exposure to luminal contents. J Pediatr Surg 1992; 27: 1061–5.
9. Gleeson MH, Cullen J, Dowling RH. Intestinal structure and function after small bowel by-pass in the rat. Clin Sci 1972; 43: 731–42.
10. Garrido AB, Freeman HJ, Kim YS. Amino acid and peptide absorption in bypassed jejunum following jejunoileal bypass in rats. Dig Dis Sci 1981; 26: 107–12.
11. Yoshino H, Kimura K, Yamazato M, Scott DH, Soper RT. The isolated bowel segment (Iowa model II): absorption studies for glucose and leucine. J Pediatr Surg 1991; 26: 1372–5.
12. Davidsson T, Carlén B, Bak-Jensen E, Månsson W. Morphological changes in intestinal mucosa with urinary contact – effects of urine or disuse? J Urol 1996; 156: 226–32.
13. Kumar V, Cotran RS, Robbins SL. Cell injury and adaptation. In: Kumar V, Cotran RS, Robbins SL. (eds). Basic Pathology, 5th edn. Philadelphia: WB Saunders, 1992: 3–24.
14. Stone J, Mukherjee TM, Hesher R. C-bodies and R-bodies in the epithelial cells of normal and diseased human rectum. Arch Path Lab Med 1977; 101: 437–41.
15. Veress B, Reinholt FP, Lindqvist K, Liljeqvist L. Different types of mucosal adaptation in the ileal reservoir after restorative proctocolectomy. A two-year follow-up study. APMIS 1990; 98: 786–96.
16. Hulthén L, Willén R, Nilsson O, Safarani N, Haboubi N. Mucosal assessment for dysplasia and cancer in the ileal pouch mucosa in patients operated on for ulcerative colitis – a 30-year follow-up study. Dis Colon Rectum 2002; 45: 448–52.
17. Rudick J, Schonholz S, Weber HN. The gastric bladder: a continent reservoir for urinary diversion. Surgery 1977; 82: 1–8.
18. Castro-Diaz D, Froemming C, Manivel JC et al. The influence of urinary diversion on experimental gastrocystoplasty. J Urol 1992; 148: 571–4.
19. Klee LW, Hoover DM, Mitchell ME, Rink RC. Long term effects of gastrocystoplasty in rats. J Urol 1990; 144: 1283–7.
20. Buson H, Diza DC, Manivel JC et al. The development of tumors in experimental gastroenterocystoplasty. J Urol 1993; 150: 730–3.
21. Little JS Jr, Klee LW, Hoover DM, Rink RC. Long-term histopathological changes observed in rats subjected to augmentation cystoplasty. J Urol 1994; 152: 720–4.
22. Close CE, Tekgul S, Ganesan GS, True LD, Mitchell ME. Flow cytometry analysis of proliferative lesions at the gastrocystoplasty anastomosis. J Urol 2003; 169: 365–8.
23. Garner JW, Goldstein AMB, Cosgrowe MD. Histological appearance of the intestinal urinary conduit. J Urol 1975; 114: 854–7.
24. Gracey M, Cay R, Bishop RF, Smith ED, Anderson CM. Mucosal morphology and bacterial flora of ileal conduits. Invest Urol 1971; 8: 596–603.
25. Deane AM, Woodhouse CRJ, Parkinson MC. Histological changes in ileal conduits. J Urol 1984; 132: 1108–11.
26. Lindell O, Mäkinen J, Nickels J, Lehtonen T. Mucosal morphology of ileal conduits with particular reference to urinary infections. Eur Urol 1986; 12: 201–6.

27. Thomas DJ, Goble NM, Gillatt DA, Hammonds JC, Smith PJB. Histological and environmental changes in longstanding ileal conduits. J R Soc Med 1990; 83: 557–8.
28. Hanke P, Hofmann M, Schneider M, Bickeböller R, Jonas D. Histological and scanning electron microscopic alterations in ileal conduit depending on the time factor. Urol Int 1990; 45: 84–7.
29. Hardy BE, Lebowitz, RL, Baez A, Colodny AH. Strictures of the ileal loop. J Urol 1977; 117: 358–61.
30. Mitchell ME, Yoder IC, Pfister RC, Daly J, Althausen A. Ileal loop stenosis, a late complication of urinary diversion. J Urol 1977; 118: 957–61.
31. Wilhelm E, Aplas G, Höhn W, Egilmez A. Die Konduitstriktur, eine Ursache der Verschlechterung des Ilealkonduits. Fortschr Röntgenstr 1980; 133: 299–305.
32. Magnusson B, Carlen B, Bak-Jensen E, Willen R, Månsson W. Ileal conduit stenosis – an enigma. Scand J Urol Nephrol 1996; 30: 193–7.
33. Hildell J. Balloon dilatation of stricture of the ileal loop after ileal conduit diversion. Am J Roentgenol 1987; 149: 993–4.
34. McLaughlin T. Crohn's disease developing in an ileal conduit. J Urol 1987; 125: 420–1.
35. Walser EM, Kopecky KK, Rowland R. Diffuse ileal conduit stenosis from Crohn's disease. Urol Radiol 1990; 12: 160–2.
36. Philipson BM, Kock NG, Jagenburg R et al. Functional and structural studies of ileal reservoirs used for continent urostomy and ileostomy. Gut 1983; 24: 392–8.
37. Höckenström T, Kock NG, Norlén LJ, Åhrén C, Philipson BM. Morphological changes in ileal reservoir mucosa after long-term exposure to urine. A study in patients with continent urostomy (Kock pouch). Scand J Gastroenterol 1986; 21: 1224–34.
38. Philipson BM, Kock NG, Höckenström T, Norlén LJ, Åhrén C, Hanson H-A. Ultrastructural and histochemical changes in ileal reservoir mucosa after long-term exposure to urine. A study in patients with continent urostomy (Kock pouch). Scand J Gastroenterol 1986; 21: 1235–44.
39. Chen KK, Ho DM, Chen MT, Chang LS. Histopathological changes in Kock pouch. Br J Urol 1993; 72: 433–40.
40. Månsson W, Willén R. Mucosal morphology and histochemistry of the continent cecal reservoir for urine. J Urol 1988; 139: 1199–201.
41. Di Tonno F, Bertoldin R, Vianfello F et al. Modificazioni fenotipiche delle cellule mucino-secernenti nella mucosa delle neovesciche ileali: lesione metaplastica o precancerosa? Chir Ital 1998; 50: 33–6.
42. Di Tonno F, Fabris C, Mazzon E, Lavelli, Milanesi C. Ultrastuctural mucosal appearance in the ileal neobladder. Eur Urol 1997; 31: 108–11.
43. Berg NO, Fredlund P, Månsson W, Olsson S-Å. Surveillance colonoscopy and biopsy in patients with ureterosigmoidostomy. Endoscopy 1987; 19: 60–3.
44. Kälble T, Tricker AR, Friedl P et al. Ureterosigmoidostomy: long-term results, risk of carcinoma and etiological factors for carcinogenesis. J Urol 1990; 144: 1110–14.
45. Iannono G, Marcheggiano A, Pallone F et al. Abnormal patterns of colo-rectal mucin secretion after urinary diversion of different types. Histochemical and lectin binding studies. Hum Pathol 1986; 17: 834–40.
46. Spence HM. Ureterosigmoidostomy: the pros and the cons. Dial Pediatr Urol 1982; 5: 3–9.
47. Brekkan E, Colleen S, Myrvold H et al. Colonic neoplasia: a late complication of ureterosigmoidostomy. Scand J Urol Nephrol 1972; 6: 197–202.
48. Filmer RB, Spencer JR. Malignancies in bladder augmentation and intestinal conduits. J Urol 1990; 143: 671–8.
49. Sooriyaarachchi GS, Johnson RO, Cartone PP. Neoplasms of the large bowel following ureterosigmoidostomy. Arch Surg 1977; 112: 1174–7.
50. Gad A. Pathophysiology of gastrointestinal mucins. Adv Physiol Sci 1981; 29: 161–84.
51. Filipe MI, Branfoot AC. Abnormal patterns of mucus secretion in apparently normal mucosa of large intestine with carcinoma. Cancer 1974; 34: 382–90.
52. Strachan JR, Rees HC, Williams G. Histochemical changes after ureterosigmoidostomy and colonic diversion. Br J Urol 1985; 57: 700–2.
53. Gilchrist KW, Uehling DT, Starling JR. Cancer surveillance after ureterosigmoidostomy: colonic microscopic changes. J Surg Res 1984; 36: 251–5.
54. Isaacson P, Attwood PRA. Failure to demonstrate specificity of the morphological and histochemical changes in mucosa adjacent to colonic carcinoma (transitional mucosa). J Clin Pathol 1979; 32: 214–18.
55. Dawson PA, Filipe MI. An ultrastructural and histochemical study of the mucous membrane adjacent to and remote from carcinoma of the colon. Cancer 1976; 37: 2388–98.
56. Shimamoto C, Hirata I, Takao Y et al. Alterations of colonic mucin after ureterosigmoidostomy. Dis Colon Rectum 2000; 43: 526–31
57. Moorcraft J, Du Boulay CEH, Isaacson P, Atwell JD. Changes in the mucosa of colon conduits with particular reference to the risk of malignant change. Br J Urol 1983; 55: 185–8.
58. Månsson W, Alm P, Ekelund L, Sundin T. Severe bleeding from urinary conduits. A case report. Scand J Urol Nephrol 1982; 16: 295–8.
59. Carlén B, Willén R, Månsson W. Mucosal ultrastructure of continent cecal reservoir for urine and its ileal nipple valve 2–9 years after construction. J Urol 1990; 143: 372–6.
60. Bjersing L. Extrophia vesicae. Long survival after operation (caecal bladder ad modum Makkas). Acta Clin Scand 1963; 125: 185–9.
61. Guerrero-Alcázar M, Gonzales-Angulo A, Oritz-Quesado F. Histochemical and ultrastructural changes observed in the mucosa of the ileal conduit. J Urol 1970; 104: 406–12.
62. Åkerlund S, Jagenburg R, Kock NG, Philipson BM. Absorption of L-phenylalanine in human ileal reservoirs exposed to urine. Urol Res 1988; 16: 321–3.
63. Hall MC, Koch MO, Halter SA, Dahlstedt SM. Morphologic and functional alterations of intestinal segments following urinary diversion. J Urol 1993; 149: 664–6.

64. Aranow JS, Fink MP. Determinants of intestinal barrier failure in critical illness. Br J Anaesth 1996; 77: 71–81.
65. McCahill PD, Whittle DI, Jacobs SC. Toxic shock syndome: a complication of continent urinary diversion. J Urol 1992; 147: 681–2
66. Davidsson T, Åkerlund S, White T, Olaisson G, Månsson W. Mucosal permeability of ileal and colonic reservoirs for urine. J Urol 1996; 78: 64–8
67. Nejdfors P, Könyves J, Davidsson T et al. Permeability of intestinal mucosa from urinary reservoirs in man and rat. BJU Int 2000; 86: 1058–63

7 Renal function considerations in bladder substitution

Jens Christian Djurhuus, Troels Munch Jørgensen and Jørgen Frøkiær

Introduction

For decades it has been known that urinary diversion is associated with impairment of kidney function which may be related to prediversion pathology, urine transport problems, infection and stone formation. Initially, with the introduction of bladder augmentation or bladder replacement, the risk of changes in kidney function was further increased due to bladder or reservoir activity, compliance and reabsorption from the larger surface incorporated into the conducting system. In recent years, however, neobladders have been optimized with significant improvement of reservoir function.

Pathogenesis of reservoir nephropathy

The relationship between urine reflux and chronic atrophic pyelonephritis was demonstrated by Hodson and Edwards in 1960,[1] and later it was substantiated that reflux nephropathy could develop in both infected and non-infected urinary systems.[2] An experimental reflux model in pigs has shown that reflux to the upper urinary tract is no threat against kidney function provided that bladder and outlet function is normal[3] but in case of bladder dysfunction and/or outlet obstruction, there is a high risk of reflux nephropathy. Pyelorenal backflow with infected urine was the most frequent case of nephropathy, with aggravation of the condition in case of bladder–urethra dysfunction, leading to increased pressure in the renal pelvis. Renal deterioration in the non-infected tract depended on the existence of increased bladder pressure transmitted with low resistance to the upper urinary system. At first it was backflow of urine aggravated by infection, especially with specific pathogens of the *Escherichia coli* type, which was thought to be necessary for the nephropathy.[4] In accordance, clinical studies showed a relation, although weak, between bladder dysfunction, functional outlet obstruction and nephropathy.[5]

Consequently, bladder augmentation or substitution function together with reflux may be deleterious for kidney function. Furthermore, alteration of bladder dynamics and reimplantation of the ureters must be regarded as a potential cause of changes in urine transport and, at least theoretically, as a hazard to kidney function following bladder substitution or reconstruction.

Urine transport and bladder substitution

The integrated contractions in the renal pelvis seem to originate in the uppermost part of the renal pelvis and traverse the renal pelvis in a very regular manner towards the ureteropelvic junction. Each upper tract has its own inherent peristaltic frequency that is controlled by the renal pelvis, and the frequency generally only varies with abrupt changes in pressure and flow. The maximum rate of peristalsis, which is equal to the frequency of calyceal activity, occurs in the transient periods of extreme changes in flow, e.g. during intravenous administration of diuretics.[6] Outside such periods of transient changes the urinary tract continues to work at its inherent frequency which may be different on the two sides. For more than a century[7] it has been known that the ureter is excitable in both directions, antegrade and retrograde. Research in recent decades has substantiated that the ureter is a paced organ, i.e. its peristaltic activity is induced either by distension or by electrical activity. Sustained peristaltic activity through the ureter requires both.

If the ureter has a so-called dry run the peristaltic activity will decrease and vanish down the course of the ureter.

Intrusion of urine into the ureter from the renal pelvis is almost passive. The pressure required is minimal.[8] A pressure less than 2 cmH_2O is sufficient to open up the ureter,[9] and thus it is evident that the pressure inside a urine bolus is low. The peristaltic contraction only ensures the conclusion of a bolus of urine and propulsive transport. The wall resistance in the ureter varies from segment to segment. The least wall resistance is found in the upper part and the maximum in the vicinity of the bladder.[10] The wall resistance follows the gradual changes in the predominant direction of fibers in the ureter. Most proximal fibers are circular to oblique, whereas they run more and more longitudinally as the ureter approaches the bladder. The resistance at the entrance into the bladder is contributed to by a valve function of the mucosal part of the ureter and external compression by the extension of the bladder musculature called Waldeyer's sheet.[11] Consequently, backflow has to overcome that resistance, but whenever it has been overcome, the backflow of urine up through the ureter into the pelvis occurs just as as easily as the antegrade flow or even more so, since the passive resistance declines in a proximal direction. Thus, prevention of deleterious backflow is a matter of creating a valve function and, perhaps even more, creating a highly compliant reservoir.

Obstruction of the ureter induces changes in its peristaltic function. The acute response to obstruction is an increase in peristaltic frequency approaching the maximum of calyceal inherent activity. Secondarily, the normal coaptive peristalsis changes to non-coaptive with progressive dilation. The high peristaltic frequency can persist as long as an acute high-pressure stimulus is present. With persistence of the obstruction, chronic morphologic and functional changes take place gradually altering the transport function. Above the site of obstruction, the muscular changes are initially hypertrophy[12] and later hyperplasia. Specific changes then take place in the muscle tissue converting the contractile fiber cells to connective tissue producing cells. Such changes are not uniform and some areas above the obstruction may look intact and non-obstructed, whereas other areas are totally changed to fibrous tissue.[13] These chronic changes decrease the conductibility between the muscles and decrease the peristaltic transport capability of the urinary tract. At first, the muscles display continuously increased frequency of peristaltic activity although with some degree of discoordination between areas. Later the peristaltic activity is almost eliminated leaving only a few scant contractions with intervals of several minutes and with discoordination from area to area.[14]

These changes occur very rapidly in total obstruction and of course with some protraction in partial obstruction. The response to obstruction in the single case is, however, unpredictable with even experimental, highly standardized total obstruction causing tremendous variation in the dilatation and wall-property changes.[15] However, in clinical cases, even very dilated systems, which on fluoroscopy seem to be discoordinated and retrograde, will still display coordinated peristalsis on electromyography in spite of significant degrees of non-coaptation.

Renal functional consequences

Following reconstructive bladder surgery, normal urine transport from the kidneys to the bladder may be disturbed. If the urine flow from the glomerulus through the rest of the nephron and the ureters is interrupted at any point, it may have important short-term and long-term consequences for kidney function. The clinical manifestation of such a restriction to urinary outflow depends on the completeness of the obstruction, the subsequent rate of distension of the collecting system, the level of obstruction, whether the obstruction is unilateral or bilateral, and whether or not the obstruction is accompanied by complications, particularly infections. If urine flow from both kidneys is restricted, the long-term consequence may be loss of control of body fluid and electrolyte homeostasis and with persistent obstruction, accumulation of waste products may be the result. If one kidney is obstructed, the result may be unilateral renal destruction and a reduction in renal ability to regulate extracellular fluid and blood pressure. As in cases where restriction of urinary drainage is caused by an increased impedance to flow, cases with vesicoureteral reflux (and intrarenal reflux) may also be considered as conditions with temporary obstruction with urine backflow caused by a sustained high bladder pressure. Consequently, 'a urinary flow restricting process' can be defined as an increase in resistance above normal which may lead to an increase in the reabsorption of salt and water, and depending on the pyeloureteral compliance to dilatation of the renal pelvis and ureter. Finally, reduction in renal blood flow and glomerular filtration rate may follow.

Possible influence on renal morphology and perfusion

Lesions in the kidneys due to obstruction or reflux in general do not look the same. Long-term partial obstruction usually damages the midportion of the kidney,[16] whereas reflux predominantly strikes the poles. The reason for these differences is still to a large extent obscure although both papillary morphology and regional variations in blood flow in the kidney seem to be some of the major factors.

Studies in kidneys with an architecture more similar to man, like the pig, also showed the presence of flow differences between different areas of the cortex and medulla.[17] The latter studies suggested that the mid-renal cortex has a higher perfusion rate than the polar areas, albeit a certain plasticity must be present in human kidneys as can be deduced from studies of kidney functional reserve. The overall plasticity of renal perfusion is to some extent also disclosed by the fact that within a week after unilateral nephrectomy, the contralateral kidney has increased its function by 50%. Also, the onset of diabetes may almost instantaneously, at least in animal experimentation, increase kidney function significantly.[18] The plasticity of kidney perfusion may be of relevance for obstruction, as discussed in detail later in this chapter. Its relevance in the development of reflux nephropathy is based on the relation between backflow of urine into the kidney causing the nephropathy and kidney perfusion.[19]

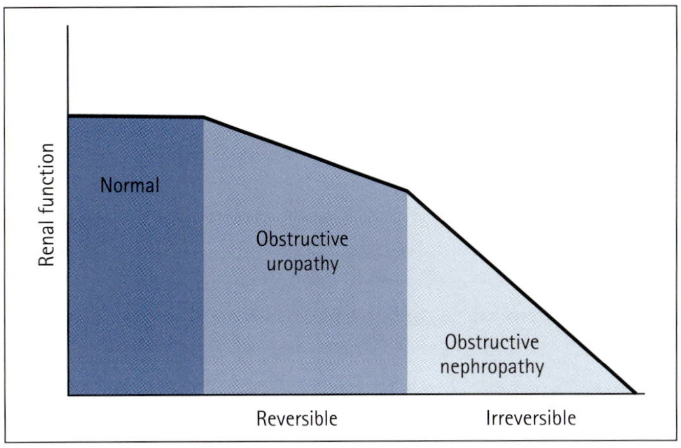

Figure 7.1 The relative course of renal function during progressive renal obstruction. Impaired urine flow causes a reversible reduction in renal function due to increased renal vascular resistance. If obstruction persists, a condition with irreversible loss of functon and parenchymal atrophy will follow.

Kidney function changes

Unilateral ureteral obstruction

It is well accepted that obstruction of the urinary tract is associated with a complex series of hormonal and hemodynamic alterations that change renal blood flow and glomerular filtration rate. Renal tubule function is altered directly due to the obstruction and secondarily due to changes in the extracellular environment. The events can be subdivided into a phase of obstructive uropathy, where primarily the anatomy of the renal transport/collecting system and urinary tract is affected and changes are reversible. Subsequently, a phase of obstructive nephropathy follows where restriction to urine flow affects nephron function and changes are irreversible (Figure 7.1).

Renal blood flow

It is documented that increased pressure in the renal pelvis and the collecting system subsequent to outflow obstruction results in a decrease in renal blood flow. In animals with unipapillary kidneys frequently used for experiments of this kind, the renal blood flow reduction is preceded by an immediate but transient increase in renal blood flow due to vasodilation.[20–22] This vasodilation concurs with an increased production of prostaglandins from the renal medulla,[23,24] which can be blocked by indomethacin.[22,25,26] However, studies of the hemodynamic changes during acute unilateral obstruction in pigs have suggested that the polypapillary kidney may react differently with a lack of the initial vasodilation.[27,28] The subsequent gradual decrease in renal blood flow is characterized by perfusion defects in both the renal cortex and medulla.[29,30] Several characteristics appear (Figure 7.2), the most prominent is an increased vascular resistance, initially on both sides of the glomerulus, and subsequently an afferent arteriolar vasoconstriction dominates. In both, awake dogs[21,31] and anesthetized pigs,[27,28] during the period of 2–5 hours following onset of obstruction, renal blood flow progressively decreases while ureteral pressure continues to rise, a finding consistent with a

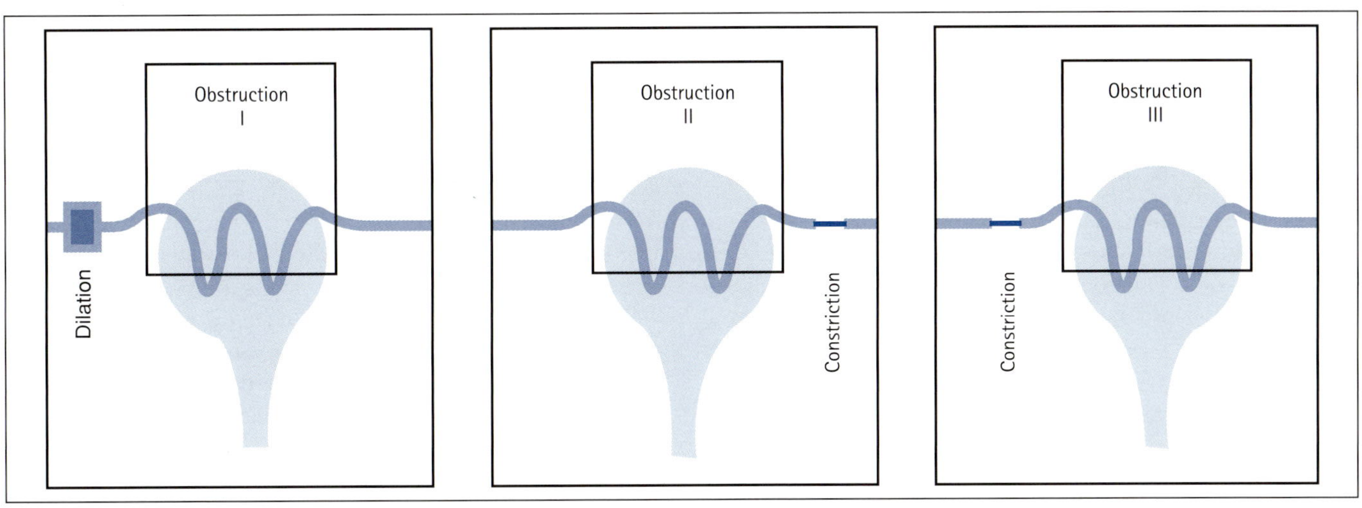

Figure 7.2 The general concept of renal hemodynamic changes during acute unilateral obstruction of the ureter. Phase I is characterized by preglomerular vasodilaton lasting 1–2 hours. Phase II is characterized by temporary postglomerular vasoconstriction which last 2–5 hours, and Phase III is dominated by constriction of primarily the preglomerular vessels.

temporary postglomerular vasoconstriction. Subsequently, renal blood flow and pelvic pressure fall in parallel, suggesting a vasoconstriction primarily of the preglomerular vasculature.[17,32–34]

Glomerular filtration rate

Very few reports exist on the glomerular filtration rate (GFR) changes in the acute phase of ureteral occlusion,[35–38] because standard clearance techniques for measuring GFR depend on continuous urine flow and hence are not applicable to a completely obstructed kidney. Consequently, most of the reported data on the effects of obstruction on GFR describe renal function after release of obstruction. By methods other than conventional clearance techniques, it has been demonstrated that filtration continues during complete obstruction of the ureter for a period of 24 hours, and probably beyond that.[36] In the anesthetized dog, GFR increased immediately by up to 20% in response to acute elevations of ureteral pressure up to 48.8 cmH_2O (30 mmHg).[35] However, in rats[36–38] and in pigs[28] the immediate response to acute ureteral obstruction appears to be a fall in filtration rate. In the study by Hvistendahl et al, GFR was maintained until the ureteral pressure exceeded 27.2 cmH_2O (20 mmHg) in pigs.[28]

Bilateral ureteral obstruction

Similar to the hemodynamic changes described for unilateral obstruction of the ureter, bilateral obstruction is accompanied by unique changes in renal blood flow.[39,40] Experimental studies in the dog have shown that bilateral obstruction is followed by an immediate increase in renal blood flow in both kidneys. However, this increase is very brief and after 1–2 hours a decrease in renal blood flow below normal appears.[39] Comparable results are seen in rats.[41] In contrast with the reduction observed in ureteral pressure following longlasting unilateral occlusion of the ureter, there are reports indicating that ureteral pressure remains elevated in the ureters following bilateral obstruction.[39,41,42] These data suggest an increase in the postglomerular vasculature during bilateral ureteral obstruction.

Glomerular filtration rate

Data regarding GFR changes following bilateral ureteral obstruction are limited to the measurement of filtration following release of obstruction. These uniformly show that GFR decreases, and more severely than after release of unilateral obstruction.[32,41,43,44]

Renal tubular function in obstructive nephropathy

Obstruction profoundly reduces the ability to concentrate and dilute the urine and reduces the ability of renal tubules to reabsorb Na^+, K^+, and H^+. The functional alterations in the renal tubules after release of obstruction depend in part on whether the obstruction is bilateral or unilateral. The major sites of abnormal function are located in distal segments of the nephron, and patients with chronic obstructive nephropathy have an impaired ability to concentrate the urine.[45] Release of obstruction in rats with either unilateral or bilateral ureteral obstruction (UUO or BUO) also showed impaired ability to concentrate the urine,[46,47] a defect not counteracted by vasopressin. Release of complete BUO is associated with a marked diuresis and natriuresis. Free water clearance is increased.[46,48–53] This is accompanied by an increase in total solute excretion.[54] The mechanisms most often proposed to explain the decrease in concentrating ability in the kidney after obstruction are an inability of the medullary interstitium to maintain its hypertonicity and insensitivity of the tubule to vasopressin.[55] The inability to establish the medullary tonicity necessary to concentrate urine comes from the inability of the thick ascending limb (TAL) of the loop of Henle to reabsorb sodium,[56] which ultimately decreases the tonicity in the medullary interstitium and, consequently, the reabsorption of water. However the molecular mechanisms involved in the urinary concentrating defect have only recently been elucidated.[57–62]

In spite of a decrease in GFR and hence in the filtered load of sodium, the excretion of sodium by the postobstructed kidney of rats with UUO has been known to be similar to that of the contralateral kidney.[47] Thus, fractional sodium excretion is greater from the postobstructed than from the contralateral kidney. Similar findings have been reported in the dog and in humans after more prolonged periods of obstruction.[63] These findings indicate significant changes in the tubular reabsorption of sodium and water by the previously obstructed kidney. After release of UUO in rats, the fraction of the filtered sodium and water that is reabsorbed in the proximal tubules (PT) of superficial nephrons is thought to be increased.[47,64] In contrast, after release of BUO, the fraction of the glomerular filtrate reabsorbed in the PT of surface nephrons has been demonstrated to be either unchanged or decreased.[46,53] Reabsorption of salt and water by the PTs of deep or juxtamedullary nephrons is decreased after the release of both BUO and UUO. The fraction of filtered water delivered to the early distal segment has been demonstrated to be increased after release of BUO,[53] indicating that both UUO and BUO diminished the ability of the TAL of Henle's loop to reabsorb salt. The effects of ureteral obstruction on collecting duct (CD) function have been explored by micropuncture and microcatheterization techniques. After release of UUO in rats fraction fluid delivery to the base of the papillae was increased.[47] This suggests that much of the salt that appears in the urine after release of UUO is derived from marked alterations in either the medullary CD function or the function of deep nephrons.

In a number of studies the fundamental role of renal aquaporins (AQP) and sodium transporters in urine concentration has been demonstrated and recently an understanding at the molecular level for the urinary concentrating defect in response to ureteral obstruction in rats is associated with significant reduction in the expression of major renal AQPs and sodium transporters along the nephron and CDs. Importantly, the expression of renal AQPs and sodium transporters was reduced, consistent with a significant impairment of tubular sodium reabsorption and decreased urine concentration. We conclude that downregulation of major renal AQPs and sodium transporters located in the nephron in rats with BUO, release of BUO, and UUO may contribute to the impaired renal tubular sodium reabsorption, increased urinary sodium excretion and decreased urine concentration during obstruction.

Intrarenal vasoactive mediators

Although the mechanisms behind the increase in vascular resistance largely remain unsolved, a number of vasoactive mediators have been demonstrated to be potentially involved in the regulation of the initial hemodynamic changes. Major interest has been devoted to the renin–angiotensin system and the prostaglandin–thromboxane system. Evidence for the renin–angiotensin system as a mediator of some of the functional and hemodynamic changes during and following release of obstruction has accumulated. Four decades ago, Vander and Miller showed that unilateral elevation of the ureteral pressure was associated with increases in the renal venous plasma renin activity.[65] This was followed by a number of studies demonstrating an increase in ipsilateral renal vein plasma renin activity during acute ureteral occlusion in dogs.[20,22,66,67] The limited data on the renin response show an initial increase in peripheral plasma renin activity with return to normal in dogs with chronic ureteral occlusion.[68,69] Although this phenomenon was transient, there was convincing evidence for the participation of the renin–angiotensin system following acute ureteral occlusion for periods of several weeks duration. Subsequent studies for additional indirect evidence for a specific role of the renin–angiotensin system was conducted with contradictory results. In dogs and rats, interference with the renin–angiotensin system was accomplished by administration of either angiotensin II receptor blockers, angiotensin I converting-enzyme inhibitors or depiction of renin by sodium loading. In some cases, improvements in renal function were found,[70–74] whereas in other cases no effect was noted.[20,69,75–77]

In several studies expression of the renin gene has been demonstrated in the ipsilateral kidney and also in the contralateral kidney of the rat during chronic obstruction.[78,79] Moreover, there is now substantial evidence to indicate that all of the components necessary for the local formation of angiotensin II exist in the kidney, and they operate in whole or in part, independently of the circulating renin–angiotensin system,[80–84] and increased secretion of renal angiotensin II has been shown during unilateral occlusion of the pig ureter.[27] Furthermore, studies have showed further evidence for an increased expression of angiotensin II during unilateral ureteral obstruction.[85–87]

The prostaglandin system represents another system which may be implicated in the hemodynamic changes following obstruction of the ureter. In addition to the prostaglandin E2-dependent vasodilation occurring immediately after the onset of obstruction in some species, it has been documented that an inhibition of the prostaglandin system is associated with detrimental reductions of renal blood flow during the late phase of acute unilateral occlusion of the ureter,[88–90] indicating that the presence of vasodilating prostaglandins is important during conditions with impaired urine flow due to obstruction. Furthermore, the decrease in renal blood flow following unilateral ureteral occlusion has been attributed to an exaggerated production of the vasoconstrictor prostaglandin thromboxane A2 (TxA2). Since the initial elegant in vitro studies by Nishikawa, Morrison and Needleman, who showed that the perfused hydronephrotic rabbit kidney maintained an exaggerated amount of the vasoconstrictor TxA2,[91,92] several studies have investigated the potential role of this compound as a mediator of obstructive nephropathy. Many of these studies have confirmed a crucial role for TxA2 in the reduction of renal blood flow,[70,93–95] whereas others have not.[96,97] Although controversial, there seems to be no doubt that TxA2, to some extent, is involved as a mediator. The underlying pathophysiological mechanism is thought to be an increased influx or proliferation of interstitial cells especially macrophages.[98] These cells in turn are believed to be responsible for the increased TxA2 synthesis since experiments following irradiation of the kidney or the administration of nitrogen mustard have shown a reduction in urinary excretion of thromboxane metabolites and a decrease in the influx of mononuclear cells.[99,100]

Several other vasoactive mediators have been suggested to participate in the renal hemodynamic and functional changes following obstruction. In the rat BUO is associated with an increase in plasma atrial natriuretic peptide (ANP) in the rat.[101–103] Patients with acute urinary retention have increased levels of plasma ANP, suggesting a role for this system in the functional adaptations to bilateral obstruction of the ureters.[104] An enhanced release of vasopressin has also been shown following stimulation of the pelvic mechanoreceptors by rapidly increasing pelvic pressure.[105] Recent studies have indicated that lipoxygenases,[106] nitrous oxide,[107] and endothelin-derived relaxing factor[108] also are involved to some extent in obstructive nephropathy. Many growth factors have recently been discovered. Among these an increased expression of transforming growth factor (TGF)-β1 has been shown to be present during chronic obstruction in the rat. It is suggested to be implicated in the renal interstitial fibrosis that is characteristic of the obstructive nephropathy.[109] Evidence for a definitive role of the renin–angiotensin system in obstruction was shown in another study by Kaneto et al, where enalapril treatment reduced the tubulointerstitial fibrosis in the obstructed kidney and the expression of collagen IV, which might implicate a reduction in the monocytes capable of secreting the profibrotic factor TGF-β1.[110] A decreased expression of the epidermal growth factor (EGF) has been shown,[111,112] suggesting a protective role for EGF in kidney apoptosis, which is the particular type of programmed cell death that develops in different organs subsequent to ischemia and reduction in blood flow, e.g. in the developing parenchymal atrophy of hydronephrosis.

Nitric oxide plays an important role in the regulation of blood flow in the normal and the diseased kidney. It is synthesized from its percursor, L-arginine, by the enzyme nitric oxide synthase (NOS). Arginine infusion 18 hours after UUO in dogs increased renal blood flow and ureteral pressure. These results sugest that the nitric oxide system of the kidney is activated in UUO.[113] In UUO, the renal vasculature remains responsive to the vasodilatory actions of nitric oxide, and blood flow changes associated with UUO involve impairment of the nitric oxide synthetic pathways in the kidney. Increased expression of both endothelial NOS and inducible NOS has been demonstrated with increasing duration of obstruction, but this probably does not correspond to a sufficient increase in enzyme activity.[114] In particular, nitric oxide is thought to exert a protective role in obstructive uropathy by ameliorating tubulointerstitial fibrosis in animal models of UUO.[115] Reyes and coworkers examined the role of NO in BUO.[116] When L-NAME, an L-arginine antagonist, was infused, there was a further decrease in the GFR and effective renal plasma flow (ERPF) compared with controls, suggesting that nitric oxide maintained GFR and ERPF during BUO.

In summary, impaired urine flow, whether unilateral or bilateral, results in reduction of renal blood flow and GFR due to an increased renal vasoconstriction. Several vasoactive mediators are potentially involved in this hemodynamic response which precedes irreversible renal parenchymal atrophy.

Clinical findings

Patients with pre-existing hepatic or renal disease are less able to compensate for the metabolic changes resulting from urinary diversion. It is thus generally accepted that serum creatinine greater than 150–200 μmol/l indicates poor risk.[117–119] Some patients may, however, have reversible renal impairment where obstruction is relieved by way of drainage for a period before surgery. Such a procedure may be indicated in ambiguous cases to assess the true renal function.

Substituting the bladder with a new reservoir formed from intestine affects the communication between the neobladder and the upper urinary tract, the urethra or other urine outlet routes. Dynamics of the bladder change: the intestinal segment used as a reservoir continues to behave as intestine, with peristaltic contractions leading to spikes of increased pressure. In order to moderate these peristaltic contractions of the intestinal reservoir, detubularization of bowel for bladder substitution was first introduced by Ekman et al in 1964,[120] improving reservoir capacity and producing a low pressure in the neobladder.[121]

Urodynamic studies of volume, capacity and pressure characteristics of continent ileal reservoirs show that during the first year after operation, the volume of the reservoir increases several hundred percent, while the spontaneous activity of the intestinal tissue is reduced.[122] If these optimal conditions are achieved, there should be no risk to the upper urinary tract and kidney function; however, even though the biomechanics of the new reservoir may mimic that of the normal bladder, a patent anastomosis to the ureters remains crucial. Initial results from clinical follow-up studies after continent urinary diversion have emphasized the importance of a good antireflux mechanism.[123,124] In these studies 40% of the patients had reflux to the upper urinary tract due to eversion or sliding of the antireflux valve. After surgical correction of the reflux no further dilatation of the upper tract occurred. However, results from the pig model[3] did indicate that reflux per se does not threaten renal function as long as the biomechanics of the bladder are normal. When constructing a neobladder, the aim is to simulate these characteristics as closely as possible.

Clinically, when doing antireflux ureteral reimplantation the rate of stenosis at the implantation site is significantly higher compared with the simple end-to-side refluxing anastomosis. Thus the stenosis rate after antireflux technique has been reported as high as 13.5% in a randomized study,[125] 13%[126] and 9%[117] compared with 3%, 1.7% and 1% with the end-to-side technique performed in the same institution. This finding appears to outweigh the theoretical benefit together with a preexistent pyelonephritis, stones or azotemia for patients undergoing large-volume, low-pressure continent diversion with antireflux technique. Still final proof from a randomized study is warranted, especially when it comes to children where the results after bladder substitution in general are more disappointing,[127] then antireflux surgery may still be recommended.

The role of ileal conduit has been declining as more continent urinary diversions and bladder augmentations have been performed in recent years. A substantial proportion of the patients with ileal conduits have upper tract dilatation and renal deterioration.[120–130] Unlike the continent reservoirs, the bowel used for the ileal conduits is not detubularized, and the intraluminal activity and pressure waves are higher. Investigations have shown a connection between these high pressures/high activity and upper tract dilatation, a condition aggravated by obstruction of the conduit.[131]

Efforts have been made to develop and analyze different designs of antireflux mechanisms,[132,133] but in colonic and ileal conduits there is no documentation of a beneficial effect of antireflux techniques. It was shown in a study where the patients were randomized prospectively to refluxing or non-refluxing ileum or colonic diversion,[134] that after a mean of 10 years there was a moderate decrease in GFR in both ileal and colonic groups and that the decline was more than could be explained by the normal age related decrease. However, the decrease in GFR was not different between refluxing and non-refluxing ureteral implantations.

It is well known that after bladder substitution or augmentation cystoplasty many patients may have to empty their reservoir by way of clean intermittent catheterization to accomplish bladder emptying that often leads to asymptomatic bacteriuria. Currently, there is an increasing number of patients with low-pressure continent urinary diversions who have considerable risk of reflux and also have a potential risk of infection caused by their intermittent catheterization and/or poor bladder emptying. Low pressure in the reservoir is not always certain and can be impeded by a functional or anatomic obstruction to drainage or overdistension due to neglect of the full bladder (because of a decrease in sensitivity as seen in neurogenic patients). The risk or renal damage in those patients remains uncertain.[135–137]

Lately, more attention has been paid on the effect of the polyuria following longstanding urinary tract obstruction. The defect in renal concentration ability can result in increased diurnal urine production and also in disappearance of the normal decrease in urine production during the night. It has been shown[138] that 24-hour urine volume greater than 2 l in boys with urethral valves and impaired bladder sensation can produce significant distension of the upper urinary tract and that it can be treated successfully with an indwelling night-time catheter.

In contrast to the patient with a normal urinary tract in whom abnormal urine volume and altered micturition pattern will be easily recognized, the patient with a urinary diversion will not necessarily notice such symptoms. Accordingly, a urinary tract obstruction from overfilling of the bladder may be completely asymptomatic. More commonly flank pain will warn of the obstruction. This is often the case, especially in neurogenic bladder disorders.

Clinical assessment of obstruction

Unlike other patients with a disorder leading to obstructive nephropathy, the patient with a urinary tract diversion is already known to the urologist and obstruction should always be suspected and excluded. Many patients coming to urinary diversion already have alterations of normal urine flow (obstruction/reflux) and have already impaired renal function and bladder disorders). For these reasons it is very important to know the level of renal function and the dynamic function of the upper urinary tract prior to urinary diversion surgery. After urinary diversion it is important to follow-up renal function. Since the most significant adverse effect of urinary diversion on renal function is related to obstruction follow-up should include visualization of urinary tract morphology by way of radiographs and magnetic resonance imaging. Renal function should be assessed by radionuclide studies. A primary intravenous urogram provides knowledge of the baseline gross anatomy of the urinary tract. Transient dilatation of the upper urinary tract is also a very common manifestation following urinary diversions. There are many possible causes and it may be associated with renal damage and if left untreated may lead to renal failure.

In patients with ileal conduits,[139] ureterosignoidostomy diversion[140] and Kock pouch diversion[141] a good correlation was reported between changes in urinary tract morphology and changes on renography. An abnormal time to peak and a prolonged third segment of the renogram indicate a dilated upper urinary tract. However, pre-existing dilatation is frequent and it should be emphasized that dilatation of the upper tract is not tantamount to obstruction. This is further complicated by difficulties in assessing the clinical diagnosis of obstruction despite the wide range of methods available for this purpose.[142–149] All efforts to refine the diagnosis of obstruction are based on the assumption that obstruction will lead to progressive destruction of the kidney. It must be stressed that no single method is available to distinguish between 'simple' dilatation and obstruction. However, in the context of renal functional measurement renal radionuclide studies by renography should be considered important and are normally very useful. Provided that the patient is well hydrated restriction to urinary flow will affect the movement of the radiopharmaceutical from the renal input to the renal output. A renographical study using ^{99m}Tc-DTPA or ^{99m}Tc-MAG will objectively reflect the accumulation, transit and elimination of the tracer activity by each individual kidney as a simple and non-invasive procedure. Today, the clinical use of renography is restricted to the use of the above two tracers. Although the kinetics of the tracers are different[150] they are all rapidly transported from the blood to the proximal tubular lumen. This has been the rationale for development of techniques which might discriminate between dilatation with and without obstruction.[140,143,151] The value of renal functional observation by renography has accordingly been demonstrated in a number of studies[138,141,152] given the limitations previously stated concerning the difficulties disclosing obstruction.

Thus, in a prospective study by Chen and co-workers, the value of renographic evaluation of patients with Kock pouch diversion was demonstrated.[141] Following urinary diversion, renal function deteriorated with development of bilateral hydronephrosis in five of six patients within the first month. No reflux was demonstrated and subsequently the hydronephrosis resolved and renal function improved, indicating that the changes are reversible and possibly attributed to the operative procedures with swelling at the sites of anastomosis.[141] Few attempts have been made to comprehensively study renal function in this patient population. Chen and associates provided data from the measurement of effective renal plasma flow and showed deterioration after 1 month. Although this is a functional parameter, it must be asked to what extent it reflects renal function. A more useful parameter is the GFR. Månsson and associates[153] showed only slight to moderate decrease in GFR in 94 patients with different urinary diversion types 2–10 years postoperatively. They concluded that it was demonstrated in this study and previous studies, that a full cecal reservoir constitutes intermittent functional obstruction to urine flow,[152] and intermittent high pressure which may occur within a full reservoir does not seem to affect renal function to any major extent.[153] However, tubular function suffers earlier and to a greater degree than GFR in chronic obstruction.[154] In addition to the electrolyte disturbance caused by the urinary diversion, this may lead to defects in the urine concentrating ability with impairment of salt and water reabsorption and urinary acidifying potential thereby expanding the metabolic consequences of a urinary diversion. GFR may well be preserved until the late stages of renal functional deterioration. Thus biochemical evaluation including serum creatinine and blood urea should be done routinely. Additionally the free water clearance and urine concentrating ability will help determine total renal capacity.

It is generally accepted that creatinine clearance is an unsuitable marker for GFR. The reason is that urine passes through an intestinal segment where urine/creatinine is reabsorbed. Therefore most of the studies evaluating GFR have applied methods based on clearance of ^{51}Cr-EDTA. Although this clearance technique is widely accepted, some reabsorption of EDTA does take place. Indeed, McDougal and Koch[155] showed that a similar glomerular filtration tracer, DTPA, correlated poorly with true glomerular filtration measured as the renal clearance of inulin in different types of urinary diversion. They found that the creatinine clearance technique modified by diuretic conditions was superior to other methods. However, the reasons for these discrepancies are not fully understood. With rapidly developing technology including software to analyze γ-camera data, it is now possible to directly calculate GFR renal plasma flow and thereby filtration fraction given the right tracer.

In summary, urinary diversions are often associated with dilatation of the upper urinary tract. The frequency of obstruction is not known, but intermittent and chronic obstruction including reflux from a high-pressure reservoir is a serious complication. Few studies have undertaken comprehensive studies of the long-term impact of urinary diversion on GFR.

Experimental models

Several groups have used experimental animal models to study renal function in individuals where bowel was used for urinary diversion. In 1978, Kock studied the changes in renal parenchyma and upper urinary tract in 12 dogs following urinary diversion via a continent reservoir made out of detubularized ileum.[156] Only the right ureter was connected to the reservoir, the left side being kept intact. In two dogs, no protection against reflux was made; in the remaining 10 an intussuscepted valve was inserted between the diverted ureter and the reservoir. The animals were followed for 12 weeks and catheterized twice a day to empty the reservoir. With no reflux protection, the upper tract dilated and pyelonephritic renal deterioration developed. With an intact antireflux mechanism, no dilatation was found, and only slight pyelonephritic changes developed. These results correlate with what has also been shown in patients with continent ileal reservoirs.[157]

Experimental models have also been used for histologic examination of kidneys drained by an ileal conduit. Other published studies have also shown very different outcomes regarding the incidence of renal deterioration in animals.[158,159] In Redman's study,[159] ileal conduits were constructed in 17 dogs. The right ureter was connected to the conduit; the left was left untouched. The animals were followed for 4 months. Only three dogs developed pyelonephritis, and the author concluded that sterile ureteral reflux alone did not seem to cause renal damage, but combined reflux and obstruction of the conduit was an important factor in development of pyelonephritis in kidneys drained by ileal conduits. Jørgensen's reflux model in pigs[3] showed the same results for kidneys drained by the pigs' native bladder.

Antireflux nipple valves have also been studied in an experimental animal model.[160] Fifteen dogs (four males, eleven females) underwent construction of a hemi-Kock reservoir with antireflux nipple valve but without an efferent valve and limb and with the reservoir anastomosed to the native bladder. The right ureters were anastomosed to the afferent limb of the reservoir; the left sides were left untouched and served as controls. Five dogs including three males died in the second postoperative week. The fourth male dog died just before the follow-up examination; all males died because of impaired urine drainage, which was not a problem in the female group. The remaining nine dogs were followed for 12–36 months. Three dogs had dilated right ureters and histologically chronic pyelonephritis, but all cystograms were normal with no evidence of reflux. The changes were found to be secondary to ureteroileal stenosis and calculus formation on staples used in the valve formation. The study emphasizes the importance of leaving no metal staples exposed to urine, if they are used in valve formation. In 1992 St Clair et al[161] studied enterocystoplasty and reflux nephropathy in a canine model. The results indicated that preoperatively present vesicoureteral reflux should be corrected in patients undergoing an enterocystoplasty. Bladder augmentation was performed using detubularized ileum and an operative procedure ensured unilateral reflux in six dogs. Fluoroscopic studies were done to ensure this, and intravesical pressure measurements and excretory cystograms excluded outflow obstruction. On follow-up, bacterial colonization of the upper tract and pyelonephritis were found in five of the six dogs with reflux. On the control side, only one upper tract was infected. Enterocystoplasty is used in an increasing number of patients suffering from neurogenic bladder hyperactivity or unexplained urge/urge incontinence. In the neurogenic group reflux is a well-known problem and the results from this study support the recommendation of correction at the time of cystoplasty operation.[162]

Conclusion

This chapter has outlined some of the important factors in the development of obstructive nephropathy with special reference to reservoirs. Changes in metabolism resulting from the differences between bladder wall function and intestinal tract wall function have been discussed and the importance of reflux and urinary tract transport function have been stressed.

In spite of the well-known fact that differences are lost even after brief episodes of obstruction, most of the mechanisms are still to be elucidated. Some of the limitations of our knowledge are due to the fact that it is difficult to mimic the clinical situation in the animal model and the fact that most of the models hitherto developed for elucidating obstruction seem to have fundamental differences from the human response. The inherent spontaneous activity of reservoirs, the hazards of reservoirs with low-compliance qualities, the established fact that reflux from reservoirs due to the spontaneous activity of the reservoir is a hazard to the kidney function and the fact that all reservoirs lead to changes in metabolism, are major challenges in the long term for diagnostics and follow-up in this fast-growing area of urologic surgery.

References

1. Hodson CJ, Edwards D. Chronic pyelonephritis and vesicoureteric reflux. Clin Radiol 1960; 11: 219–31.
2. Hodson CJ, Malling TMJ, McManarnon LM. The pathogenesis of reflux nephropathy. Br J Radiol 1975; Suppl 13: 1–26.
3. Jørgensen TM. Dynamics of the urinary tract during induced vesico-ureteric reflux in pigs. II. Scand J Urol Nephrol 1985; 19: 173–82.
4. Ransley PG, Risdon RA. Reflux and renal scarring. Br J Radiol 1978; Suppl 14.
5. Nielsen JB, Nørgaard JP, Djurhuus JC. Continuous overnight monitoring of bladder activity in vesico, ureteral reflux patients. II. Bladder activity types. Neurourol Urodyn 1984; 3: 7–21.
6. Djurhuus JC, Nerstrøm B, Iversen Hansen R, Gyrd-Hansen N, Rask-Andersen H. Dynamics of upper urinary tract. II. An electrophysiologic in vivo study of renal pelvis in pigs: analysis of the modality of pelvic activity during normal hydration and diuresis. Invest Urol 1977; 14: 469–74.
7. Engelmann TW. Zur Physiologie des Ureters. Pflügers Arch 1969; 2: 243.
8. Bisballe S, Djurhuus JC, Mortensen J, Jørgensen TM. Pyeloureteral hydrodynamics. The pelviureteral junction resistance in the pig. Urol Int 1983; 38: 55–7.
9. Griffiths DJ, Notschaele C. The mechanics of urine transport in the upper urinary tract. 1. The dynamics of the isolated bolus. Neurourol Urodyn 1983; 2: 155–66.
10. Knudsen L, Gregersen H, Eika B, Frøkiær J. Elastic wall properties and collagen content in the ureter. Neurourol Urodyn 1994; 13: 597–608.
11. Coolsaet BLRA, van Venrooij GEPM, Blok C. Detrusor pressure versus wall stress in relation to ureterovesical resistance. Neurourol Urodyn 1982; 1: 105–12.
12. Gee WF, Kiviat MD. Ureteral response to partial obstruction. Smooth muscle hyperplasia and connective tissue proliferation. Invest Urol 1975; 12: 309–16.
13. Ladefoged O, Djurhuus JC. Morphology of the upper urinary tract in experimental hydronephrosis in pigs. Acta Chir Scand 1976; 472: 29–35.
14. Djurhuus JC, Nerstøm B, Gyrd-Hansen N, Rask-Andersen J. Experimental hydronephrosis. An electrophysiologic investigation before and after release of obstruction. Acta Chir Scand (Suppl) 1978, 472: 17–28.
15. Mortensen J, Djurhuus JC, Møller JCF, Laursen H, Taagehoj-Jensen F. The pressure-volume relationship of the renal pelvis in total obstruction in pigs. Urol Res 1983; 11: 251–3.
16. Møller JC, Djurhuus JC. Obstructive disease of the kidney (hydronephrosis) and the urinary tract. In: Tisher CC, Brenner BM (eds). Renal Pathology: With Clinical and Functional Correlations. Philadelphia: JB Lippincott, 1994; 863–94.
17. Frøkiær J, Flø C, Knudsen L, et al. Regional blood flow in the normal pig kidney. Nucl Med Commun 1992; 13: 379(A).
18. Seyer-Hansen K, Hansen J, Gundersen HJG. Renal hypertrophy in experimental diabetes. Diabetologia 1980; 18: 501–5.
19. Thomsen HS, Dorph S, Olsen S. Pyelorenal backflow in normal and ischemic rabbit kidneys. Invest Radiol 1981; 16: 206–14.
20. Vaughan ED, Shenasky JH, Gillenwater JY. Mechanisms of acute hemodynamic response to ureteral occlusion. Invest Urol 1971; 9: 109–18.
21. Moody TE, Vaughan ED, Gillenwater JY. Relationships between renal blood flow and ureteral pressure during 18 hours of total unilateral ureteral obstruction. Invest Urol 1975; 13: 246–51.
22. Cadnapaphornchai P, Aisenbrey G, McDonald K, Burke TJ, Schrier RW. Prostaglandin mediated hyperemia and renin-mediated hypertension during acute ureteral obstruction. Prostaglandins 1978; 16: 965–71.
23. Olsen UB, Magnussen MP, Eilersten E. Prostaglandins, a link between renal hydro- and hemodynamics in the dog. Acta Physiol Scand 1976; 97: 369–76.
24. Anggaard E, Bohman SO, Griffin JE, Larsson C, Maunsbach AB. Subcellular localization of the prostaglandin system in the rabbit papilla. Acta Physiol Scand 1972; 84: 231–6.
25. Dal Canton A, Stanziale R, Corradi A, Andreueei VE, Migone I. Effects of acute ureteral obstruction on glomerular hemodynamics in rat kidneys. Kidney Int 1977; 12: 403–11.
26. Allan JT, Vaughan ED, Gillenwater JY. The effect of indomethacin on renal blood flow and ureteral pressure in unilateral ureteral obstruction in awake dogs. Invest Urol 1978; 15: 324–7.
27. Frøkiær J, Knudsen L, Nielsen AS, Pedersen EB, Djurhuus JC. Enhanced intrarenal angiotensin II generation in response to obstruction of the pig ureter. Am J Physiol 1992; 263: F527–F533.
28. Hvistendahl JJ, Pedersen TS, Jørgensen HH et al. Renal hemodynamic response to graduated unilateral obstruction of the pig ureter. Nephron (In press).
29. Bay WH, Stein JH, Rector JB, Osgood RW, Ferris TF. Redistribution of renal cortical blood flow during elevated ureteral pressure. Am J Physiol 1972; 222: 33–7.
30. Miyazaki M, McNay J. Redistribution of renal cortical blood flow during ureteral occlusion and renal venous constriction. Proc Soc Exp Biol Med 1971; 138: 454–9.
31. Vaughan ED, Sørensen EJ, Gillenwater JY. The renal hemodynamic response to chronic unilateral complete ureteral occlusion. Invest Urol 1970; 9: 78–90.

32. Harris RH, Yarger WE. Renal function after release of unilateral ureteral obstruction in rat. Am J Physiol 1974; 227: 806–15.
33. Yarger WE, Griffith LD. Intrarenal hemodynamics following chronic unilateral ureteral obstruction in the dog. Am J Physiol 1974; 227: 816–26.
34. Arendshorst WJ, Finn WF, Gottschalk CW. Nephron stop-flow pressure response to obstruction on glomerular function in the rat kidney. J Clin Invest 1974; 53: 1497–500.
35. Navar LG, Baer PG. Renal autoregulatory and glomerular filtration responses to graduated ureteral obstruction. Nephron 1970; 7: 301–16.
36. Harris RH, Gill JM. Changes in glomerular filtration rate during complete ureteral obstruction in rats. Kidney Int 1981; 19: 603–8.
37. Provoest AP, Molenaar JC. Renal function during and after a temporary complete unilateral ureter obstruction in rats. Invest Urol 1981; 18: 242–6.
38. Dal Canton A, Corradi A, Stanziale R, Maruccio G, Migone L. Effects of 24-hour unilateral ureteral obstruction on glomerular hemodynamic in rat kidney. Kidney Int 1979; 15: 457–62.
39. Moody TE, Vaughan ED Jr, Gillenwater JY. Comparison of the renal hemodynamic response to unilateral and bilateral ureteral occlusion. Invest Urol 1977; 14: 455–9.
40. Nascimento L, Harris AP, Ayala JM, Opava-Stitzer S, Martinez-Maldonado M. Renin release. Effects of vasodilators and bilateral ureteral obstruction. J Pharmacol Exp Ther 1980; 212, 481–6.
41. Dal Canton A, Coradil A, Stanziale R, Maruccio G, Migone L. Glomerular hemodynamics before and after release of 24-hour bilateral ureteral obstruction. Kidney Int 1980; 17: 491–6.
42. Tanner GA. Effects of kidney tubule obstruction on glomerular function in rats. Am J Physiol 1979; 237: F379–F385.
43. McDougal WS, Wright FS. Defect in proximal and distal sodium transport in post-obstructive diuresis. Kidney Int 1972; 2: 304–17.
44. Yarger WE, Aynedjian HS, Bank N. A micropuncture study of the postobstructive diuresis in the rat. J Clin Invest 1972; 51: 625–37.
45. Curhan GC, Zeidel ML. Urinary tract obstruction. In: Brenner BM (ed). The Kidney. WB Saunders Company 1996; 1936–58.
46. Buerkert J, Head M, Klahr S. Effects of acute bilateral ureteral obstruction on deep nephron and terminal collecting duct function in the young rat. J Clin Invest 1977; 59: 1055–65.
47. Buerkert J, Martin D, Head M, Prasad J, Klahr S. Deep nephron function after release of acute unilateral ureteral obstruction in the young rat. J Clin Invest 1978; 62: 1228–39.
48. Peterson LJ, Yarger WE, Schocken DD, Glenn JF. Post-obstructive diuresis: a varied syndrome. J Urol 1975; 113: 190–4.
49. Vaughan ED Jr, Sweet RE, Gillenwater JY. Unilateral ureteral occlusion: pattern of nephron repair and compensatory response. J Urol 1973; 109: 979–82.
50. Dal Canton A, Corradi A, Stanziale R, Maruccio G, Migone L. Glomerular hemodynamics before and after release of 24-hour bilateral ureteral obstruction. Kidney Int 1980; 17: 491–6.
51. Harris RH, Yarger WE. The pathogenesis of post-obstructive diuresis. The role of circulating natriuretic and diuretic factors, including urea. J Clin Invest 1975; 56: 880–7.
52. Sonnenberg H, Wilson DR. The role of the medullary collecting ducts in postobstructive diuresis. J Clin Invest 1976; 57: 1564–74.
53. Yarger WE, Aynedjian HS, Bank N. A micropuncture study of postobstructive diuresis in the rat. J Clin Invest 1972; 51: 625–37.
54. McDougal WS, Wright FS. Defect in proximal and distal sodium transport in post-obstructive diuresis. Kidney Int 1972; 2: 304–17.
55. Wilson DR, Klahr S. Urinary tract obstruction. In: Schrier RW (ed). Diseases of the Kidney. Boston: Little, Brown, 1993: 657–88.
56. Hanley MJ, Davidson K. Isolated nephron segments from rabbit models of obstructive nephropathy. J Clin Invest 1982; 69: 165–74.
57. Frøkiær J, Marples D, Knepper MA, Nielsen S. Bilateral ureteral obstruction downregulates expression of vasopressin-sensitive AQP-2 water channel in rat kidney. Am J Physiol 1996; 270: F657–F668.
58. Frøkiær J, Christensen BM, Marples D et al. Downregulation of aquaporin-2 parallels changes in renal water excretion in unilateral ureteral obstruction. Am J Physiol 1997; 273: F213–F223.
59. Li C, Wang W, Kwon TH et al. Downregulation of AQP1, -2 and -3 after ureteral obstruction is associated with a long-term urine-concentrating defect. Am J Physiol 2001; 281: F163–F171.
60. Li C, Wang W, Kwon TH et al. Altered expression of major renal Na transporters in rats with bilateral ureteral obstruction and release of obstruction. Am J Physiol 2003; 285: F889–F901.
61. Li C, Wang W, Knepper MA, Nielsen S, Frøkiær J. Downregulation of renal aquaporins in response to unilateral ureteral obstruction. Am J Physiol 2003; 284: F1066–F1079.
62. Li C, Wang W, Knepper MA, Nielsen S, Frøkiær J. Altered expression of major renal Na transporters in rats with unilateral ureteral obstruction. Am J Physiol 2003; 284: F155–F166.
63. Gillenwater JY, Westervelt FBJ, Vaughan EDJ, Howards SS. Renal function after release of chronic unilateral hydronephrosis in man. Kidney Int 1975; 7: 179–86.
64. Harris RH, Yarger WE. Renal function after release of unilateral ureteral obstruction in rats. Am J Physiol 1974; 227: 806–15.
65. Vander AJ, Miller R. Control of renin secretion in the anaesthetized dog. Am J Physiol 1964; 207: 537–46.
66. Vander EJ. Renin secretion during mannitol diuresis and ureteral occlusion. Proc Soc Exp Biol Med 1968; 128: 518–20.
67. Blackshear JL, Wathen RL. Effects of indomethacin on renal blood flow and renin secretory responses to ureteral occlusion in the dog. Min Electrol Metab 1978; 1: 271–8.
68. Vaughan ED Jr, Sweet RC, Gillenwater JY. Peripheral renin and blood pressure changes following complete unilateral ureteral occlusion. J Urol 1970; 104: 89–92.
69. Moody TE, Vaughan ED, Wykder AT, Gillenwater JY. The role of intrarenal angiotensin II in the hemodynamic response to unilateral obstructive uropathy. Invest Urol 1977; 14: 390–7.
70. Yarger WE, Schocken DD, Harris RH. Obstructive nephropathy in the rat. Possible roles for renin–angiotensin system, prostaglandins, and thromboxane in postobstructive renal function. J Clin Invest 1980; 65: 400–12.
71. McDougal WS. Pharmacologic preservation of renal mass and function in obstructive uropathy. J Urol 1982; 128: 418–21.
72. Carmines PK, Tanner GA. Angiotensin in the hemodynamic response to chronic nephron obstruction. Am J Physiol 1983; 245: F75–F82.

73. Chevalier RL, Peach MJ. Hemodynamic effects of enalapril on neonatal chronic partial ureteral obstruction. Kidney Int 1985; 28: 891–8.
74. Chevalier RL, Iones CE. Contribution of endogenous vasoactive compounds to renal vascular resistance in neonatal chronic partial ureteral obstruction. J Urol 1986; 136: 532–5.
75. Huland H, Leichtweiss HP, Augustin HJ. Effect of angiotensin II agonist, alpha-receptor blockade and denervation on blood flow reduction in experimental hydronephrosis. Invest Urol 1980; 18: 46–9.
76. Vaughan ED Jr, Marion D, Felsen D. Evidence against angiotensin II (AII) or thromboxane A_2 (TxA2) as mediators of the increased renal vascular resistance (RVR) found following unilateral ureteral occlusion (UUO). Kidney Int 1986; 30: 237A.
77. Huguenin M, Ott CE, Romero JC, Knox FG. Influence of renin depletion on renal function after release of twenty-four hour ureteral obstruction. J Lab Clin Med 1976; 87: 58–63.
78. El-Dahr SS, Gomez RA, Gray MS et al. In situ localization of renin and its mRNA in neonatal ureteral obstruction. Am J Physiol 1990; 258: F854–F862.
79. El-Dahr SS, Gomez RA, Khare G et al. Expression of renin and its mRNA in the adult rat kidney with chronic ureteral obstruction. Am J Kidney Dis 1990; 15: 575–82.
80. Campbell DJ. Circulating and tissue angiotensin systems. J Clin Invest 1987; 79: 1–6.
81. Rosivall L, Narkates AJ, Oparil S, Navar LG. De novo intrarenal formation of angiotensin II during control and enhanced renin secretion. Am J Physiol 1987; 252: F1118–F1123.
82. Inagami T, Mizuno K, Naruse K, Okamura T, Kawamutel M. Intracellular formation and release of angiotensins from juxtaglomerular cells. Kidney Int 1990; 38 (Suppl 30): S33–S37.
83. Mitchell KD, Navar LG. Interactive effects of angiotensin II on renal hemodynamics and tubular reabsorptive function. Kidney Int 1990; 38 (Suppl 30): 869–73.
84. Ichikawa I, Harris RC. Angiotensin actions in the kidney: renewed insight into the old hormone. Kidney Int 1991; 40: 583–96.
85. El-Dahr SS, Gee J, Dipp S et al. Upregulation of reninangiotensin system and downregulation of kallekrein in obstructive nephropathy. Am J Physiol 1993; 264: F874–F881.
86. Pimentel JL Jr, Martinez-Maldonado M, Wilcox JN, Wang S, Luo C. Regulation of renin-angiotensin system in unilateral ureteral obstruction. Kidney Int 1993; 44: 390–400.
87. Pimentel JL Jr, Wang S, Martinez-Maldonado M. Regulation of the renal angiotensin II receptor gene in acute unilateral ureteral obstruction. Kidney Int 1994; 45: 1614–21.
88. Allen JT, Vaughan ED Jr, Gillenwater JY. The effect of indomethacin on renal blood flow and ureteral pressure in unilateral ureteral obstruction in awake dogs. Invest Urol 1978; 15: 324–7.
89. Frøkiær J, Nielsen AS, Knudsen L, Djurhuus JC, Pedersen EB. The effect of indomethacin infusion on renal hemodynamics and on the renin-angiotensin system during unilateral ureteral obstruction of the pig. J Urol 1993; 150: 1557–63.
90. Perlmutter A, Miller L, Trimble L et al. Toradol, a NSAID used for renal colic, decreases renal perfusion and ureteral pressure in a canine model of unilateral ureteral obstruction. J Urol 1993; 149: 926–32.
91. Nishikawa K, Morrison AR, Needleman P. Exaggerated prostaglandin biosynthesis and its influence on renal resistance in isolated hydronephrotic rabbit kidney. J Clin Invest 1977; 59: 1143–50.
92. Morrison AR, Nishikawa K, Needleman P. Unmasking of thromboxane A2 synthesis by ureteral obstruction in rabbit kidney. Nature 1977; 267: 259–60.
93. Strand JC, Edwards BS, Anderson ME, Romero JC, Knox FG. Effect of imidazole on renal function in renal function in unilateral ureteral obstructed rat kidneys. Am J Physiol 1981; 240: F508–F514.
94. Kawasaki A, Needleman P. Contribution of thromboxane to renal resistance changes in the isolated perfused hydronephrotic rabbit kidney. Circ Res 1982; 50: 486–90.
95. Purkerson ML, Klahr S. Prior inhibition of vasoconstrictors normalizes GFR in postobstructed kidneys. Kidney Int 1989; 35: 1306–14.
96. Loo MH, Marion DN, Vaughan ED Jr, Felsen D, Athanese CT. Effect of thromboxane inhibition on renal blood flow in dogs with complete unilateral ureteral obstruction. Urology 1986; 136: 1343–47.
97. Loo MH, Egan D, Vaughan ED Jr, Marion DN, Felsen D, Weisman SM. The effect of thromboxane A_2 synthesis inhibitor OKY-046 on renal function in rabbits following release of unilateral ureteral obstruction. J Urol 1987; 137: 571–6.
98. Okegawa T, Jonas PE, DeSchryver K, Kawasaki A, Needleman P. Metabolic and cellular alterations underlying the exaggerated renal prostaglandin and thromboxane synthesis in ureter obstructed rabbits. Inflammatory response involving fibroblasts and mononuclear cells. J Clin Invest 1983; 71: 81–90.
99. Lefkowith JB, Okegawa T, DeSchryver K, Needleman P. Macrophage-dependent arachidonate metabolism in hydronephrosis. Kidney Int 1984; 26: 10–17.
100. Harris KPG, Schreiner GF, Klahr S. Effect of leucocyte depletion on the function of the postobstructed kidney in the rat. Kidney Int 1989; 36: 20–215.
101. Himmelstein SI, Coffman TM, Yarger WE, Klotman PE. Atrial natriuretic peptide-induced changes in renal prostacyclin production in ureteral obstruction. Am J Physiol 1990; 258: F281–F286.
102. Purkerson ML, Blaine EH, Stokes TJ, Klahr S. Role of atrial peptide in the natriuresis and diuresis that follows relief of obstruction in rat. Am J Physiol 1989; 256: F583–F589.
103. Freid TA, Lau AT, Ayon MA, Stein JH. Elevation of ANP levels in ureteral obstruction in the rat. Clin Res 1986; 34: 204A.
104. Gulmi FA, Mooppan UMM, Chou S, Kim H. Atrial natriuretic peptide in patients with obstructive uropathy. J Urol 1989; 142: 268–72.

105. Yamamoto A, Keil LC, Reid IA. Activation of renal mechanoreceptors increases vasopressin release in rabbits. Am J Physiol 1991; 261: R484–R490.
106. Reyes AA, Lefkowith JB, Pippin J, Klahr S. Role of the 5-lipoxygenase pathway in obstructive nephropathy. Kidney Int 1992; 41: 100–6.
107. Chevalier RL, Thornhill BA, Gomez RA. EDRF modulates renal hemodynamics during unilateral obstruction in the rat. Kidney Int 1992; 42: 400–6.
108. Reyes AA, Klahr S. Renal function after release of ureteral obstruction: role of endothelin and the renal artery endothelium. Kidney Int 1992; 42: 632–8.
109. Kaneto H, Morrissey J, Klahr S. Increased expression of TGF-β1 mRNA in the obstructed kidney of rats with unilateral ureteral ligation. Kidney Int 1993; 44: 313–21.
110. Kaneto H, Morrissey J, McCracken R, Reyes AA, Klahr S. Enalapril reduces collagen type IV synthesis and expansion of the interstitium in the obstructed rat kidney. Kidney Int 1994; 45: 1637–47.
111. Storch S, Saggi S, Megyesi J, Price PM, Safirstein R. Ureteral obstruction decreases renal prepro-epidermal growth factor and Tamm-Horsfall expression. Kidney Int 1992; 42: 89–94.
112. Walton G, Buttayn R, Garcia-Montes E et al. Renal growth factor expression during the early phase of experimental hydronephrosis. J Urol 1992; 48: 510–14.
113. Felsen D, Schulsinger D, Gross SS et al. Renal hemodynamic and ureteral pressure changes in response to ureteral obstruction: the role of nitric oxide. J Urol 2003; 169: 373–6.
114. Klahr S. Urinary tract obstruction. Semin Nephrol 2001; 21: 133–45.
115. Trachtman H, Futterweit S, Garg P, Reddy K, Singhal PC. Nitric oxide stimulates the activity of a 72-kDa neutral matrix metalloproteinase in cultured rat mesangial cells. Biochem Biophys Res Commun 1996; 218: 704–8.
116. Reyes AA, Martin D, Settle S, Klahr S. EDRF role in renal function and blood pressure of normal rats and rats with obstructive uropathy. Kidney Int 1992; 41: 403–13.
117. Hautmann RE. Urinary diversion: ileal conduit to neobladder. J Urol 2003; 169: 834–42.
118. Mills RD, Studer UE. Metabolic consequences of continent urinary diversion. J Urol 1999; 161: 1057–66.
119. Skinner DG, Studer UE, Okada K et al. Which patients are suitable for continent diversion or bladder substitution following cystectomy or other definitive local treatment? Int J Urol 1995; Suppl 2: 105.
120. Ekman H, Jacobsen G, Kock NG, Sundin T. The functional behavior of different types of intestinal urinary bladder substitutes. Paris, XIII Cong Soc Int d'Ueol 1964; 11: 213.
121. Wenderoth, UK, Bachor, R, Egghart G et al. The ileal neobladder: experience and results of more than 100 consecutive cases. J Urol 1990; 143: 492–7.
122. Berglund B, Kock NG, Norlén L, Philipson BM. Volume capacity and pressure characteristics of the continent ileal reservoir used for urinary diversion. J Urol 1987; 137: 29–34.
123. Kock NG, Nilson AE, Nicisson LO, Norldn LJ, Philipsson BM. Urinary diversion via a continent ileal reservoir: clinical results in 12 patients. J Urol 1982; 128: 469–75.
124. Kock NG, Ghoncim MA, Lycke KG, Mahran MR. Replacement of the bladder by the urethral Kock pouch: functional results, urodynamics and radiological features. J Urol 1989; 141: 1111–16.
125. Studer UE, Danuser H, Thalmann GN, Springer JP, Turner WH. Antireflux nipples or afferent tubular segments in 70 patients with ileal low pressure bladder substitutes: long-term results prospective randomized trial. J Urol 1996; 156: 1913–17.
126. Pantuck AJ, Han KR, Perrotti M, Weiss RE, Cummings KB. Ureteroenteric anastomosis in continent urinary diversion: long-term results and complications of direct versus nonrefluxing techniques. J Urol 2000; 163: 450–5.
127. Abd-el-Gawad G, Abrahamsson K, Hanson E. Kock urinary reservoir maturation in children and adolescents: consequences for kidney and upper urinary tract. Eur Urol 1999; 36: 443–9.
128. Neat DE, Hawkins T, Gailaugher AS, Ewnhigh DM, Hall RR. The role of ileal conduit in the development of upper tract dilatation. Br J Urol 1985; 57: 520–4.
129. Pitts WR Jr, Muecke EC. A 20-year experience with ileal conduits: the fate of the kidneys. J Urol 1979; 122: 154–7.
130. Madersbacher S, Schmidt J, Eberle JM et al. Long-term outcome of ileal conduit diversion. J Urol 2003; 169: 985–90.
131. Neal DE. Urodynamic investigation of the ileal conduit: upper tract dilatation and the effects of revision of the conduit. J Urol 1989; 142: 97–100.
132. Kock NG. Continent ileostomy. Progr Suig 1973; 12: 180.
133. Noll E, Schreiter E, Borkowsky J, Schweim FRG. Is Kock's nipple valve really antirefluxive? J Urol 1989; 141: 304A.
134. Kristjansson A, Wallin L, Mansson W. Renal function up to 16 years after conduit (refluxing or antireflux anastomosis) or continent urinary diversion. 1. Glomerular filtration rate and patency of uretero-intestinal anastomosis. Br J Urol 1995; 76: 539–45.
135. Paiss T, Gschwend J, Gottfried W, Hautmann RE. Die Signifikanz der Bakteriuria bei der Ileum-Neoblase. Der Urologe, 1995; 1: 49.
136. Åkerlund S, Campanello M, Kaijser B, Jonsson O. Bacteriuria in patients with a continent ileal reservoir for urinary diversion does not regularly require antibiotic treatment. Br J Urol 1994; 74: 177–81.
137. Wullt B, Holst E, Colleen S, Månsson W. Microbial ecology of the lower urinary tract on patients with colonic neobladders. J Urol 1997; 157: 235.
138. Koff SA, Mutabagani KH, Jayanthi VR. The valve bladder syndrome: pathophysiology and treatment with nocturnal bladder emptying. J Urol 2002; 167: 291–7.
139. Soloway MS, Meyers GH Jr, Johnston G, Ketcham A. Renography in the evaluation of patients with ileal conduits. Surg Gynecol Obstet 1972; 135: 521–5.
140. Wilson KS, Doig A, Fowler JW. Renography in the assessment of patients with uretero-sigmoid diversion. Br J Urol 1977; 49: 195–8.

141. Chen KK, Chang LS, Chen MT, Yeh SH. Prospective radionuclide renal function evaluation and its correlation with radiological findings in patients with Kock pouch urinary diversion. J Urol 1991; 145: 952–5.
142. Britton KE, Nimmon CC, Whitfield HN, Hendry WE. Obstructive nephropathy: successful evaluation with radio nuclides. Lancet 1979; i: 905–7.
143. Whitfield HN, Britton KE, Kelsey I et al. The obstructed kidney: correlation between renal function and urodynamical assessment. Br J Urol 1977; 49: 615–19.
144. Hay AM, Norman W, Rice ML, Stevenson RD. A comparison between diuresis renography and the Whitaker test in 64 kidneys. Br J Urol 1984; 56: 561–4.
145. Djurhuus JC, Sørensen SS, Jørgensen TM, Jensen ET. Predictive value of pressure flow studies for the functional outcome of reconstructive surgery for hydronephrosis. Br J Urol 1985; 57: 6–9.
146. Poulsen EU, Frøkiær J, Jensen ET et al. Diuresis renography and simultaneous renal pelvic pressure in hydronephrosis. J Urol 1987; 138: 272–5.
147. Neal DE, Simpson W, Bartholomew P, Keavey PM. Comparison of dynamic computed tomography, diuresis renography and DTPA parenchymas transit time in the assessment of dilation of the upper urinary tract. Br J Urol 1985; 57: 515–19.
148. Piepsz A, Ham HR, Thoua JL. Sensitivity of cortical transit and furosemide response in the diagnosis of renal obstruction. An experimental model. Uremia Invest 1986; 9: 245–8.
149. Hunter GJ, Gordon I, Sweeney L, Tood-Pokropek A, Ransly PG. ^{99m}Tc-DTPA scanning with diuretic washout. Is it useful in the investigation of obstruction in the presence of gross renal tract dilatation. Br J Urol 59: 208–10.
150. Rehling M, Frøkiær J, Poulsen EU et al. ^{99m}Tc-MAG$_3$ kinetics in the normal pig. A comparison to ^{131}I-Iothalamate after single and during continuous infusion. Clin Physiol 1995; 15: 57–71.
151. O'Reilly PH, Testa T, Lawson RS, Farrar DJ and Chariton Edwards E. Diuresis renography in equivocal urinary tract obstruction. Br J Urol 1978; 50: 76–80.
152. Månnson W, Mattiasson A, White T. Acute effects of full urinary bladder and full caecal urinary reservoir on regional renal function. Scand J Urol Nephrol 1984; 18: 299–306.
153. Månsson W, Ahlgren G, White T. Glomerular filtration rate up to 10 years after urinary diversion of different types. Scand J Urol Nephrol 23: 195–200.
154. Yarger WE. Urinary tract obstruction. In: Brenner BM, Rector EC Jr (eds). The Kidney. 4th edn. Philadelphia: WB Saunders, 1991: 1765–1808.
155. McDougal WS, Koch MO. Accurate determination of renal function in patients with intestinal urinary diversions. Urology 1986; 135: 1175–8.
156. Kock NG, Nilsson AE, Norlén L, Sundin T, Trasti H. Changes in renal parenchyma and the upper urinary tracts following urinary diverson via a continent ileum reservoir. An experimental study in dogs. Scand J Urol Nephrol 1978; (Suppl 49): 11–22.
157. Richie JP, Skinner, DG, Waisman J. The effect of reflux on the development of pyelonephritis in urinary diversion: and experimental study. J Surg Res 1974; 16: 256.
158. Richie JR, Skinner DO. Urinary diversion: the physiological rationale for non-refluxing oolonic conduits. Br J Urol 1975; 47: 269–75.
159. Redman JF. Histologic study of kidneys drained by short ileal conduits in dogs. Invest Urol 24: 185–8.
160. Boyd SD, Skinner DG, Lieskovsky G, Kawachi MH, Ahlering TE. Study of antireflux nipple valves of Kock ileal urinary reservoir. Invest Urol 1991; 37: 80–7.
161. St Clair SR, Hixson CJ, Ritchey ML. Enterocystoplasty and reflux nephropathy in the canine model. J Urol 1992; 148: 728–32.
162. Nasrallah PE, Aliabadi HA. Bladder augmentation in patients with neurogenic bladder and vesicoureteral reflux. J Urol 1991; 146: 563–6.

8 Bone mineralization after urinary diversion

Thomas Davidsson, Karl Obrant, Birger Lindergård

Introduction

Metabolic bone disease following urinary diversion seems to have been first described by Turner,[1] who in 1929 reported an 18-year-old boy with generalized rickets developing 10 years after implantation of the ureters into the sigmoid colon because of congenital bladder defect. Turner, however, was unaware of a link between the rickets and the urinary diversion. The possibility of bone complications in patients with urinary diversion was first recognized by Boyd[2] when in 1931 he reported a 10-year-old boy who 3 years previously had undergone similar ureteric transplantation due to exstrophy of the bladder and 2 years later had developed active rickets as well as chronic acidosis, hypocalcemia, hypophosphatemia and nitrogen retention. The rickets resisted treatment with vitamin D until it was combined with large doses of sodium bicarbonate. Rickets and osteomalacia belong to a group of metabolic bone diseases with varying pathogenesis and characterized by deficient mineralization of osteoid (Box 8.1). Rickets involves widening of the growth plate in the distal ends of long bones, whereas in osteomalacia, mineralization is impaired in the cortical and cancellous bone when growth has ceased (Figure 8.1).

Utilization of relatively long bowel segments for reconstructive surgery of the urinary tract in children or adults has focused interest on anticipated metabolic disturbances due to absorption of solutes across the gut mucosa. Although no clinical problems seem to arise while renal function remains normal, careful metabolic study of patients with bowel segments incorporated into the urinary tract reveals compensated chronic hyperchloremic metabolic acidosis.[3] Even subtle changes in electrolytes and acid–base balance can have negative long-term

BOX 8.1 PATHOGENESIS OF OSTEOMALACIA AND RICKETS

Abnormal vitamin D metabolism
- Vitamin D deficiency
- Inadequate dermal production of vitamin D_3
- Inadequate hepatic synthesis of 25-hydroxyvitamin D_3
- Defective renal synthesis of 1,25-dihydroxyvitamin D_3
- Defective end-organ response to 1,25-dihydroxyvitamin D_3
- Renal loss of vitamin D-binding protein

Phosphate deficiency
- Diminished phosphate intake
- Impaired renal tubular absorption of phosphate

Defects in mineralization
- Enzyme deficiency
- Circulating inhibitors of calcification
- Abnormal bone collagen or matrix

States of rapid bone formation

Miscellaneous
- Parenteral alimentation
- Gastrectomy
- Hyperchloremic metabolic acidosis

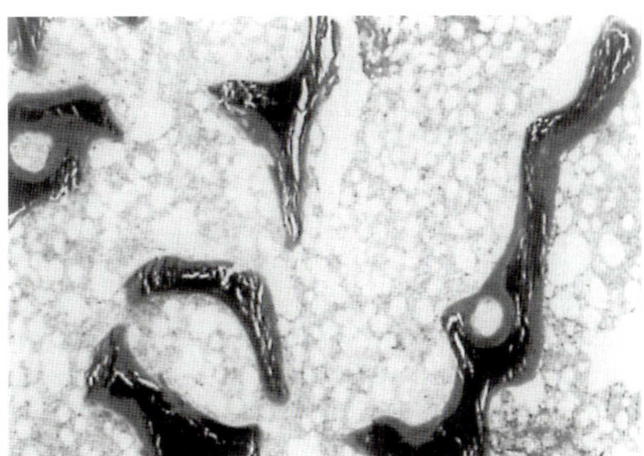

Figure 8.1 Light microscopy of undecalcified stained bone biopsy, showing amounts of osteoid (grey) close to the mineralized bone (black) in a patient with intestinal urinary diversion and osteomalacia. The light large areas are fat.

effects. The acid–base homeostatic functions in such patients and the associated metabolic derangements are not fully understood. Increased incidence of complications in orthopedic manipulations and effects on linear growth and skeletal development have been described.[4,5] Understanding of the pathophysiology of metabolic bone disease following urinary diversion requires knowledge of both normal bone metabolism and normal systemic acid–base homeostasis.

Bone physiology

Bone consists of an inorganic, or mineral, component and an organic, non-mineral, component. The mineral component provides structural stability for the skeleton and has well-known and important ionic homeostatic functions in the body.[6] The organic component consists of a matrix with dispersed osteoid and various types of bone cells. The mineral phase, comprising about two-thirds of the total bone volume, contains small crystals with an X-ray diffraction pattern of hydroxyapatite, structural formula $Ca_{10}(PO_4)_6(OH)_2$.[6] The surface area of these crystals, ~200 m^2/g,[7] is a prerequisite for ready participation of bone tissue in many physiological processes.[8,9] Hydroxyapatite is thought to be the final product of the complex and incompletely understood process of bone mineralization. The mineral phase of bone contains 99% of the body's calcium, 85% of its phosphorus and 40–60% of the total body sodium and magnesium.[10] Ion fluxes in and out of bone are therefore an important factor in the homeostatic regulation of these vital minerals.[9,11–13] The bone carbonic dioxide store, together with the surface bonded ions, sodium and potassium, have crucial roles in buffering of hydrogen ions during metabolic acidosis,[9,14,15] as has bone-derived phosphate when utilized by the kidneys for buffering hydrogen ions in urine.

Osteoid, which is mostly young bone tissue, consists mainly of type I collagen, but also of non-collagen proteins such as osteocalcin and osteonectin. Because the concentration of these proteins increases with activity of bone formation, they can be used as markers of bone metabolism.

The bone cells of the organic phase are of four principal types – osteoclasts, osteoblasts, osteocytes and lining cells.[16–18] The osteoclasts are giant multinucleated cells, derived from hematopoietic stem cells, which can reabsorb bone at the ruffled borders, after which release of calcium from the mineralized bone matrix (cell-mediated calcium release) and degradation of collagenous matrix occur. Many systemic and local factors can influence osteoclast function. Parathyroid hormone stimulates osteoclasts and resorption of mineral bone and calcitonin inhibits this function.[17–19]

The osteoblasts are mononucleated cells derived from stromal precursors of the bone marrow. They synthesize bone matrix – osteoid – which in time becomes mineralized. In bone biopsies, osteoblasts are seen close to osteoid seams. Differentiation from preosteoblasts to mature cells is stimulated by thyroid, parathyroid and growth hormones and prostaglandins, but inhibited by estrogen and corticosteroids. The mature osteoblast is stimulated by the same hormones[17,18] as the preosteoblasts but also by estrogen. The osteocytes arise from active osteoblasts, which during the period of bone matrix synthesis and mineralization, become surrounded by, or incorporated into, the bone matrix. The osteocytes occupy spaces within bone and are linked together by numerous cytoplasmic processes which pass through canaliculi. The mineral phase immediately around the osteocytes is thought to be amorphous, thus facilitating transport of calcium and other ions. The main function of osteocytes appears to be utilization of the amorphous mineral phase as a calcium reservoir, but they also contribute to initiation of bone resorption and to the repair of microfractures.[18,20,21]

The bone-lining cells form a continuous flat layer on the inner surface of bone, surrounding marrow and blood vessels. The exact function of these cells is not known, but they are thought to assist in the interchange of water and ions between the mineral and marrow compartments.[16]

Macroscopically, bone has cancellous and cortical components. Cancellous bone contains a network of trabeculae and predominates in areas such as vertebrae, osseous pelvis, distal radius and the femoral neck. The shaft of long bones is cortical bone. Although the bony skeleton is only 20% cancellous, the skeletal metabolism is evenly distributed between the two types, as cancellous bone is metabolically more active. The response to metabolic and other forms of stress differs accordingly. In periods of high bone turnover, as in fracture healing, the normal lamellar bone is replaced by woven bone, in which the collagen fibrils are disorganized and the mechanical properties consequently inferior.[18,22] Normal formation of new bone is complex and not yet fully understood. The osteoblasts synthesize the organic matrix, or osteoid. This matrix then undergoes a 10–15 day maturation process, after which mineralization of the osteoid occurs in the vicinity of previously mineralized bone. For normal mineralization, the osteoid must be quantitatively and qualitatively normal. Calcium and phosphate are thought to be present in supersaturated state in the extracellular fluid, but it is not known if the formed mineral results from phase transformation of this amorphous matrix or from a physicochemical process with formation of amorphous calcium phosphate. Normal mineralization is regulated by numerous local and systemic factors – ion concentrations, calciotrophic hormones, growth factors and pH at the mineralization site,[6,16,23] and any deviation from physiologic norms will influence the process. Thus decreased availability of calcium or phosphates, or both, can lead to derangement of mineralization and ultimately metabolic bone disease, the sites most affected being those with highest bone turnover. Throughout life the skeleton constantly undergoes renewal and repair.[24] The modeling process in childhood and adolescence, when the skeleton is growing and rapidly reshaping, gives way to remodeling when growth has ceased. This remodeling is a continuous process, responsible for maintenance of the normal structure and mechanical integrity of the osseous structure. In the adult skele-

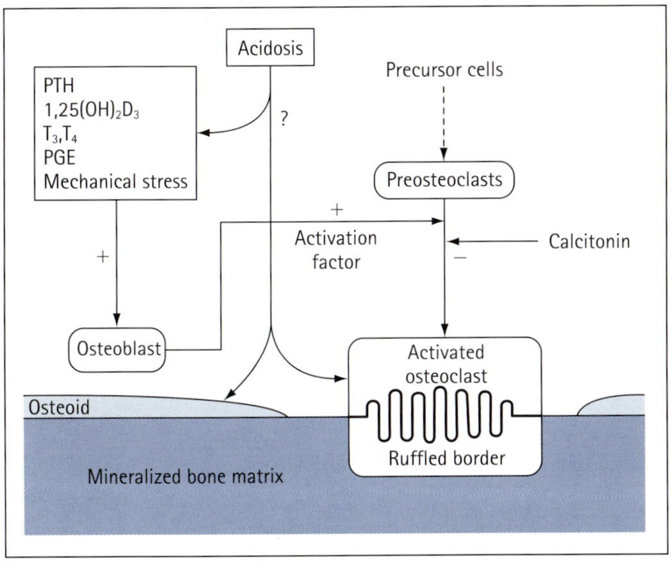

Figure 8.2 Hypothetical overview of the interactive factors influencing bone metabolism. PTH, parathyroid hormone; $1{,}25(OH)_2D_3$, 1,25-dihydroxyvitamin D_3; T_3, triiodothyronine; T_4, thyroxine. PGE, prostaglandin E. (Adapted from Vaes G. Clin Orthop 1988; 231: 239–71[19] with permission from Lippincott Williams & Wilkins)

ton, about 20% of the bone is involved in the remodeling process each year. Defective mineralization can therefore be manifest in both children and adults.

Normal coupling between resorption and formation of bone guarantees balance between the amount removed and the amount produced. Imbalance of this physiologic coupling, the mechanism of which is not clear, can damage, or even enhance, the skeletal structure. Cortical bone is bounded exteriorly by periosteum and interiorly by endosteum. As periosteal bone accretion exceeds bone resorption, while the reverse applies to the endosteum, there is a net increase of outer diameter and of bone marrow with age.[25] Since bone contains almost all of the body's calcium, all factors that affect calcium homeostasis will directly or indirectly influence bone-cell metabolism and thereby modeling and remodeling. Regulation of these functions is intricate, due to profound interactions, many of which seem to be influenced by changes in acid–base balance (Figure 8.2).

Bone mineral assessment

Densitometry – measurement of bone mass – is useful for assessing bone mineralization and estimating fracture risk at specific sites in individual patients. The method is also helpful for evaluating changes in skeletal mineralization in various bone and metabolic diseases. The findings are expressed as bone mineral content (BMC) g/cm of ashed bone/cm of axial length, or normalized for bone diameter as bone mineral density (BMD) g/cm^2.[26,27]

The original standard method for densitometry measured the attenuation of a photon beam from an isotopic source passing through bone. Single photon absorptiometry (SPA) utilizes attenuation of a single photon beam, and is most useful for measurements at the distal appendicular skeleton, where soft tissue is negligible and controllable. To overcome the problem of soft tissues, a technique utilizing two photon beams with two different wavelengths has been developed, one beam absorbed mainly by the soft tissue and the other by bone mineral. This technique is known as dual photon bone absorptiometry (DPA). A major advance on SPA and DPA technology was achieved by substituting an X-ray source for the isotopic source. The advantages of these new techniques – single-energy and dual-energy X-ray absorptiometry (SXA and DEXA, respectively) – are greater precision and accuracy, together with lower radiation dose and shorter scanning times.[26,28,29]

In densitometric assessment the mineral component of skeletal bone is 99% calcium. The total body calcium increases from 20–30 g at birth to around 1500 g at the age of 20 years. Illness or other factors that interfere with normal growth and mineral deposition may result in deficit bone mass, and consequently of calcium, in the growing skeleton.[30] Reduced peak bone mass can predispose to skeletal problems later in life.[31] The main usefulness of bone-mineral measurements is in adult life after peak bone mass has been reached. Most metabolic bone disorders affect cancellous bone more than cortical bone, due to higher turnover and metabolic activity in the former type. Densitometry can provide good estimates of bone mineral content in different sites, depending on the type of equipment. It is useful in surveillance of patients at risk of metabolic bone problems,[32] for evaluating their response to treatment, and for estimating the risk of fracture at specific sites.[33] Although the information on bone mineral content does not include changes in bone-cell function or in the mechanical properties of bone related to age or disease, it is helpful for investigating in vivo bone function at organ level.

Bone histomorphometry

The cornerstone in study of metabolic bone disease at cellular level is histomorphometric analysis of bone. Biopsies are usually taken under local anesthesia from the iliac crest, following double tetracycline labeling. The bone core is fixed in alcohol and then embedded in plastic to facilitate cutting with a heavy-duty microtome. The sections are stained and studied under the light microscope (see Figure 8.1). Unstained sections are examined with fluorescent microscopy to judge the tetracycline labeling. The aims of the analysis are systematic morphological and quantitative evaluation of bone cells, detection of possible imbalance in the resorption–formation coupling process, and estimation of the percentage distribution of unmineralized/mineralized bone.[34] Incorporation of tetracycline as a time marker provides information on the dynamic processes of the remodeling system in bone disease.[35]

The primary static parameters in bone histomorphometry include the following: trabecular bone volume (BV), expressed as mm^3/mm^3, i.e. the amount of mineralized/unmineralized trabecular bone; the osteoid volume (OV) as a percentage or mm^3/mm^3, describing the fraction of a given BV which is osteoid; the osteoid surface (OS), expressed as a percentage of BV surface covered with osteoid, i.e. unmineralized bone matrix; and the resorption surface (RS), which is the fraction (%) of bone surface covered with resorption lacunae and osteoclasts or with osteoclasts only.

The dynamic parameters include the mineral apposition rate (MAR), expressed in mm/day, measuring the average distance between the tetracycline double-labeled surfaces, i.e. where tetracycline stains the mineralization front, because of its affinity for newly formed bone mineral. In addition to the static and dynamic primary measurements, many derived indices can be calculated which can be useful for highlighting specific concerns.[36]

Acid–base physiology

To maintain a stable acid–base balance the kidney must excrete the net acid generated in metabolic production of non-volatile acid. The net acid excretion in the urine averages 1 mmol H^+/kg bodyweight daily. To stabilize serum pH and serum bicarbonate concentration, the kidney has two main mechanisms in acidification of the urine. One is reabsorption of about 75% of the filtered HCO_3^- from the lumen of the proximal tubules, and the other is to regenerate new HCO_3^- to replace that used in the extrarenal buffering of acid. The latter process takes place in the distal tubular cells by the influence of carbonic anhydrase, and the H^+ produced is secreted along the collecting tubule. This H^+ is excreted in urine as free hydrogen ion, ammonium and titrable acid. The free hydrogen excretion is negligible, and in normal conditions the ammonium excretion accounts for two-thirds and the titrable acid for one-third of the acid excretion. Titrable acids include the phosphate buffers, creatinine and other weak organic acids, with phosphate predominating. In the tubular lumen dihydrogen phosphate is formed, due to excess of H^+. Ammonia (NH_3) diffuses readily into the tubular lumen, where it binds to H^+ to form ammonium (NH_4^+). Both $H_2PO_4^-$ and NH_4^+ permeate poorly across the renal tubular cell membrane and therefore remain in the urine.[37–39]

Urinary diversion and acid–base homeostasis

The mucosa of ileal and colonic intestinal segments incorporated into the urinary tract undergoes atrophic changes.[40,41] Although the absorptive capacity of this atrophic mucosa is thought to undergo time-related decrease, considerable absorptive function remains.[42–44] Studies have even negated the effect of histological changes on the reabsorption of ions.[43] Patients with urinary diversion are therefore predisposed, both in the short term and in the long term, to complications arising from reabsorption of solutes and waste products from the urine. The risk of hyperchloremic metabolic acidosis associated with urinary diversion has been recognized since the early 1950s.[45–47] The endogenous chronic load derives mainly from reabsorption of NH_4^+ from urine, probably through potassium pathways in the intestinal mucosa.[48,49] Chloride reabsorption from urine balances the ammonium transport, thereby maintaining electrical neutrality. Reabsorption of hydrogen ions, organic acids and mucosal bicarbonate secreted into the urine accounts for only a minor portion of the acid load. If the renal function is normal, the acidosis seems clinically to be well compensated, but closer study shows variably compensated hyperchloremic metabolic acidosis.[3] Base excess is usually within normal range when renal function is normal, but hyperchloremia is often found when intestinal segments of considerable length are incorporated into the urinary tract.[3,50] The handling of solutes by interposed gut can vary according to the origin of the segment.

Because of the constant endogenous acid load in patients with urinary intestinal diversion, the normal mechanism for excretion of non-volatile acids is impaired, thus increasing the importance of the titrable acids in acid–base homeostasis.[39,48] During acidosis parathyroid hormone may enhance the clearance of phosphate and so increase the amount of titrable acid.[51] In the acute situation, metabolic acidosis is modified by serum and bone buffers and renal excretion of titrable acids.[14,48,52] The chronic acid load, causing increased excretion of titrable acids (phosphates) derived from bone mineral, may result in depletion of bone buffer stores, and this may influence the normal mineralization process. If the renal function is impaired, overt osteomalacia can develop. Fall in systemic pH can also influence the regulating processes of normal bone metabolism, as can a pH fall (i.e. reduced HCO_3^- concentration) in close proximity to the bone cells, affecting cell metabolism and hence mineralization.

Bone buffers

During acute metabolic acidosis about 60% of the acid load is buffered outside the extracellular fluid by soft tissues and by bone.[14] As bone contains large stores of sodium, potassium and phosphate and also approximately 80% of the body's total carbon dioxide in the form of CO_3^{2-} and HCO_3^-, these bone buffers obviously play an important part in the maintenance of stable acid–base homeostasis.[53]

The bone surface normally is coated with negative sites, which are occupied by positive ions – sodium, potassium and protons. Sodium and potassium are freely accessible to the surrounding fluid. In systemic acidosis with proton increase, sodium and potassium from the bone surface are thought to be exchanged for protons, thereby buffering the acidity.[53] In this way, bone acts as a direct hydrogen-ion buffer during acute acidotic load.[9,54]

The skeletal CO_2 store, the largest in the human body, is thought to be composed of two separate pools. Two-thirds of the bone carbonate is in the relatively inaccessible form of CO_3^{2-} and may be located in the lattice of bone crystals, with complex bonding to calcium, sodium and other cations. Its utilization is believed to require dissolution of bone, simultaneously releasing CO_3^{2-} and calcium. The other, more readily exchangeable third of the bone carbonate is presumed to be located in a hydration shell around the bone crystals, where it is available to the systemic circulation.[13,55] How the balance between CO_3^{2-} and HCO_3^- in bone mineral is maintained is unknown.

In acute metabolic acidosis, the extracellular HCO_3^- declines, due to buffering of the increased hydrogen-ion concentration. A fall in systemic HCO_3^- directly influences the concentration in the skeleton, as more HCO_3^- is needed for buffering. The readily exchangeable pool is thought to be first used for this short-term buffering, and little mineral is dissolved from bone. Experimental studies[9,56] have confirmed the depletion of skeletal CO_2 and surface sodium during increased hydrogen-ion concentration (Figure 8.3), although the buffering capacity of this mechanism and the exchangeable content of the ions in bone mineral remain to be determined.

In chronic metabolic acidosis, systemic pH and HCO_3^- can remain stable for long periods. The main buffer is thought to be HCO_3^-/CO_3^{2-}, derived from the CO_2 reservoir in skeletal bone. Utilization of HCO_3^-/CO_3^{2-} for buffering is accompanied by an efflux of calcium, due to dissolution of the mineral phase of bone. The mechanism by which acidosis induces dissolution of skeletal mineral is not fully known. It may be either a direct physicochemical effect of H^+ on bone, or an osteoclast-mediated mechanism[13] dependent on parathyroid hormone[57] and inhibited by calcitonin.[58] Further, it seems that HPO_4^- to some extent replaces the released CO_3^{2-}.[15] Calcium efflux from bone has also been suggested to depend on decreased bicarbonate concentration, and not only on reduced pH.[59] This assumption implies that patients with compensated chronic metabolic acidosis and low bicarbonate levels may be predisposed to bone calcium and phosphate depletion in the long term.

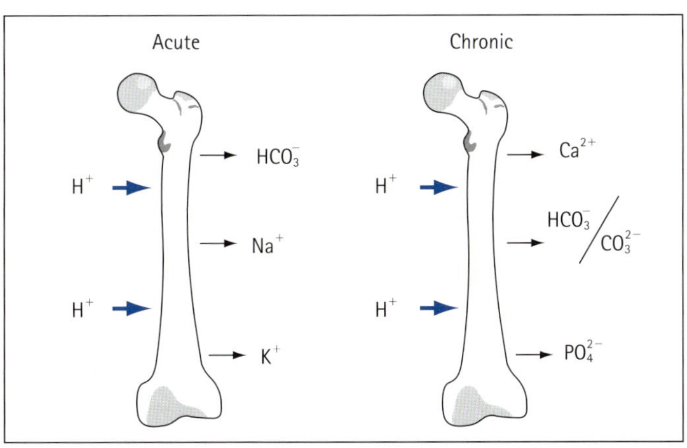

Figure 8.3 Schematic representation of skeletal bone response in acute and chronic metabolic acidosis.

Acidosis and bone mineralization

Osteomalacia and rickets have long been known to complicate chronic metabolic acidosis.[60] Three main causes of such acidosis can be associated with metabolic bone disease in humans, that is chronic uremia, defective tubular function (renal tubular acidosis) and urinary diversion utilizing bowel. Osteomalacia and rickets have been recognized in all three conditions.[61,62]

In chronic uremia the acid secretion is reduced by defective glomerular and tubular function, and histologic findings can include osteomalacia and osteitis fibrosa together with aplastic changes.[63] The etiology of uremic osteodystrophy is highly complex, involving metabolic acidosis, impaired metabolism of vitamin D and phosphates, and also secondary hyperparathyroidism. In renal tubular acidosis the defective acid secretion caused by tubular damage can lead to hyperchloremic metabolic acidosis.[37]

Osteomalacia and rickets can occur in patients with renal tubular acidosis but normal renal function.[64] If the GFR falls in these patients, however, the bones undergo changes resembling uremic osteodystrophy. The chronic endogenous acid load in patients with an intestinal segment incorporated into the urinary tract predisposes to hyperchloremic metabolic acidosis with electrolyte values similar to those in renal tubular acidosis.[65] If clinical signs of osteomalacia appear, the patient usually is severely acidotic, often as a result of impaired renal function.[66,67] These observations indicate that patients with urinary diversion can cope with the increased acid load as long as the renal function is normal, or that severe acidosis is required for production of bone disease. However, decreased appositional rate and increased trabecular bone volume has been found in cecal reservoir patients with normal renal function and normal pH implying that even compensated chronic metabolic acidosis can influence bone metabolism.[68] As mineralization of osteoid presumably occurs with calcium and phosphorus in supersaturated state,[6] any factor that alters the availability of these substances will influence the mineralization process. Metabolic bone disease is thought to be produced by diminished conversion from amorphous calcium phosphate to hydroxyapatite at the mineralization front.[69] In acidosis the critical factor for calcium efflux from bone mineral seems to be not the lowered pH per se, but the decrease in serum bicarbonate.[59] As mentioned earlier, the bicarbonate in bone is exchangeable with serum HCO_3^-/CO_3^{2-} and thus participates in the acid–base homeostasis.[15] Adequate mineralization requires quantitatively and qualitatively normal osteoid.[23] Although acidosis has been shown to impair bone formation,[70] its effect on osteoid is not known. Normal bone mineral metabolism also requires sufficient amounts of sodium, potassium, magnesium, zinc and fluoride incorporated in the bone crystals or bonded to their surface.

In patients with chronic metabolic acidosis but no intestinal segment in the urinary tract, the urinary excretion of calcium is increased,[71] while the intestinal absorption of calcium is normal or reduced. The hypercalciuria lowers the plasma calcium, which leads to increase of parathyroid hormone with resultant enhanced release of calcium and phosphate from bone.[51] Parathyroid hormone seems to augment the effect of chronic acidosis on calcium release from bone,[72] an effect that may be mediated by activation of carbonic anhydrase at the ruffled border of the osteoclasts. The action of parathyroid hormone on the kidney gives rise to hyperphosphaturia and hypophosphatemia, further impeding the attainment of calcium and phosphate supersaturation in bone matrix. Whether or not chronic acidosis disturbs the metabolism of vitamin D in the human kidney is still controversial.[73–75] Normal metabolism of vitamin D, however, is dependent on the renal function, as conversion of 25-hydroxyvitamin D_3 formed in the liver to 1,25-dihydroxyvitamin D_3 takes place in the proximal tubules.[76] Parathyroid hormone, calcium, phosphate and 1,25-dihydroxyvitamin D_3 are regarded as the main controlling factors of this renal conversion.

Urinary diversion and bone mineralization

Since the first report in 1929,[1] metabolic bone disease in patients with urinary intestinal diversion has attracted much interest.[2,65–67,77–80] The mechanism which induces rickets in children and osteomalacia in adults is not clear. As changes in acid–base balance influence the bone mineral metabolism, the hyperchloremic metabolic acidosis often seen in patients with such urinary diversion has been attributed a crucial role in the pathogenesis of defective mineralization.[13,65,81,82] The clinical features of overt disease include bone pain, proximal muscle weakness, waddling gait, fractures or pseudofractures, swelling of costochondral junctions (rachitic rosary) in children, bowing of the long bones and widening of the growth plate.[77,78,80] The spectrum of bone histomorphology runs from decreased bone turnover[68] without clinical problems to overt rickets or osteomalacia.[62,65–67,83] Recognition of the metabolic, electrolyte and acid–base balance complications associated with urinary intestinal diversion has minimized their occurrence, and overt osteomalacia is now rare. Early correction of a negative base excess with alkali only in patients with decreased renal function has shown good influence with no decrease in the bone mineral content in patients with ileal or colonic segments incorporated in the urinary tract.[84,85]

Despite the present rarity of serious effects on bone metabolism, it is possible that subtle disturbances of the normal mineralization process over a long period in patients with intestinal urinary diversion can lead to a reduced skeletal mineral content. The risk probably is greatest in children and women. Delayed linear growth was observed in children with enterocystoplasty.[86] Abnormal linear bone growth was more common in myelomeningocele patients with ileal or colonic conduit urinary diversion than in a group managed with clean intermittent catheterization, and the proportion of patients requiring surgical correction of spinal curvature and the incidence of complications from orthopedic procedures were higher in the conduit group.[4]

In patients with cecal reservoir or ileal or colonic conduit, bone biopsies showed histomorphological derangements.[68] Decreased appositional rate and increased trabecular bone volume in the cecal reservoir group compared with a reference group implicate decreased bone turnover. No effects were found on bone mineralization parameters or on the resorption surface (Table 8.1). In patients with ileal Kock urinary reservoir,[87] short-term longitudinal evaluation of the bone mineral status showed significantly reduced mineral content in spine and distal forearm – areas in which cancellous bone predominates – in the first postoperative year. In another study patients with the same type of urinary reservoir did not reveal any decrease in bone mineralization when followed up to 17 years,[88] but patients with a moderately reduced GFR may be at risk in the long term.[89]

The type of intestine utilized in the reconstruction of the urinary tract and its influence on the bone mineral content has also been evaluated. In a rat study it was shown that enterocystoplasty utilizing an ileal or a colonic segment neither impairs skeletal growth or bone quantity, but leads to loss of bone mass when combined with resection of the ileocecal segment. The rarefaction of the cancellous bone, which is the most metabolically active part of bone tissue, may therefore be attributed to intestinal malabsorption, and not only the difference in handling of urinary solutes by the intestinal segments incorporated.[90] However, in another study gastrocystoplasty-operated rats showed little influence on bone metabolism when compared to ileal enterocystoplasties indicating a difference in handling of urinary solutes by different intestinal segments incorporated in the urinary tract.[91–93] Even if renal function and the acid–base balance is within normal limits there might be a

Table 8.1 Bone biopsy histomorphometric analysis (mean ± SD)[68]

	Conduit	Reservoir	Normal values
Parameter	(n = 17)	(n = 18)	Reference group values
Trabecular bone volume (%)	24 ± 5.7	27 ± 8.0[a]	22 ± 6.5[a]
Osteoid volume (%)	2.2 ± 2.9	1.6 ± 1.2	2.2 ± 2.4
Osteoid surface (%)	12.4 ± 9.8	14.7 ± 8.2	16.2 ± 11.0
Resorption surface (%)	0.18 ± 0.73	0.44 ± 1.04	0.03 ± 0.17
Appositional rate (mm/day)	0.57 ± 0.02[b]	0.49 ± 0.03[c]	0.65 ± 0.12[b,c]

[a,b,c] $P < 0.05$.

Reproduced from Salahudeen et al. J Urol 1984; 131: 335–7[68] with permission from Lippincott Williams & Wilkins.

decrease in bone mineral density of the growing skeleton in the long term,[94] increasing the risk of osteoporosis later in life.[30,31]

Overt rickets or osteomalacia in patients with urinary diversion showed clinical and histomorphometric regression in response to treatment with alkali alone or combined with vitamin D.[62,66,67,82] Infants and children with classic renal tubular acidosis and accompanying hyperchloremic metabolic acidosis were given alkali 5–14 mEq/kg per day over long periods. Stature was initially stunted in all the children, but increased during the treatment time substantially more than expected for their age. The alkali dosage was much greater than that normally required for simple correction of acidosis.[95] In a patient with renal tubular acidosis and osteomalacia, bone formation was stimulated and cure effected by administration of potassium and sodium citrate.[64] In animals with urinary intestinal diversion, bone demineralization was prevented with bicarbonate and vitamin C,[81,93] and in animals fed a low calcium diet, sodium and potassium bicarbonate had similar effect.[96] A preventive effect was also noticed when calcitonin was administered.[97]

The data presented indicate that treatment aiming to reduce metabolic acidosis and thereby acidotic influence on bone mineralization can be appropriate in patients with urinary intestinal diversion and rapid skeletal growth, i.e. children and postfracture patients, even if the acidosis seems clinically to be well balanced. Defective mineralization in childhood, and especially in adolescence, will predispose to skeletal problems later in life, as the established peak bone mass will be inadequate. Optimal peak bone mass reduces the risk of osteopenia and fractures when bone loss occurs with age.[31] Inferior or insufficient bone mass will not be compensated later, even if the metabolic bone disorder is cured.[98] Women with urinary intestinal diversion will probably benefit from treatment, because of their risk for osteoporosis with increasing age. Administration of alkali and vitamin C to patients in growth phase and alkali only to others has been suggested.[50] Estrogen replacement therapy should be considered for women to counteract menopausal acceleration of bone loss. The rationale for treatment with agents that inhibit reabsorption of ammonium,[50] thereby reducing the endogenous acid load, remains to be established.

Acknowledgements

Some of the studies in this chapter were supported by grants from the Swedish Cancer Society, the Medical Faculty of Lund University and the Gunnar, Arvid and Elisabeth Nilsson Fund, Helsinborg, Sweden.

References

1. Turner GG. The treatment of congenital defects of the bladder and urethra by implantation of the ureters into the bowel: with a record of 17 personal cases. Br J Surg 1929; 17: 114–78.
2. Boyd JD. Chronic acidosis secondary to ureteral transplantation. Am J Dis Child 1931; 42: 366–71.
3. Nurse DE, Mundy AR. Metabolic complications of cystoplasty. Br J Urol 1989; 63: 165–70.
4. Koch MO, McDougal WS, Hall MC, Hill DE, Braren HV, Donofrio MN. Long-term metabolic effects of urinary diversion: a comparison of myelomeningocele patients managed by clean intermittent catheterization and urinary diversion. J Urol 1992; 147: 1343–7.
5. Mundy AR, Nurse DE. Calcium balance, growth and skeletal mineralisation in patients with cystoplasties. Br J Urol 1992; 69: 257–9.
6. Posner AS. The mineral of bone. Clin Orthop 1985; 200: 87–99.
7. Weiner S, Price PA. Disaggregation of bone into crystals. Calcif Tiss Int 1986; 39: 365–75.
8. Rowland RE. Exchangeable bone calcium. Clin Orthop Rel Res 1966; 49: 233–48.
9. Chabala JM, Levi-Setti R, Bushinsky DA. Alteration in surface ion composition of cultured bone during metabolic, but not respiratory, acidosis. Am J Physiol 1991; 261(1 Pt 2): F76–F84.
10. Glimcher MJ. The nature of the mineral component of bone and the mechanism of calcification. Instr Course Lect 1987; 36: 49–69.
11. Bushinsky DA, Krieger NS. Role of the skeleton in calcium homeostasis. In: Seldin DW, Giebisch G (ed). The Kidney: Physiology and Pathophysiology. 2nd edn. New York: Raven Press, 1992: vol 2.
12. Nichols Jr G, Rogers P. Bone cell calcium stores: their size, location and kinetics of exchange. Calcif Tiss Res 1972; 9: 80–94.
13. Green J, Kleeman CR. The role of bone in the regulation of systemic acid-base balance. Contrib Nephrol. 1991; vol 91: 61–76.
14. Swan RC, Pitts RF, Madisso H. Neutralization of infused acid by nephrectomized dogs. J Clin Invest 1954; 34: 205–12.
15. Biltz RM, Pellegrino ED, Letteri JM. Skeletal carbonates and acid-base regulation. Mineral Electrolyte Metab 1981; 5: 1–7.
16. Marks SC, Popoff SN. Bone cell biology: the regulation of development, structure and function in the skeleton. Am J Anat 1988; 183: 1–44.
17. Martin TJ, Ng KW, Suda T. Bone cell physiology. Endocrin Metab Clin North Am 1989; 118: 833–58.
18. Eriksen EF. Osteoporosis Pathogenesis and Treatment. Aarhus: Novo Nordisk A/S, 1992.
19. Vaes G. Cellular biology and biochemical mechanism of bone resorption. Clin Orthop 1988; 231: 239–71.
20. Matthews JL, Martin JH. Intracellular transport of calcium and its relationship to homeostasis and mineralisation. Am J Med 1971; 50: 589–97.
21. Jande SS, Bélanger LF. Life cycle of the osteocyte. Clin Orthop Rel Res 1973; 94: 281–305.
22. Eriksen EF, Axelrod DW, Melsen F. Bone Histomorphometry. An Official Publication of the American Society for Bone and Mineral Research. New York: Raven Press, 1994.
23. Christoffersen J, Landis WJ. A contribution with review to the description of mineralization of bone and other calcified tissues in vivo. Anat Rec 1991; 230: 435–50.

24. Eriksen EF. Normal and pathological remodeling of human trabecular bone: three dimensional reconstruction of the remodeling sequence in normals and metabolic bone disease. Endocr Rev 1986; 7: 379–408.
25. Epker BN, Kelin M, Frost HM. Magnitude and location of cortical bone loss in human rib with aging. Clin Orthop 1965; 41: 198–203.
26. Wahner HW, Dunn WL, Riggs BL. Assessment of bone mineral. Part 2. J Nucl Med 1984; 25: 1241–53.
27. Desforges JF. Clinical use of bone densitometry. N Engl J Med 1981; 324: 1105–9.
28. Health and Public Policy Committee ACoP. Radiologic methods to evaluate bone mineral content. Ann Int Med 1984; 100: 908–11.
29. Delmas PD. Bone mass measurement: how, where, when and why? Int J Fertil 1993; 38 (Suppl 2): 70–6.
30. Matkovic V. Calcium and peak bone mass. J Intern Med 1992; 231: 151–60.
31. Chestnut CH. Theoretical overview: bone development, peak bone mass, bone loss and fracture risk. Am J Med 1991; 91(Suppl 5B): 5B-2S–5B-4S.
32. Graversen PH, Gasser TC, Friedman AL, Bruskewitz RC. Surveillance of long-term metabolic changes after urinary diversion. J Urol 1988; 140: 818–19.
33. Krølner B, Pors Nielsen S. Bone mineral content of the lumbar spine in normal and osteoporotic women: cross-sectional and longitudinal studies. Clin Sci 1982; 62: 329–36.
34. Melsen F, Mosekilde L. The role of bone biopsy in the diagnosis of metabolic bone disease. Orthop Clin North Am 1981; 12: 571–601.
35. Frost HM. Tetracycline-based histological analysis of bone remodeling. Calcif Tiss Res 1969; 3: 211–37.
36. Parfitt AM, Drezner MK, Glorieux FH et al. Bone histomorphometry: standardization of nomenclature, symbols and units. J Bone Min Res 1987; 2: 595–610.
37. Rothstein MR, Obialo C, Hruska KA. Renal tubular acidosis. Endocr Met North Am 1990; 19: 869–87.
38. Alpern RJ, Stone DK, Rector FC. Renal acidification mechanisms. In: Brenner BM, Rector FC (ed). The Kidney, 4th edn. Philadelphia: WB Saunders Company, 1991; vol 1: 318–79.
39. Culpepper RM, Schoolwerth AC. Contribution of urinary titrable acid to acid-base homeostasis. Am J Kidney Dis 1992; XIX: 192–5.
40. Philipson BM, Kock NG, Höckenström T et al. Ultrastructural and histochemical changes in ileal reservoir mucosa after long-term exposure to urine. A study in patients with continent urostomy (Koch pouch). Scand J Gastroenterol 1986; 21: 1235–44.
41. Carlén B, Willén R, Månsson W. Mucosal ultrastructure of continent cecal reservoir for urine and its ileal nipple valve 2–9 years after construction. J Urol 1990; 143: 372–6.
42. Åkerlund S, Jagenburg R, Kock NG, Philipsson BM. Absorption of L-phenylalanine in human ileal reservoirs exposed to urine. Urol Res 1988; 16: 321–3.
43. Hall MC, Koch MO, Halter SA, Dahlstedt SM. Morphologic and functional alterations of intestinal segments following urinary diversion. J Urol 1993; 149: 664–6.
44. Davidsson T, Åkerlund S, Forsell-Aronsson E, Kock NG, Månsson W. Absorption characteristics of 22Na and 36Cl in continent reservoirs for urine: a comparative study of ileal and colonic reservoirs. J Urol 1994; 151: 335–7.
45. Hall MC, Koch MO, Halter SA, Dahlstedt SM. Morphologic and functional changes of intestinal segments following urinary diversion. J Urol 1992; 147: 430A.
46. Ferris DO, Odel HM. Electrolyte pattern of the blood after bilateral ureterosigmoidostomy. JAMA 1950; 142: 634–41.
47. Eiseman B, Bricker EM. Electrolyte absorption following bilateral ureterostomy into an isolated intestinal segment. Ann Surg 1952; 136: 761–9.
48. Stamey TA. The pathogenesis and implications of the electrolyte imbalance in ureterosigmoidostomy. Surg Gynecol Obst 1956; 103: 735–58.
49. Koch MO, McDougal WS. The pathophysiology of hyperchloremic metabolic acidosis after urinary diversion through intestinal segments. Surgery 1985; 98: 561–70.
50. Hall CM, Koch MO, McDougal WS. Mechanism of ammonium transport by intestinal segments following urinary diversion: evidence for ionized NH_4^+ transport via K^+-pathways. J Urol 1992; 148: 453–7.
51. McDougal WS. Metabolic complications of urinary intestinal diversion. J Urol 1992; 147: 1199–208.
52. Wachman A, Bernstein DS. Parathyroid hormone in metabolic acidosis. Clin Orthop Rel Res 1970; 69: 252–63.
53. Lemann J, Litzow JR, Lennon EJ. The effects of chronic acid load in normal man: further evidence for the partition of bone mineral in the defence against chronic metabolic acidosis. J Clin Invest 1966; 45: 1608–14.
54. Bushinsky D. Internal exchanges of hydrogen ions: bone. In: Seldin DW, Giebisch G (eds). The Regulation of Acid–Base Balance. New York: Raven Press, 1989: 69–88.
55. Bushinsky DA. Net proton influx into bone during metabolic, but not respiratory, acidosis. Am J Physiol 1988; 256(3 Pt 2): F306–F310.
56. Poyart CF, Bursaux E, Fréminet A. The bone CO_2 compartment: evidence for a bicarbonate pool. Respir Physiol 1975; 25: 89–99.
57. Bettice JA. Skeletal carbon dioxide stores during metabolic acidosis. Am J Physiol 1984(2 Pt 2): F326–F330.
58. Kraut JA, Gordon EM, Ransom JC, Coburn JW, Kurokawa K. The effect of chronic metabolic acidosis on the end organ responsiveness to parathyroid hormone in man. J Clin Endocrinol Metab 1983; 56: 619–22.
59. Kraut JA, Mishler DR, Kurokawa K, Warech E. Effect of colchicine and calcitonin on calcemic response to metabolic acidosis. Kidney Int 1984; 25: 608–12.
60. Bushinsky DA. Net calcium efflux from live bone during chronic metabolic, but not respiratory, acidosis. Am J Physiol 1989; 256(5 Pt 2): F836–F842.
61. Albright F, Burnett CH, Parson W, Reifenstein EC, Roos A. Osteomalacia and late rickets. Medicine 1946; 25: 399–479.

62. Rosenberg AE. The pathology of metabolic bone disease. Radiol Clin North Am 1991; 29: 19–36.
63. Cunningham J, Fraher LJ, Clemens TL, Revell PA, Papapoulos SE. Chronic acidosis with metabolic bone disease. Effect of alkali on bone morphology and vitamin D metabolism. Am J Med 1982; 73: 199–204.
64. Malluce HH, Ritz E, Lange HP et al. Bone histology in incipient and advanced renal failure. Kidney Int 1976; 9: 355–62.
65. Mautalen C, Montoreano R, Labarrere C. Early skeletal effect of alkali therapy upon the osteomalacia of renal tubular acidosis. J Clin Endocrinol Metab 1976; 42: 875–81.
66. Leite CA, Frame B, Frost HM, Arnstein AR. Osteomalacia following ureterosigmoidostomy, with observations on bone morphology and remodeling rate. Clin Orthop 1966; 49: 103–8.
67. Perry W, Allen LN, Stamp TCB, Walker PG. Vitamin D resistance in osteomalacia after ureterosigmoidostomy. N Engl J Med 1977; 297: 1110–12.
68. Salahudeen AK, Elliott RW, Ellis HA. Osteomalacia due to ileal replacement of ureters: report of 2 cases. J Urol 1984; 131: 335–7.
69. Davidsson T, Lindergård B, Obrant K, Månsson W. Long-term metabolic effects of urinary diversion on skeletal bone: histomorphometric and mineralogic analysis. Urology 1995; 46: 328–33.
70. Hutchison FN, Bell NH. Osteomalacia and rickets. Semin Nephrol 1992; 12: 127–45.
71. Kraut JA, Mishler DR, Singer FR, Goodman WG. The effects of metabolic acidosis on bone formation and bone resorption in the rat. Kidney Int 1986; 30: 694–700.
72. Lemann J, Litzow JR, Lennon EJ, Kelly OA. Studies of the mechanism by which chronic metabolic acidosis augments urinary calcium excretion in man. J Clin Invest 1967; 46: 1318–28.
73. Beck N, Webster SK. Effects of acute metabolic acidosis on parathyroid hormone action and calcium mobilization. Am J Physiol 1976; 230: 127–31.
74. Cunningham J, Bikle DD, Avioli LV. Acute, but not chronic, metabolic acidosis disturbs 25-hydroxyvitamin D_3 metabolism. Kidney Int 1984; 25: 47–52.
75. Kraut JA, Gordon EM, Ransom JC et al. Effect of chronic metabolic acidosis on vitamin D metabolism in humans. Kidney Int 1983; 24: 644–8.
76. Reddy SG, Jones G, Kooh SW, Fraser D. Inhibition of 25-hydroxyvitamin D_3-1-hydroxylase by chronic metabolic acidosis. Am J Physiol 1982; 243(Endocrinol Metab 6): E265–E271.
77. Brunette MG, Chan M, Ferriere C, Roberts KD. Site of 1,25$(OH)_2$ vitamin D_3 synthesis in the kidney. Nature 1978; 276: 287–9.
78. Specht EE. Rickets following ureterosigmoideostomy and chronic hyperchloremia. J Bone Joint Surg (Am) 1967; 49: 1422–30.
79. Siklos P, Davie M, Jung RT, Chalmers TM. Osteomalacia in ureterosigmoidostomy: healing by correction of the acidosis. Br J Urol 1980; 52: 61–2.
80. Bailey RR. Chronic acidosis with metabolic bone disease. N Z Med J 1985; 98: 483–4.
81. Levin EJ, Frank DF. Bone changes following ureteroileostomy. Am J Roentgenol Radium Ther Nucl Med 1973; 118: 347–55.
82. Cunningham J, Fraher LJ, Clemens TL, Revell PA, Papapoulos SE. Chronic acidosis with metabolic bone disease. Effect of alkali on bone morphology and vitamin D metabolism. Am J Med 1982; 2: 199–204.
83. McDougal WS, Koch MO, Shands CI, Price RR. Bony demineralization following urinary intestinal diversion. J Urol 1988; 140: 853–5.
84. Stein R, Fisch M, Andreas J et al. Whole-body potassium and bone mineral density up to 30 years after urinary diversion. Br J Urol 1998; 82: 798–803.
85. Hochstedtler JA, Flanigan MJ, Kreder KJ. Impaired bone growth after ileal augmentation cystoplasty. J Urol 1998; 159: 1310–11.
86. Phelps KR, Einhorn TA, Vigorita VJ, Lieberman RL, Uribarri J. Acidosis-induced osteomalacia: metabolic studies and skeletal histomorphometry. Bone 1986; 7: 171–9.
87. Wagstaff KE, Woodhouse CRJ, Duffy PG, Ransley PG. Delayed linear growth in children with enterocystoplasties. Br J Urol 1992; 69: 314–17.
88. Campanello A, Herlitz H, Lindstedt G et al. Bone mineral and related biochemical variables in patients with Kock ileal reservoir or Bricker conduit for urinary diversion. J Urol 1996; 155: 1209–13.
89. Campanello A, Herlitz H, Lindstedt, G et al. Determinants of bone loss in patients with Kock ileal urinary reservoir. Scand J Urol Nephrol 1999; 33: 312–16.
90. Gerharz EW, Gasser JA, Mosekilde L et al. Skeletal growth and long-term bone turnover after enterocystoplasty in a chronic rat model. Br J Urol 2003; 92: 306–13.
91. Brkovic D, Seibel M, Kissling C et al. Impaired bone metabolism following augmentation cystoplasty in growing rats. Eur Urol 2000; 38: 766–73.
92. Davidsson T, Åkerlund S, Forssell-Aronsson E, Kock NG, Månsson W. Absorption of sodium and chloride in continent reservoirs for urine comparison of ileal and colonic reservoirs. J Urol 1994; 151: 335–7.
93. Vajda P, Pinter AB, Harangi F et al. Metabolic findings after colocystoplasty in children. Urology 2003; 62: 542–6.
94. Hafez AT, McLorie G, Gilday D et al. Long-term evaluation of metabolic profile and bone mineral density after ileocystoplasty in children. J Urol 2003; 170: 1639–42.
95. Poulsen AL, Overgaard K, Christiansen C, Thode J, Steven K. Bone mineral status following urinary diversion with the ileal kock reservoir. The European Association of Urology Xth Meeting, Genoa, Italy, 1992. Abstracts: 411, P 335.
96. McSherry E, Morris RC. Attainment and maintenance of normal stature with alkali therapy in infants and children with classic renal tubular acidosis. J Clin Invest 1978; 61: 509–27.
97. Barzel US, Jowsey J. The effects of chronic acid and alkali administration on bone turnover in adult rats. Clin Sci 1969; 36: 517–24.
98. Parfitt AM, Sudhakar Rao D, Stanciu J et al. Irreversible bone loss in osteomalacia. Comparison of radial absorptiometry with iliac bone histomorphometry during treatment. Am Soc Clin Invest 1985; 76: 2403–12.

9 Problem of secondary malignancy after urinary diversion and cystoplasty

Jerilyn M Latini and Karl J Kreder

Introduction

The use of gastrointestinal segments in urinary diversion and urinary tract reconstruction dates back to 1852.[1] Since that time, every gastrointestinal segment has been fashioned into conduits and reservoirs. With the introduction and success of clean intermittent catheterization, and with improved surgical techniques, the use of gastrointestinal segments for urine transport and storage has increased tremendously. Indications for urinary diversion and reconstruction encompass benign and malignant conditions in both the pediatric and adult populations.

Chronic interposition of gastrointestinal segments within the urinary tract is not without risk. Most of the postoperative morbidities associated with urinary diversion and reconstruction are identifiable and manageable, including infection, obstruction and metabolic abnormalities. However, the small but significant, risk of malignant degeneration remains a growing concern. The long latency period and relatively short-term follow-up of many patients contribute to the difficulty in determining the true incidence of malignant change. A summary of the reported malignancies following urinary diversion and reconstruction is presented in Table 9.1.

In this chapter the epidemiology, histologic and biochemical changes, pathophysiology, treatment and surveillance protocols for patients undergoing urinary diversion and/or reconstruction of the urinary tract using gastrointestinal segments will be discussed.

Epidemiology and clinical experience

Primary intestinal carcinoma

An understanding of the epidemiology of primary intestinal carcinoma is essential in the discussion of the incidence of neoplasia associated with urinary diversion and reconstruction using gastrointestinal segments. Colorectal carcinoma is the third most common site of new cases of cancer in adults and cause of cancer mortality in the USA in both males and females.[2] Colorectal cancer accounted for 11% of cancers in males and 12% in females in 2002, and 10% of cancer deaths in males and 11% in females. Overall incidence and mortality have declined following a peak in 1985,[3] and colorectal cancer deaths have decreased in the USA by 1.8% per year from 1992 through 1998.[4] The lifetime risk of developing colorectal carcinoma is about 6%, and the risk is age dependent, with over 90% of cases occurring after the age of 50 years.[5] The probability of developing invasive colorectal cancer over selected age intervals by sex, based on cancers diagnosed during 1996 through 1998 is shown in Table 9.2. Tumor location is age dependent as well, with right-sided tumors (cecal and ascending colon) predominantly diagnosed in older patients,[6] especially in elderly women.[7]

Sex, geographic location and diet also influence the incidence of colorectal carcinoma.[8–11] Changes in the bioavailability of circulating sex hormones may play a role. A diet high in fiber directly reduces the exposure time of secondary carcinogens. Diets low in fat reduce the generation of secondary carcinogens and the amount of non-protein-bound estradiol and testosterone,[12,13] suggesting a relationship between diet and sex.

Table 9.1 Summary of reported secondary malignancies following urinary diversion

Details	Ureterosigmoidostomy	Intestinal conduit	Rectal bladder	Cystoplasty	Continent diversion
First case performed	1852[a]	1950 (ileal) 1960 (colon)	1912 (Heitz-Boyer) 1950 (Boyce-Vest)	1900[b]	
First carcinoma reported (no. of cases reported)	1929 (>90)	1978 (ileal 9) 1982 (7)	1989 (8)	1971 (ileal 31; ileocecal 10; colon 7)	1997 (orthotopic neobladder 1; Indiana/right colon pouch 5)
Type of gastrointestinal segment	Sigmoid colon	Ileum, colon	Rectosigmoid colon	Ileum, ileocecum, colon	Ileocecum, right colon
Tumor histology	Adenocarcinoma	Adenocarcinoma, squamous cell, TCC	Adenocarcinoma, adenoma	Adenocarcinoma, TCC, sarcoma, small cell, signet ring adenocarcinoma	Adenocarcinoma, adenoma, squamous cell carcinoma
Tumor location	Ureterointestinal anastomosis	Ureterointestinal anastomosis, stoma	Ureterointestinal anastomosis	Ureterointestinal anastomosis	Ureterointestinal anastomosis, ileal segment
Latency (years)	20-26	Ileal 4-36 Colon 1-26	6-25	5-40	2-22

[a]General use began in 1920s.
[b]General use began in 1950s.
TCC, transitional cell carcinoma

Table 9.2 Probability of developing invasive colorectal cancer over selected age intervals by sex based on cancers diagnosed in 1996-1998[a]

	Birth-39 years	40-59 years	60-79 years	Birth-death
Males	0.07 (1:1508)	0.87 (1:115)	4.0 (1:25)	5.88 (1:17)
Females	0.06 (1:1719)	0.69 (1:145)	3.03 (1:33)	5.55 (1:18)

[a]Adapted from American Cancer Society. Surveillance Research 2002. Cancer Facts and Figures 2002.[2]

Risk factors for colorectal cancer and their relative risks (RR) include: family history with an affected first-degree relative (RR 1.8), physical activity of less than 3 hours per week (RR 1.7), inflammatory bowel disease, Crohn's disease, ulcerative colitis or pancolitis (RR 1.5), obesity (RR 1.5), red meat (RR 1.5), smoking (RR 1.5), alcohol intake of more than one drink per day (RR 1.4), high vegetable consumption of five or more servings per day (RR 0.7), oral contraceptive use for more than 5 years (RR 0.7), estrogen replacement for more than 5 years (RR 0.8) and use of multivitamins with folic acid (RR 0.5).[14]

Primary malignant tumors of the small intestine are rare. Large autopsy series report a 0.1–0.5% prevalence,[15,16] with 60–75% being benign lesions, usually leiomyomas or adenomas.[16–21] Adenocarcinomas, followed by lymphomas, carcinoid tumors and leiomyosarcomas, comprise the majority of the remaining 25–40% of small intestinal carcinomas. The majority of primary small intestinal tumors are located in the duodenum near the ampulla of Vater, followed by the jejunum and then the ileum.[15] Adenocarcinomas and lymphomas of the small bowel are associated with diseases that appear to increase the risk of these malignancies, such as immunoproliferative small intestinal disease (IP-SID) or Mediterranean lymphoma, celiac sprue, immunodeficiency syndromes (HIV, AIDS), Crohn's disease, nodular lymphoid hyperplasia, gastrointestinal polyposis syndromes (familial adenomatous polyposis, Gardner's syndrome), hereditary non-polyposis colon cancer and neurofibromatosis.[22]

Adenomatous polyps and other premalignant lesions have been identified in patients at risk for and with colorectal carcinoma.[23–26] As adenomatous polyps increase in size, degree of dysplasia and villous component, the probability of malignancy increases. Malignant progression within 11.4 years has been reported for adenomatous polyps with mild atypia compared with 3.6 years for polyps with severe dysplasia.[27] As with primary colorectal carcinomas, a number of premalignant lesions have been identified in patients with urinary diversions and reconstructed urinary tracts using gastrointestinal segments.[28–31]

Secondary malignancies

Long-term outcome data are available for patients with ureterosigmoidostomy and ileal conduits. Since the first report of colon cancer as a late complication of ureterosigmoidostomy by Hammer,[32] there have been many reported occurrences. Malignant potential in these patients has been determined.[33,34] The majority of the malignancies are adenocarcinomas originating at the urointestinal anastomotic junction approximately 15–25 years following the original reconstruction/diversion,[34] with a mean latency period between ureterosigmoidostomy and the diagnosis of tumor being 26 years (range 3–53 years).[33] The reported risk of developing carcinoma of the colon following ureterosigmoidostomy is about 5%, and at least 16–41% of patients develop a benign polyp.[35] There are similarities in the histology, location and latency period of many of these malignancies, independent of the intestinal segment employed. Compared with similar series of primary intestinal malignancies, malignancies occurring at the uro-intestinal junction were of higher stage and associated with an increased mortality rate (up to 50%).[3,33,36]

Since the first reported cystoplasty around 1900, and the initial reports of ileal conduits in the 1950s and colon conduits in the 1960s, these diversion techniques have gained significant utility and popularity. Outcome data for intestinal conduits and augmentation cystoplasty are becoming available. Unfortunately, only limited long-term data are available for other types of urinary diversion including continent diversion, undiversion, orthotopic neobladders and ileal ureters. The true incidence of malignant change associated with these newer and increasingly popular procedures remain speculative, based on animal studies, small patient populations and experience extrapolated from ureterosigmoidostomy patients. Nevertheless, patients who undergo urinary reconstructive procedures using intestinal segments should be regarded as being at increased risk for late malignant transformation.[34,37]

Ureterosigmoidostomy

Simon performed the first ureterosigmoidostomy in 1852, but it was not until the 1920s that this procedure gained popularity.[38] In 1929, the first case of malignancy following ureterosigmoidostomy was reported.[32] In the next four decades, sporadic cases of benign and malignant lesions after ureterosigmoidostomy were reported. The true incidence remained unknown. Benign polyps are more common than malignant tumors, and evidence suggests that tumors follow the progression of adenocarcinoma similar to that in usual colorectal tumors.

Kalbe et al performed colonoscopy in 31 patients in a series of 104 who had undergone ureterosigmoidostomy.[39] Three (9.7%) were found to have adenocarcinoma at the urointestinal anastomosis. Mean surveillance time was 14.6 years (23/31 patients followed for less than 20 years). Others have also found evidence of polyps at or near the urointestinal anastomosis at the time of screening colonoscopy in 17.6–31% of patients with ureterosigmoidostomy.[28,40] Most of the tumors in these series were adenomas, diagnosed with a mean latency time of 19.8 years. This is in contrast to the mean latency period for carcinoma development, that is 26 years.

Several large series have estimated the incidence of colon carcinoma following ureterosigmoidostomy to be 3.5–19%.[41–43] A Medline review of reported tumors in ureterosigmoidostomies revealed the incidence of these secondary carcinomas to range from 2 to 15%.[44] These malignancies occurred in the area of the urointestinal anastomosis, at a rate 100–7000 times more frequently than the incidence of primary colorectal carcinoma in age-matched controls with no history of ureterosigmoidostomy.[33,45–49]

A series of 94 colonic neoplasms occurring after ureterosigmoidostomy in patients with exstrophy was reviewed by Husmann and Spence.[33] In 70% the diversions were performed before the age of 12 years. The average interval to identification of a colonic neoplasm was 26 years (range 3–53 years), with adenocarcinoma being the most common. A review by Fichtner revealed an incidence of tumor at the urointestinal anastomosis to be 2–29%.[50] Polypoid benign adenomas were most frequent, with the most common tumor being adenocarcinoma. The development of polyps or tumors in up to 40% of these patients has been documented, when followed long-term.[51] The time between surgery and tumor development ranged from 10 to 46 (mean 25) years.[52] More recently reviewed, the latent period appears to be between 20 and 26 years following ureterosigmoidostomy.[44]

As is evident in the following discussion, case reports are the primary means of information on malignancies developing in urinary diversions and reconstructions. Data have been compiled indicating that secondary malignancies can indeed occur in complete absence of fecal material. It has been recognized that both isolated small and large bowel interposed in the urinary tract can be affected by malignant transformation; however it is unclear how gastric segments will evolve over time.

Intestinal conduit

Carcinomas in intestinal conduits isolated from the fecal stream are rare. Theories of carcinogenesis include chronic irritation, mechanical trauma, excessive concentration of electrolytes and the presence of nitrate-reducing bacterial flora.[37,42]

The ileal conduit was originally described in 1950 by Bricker and has been used extensively ever since.[53] To date, nine cases of primary neoplasms have been reported.[54–62] Most patients (five of nine) developed adenocarcinoma in the region of the urointestinal anastomosis. One case of squamous cell carcinoma[61] and one of transitional cell carcinoma[62] have been reported. In the other patients adenomatous polyps developed within the ileal conduit. The polyps were excised with either revision of the conduit or creation of a second conduit without further difficulties.[56,57] Tumors developing in ileal conduits were originally thought to have the same histopathology as the primary tumor for which urinary diversion was indicated.[63–65] Transitional cell carcinomas arising within the intestinal conduit have been reported,[62] but may represent disseminated primary disease or seeding at the time of the original oncologic surgery.[66–69]

Seven cases of neoplasms arising within colon conduits have been reported according to a review of the literature.[70–73] Histologically, all were adenocarcinomas with latency periods of 1–31 years. Six tumors involved sigmoid colon conduits, and one involved a transverse colon[72] conduit. The true incidence of the neoplastic potential of colon conduits is not known. Longer follow-up and larger series of patients are needed, given that colon conduits have become more popular primarily during the past two decades.

Augmentation cystoplasty

Augmentation cystoplasty was initially described in 1900 in humans but did not become popular until the 1950s. Following the introduction and acceptance of clean intermittent catheterization, augmentation cystoplasty using gastrointestinal segments became popular. Current techniques utilize gastric patches and detubularized segments of ileum and/or colon.

A review of 14 cases of neoplasms associated with augmentation cystoplasties included procedures performed for tubercular cystitis, chronic cystitis, radiation cystitis and neurogenic bladder using non-detubularized ileum, colon or cecum.[74] Tumors developed in nine ileocystoplasties, two cecocystoplasties and three colocystoplasties. Mean patient age at surgery was 31.3 years (range 13–49 years) with the mean latency period to neoplasm being 18 years (range 5–29 years). The tumors occurred at the urointestinal anastomotic junction and were primarily adenocarcinomas (64%), but others types were also reported: transitional cell carcinoma, oat cell carcinoma and undifferentiated sarcoma. Many patients had history of recurrent infection, implying a poorly emptying augmented bladder. As with tumors following ureterosigmoidostomy, tumors following augmentation cystoplasties are associated with high mortality (36%) and a long latency period.

Most of the tumors reported to date involving enterocystoplasties are adenocarcinomas, although adenomas, squamous cell carcinomas, sarcomas and transitional cell carcinomas have also been reported. To the best of our knowledge, malignancies have been reported in 31 ileocystoplasties,[62,74–96] 7 colocystoplasties,[37,97–102] and 10 ileocecal or cecocystoplasties.[102–111]

Rectal bladder

Although not currently used as often nor as popular as other forms of urinary diversions, rectal bladders have been performed for over 80 years. Eight cases of neoplasia have been reported in patients with rectal bladders, including the Heitz–Boyer, Gersuny and Boyce–Vest procedures.[37,100,112–116] Six developed adenocarcinomas 6–25 years after their urinary diversion.[37,100,113–116] Chronic infection of the rectal bladder and/or subsequent conduit diversion with re-exposure of the ureteral stumps to feces may have contributed to the neoplastic transformation in two of these patients.[113,114] The other two of the eight patients included an 82-year-old male who developed an adenomatous polyp 4 months after urinary diversion,[115] and a 25-year-old female who developed a benign colonic polyp 17 years following surgery.[112]

The most comprehensive data on rectal bladders and malignancy have been reported for 22 patients followed for at least 12 years after a Boyce–Vest diversion (proximal diversion and rectal pouch).[117] Patients were followed with urine cultures and cytologies, biopsies and sigmoidoscopies. No evidence of infection, premalignant or malignant lesions was reported. Longer follow-up and larger series of patients are needed, as with other types of diversions and reconstructive procedures.

Other diversions

Continent diversions and orthotopic neobladders have been popular over the past 10–15 years. Ileal replacement of the ureter is a well-known technique for reconstruction of a long segment of ureteral stricture. Mitrofanoff operations such as the appendicovesicostomy have proved invaluable in the urinary reconstruction of both pediatric and adult patients. Gastrointestinal segments, specifically, gastric, ileal and colonic, have been incorporated in numerous configurations. To date, there have been few reports of premalignant or malignant lesions occurring in these modern, detubularized urinary diversions.

Ileal replacement of the ureter involving squamous cell carcinoma (one case)[37] and adenocarcinoma (two cases)[62] has been reported. Malignant transformation of the ileal segment used as the nipple valve in a right colon reservoir into adenocarcinoma has been found.[118] Adenocarcinoma arising in an Indiana pouch following cystectomy for transitional cell carcinoma has been reported by four groups.[119–122] One patient has been reported with adenomas involving a right colon orthotopic neobladder 5 and 6 years following urinary diversion for invasive transitional cell carcinoma of the bladder in 1989.[123] Transurethral resection of the two adenomas (at 5 years post-diversion) and a recurrent adenoma (at 6 years post-diversion) was performed without reported incident.

In another study, mucosal histopathology was studied in 100 patients who underwent sigmoidocolocystoplasty at a mean age of 10.6 years, over the short term (less than 5 years) in 44 cases, medium term (5–10 years) in 48 cases and long term (over 10 years) in 8 cases.[124] Hyperplasia was found in two patients and metaplasia in five. No dysplastic or malignant changes were identified in any patient.

The need for preoperative colorectal screening is debated by some, but it seems prudent to rule out pre-existing dysplastic, premalignant or malignant disease. In patients with hereditary non-polyposis colon cancer syndrome the possible influence of the syndrome on using the colon remains to be determined. Given the experience with other forms of urinary diversions, it is not surprising that malignancy has been documented in ileal ureters, continent diversions and orthotopic neobladders. Longer-term follow-up of larger populations of patients will allow determination of the true potential risk for malignancy.

Histologic and biochemical changes

When gastrointestinal tissue is exposed to urine or a urine/feces combination, various histologic and biochemical changes have been reported to occur in human and animal studies. To what extent these changes represent progression to neoplastic growth remains unknown. Data support the findings that malignancy can occur in patients who have undergone urinary diversion or reconstruction using intestinal segments in the absence of the fecal stream.[37]

Histology

A variety of histopathologic changes have been reported. These changes are variable within the conduit or reservoir, between patients, within the gastrointestinal tract segment and depending on the length of time following surgery.[125] The severity of these histologic changes is also influenced by the presence of bacteriuria, calculi, catheters and feces.

Villous atrophy, chronic mucosal inflammation, fragmentation and thickening of the muscularis mucosa, and submucosal edema are seen in intestinal segments chronically exposed to urine. Ileal conduits will show progressive villous atrophy starting as early as 1 week following surgery[125–128] with goblet cell hyperplasia.[129–135] These chronic mucosal inflammatory changes are more prominent near the ureteral orifices and stoma, being more severe in older conduits.[125] Similar atrophic and inflammatory changes have been described for canine and rat ileal patch cystoplasties and ileal reservoirs such as the Kock pouch.[136–138] Ileal orthotopic neobladders show marked villous shortening and goblet cell hyperplasia up to 3 years postoperatively.[139] After 3 years, the mucosa progressively flattens and after 6 years, the epithelium is flat and avillous. In this study, no epithelial dysplasia, mucosal erosion or malignancy developed during 8 years of follow-up. These morphological changes of ileal neobladder segments (progressive villous and microvillous atrophy, inflammatory infiltration of the lamina propria and goblet cell hyperplasia) have been well reported in humans and animal models.[129–135] The histomorphology of an orthotopic ileal neobladder created 24 years before was reported to show similar changes as those stated above, including changes often found in colonic tissues with villous atrophy and goblet cell hypertrophy.[140]

Mucosal morphology is well maintained in cecal and colon segments when used as conduits, reservoirs, ureterosigmoidostomies or colocystoplasties.[141–146] In ureterosigmoidostomy patients, inflammatory granulomas are observed histologically in endoscopically biopsied protruding lesions found at the urointestinal anastomosis.[147,148] Secretory function is maintained but there are variations in the type of mucus produced. The abnormal pattern of mucin secretion has been associated with an increased risk of malignant transformation.[149–152] Increased lymphocytes and eosinophils are present throughout the colon segment but unlike inflammatory bowel disease, crypt abscesses and mucosal ulcerations are not prevalent unless acute infection or calculi exist. Unlike ulcerative colitis, this chronic, global inflammatory response does not seem to lead to the same dysplastic and malignant changes, despite comparable latency periods.

There have been few human studies of the histologic changes in gastric segments used in urinary diversion. Metaplastic, hyperplastic and dysplastic mucosal changes with glandular hypertrophy have been demonstrated in rats following gastrocystoplasty.[153] In contrast with intestinal segments, inflammatory changes were not seen.

Some metaplastic and most dysplastic changes are considered premalignant lesions. However, the role that hyperplasia and inflammation may play in neoplastic degeneration or transformation is not clear. Hyperplasia and inflammation are present throughout any given conduit or reservoir but have been found to be more prominent at the urointestinal anastomosis. These factors may contribute to or promote neoplastic degeneration or transformation, but it seems that other factors are necessary to initiate the process. The histologic, morphologic and inflammatory changes seen in urinary diversion and urinary tract reconstruction may represent a defense mechanism of the intestinal mucosa exposed to urine, or they may indeed represent potential preneoplastic lesions.

Urothelium has been shown to exhibit plasticity and changes phenotypically in response to stromal–epithelial interactions with gastrointestinal tissues.[154] With tissue recombination techniques rat and mouse urothelium changed into an intestinal-like epithelium, in response to mesenchymal/stromal stimulation by gastrointestinal mesenchymal tissues. The urothelial transdifferentiation into intestinal glandular epithelium may be pertinent in the heterotypic stromal–epithelial interactions created in patients with urinary diversions and reconstructions.

The cellular ploidy of bowel segments used for ileal and colon conduits, cystoplasties and Kock pouches was studied and compared with normal ileal histograms using DNA flow cytometry.[155] No statistically significant difference in hyperploidy was found, although hyperploidy did increase slightly with increased time of urine exposure. Further evaluation is needed to determine if longer latency periods will influence cellular ploidy and potentially lead to metaplastic transformation.

Mucin

Goblet cells of the colonic mucosa normally produce both neutral and acidic (sialomucins and sulfomucins) mucins. Sulfomucins predominate in the cecum and sigmoid colon throughout the length of the mucosal crypts, whereas sialomucins are typically only present in the upper third of the crypts.[142,156] Early in carcinogenesis, there is a histochemical change in which sialomucins dominate, which are present throughout the length of the crypts. In patients with colon carcinoma, changes in the composition of colonic mucus have been demonstrated in the mucosa adjacent to the tumor, with sialomucins throughout the crypts.[157] Animals exposed to colonic carcinogens developed a similar change in mucin production before tumor development.[158,159] This was later termed 'transitional' mucosa and theorized to be a possible premalignant lesion. In colonic mucosa, abnormal variations in the histochemical phenotype of the secreted mucin have been related to an increased risk of malignant transformation.[149–152]

A similar pattern and increase in sialomucin production has been identified in patients with colonic conduits, ureterosigmoidostomies, augmentation cystoplasties and continent colon reservoirs.[142–146,148] Although thought to represent a premalignant lesion, this change may represent a non-specific defense mechanism of the intestinal mucosa exposed to irritants such as urine[143] with chronic inflammatory reaction,[156] and may not increase the risk of carcinoma. Changes in the pattern of colonic mucin production may not be useful as a marker for malignant transformation, as similar global changes are evident throughout intestinal segments in patients with ureterosigmoidostomies, colon conduits and continent diversions.[143,155] Study of the variation in the histochemical phenotype of the mucin secreted by the increased numbers of goblet cells found in ileal orthotopic neobladders has shown a predominance of sulfomucins up to 3 years following surgery. After 3 years, the mucosa progressively atrophies and mucin production decreases until after 6 years, when there is no evidence of mucin secretion.[139] An increase in sialomucins has not been demonstrated in rectal bladders.[160]

Conversely, these alterations in colonic mucin after urinary diversion, especially ureterosigmoidostomy, may represent a premalignant lesion. In addition to demonstrating increased sialomucin production at the urointestinal anastomosis following ureterosigmoidostomy, the proportion of peanut-agglutinin binding mucin, not found in normal mucosa but seen in premalignant and malignant mucosa, was increased.[148] This may represent an association with carcinogenesis.

For 1–3 months following anastomosis in the small bowel,[161] transverse colon[162] and descending colon,[163] stimulated crypt-cell proliferation occurs. The stem cells within the crypts are increased during this healing period, and appear to be the cells at risk for malignant transformation.[164,165] Carcinomas with similar histology and latency period to those found in association with urinary diversions are also identified in other disease states with increased cellular proliferation, such as ulcerative proctocolitis[25,166] and possibly pelvic irradiation.[167,168]

Ornithine decarboxylase

Ornithine decarboxylase (ODC) is a catalytic enzyme that converts ornithine to putrescine. It is the first and rate-limiting step in the biosynthesis of polyamines, necessary for normal cell growth.[169,170] Increased ODC activity is associated with cellular proliferation,[171,172] and conversely, inhibiting the activity of ODC has been shown to suppress mucosal growth in rats.[173] Inhibition of ODC in human tumor cell lines in vivo and in vitro, including a colonic adenocarcinoma cell line, suppressed cellular growth.[170,174] Colonic ODC activity in animals exposed to colon carcinogens is increased and precedes neoplastic growth.[175] Inhibiting ODC has been shown to prevent carcinogen-induced tumors.[176,177]

The enzymatic activity of ODC was measured in patients with familial polyposis who are at risk for colon carcinoma.[178] Mucosal ODC activity was elevated and increased steadily in colonic biopsies from morphologically normal, flat mucosa to adenomatous polyps and dysplastic polyps in patients with colonic polyposis compared with normal controls. This lends evidence to the hypothesis that enhanced ODC activity may exist even before tumors are detected on the urointestinal mucosa.

N-nitroso compounds[179] and fatty acids[180] are known colonic carcinogens and have been shown to induce increased ODC activity. Bile salts are known promoters of colon carcinogenesis, and may induce ODC activity in rat colonic cells.[181] ODC activity has been shown to be increased in human colorectal adenomas and adenocarcinomas, as well as at the urointestinal anastomosis in rats.[182]

ODC activity is increased at the urointestinal anastomosis compared with the proximal colon in animals with vesicosigmoidostomies.[183] Inhibition of ODC inhibited neoplastic growth in rats with nitrosamine-induced bladder cancer.[179] In rats treated with a colonic carcinogen and followed for 35 weeks, increased ODC activity was present throughout the small intestine, especially ileum, but no macroscopic tumors were found in the small intestine. There was, however, a biphasic increase and presence of concurrent colonic tumors.[175]

Pathophysiology

The pathophysiology of malignant transformation associated with the interposition of intestinal segments in the urinary tract remains an enigma. The identification of the exact mechanism of tumorigenesis is challenging because of the long latency period between carcinogen exposure and the recognition of tumor development. Experience and data from other tumor models, as well as available human and animal data support the hypothesis that the initiation, promotion and progression of neoplastic transformation and growth of the neoplasms are multifactorial and multistaged. The pathogenesis of most malignancies associated with urinary diversion may be similar given the similarities in the latency period, histologic type and tumor location.

Animal studies

A reliable animal model was necessary to study the pathogenesis of secondary malignancies following urinary diversion and cystoplasty because of the long latency associated with the tumors in humans. Wistar-Furth rats that underwent vesicosigmoidostomies were found to develop adenomas and adenocarcinomas at the urointestinal anastomosis with a latency period of 8–11 months.[47] One rat year is approximately equal to 30 human years, thus the latency period in the animal model was similar to that reported in human studies.[184] Further work with Wistar rats provided another reproducible animal model.[185–188] Tumor histology in the animal models was variable, including adenocarcinoma, adenoma, adenocarcinoma-like transitional cell carcinomas and polyploid squamous cell metaplasia. The wide range of histological tumor types identified may be the result of variability and discrepancies in the interpretation of the histology.

Modifications of the ureterosigmoidostomy animal models were carried out to study the neoplastic effects of urine, feces and the urine/feces mixture on the urothelium and intestinal segments. Gittes reported that urine and colonic epithelium alone did not produce tumors when the fecal stream was diverted from the urointestinal anastomosis.[189] If the proximal colostomy was delayed for a number of months, allowing feces and urine to mix and contact the healing urointestinal anastomosis, tumors developed but were smaller than those identified in animals without fecal diversion. When the proximal colostomy was performed at the time of urinary diversion, then later reversed at 1 or 3 months, small tumors were identified in the 1-month but not the 3-month models. Gittes hypothesized that a factor related to the mixing of urine and feces was necessary for carcinogenesis to occur. It appeared that this factor might be most pronounced on fresh, healing, urointestinal anastomoses.

Ileal[189] or colon[186] segments interposed between the bladder and sigmoid colon revealed an absence or decrease in the number of tumors present, respectively. Tumors that developed in the animal models with the sigmoid interposition were located at the urointestinal anastomosis, and not at the colocolonic anastomosis where the urinary and fecal streams converged.[186] In rats with augmentation cystoplasty, hyperplastic, metaplastic and early neoplastic growths were identified at the urointestinal anastomosis, in both ileal and colonic cystoplasties.[190] The role of fecal involvement was subject to debate.

Others have postulated that the tissue of origin might be the urothelium and not the colon.[191] Studies have been designed to address this issue, but gave mixed results. Animal models with an isolated urothelial patch implanted into the intact colon were found to have no evidence of tumor formation[189] whereas others found that two of 17 rats developed tumors.[191] Inherent differences between rat strains and variability in tumor development may be responsible for these results.

Several points may be drawn from the results of the available animal studies, despite the inconsistencies. Urointestinal anastomoses are susceptible to neoplastic transformation, and urothelium is a crucial factor either as the source or initiator of neoplastic transformation and carcinogenesis. The presence of feces may promote neoplastic growth, but it does not appear to be a vital factor in the pathogenesis of carcinogenesis, as both premalignant and malignant neoplasms developed in its absence. Caution must be used when extrapolating the available animal data to humans.

Chromosomal aberrations

Neoplastic transformation and tumor formation involve a series of carcinogenic events at the genetic level, which lead to structural and chromosomal aberrations. Endogenous or exogenous carcinogens may act as initiators, causing irreversible structural changes in deoxyribonucleic acid (DNA). Promoters enhance the effects of the initiators. These initiating and promoting events lead to changes in the DNA sequence causing an increase (oncogene) or decrease (tumor suppressor gene) in the expression of the gene product. Oncogenes and tumor suppressor genes have been identified in many genitourinary, gastrointestinal and other premalignant and malignant neoplasms.

p53 is a well-characterized tumor suppressor gene located on chromosome 17 involved in both urothelial and colorectal neoplasms. The protein product of *p53* is a cell-cycle regulatory protein possibly involved in apoptosis, and which may mediate the transition from a premalignant to a malignant condition.[192] Mutation of one allele could lead to decreased functional protein product, potentially leading to abnormal growth.[193] If loss of the remaining allele then occurred, the premalignant abnormal growth might progress to a true neoplasm. Allelic loss of 17p has been identified in over 75% of colon carcinomas[194] and in 63% of transitional cell carcinomas of the bladder.[195]

Structural changes in chromosomes 9q and 11q have been identified in transitional cell carcinomas of the bladder.[196,197] Numerous other chromosomal abnormalities have been reported in in vitro studies of transitional cell carcinoma cell lines including loss of 1p, 1q, 3p, 5p, 5q, 6q, 9q, 11q, 15q and 18q.[198] Aberrations in chromosomes 5q and 18q have been identified in colorectal carcinomas.[194] The genetic factors and chromosomal mutations that are involved, their exact mechanisms, significance and contribution to the neoplastic process is the focus of ongoing research. If identified, the chromosomal mutations involved may provide insight not only into the mechanism and pathophysiology of malignancy, but may also provide exciting opportunities for diagnostic and treatment strategies, as well as surveillance.

N-nitrosamines

Compounds containing the *N*-nitroso group have been long recognized to be highly tumorigenic, having initially been shown to induce tumorigenesis in animal models in 1956.[199] The role of *N*-nitrosamines in urologic and urointestinal malignancies has been hypothesized.[200] *N*-nitrosamines and their analogs alkylate and methylate DNA, and cause single strand breaks in the DNA,[201–204] resulting in cell damage, mutagenesis and possible tumorigenesis. The changes that occur at the DNA level are species- and organ-specific, influenced by organ-specific metabolism rate, distribution of carcinogen and effectiveness of cellular DNA repair mechanisms.[205,206] Some of these compounds are procarcinogens, requiring enzymatic activation to exert a mutagenic effect; others can act directly.[207] *N*-nitroso compounds can induce tumors in animal models, including lung, trachea, nasal cavity, esophagus, pancreas, liver and urinary bladder.[206,208–210] Epidemiologic studies in humans have provided evidence that *N*-nitrosamines may play a role in the tumorigenesis of gastric, esophageal, nasopharynx, lung and bladder cancer.[211–213] *N*-nitroso compounds can cause chromosomal changes on 17p (*p53*).[214]

N-nitrosamines are endogenously generated from nitrates and secondary amines,[215] and found in the diet[216] and the environment.[217] Nitrosamines are not found in appreciable amounts in sterile urine[218] or feces.[219] Under normal conditions, 60–70% of dietary nitrates are excreted in the urine (0.8–1.9 mmol/day).[220,221] Normal fecal nitrate (0–14 µmol/kg feces) and nitrite (5–19 µmol/kg feces) concentrations are much lower.[222] Small quantities of dietary secondary amines are present, but the majority is produced in the gastrointestinal tract by bacterial decarboxylation of amino acids,[223] metabolism of creatinine[224] and choline to methylamine.[225] Secondary amines are found in the highest concentration in urine, as are nitrates,[226] and are almost completely absorbed, leaving low concentrations in the feces.[227] They are also present normally in saliva, gastric juice and blood.

The formation of *N*-nitroso compounds (*N*-nitrosation) from nitrates and urinary secondary amines normally occurs in an acidic environment, and cannot occur under basic conditions or in the absence of nitrate-reducing bacteria (*Escherichia coli*, *Proteus*, *Klebsiella* and *Pseudomonas*) or activated macrophages.[215,228–232] *N*-nitrosamine formation is catalyzed by macrophages stimulated by bacterial lipopolysaccharide or interferon.[231] Inflammation following surgery may be in part responsible for an increased risk of malignant transformation at the urointestinal anastomosis.[48]

Many Gram-negative bacteria reduce nitrate to nitrite and catalyze the formation of *N*-nitroso compounds. These bacteria are usual urologic pathogens and also inhabit the colon. In addition, *Peptostreptococcus* spp. have been identified in high concentrations in the rectal slurry of patients with ureterosigmoidostomies.[41] This bacterium catalyzes the first step in the production of nitrate from urea.

N-nitroso compounds found in infected, static urine are directly associated with an increased risk of transitional cell carcinoma of the bladder in humans[233] and carcinogenesis in rats.[234] The presence of these bacteria in the colon, with the addition of urinary nitrates and secondary amines, led Stewart et al. to hypothesize that *N*-nitrosamines may play a role in the tumorigenesis of urinary diversion.[200] High concentrations of nitrate, nitrite and *N*-nitrosamines were found in the rectal slurry of patients with ureterosigmoidostomies in subsequent studies.[200,235,236] The urine of patients with infection,[215,237–239] bilharzia[239,240] and paraplegic patients[241] has been found to contain nitrate-reducing bacteria, nitrates and *N*-nitrosamines. Epidemiologic studies provide evidence that these patients are at higher risk for carcinogenesis. *N*-nitrosamines may play a role. Elevated urine levels of *N*-nitrosamines have also been found in patients with ileal and colon conduits,[235] augmentation cystoplasties,[146,242] ileal reservoirs[243] and rectal bladders.[235] Numerous factors correlate with the variable urinary levels of these compounds including bacteriuria, inflammation, gastrointestinal tract segment, mucosal contact time and others (calculi, catheterization). These factors and others that have yet to be identified may be responsible for the variation in tumorigenic potential and latent periods seen with these malignancies.

The microbiologic characteristics of urine from enterocystoplasty patients were assessed and correlated with the effect of prophylactic and therapeutic antibiotics on urinary nitrosamine levels.[244] Mean nitrosamine levels were highest in patients with urine infection, and fell with antibiotic treatment to those found in unoperated controls. Antibiotic prophylaxis reduced the nitrosamine levels to control levels as well. Similar results were found in enterocystoplasty patients with significant bacteriuria or higher white cell counts, when compared with patients with interstitial cystitis, infective cystitis and normal unoperated controls.[242]

Patients with enterocystoplasty have significantly higher urinary nitrosamine levels than unoperated controls.[245] Those with enterocystoplasty and infected urine had even higher levels of urinary nitrosamines, when those with sterile pyuria were excluded from the analysis. In addition, all patients with sterile pyuria, those on clean intermittent catheterization and those not taking prophylactic antibiotics had higher urine nitrosamine levels compared with controls. Similar results have been reported in patients with ureterosigmoidostomy,[246] rectal bladder, ileal or colon conduit,[200] ileal reservoir[243] and enterocystoplasty.[242] If elevated urinary nitrosamine levels are considered a risk factor for malignant transformation, then urinary reconstruction using intestinal segments, such as enterocystoplasty, are at risk; as well as urinary diversion.

The role of *N*-nitrosamines in neoplastic transformation and growth in urinary diversion has been challenged.[186,188] Although others had identified *N*-nitrosamines in rats with ureterosigmoidostomies,[236] Kalble and colleagues did not, but did identify the presence of nitrate, nitrate-reducing bacteria and urocolonic neoplasms in these animals.[188] When ascorbic acid, a known inhibitor of *N*-nitrosamine formation, was given to the animals, there was a decrease in *N*-nitrosamine, but there was no effect on the frequency of tumor formation.[184,247] Tumorigenesis is clearly a multifactorial process and other, as yet unidentified, procarcinogens and carcinogens are likely to be involved.

Oxygen radicals and inflammatory reaction

The inflammatory response to infection or tissue injury may contribute to neoplastic change.[163,233] Bacterial colonization of the urine is present in 85% of patients with colocystoplasties and in 57% with ileal cystoplasties.[146] Not only can urinary pathogens directly produce carcinogens, but the host inflammatory response also produces potential mutagens such as cytokines, free radicals and other *N*-nitrosamines.[232,248] Stimulated macrophages can generate nitrosamines by nitrosation of secondary amines when exposed to interferon or *E. coli* lipopolysaccharide.[249] Bacterial catalysis of nitrosamine formation from nitrate may play a role in tumorigenesis.[48,238,250,251] When nitrosamines are combined with oxygen-free radicals in vitro, single strand DNA breakage increases by 50%.[213] Animal studies have demonstrated the importance of superoxide in tumorigenesis.[232]

Following tissue injury, an inflammatory response removes cellular debris and promotes tissue healing. Macrophages, phagocytes, lymphocytes and fibroblasts are some of the mediators of this response, producing substances that stimulate cell division and tissue healing. Areas of rapid cellular proliferation in this environment appear to be at risk for malignant transformation.[163] Tumors associated with urinary diversions tend to be located at or near the urointestinal anastomosis. It is possible that the initiating tumorigenic event occurs early, during postoperative healing, in association with the inflammatory response.[48] Oxygen free-radical production by activated phagocytes during the inflammatory response at the urointestinal anastomosis may play a role in tumorigenesis.[232]

Many factors are suspected as mechanisms for inducing colon carcinogenesis at the urointestinal anastomosis including chronic irritation of the colonic mucosa by prolonged contact with urine[251] and mechanical trauma by feces.[252] Other potential promotors of tumorigenesis include epidermal growth factor,[253] urinary metabolites (Na^+, K^+, alkaline urine),[254] sutures,[255–257] calculi[258] and catheters.[258]

Serum markers

Serum carcinoembryonic antigen (CEA), a polysaccharide–protein complex, is one of the most valuable tools in the management of colorectal carcinoma. Serum CEA is useful in diagnosing, staging, estimating prognosis and in the surveillance of colorectal carcinoma. It is currently the most reliable marker for adenocarcinoma arising in the digestive tract. CEA levels in the serum and urine of colon and ileal neobladder as well as ileal conduit patients have been studied.[259] Colon neobladder patients had significantly elevated serum CEA levels compared with ileal neobladders or conduits. Elevated serum CEA levels correlated with urinary CEA levels in colonic neobladder patients. The elevated serum levels may be due to reabsorption of CEA from urine, as opposed to an association with malignant changes in the interposed intestinal segments. Further studies are needed to better address the association and clinical utility of serum/urine CEA in patients following urinary diversion.

Patient management

Patients being considered for and who have undergone urinary diversion or reconstruction using gastrointestinal segments should undergo evaluation and surveillance according to current protocols, over their lifespan.[31,33,34] Preoperatively, patients should be counseled regarding the potential risk of malignant degeneration and the necessity for lifelong surveillance. Preexisting colorectal carcinoma must be ruled out in those patients at risk prior to performing urinary diversion or reconstruction. If dysplasia, polyp or carcinoma is found, then the involved intestinal segment must not be used in diversion/reconstruction.

Postoperative surveillance will vary depending on the type of urinary diversion performed. Assimilating the available data, patients with functional ureterosigmoidostomies should undergo annual fecal occult blood testing and sigmoidoscopy in an effort to identify potentially treatable lesions as early as possible, beginning soon after the ureterosigmoidostomy. Those with an intact urointestinal anastomosis, even if defunctionalized, still require continued surveillance, as they remain at risk for malignancy despite early defunctionalization.[33,260] Any patient who develops obstructive urinary symptoms more than 2 years after ureterosigmoidostomy should be evaluated for possible malignancy. Recommendations include urine cytology and occult blood tests, abdominopelvic computed tomography scan, colonoscopy and barium enema.[44] If a benign tumor is identified, snare polypectomy is acceptable. In the case of dysplasia, suspicious polyps or carcinoma, the lesion with the urointestinal anastomosis and its lymphatic drainage should be excised and the urinary diversion reconstructed to a conduit, most typically.

Given the available data that malignancy has been reported in patients with rectal bladders, intestinal cystoplasty, intestinal conduits, continent diversions, ileal ureters and in an orthotopic neobladder (see Table 9.1) it is recommended that these patients undergo annual cystologies and endoscopy with biopsy starting 10 years following the operation.

Experience with gastric diversions and augmentation is limited. As *N*-nitrosamines have been identified as carcinogens in gastric carcinoma, it seems prudent to place these patients on a similar surveillance protocol with cytologic examination and endoscopy with biopsy. Those with sterile pyuria, infected urine and those on clean intermittent catheterization have the highest urinary nitrosamine levels. If *N*-nitrosamine carcinogenesis is thought to be significant, then these patients, who appear to be at greatest risk, should be considered for antibiotic prophylaxis.

Identification of chromosomal abnormalities has yet to be determined for patients at risk for neoplastic transformation following urinary diversion and reconstruction using gastrointestinal segments. The identification and role of oncogenes and tumor suppressor genes will become a reality given the molecular genetic technology available at the present time and in the future.

Conclusion

The potential for carcinogenesis exists in any patient who has undergone urinary diversion or reconstruction using intestinal segments. The process is complex and multifactorial, involving initiators and promoters, some of which are not yet identified or recognized. Possible initiators are the inflammatory response following surgery and oxygen radicals; enteric bacteria in the urine catalyzing *N*-nitrosation and urinary stasis with infection; and increased cell proliferation at the urointestinal anastomosis. Promoters such as ornithine decarboxylase and *N*-nitroso compounds may enhance these initiators.

Neoplastic transformation may begin with or without the interaction of urine and feces with the healing urointestinal anastomosis. DNA damage by reactive oxygen species synthesized by activated neutrophils at the healing anastomosis, and the production of *N*-nitrosamines by bacteria in the urine, have both been implicated in the pathogenesis of carcinogenesis.

Patients with urinary diversions and reconstruction of the urinary tract using intestinal segments should be followed for their entire lifespan. The goal of surveillance is to identify and effectively treat before forthright malignancy develops. This is in an effort to ultimately improve survival.

References

1. Simon J. Ectopia vesicae (absence of the anterior walls of the bladder and pubic abdominal parietes): operation for diverting the orifices of the ureters into the rectum, temporary success, subsequent death, autopsy. Lancet 1852; 2: 568–70.
2. American Cancer Society, Surveillance Research 2002. Cancer Facts and Figures. DevCan, Probability of Developing or Dying of Cancer Software, Version 4.1. http://www.cancer.org/docroot/STT/SH_0_2002.asp?sitearea=STT&level=1.
3. Seidman H, Mushinski MH, Gelb SK, Silverberg E. Probabilities of eventually developing or dying of cancer: 1985. CA Cancer J Clin 1985; 35: 36–56.
4. Howe H, Wingo P, Thun M et al. Annual report to the nation on the status of cancer (1993 through 1998) featuring cancers with recent increasing trends. J Natl Cancer Inst 2001; 93: 824–42.
5. Burt RW. Colon cancer screening. Gastroenterology 2000; 119: 837–53.
6. Butcher D, Hassanein K, Dudgeon M, Rhodes SJ, Holmes FF. Female gender is a major determinant of changing subsite distribution of colorectal cancer with age. Cancer 1985; 56: 714–16.
7. Alley PG, McNee RK. Age and sex differences in right colon cancer. Dis Colon Rectum 1986; 29: 227–9.
8. Miller BA, Ries LAG, Hankey BF et al. Cancer Statistics Review 1973–89. NIH Publication No. 92-2789. Bethesda, MD: National Cancer Institute, 1992.
9. Greenwald P, Lanza E, Eddy GA. Dietary fiber in the reduction of colon cancer risk. J Am Diet Assoc 1987; 87: 1178–88.
10. Willett WC, Stampfer ML, Colditz GA, Rosner BA, Speizer RE. Relation of meat, fat, and fiber intake to the risk of colon cancer in a prospective study among women. N Engl J Med 1990; 323: 1664–72.
11. Wynder EL. Primary prevention of cancer. Planning and policy consideration. J Natl Cancer Inst 1991; 83: 475–9.
12. Rose DP, Goldman M, Connolly JM, Strong LE. High-fiber diet reduces serum estrogen concentrations in pre-menopausal women. Am J Clin Nutr 1991; 54: 520–5.
13. Ingram DM, Bennett FC, Willcox D, deClerk N. Effect of low-fat diet on female sex hormone levels. J Natl Cancer Inst 1987; 79: 1225–9.
14. Colditz G, Atwood K, Emmons R et al. Harvard report on cancer prevention. Vol. 4: Harvard cancer risk index. Cancer Causes Control 2000; 11: 477–88.
15. Perlin KH, Bridge MF. Adenomas of the small intestine: a clinicopathologic review of 51 cases and a study of their relationship to carcinoma. Cancer 1984; 48: 799–819.
16. Darling RC, Welch CE. Tumors of the small intestine. N Engl J Med 1959; 260: 397–408.
17. Elias WS, Lund CC, Yonemoto R. Neoplasms of the small intestine. Am J Surg 1954; 88: 384–9.
18. Good CA. Tumors of the small intestine. Am J Roentgenol 1963; 89: 685–705.
19. Hoffman BP, Grayzel DM. Benign tumors of the duodenum. Am J Surg 1945; 70: 394–400.
20. Raiford TS. Tumors of the small intestine. Arch Surg 1932; 25: 122–77, 321–55.
21. River L, Silverstein J, Tope JW. Collective review: benign neoplasms of the small intestine. A critical comprehensive review with reports of 20 new cases. Surg Gynecol Obstet 1956; 102: 1–38.
22. Ryan JC. Premalignant conditions of the small intestine. Semin Gastrointest Dis 1996; 7: 88–93.

23. Morson B. President's address: the polyp-cancer sequence in the large bowel, Proc R Soc Med 1974; 67: 451–7.
24. DeCrosse JJ, Tsioulias GJ, Jacobson JS. Colorectal cancer: detection, treatment and rehabilitation. CA Cancer J Clin 1994; 44: 27–42.
25. Lennard-Jones JE, Melville DM, Morson BC, Ritchie JK, Williams CB. Precancer and cancer in extensive ulcerative colitis: findings among 401 patients over 22 years. Gut 1990; 31: 800–6.
26. Tierney RP, Ballantyne GH, Modlin IM. The adenoma to carcinoma sequence. Surg Gynecol Obstet 1990; 171: 81–94.
27. Kozuka S, Nogaki M, Ozeki T, Masumori S. Premalignancy of the mucosal polyp in the large intestine. II. Estimation of the periods required for malignant transformation of mucosal polyps. Dis Colon Rectum 1975; 18: 494–500.
28. Stewart M, Macrae EA, Williams CB. Neoplasia and ureterosigmoidostomy: a colonoscopy survey. Br J Surg 1982; 69: 414–16.
29. Berg NO, Fredlund P, Mansson W, Olsson SA. Surveillance colonscopy and biopsy in patients with ureterosigmoidostomy. Endoscopy 1987; 19: 60–3.
30. Ferguson CJ, Balfour TW, Padfield JH. Uretersigmoidostomy complicated by polyp formation: report of two cases. Dis Colon Rectum 1988; 31: 961–4.
31. Spencer JR, Filmer RB. Malignant potential of lower urinary tract reconstruction using bowel. AUA Update 1993; 12: 297–304.
32. Hammer E. Cancer du colon sigmoide dix ans apres implantation des ureteres d'une vessie exstrophique. J Urol Nephrol (Paris) 1929; 28: 260–3.
33. Husmann DA, Spence HM. Current staus of tumor of the bowel following ureterosigmoidostomy: a review. J Urol 1990; 144: 607–10.
34. Filmer RB, Spencer JR. Malignancies in bladder augmentations and intestinal conduits. J Urol 1990; 143: 671–8.
35. Rainwater LM, Segura JW, Ureterosigmoidostomy. In: Rowland RG (ed). Problems in Urology: Use of Gastrointestinal Segments in Urologic Surgery, Vol 5. Philadelphia: JB Lippincott, 1991: 299–306.
36. Leadbetter GW, Zickerman P, Pierce E. Ureterosigmoidostomy and carcinoma of the colon. J Urol 1979; 121: 732–5.
37. Shokeir AA, Shamaa M, El-Mekresh MM, El-Baz M, Ghoneim MA. Late malignancy in bowel segments exposed to urine without the fecal stream. Urology 1995; 46: 657–61.
38. Treiger BFG, Marshall FF. Carcinogenesis and the use of intestinal segments in the urinary tract. Urol Clin North Am 1991; 18: 737–2.
39. Kalbe T, Tricker AR, Mohring K et al. The role of nitrate, nitrite and N-nitrosamines in the carcinogenesis of colon tumors following ureterosigmoidostomy. Urol Res 1990; 18: 123–9.
40. Berg NO, Fredlund P, Mansson W, Olsson SA. Surveillance colonoscopy and biopsy in patients with ureterosigmoidostomy. Endoscopy 1987; 19: 60–3.
41. Silverman SH, Woodhouse CR, Strachen JR, Cumming J, Keighley MRB. Long-term management of patients who have had urinary diversions into colon. Br J Urol 1986; 58: 634–9.
42. Stewart M. Urinary diversion and bowel cancer. Ann R Coll Surg (Engl) 1986; 68: 98–102.
43. Strachen JR, Woodhouse CRJ. Malignancy following ureterosigmoidostomy in patients with exstrophy. Br J Surg 1991; 78: 1216–18.
44. Azimuddin K, Khubchandani IT, Stasik JJ, Rosen L, Riether RD. Neoplasia after ureterosigmoidostomy. Dis Colon Rectum 1999; 42: 1632–8.
45. Sooriyaarachchi GS, Johnson RO, Carbone PP. Neoplasms of the large bowel following ureterosigmoidostomy. Arch Surg 1977; 112: 1174–7.
46. Urdaneta LF, Duffell D, Creevy CD, Aust JB. Late development of primary carcinoma of the colon following ureterosigmoidostomy: report of three cases and literature review. Ann Surg 1966; 164: 503–13.
47. Crissey MM, Steele GD, Gittes RF. Rat model for carcinogenesis in ureterosigmoidostomy. Science 1980; 207: 1079–80.
48. Gittes RF. Carcinogenesis in ureterosigmoidostomy. Urol Clin North Am 1986; 13: 201–5.
49. Kalble T, Tricker AR, Friedl P et al. Ureterosigmoidostomy: long-term results, risk of carcinoma and etiological factors for carcinogenesis. J Urol 1990; 144: 1110–14.
50. Fichtner J. Follow-up after urinary diversion. Urol Int 1999; 63: 40–5.
51. Starling JR, Uehling DT, Gilchrist KW. Value of colonoscopy after ureterosigmoidostomy. Surgery 1984; 96: 784–7.
52. Spence HM, Hoffman WW, Fosmire GP. Tumor of the colon as a late complication of ureterosigmoidostomy for exstrophy of the bladder. Br J Urol 1979; 51: 466–70.
53. Bricker EM. Bladder substitution after pelvic evisceration. Surg Clin North Am 1950; 30: 1511.
54. Shousha S, Scott J, Polak J. Leal loop carcinoma after cystectomy for bladder exstrophy. BMJ 1978; ii: 397–8.
55. Kochevar J. Adenocarcinoid tumor, goblet cell type, arising in a ureteroileal conduit: a case report. J Urol 1984; 131: 957–9.
56. Tomera KM, Krishnan KU, Utz DC. Adenomatous polyp in ileal conduit. J Urol 1982; 125: 1025–6.
57. Peterson NE. Adenoma of ileal conduit. J Urol 1984; 131: 1171–2.
58. Sakano S, Yoshihiro S, Joko K et al. Adenocarcinoma developing in an ileal conduit. J Urol 1995; 153: 146.
59. Tsuboniwa N, Miki T, Kuroda M et al. Primary adenocarcinoma in an ileal conduit. Int J Urol 1996; 3: 64–6.
60. Ng FC, Woodhouse CR, Parkinson MC. Adenocarcinoma in an ileal conduit. Br J Urol 1996; 77: 321–2.
61. Yamada Y, Fujisawa M, Nakagawa H et al. Squamous cell carcinoma in an ileal conduit. Int J Urol 1998; 5: 613–14.
62. Ali-el-Dein B, El-Tabey N, Abdel-Latif M, Abdel-Rahim M. El-Bahnasawy M. Late uro-ileal cancer after incorporation of ileum into the urinary tract. J Urol 2002; 167: 84–8.
63. Meretyk S, Landau EH, Okon E et al. Adenocarcinoma in an ileal conduit: a late recurrence of urethral adenocarcinoma. J Urol 1987; 138: 859–60.
64. Rosvanis TK, Rohner TJ, Abt AB et al. Transitional cell carcinoma in an ileal conduit. Cancer 1989; 63: 1233–6.
65. Roberts SD, Williams HJ, Resnick MI. Metastatic transitional cell carcinoma in an ileal conduit following cystectomy. J Urol 1987; 137: 734–5.

66. Beniao OA, Waisman J, Kaufman JJ. Papillary (transitional) carcinoma in an ileal conduit. J Urol 1975; 114: 626–7.
67. Allan DM. Recurrent transitional cell carcinoma complication ileal conduit. Br J Urol 1976; 48: 60.
68. Wajsman Z, Baumgartner G, Mervin C. Transitional cell carcinoma of ileal loop following cystectomy. Urology 1975; 5: 255–6.
69. Grabstald H. Carcinoma of ileal bladder stoma. J Urol 1974; 112: 332–4.
70. Chiang MS, Minton JP, Clausen K, Clatworthy HW, Wise HA. Carcinoma in colon conduit urinary diversion. J Urol 1982; 127: 1185–7.
71. Marchetti DL, Piver MS, Tsukada Y. Adenocarcinoma in an isolated sigmoid urinary conduit. Obstet Gynecol 1984; 63 (Suppl 3): 54S–56S.
72. Wilson JWL, Morales A. Development of adenocarcinoma in transverse colon conduit. Urology 1982; 20: 182–3.
73. Pelaez C, Leslie JA, Thompson IM. Adenocarcinoma in a colon conduit. J Urol 2002; 167: 1780.
74. Filmer RB, Spencer JR. Malignancies in bladder augmentations and intestinal conduits. J Urol 1990; 143: 671–8.
75. Leedham PW, England HR. Adenocarcinoma developing in an ileocystoplasty. Br J Surg 1973; 60: 158–60.
76. Egbert BM, Kraft JK, Perkash I. Undifferentiated sarcoma arising in an augmented ileocystoplasty patch. J Urol 1980; 123: 272–4.
77. Takasaki E, Murahashi I, Toyoda M, Honda M, Waku S. Signet ring adenocarcinoma of ileal segment following ileocystoplasty. J Urol 1983; 130: 562–3.
78. Kamidono S, Arakawa S, Umezu K, Ishigami J, Maeda A. A rare case of adenocarcinoma of bladder following augmentation enterocystoplasty. Hinyokika Kiyo 1985; 31: 315–18.
79. Hasegawa S, Ohshima S, Kinukawa T et al. Adenocarcinoma of the bladder 29 years after ileocystoplasty. Br J Urol 1988; 61: 162.
80. Stone AR, Davies N, Stephenson TP. Carcinoma associated with augmentation cystoplasty. Br J Urol 1987; 60: 236–8.
81. Smith P, Hardy GJ. Carcinoma occurring as a late complication of ileocystoplasty. Br J Urol 1971; 43: 576–9.
82. Kawamura S, Takata K, Yoshida I, Seino K. A rare case of adenocarcinoma following ileocystoplasty. Hinyokika Kiyo 1987; 33: 1455–8.
83. Takashashi A, Tsukamoto T, Kumamoto Y et al. Adenocarcinoma arising in the ileal segment of a defunctionalized ileocystoplasty. Hinyokika Kiyo 1993; 39: 753–5.
84. Jung JL, Abouelfadel Z, Dettloff H. Adenocarcinoma developing on an ileal loop after augmentation cystoplasty. Ann Urol (Paris) 1996; 30: 69–71.
85. Fernandez-Arjona M, Herrero L, Romero JC et al. Synchronous signet ring cell carcinoma and squamous cell carcinoma arising in an ileocystoplasty. Case report and review of the literature. Eur Urol 1996; 29: 125–8.
86. Barrington JW, Fulford S, Griffiths D, Stephenson TP. Tumors in bladder remnant after augmentation cystoplasty. J Urol 1996; 157: 482–6.
87. Carr LK, Herschorn S. Early development of adenocarcinoma in a young woman following augmentation cystoplasty for undiversion. J Urol 1997; 157: 2255–6.
88. Ishida T, Koizumi H. A case of adenocarcinoma of the reconstructed bladder following ileocystoplasty. Nippon Hinyokika Gakkai Zasshi 1997; 88: 439–42.
89. Monnerat R, Pesqueira Santiago D, Pereiro-Alvarez M et al. Adenocarcinoma in ileocystoplasty. Acta Urol Esp 1997; 21: 614–16.
90. Louis L, Vanegas JP, Schulamn CC, Simon J. Carcinoma of urinary derivation. A case and review of the literature. Acta Urol Belg 1997; 65: 81–3.
91. Yoshida T, Kom CJ, Konishi T et al. Adenocarcinoma of the bladder 19 years after augmentation ileocystoplasty: report of a case. Nippon Hinyokika Gakkai Zasshi 1998; 89: 54–7.
92. Sato M, Fukui S, Fujita I et al. Adenocarcinoma of the ileal segment with transitional cell carcinoma of the bladder following ileocytoplasty: a case report. Hinyokika Kiyo 2000; 46: 33–6.
93. Ulmer M, Cormieu L, Hubert J. Carcinomatous degeneration of augmentation enterocystoplasty. Prog Urol 2000; 10: 450–5.
94. Lane T, Shah J. Carcinoma following augmentation ileocystoplasty. Urol Int 2000; 64: 31–2.
95. Koizumi S, Johnin K, Kataoka A, Nakai M, Tomoyoshi T. Adenocarcinoma occurring 37 years after augmentation ileocystoplasty for tuberculous bladder atrophy: report of a case. Hinyokika Kiyo 1997; 43: 743–5.
96. Docimo SG, Chow NH, Steiner G et al. Detection of adenocarcinoma by urinary microsatellite analysis after augmentation cystoplasty. Urology 1999; 54: 561.
97. Bono Arino A, Sanz Velez JI, Esclarin Duny MA, Berne Manero JM, Vera Alvarez J. Signet ring-cell adenocarcinoma in colocystoplasty. Acta Urol Esp 2001; 25: 312–14.
98. Llarena Ibarguren R, Pertusa Pena C, Zabala Egurrola JA, Olaizola Fuertes G. Adenocarcinoma of the colon. Occurrence on colonocystoplasty. Arch Esp Urol 1989; 45: 459–61.
99. Gepi-Attee S, Ganabathi K, Abrams PH, MacIver AG. Villous adenoma in augmentation colocystoplasty: a case report and discussion of the pathogenesis. J Urol 1992; 147: 128–30.
100. Harzmann R, Kopper B, Carl P. Cancer induction by urinary drainage or diversion through intestinal segments. Urologe A 1986; 25: 198–203.
101. Steg A, Conquy S, Teyssier P, Amar E, Schrameck E, Boiteux JP. Cancer of the colon following ureterosigmoidostomy or following bladder enlargement using a colonic graft. Ann Urol (Paris) 1985; 19: 283–7.
102. Golomb J, Klutke CG, Lewin KJ et al. Bladder neoplasms associated with augmentation cystoplasty: report of 2 cases and literature review. J Urol 1989; 142: 377–80.
103. Lamm DL, Gittes RF. Inflammatory carcinoma of bladder and interstital cystitis. J Urol 1977; 117: 49.
104. Kirby RS, Lloyd-Davies RW. Adenocarcinoma occurring within a caeococystoplasty. Br J Urol 1985; 57: 357–8.
105. Grainger R, Kenny A, Walsh A. Adenocarcinoma of the cecum occurring in a caecocystoplasty. Br J Urol 1988; 61: 164–5.
106. Nahas WC, Iizuka FH, Mazzucchi E et al. Adenocarcinoma of an

augmented bladder 25 years after ileocystoplasty and 6 years after renal transplantation. J Urol 1999; 162: 490–1.
107. Kadow C, Heaton ND, Paes T, Yates-Bell AJ, Packham DA. Adenocarcinoma in a substitution cystoplasty. Br J Urol 1989; 63: 649–50.
108. Gregoire M, Kantoff P, deWolf WC. Synchronous adenocarcinoma and transitional cell carcinoma of the bladder associated with augmentation: case report and review of the literature. J Urol 1993; 149: 115–18.
109. Telle Z, Martinez-Fornes M, Burgos Reville FJ et al. Metastasizing adenocarcinoma of the colon in a patient with caecocystoplasty. Acta Urol Esp 1993; 17: 80–3.
110. Khawaja MA, Thompson EM, Williams G. Adenocarcinoma of the residual bladder following caecocystoplasty for cyclophosphamide-induced cystitis. Br J Urol 1996; 78: 465–6.
111. Gousse AE, Safir MH, Cortina G, Safman K, Raz S. Tubulovilloud adenoma in the cecal segment after cecocystoplasty. J Urol 1998; 160: 490–1.
112. Phillips TH, Ritchey ML, Dunn CD, Sarosdy MF. Complications of the Heitz-Boyer urinary diversion: case report of late development of malignancy. J Urol 1991; 146: 159–61.
113. Metzger PP. Adenocarcinoma developing in a rectosigmoid conduit used for urinary diversion. Report of a case. Dis Colon Rectum 1989; 32: 247–1.
114. Shaaban AA, Sheir KZ, El-Baz MA. Adenocarcinoma in an isolated rectosigmoid bladder: case report. J Urol 1992; 147: 457–8.
115. Stillwell TJ, Meyers PR. Adenomatous polyp in defunctionalized colonic segment used as a urinary bladder. Urology 1988; 32: 538–40.
116. Kotanagi H, Ito M, Koyama K, Sato K, Kato T. Colon cancer in rectal bladder. J Gastroenterol 2001; 36: 718–22.
117. Boyce WH, Kroovand RL. The Boyce-Vest operation for exstrophy of the bladder: 35 years later. Urol Clin North Am 1986; 13: 307–20.
118. Ahlstrand C, Herder A. Primary adenocarcinoma of distal ileum used as outlet from a right colonic urinary reservoir. Scand J Urol Nephrol 1998; 32: 70–2.
119. Lisle D, Cataldo P, Bibawi SE, Wood M. Colonic adenocarcinoma occurring in an Indiana pouch: report of a case and review of the literature. Dis Colon Rectum 2000; 43: 864–7.
120. L'Esperance JO, Lakshmanan Y, Trainer AF et al. Adenocarcinoma in an Indiana pouch after cystectomy for transitional cell carcinoma. J Urol 2001; 165: 901–2.
121. Gazzaniga MS, Turbow B, Ahlering TE, Shanberg AM. Adenocarcinoma in an Indiana pouch urinary diversion. J Urol 2000; 163: 900.
122. Albertini JJ, Sujka SK, Helal MA, Seigne JD, Lockhart JL. Adenocarcinoma in a continent colonic urinary reservoir. Urology 1998; 51: 499–500.
123. Okada H, Yamada Y, Nakamura I et al. Adenoma in the orthotopic neobladder. J Urol 1997; 157: 1358.
124. Miyano T, Yamataka A, Iwashita K et al. Histology of the neobladder mucosa after sigmoidocolocystoplasty. J Pediatr Surg 2000; 35: 104–8.
125. Deane AM, Woodhouse CRJ, Parkinson MC. Histological changes in ileal conduits. J Urol 1984; 132: 1108–11.
126. Gamer JW, Goldstein AMB, Cosgrove MD. Histology appearance of the intestinal urinary conduit. J Urol 1975; 114: 854–7.
127. Goldstein MJ, Melamed MR, Grabslatel H, Sherlock, P. Progressive villous atrophy of the ileum used as a urinary conduit. Gastroenterology 1967; 52: 859–64.
128. Gracey M, Kay R, Bishop RF, Smith ED, Anderson CM. Mucosal morphology and bacterial flora of ileal conduits. Invest Urol 1971; 8: 596–603.
129. Hall MC, Koch MO, Halter SA, Dahlstedt SM. Morphologic and functional alterations of intestinal segmenst following urionary diversion. J Urol 1993; 149: 664–6.
130. Davidsson T, Carlen B, Bak-Jensen E, Willen R, Mansson W. Morphologic changes in intestinal mucosa with urinary contact. Effects of urine or disuse? J Urol 1996; 156: 226–32.
131. Philipson BM, Kock NS, Hockenstrom T et al. Ultrastructrural and biochemical changes in ileal reservoir mucosa after long-term exposure to urine. Study in patients with continent urostomy (Kock pouch). Scand J Gastroenterol 1986; 21: 1235–44.
132. Willen R. Morphological changes in intestinal mucosa in contact with urine. Scand J Urol Nephrol Suppl 1992; 142: 26–30.
133. Chen KK, Ho DM, Chen MT, Chang LS. Histological changes in the Kock pouch. Br J Urol 1993; 72: 433–40.
134. DiTonno F, Fabris C, Mazzon E, Lavelli D, Milanesi C. Ultrastructural mucosal appearance in the ileal neobladder. Eur Urol 1997; 31: 108–11.
135. Aragona F, De Caro R, Parenti A et al. Structural and ultrastructural changes in ileal neobladder mucosa: a 7-year follow-up. Br J Urol 1998; 81: 55–61.
136. Watson DW, Cockett ATK. Intestinal mucosa of dogs with ileocystoplasties. Urology 1973; 2: 385–8.
137. Hansson HA, Kock NG, Norlen L et al. Morphological observations in pedicled ileal grafts used for construction of continent reservoirs for urine. Scand J Urol Nephrol Suppl 1978; 49: 49–61.
138. Philipson BM, Kock NG, Jagenburg R et al. Functional and structural studies of ileal reservoirs used for continent urostomy and ileostomy. Gut 1983; 24: 392–8.
139. Parenti A, Aragona F, Bortuzzo G, De Caro R. Abnormal patterns of mucin secretion in ileal neobladder mucosa: evidence of preneoplastic lesion? Eur Urol 1999; 35: 98–101.
140. Gatti R, Ferretti S, Bucci G, Simonazzi M, Orlandini G. Histomorphology of an ileal orthotopic neobladder: 24 years' follow-up. Acta Anat (Basel) 1998; 163: 179–83.
141. Gilchrist KW, Uehling DT, Starling JR. Cancer surveillance after ureterosigmoidostomy: colonic microscopic changes. J Surg Res 1984; 36: 251–5.
142. Marcheggiano A, Iannoni C, Pallone F et al. Abnormal patterns of colonic mucin secretion after ureterosigmoidostomy. Hum Pathol 1984; 15: 647–50.
143. Srrachen JR, Rees HC, Williams G. Histochemical changes after ureterosigmoidostomy and colonic diversions. Br J Urol 1985; 57: 700–2.

144. Mansson W, Willen R. Mucosal morphology and histochemistry of continent cecal reservoirs for urine. J Urol 1988; 139: 1199–201.
145. Tomasino RM, Morello V, Latteri MA et al. Histological and histochemical changes in the colon mucosa after ureterosigmoidostomy or colonic conduit. Eur Urol 1988; 15: 248–51.
146. Nurse DE, Mundy AR. Assessment of the malignant potential of cystoplasty. Br J Urol 1989; 64: 489–92.
147. Bristol JB, Williamson RC. Ureterosigmoidostomy and colon carcinogenesis. Science 1981; 214: 351.
148. Shimamoto C, Hirata I, Takao Y et al. Alteration of colonic mucin after ureterosigmoidostomy. Dis Colon Rectum 2000; 43: 526–31.
149. Filipe MI, Branfoot AC. Abnormal patterns of mucus secretion in apparently normal mucosa of large intestine with carcinoma. Cancer 1974; 34: 382–90.
150. Filipe MI, Munoz N, Matko I. Intestinal metaplasia types and the risk of gastric cancer. Int J Cancer 1994; 57: 324–9.
151. Boland CR, Montgomery CK, Kim YS. Alterations in human colonic mucin occurring with cellular differentiation and malignant transformation. Proc Natl Acad Sci USA 1982; 79: 2051–5.
152. Stemmermann GN. Intestinal metaplasia of the stomach. A status report. Cancer 1994; 74: 556–64.
153. Klee LW, Hoover DM, Mitchell ME, Rink RC. Long-term effects of gastrocystoplasty in rats. J Urol 1990; 144: 1283–7.
154. Li Y, Liu W, Hayward SW, Cunha GR, Baskin LS. Plasticity of the urothelial phenotype: effects of gastro-intestinal mesenchyme/stroma and implications for urinary tract reconstruction. Differentiation 2000; 66: 126–35.
155. Broderick GA, MacDermott JP, Stone AR, Deitch AD, deVereWhite R. Bowel segments exposed to urine: the role of DNA flow cytometry in surveillance [Abstract]. J Urol 1990; 280A, no. 367.
156. Niv Y, Turani H, Fraser GM. Histochemical characterization of mucosal mucin in serial biopsies along the human colon. Digestion 1996; 57: 109–12.
157. Filipe MI, Branfoot AC. Mucin histochemistry of the colon. Curr Top Pathol 1976; 63: 143–78.
158. Filipe MI. Mucous secretion in rat colonic mucosa during carcinogenesis induced by dimethylhydrazine. A morphological and histochemical study. Br J Cancer 1975; 32: 60–77.
159. McGarrity TJ, Via EA, Colony PC. Qualitative and quantitative changes in sialomucins during 1,2-dimethylhydrazine-induced colon carcinogenesis in the rat. J Natl Cancer Inst 1987; 79: 1375–82.
160. Iannoni C, Marcheggiano A, Pallone F et al. Abnormal patterns of colorectal mucin secretion after urinary diversion of different types: histochemical and lectin binding studies. Hum Pathol 1986; 17: 834–40.
161. Sharp JG, Hanson WR, Osborne JW. The relationship between the compensatory response in the stomach and colon and the extent of small bowel resection in the rat. Virchows Arch B Cell Pathol 1983; 44: 295–304.
162. Barkla DH, Tutton PM. The influence of surgical transection and anastomosis on the rate of cell proliferation in the colonic epithelium of normal and DMH-treated rats. Carcinogenesis 1983; 4: 1323–5.
163. Roe R, Fermor B, Williamson RCN. Proliferarive instability and experimental carcinogenesis at colonic anastomoses. Gut 1987; 28: 808–15.
164. Chang WL. Pathogenesis and biological behaviour of 1,2 dimethylhydrazine-induced colonic neoplasms in the mouse. In: Appleton DR, Sunter JP, Watson AJ (eds). Cell Proliferation in the Gastrointestinal Tract. London: Pitman Medical, 1980: 278–97.
165. Bykorez AJ, Ivashchenko YD. Gastrointestinal stem cells and their role in carcinogenesis. Int Rev Cytol 1984; 90: 309–73.
166. Maratka Z, Nedbal J, Kocianova J, Kudrmann J, Hendl J. Incidence of colorectal cancer in proctocolitis: a retrospective study of 959 cases over 40 years. Gut 1985; 26: 43–9.
167. Sandler RS, Sandler DP. Radiation-induced cancers of the colon and rectum: assessing the risk. Gastroenterology 1983; 84: 51–7.
168. Umpleby HC, Bristol JB, Rainey JB, Williamson RCN. Survival of 727 patients with single carcinomas of the large bowel. Br J Surg 1984; 27: 803–9.
169. Williams-Ashman HG, Canellakis IN. Polyamines in mammalian biology and medicine. Perspect Biol Med 1979; 22: 421–53.
170. Pegg AE, McCann PP. Polyamine metabolism and function. Am J Physiol 1982; 243: C212–21.
171. Luk GD, Marton LJ, Baylin SB. Ornithine decarboxylase is important in intestinal mucosal maturation and recovery from injury in rats. Science 1980; 210: 195–8.
172. Luk GD, Baylin SB. Ornithine decarboxylase in intestinal maturation, recovery and adaptation. In: Robinson JWL, Dowling RH, Riecken E-O (eds). Mechanisms of Intestinal Adaptation. Lancaster: MTP Press, 1982: 65–80.
173. Luk GD, Baylin SB. Polyamines and intestinal growth-increased polyamine biosynthesis after jejunectomy. Am J Physiol 1983; 245: G656–60.
174. Kingsnorth AN, Russell WE, McCann PP, Diekeman KA, Malt RA. Effects of alpha-difluoromethylornithine and 5-fluorouracil on the proliferation of a human colon adenocarcinoma cell line. Cancer Res 1983; 43: 4035–8.
175. Luk GD, Hamilton SR, O'Ceallaigh D et al. Azoxymethane (AOM) induces a generalized biphasic increase in intestinal ornithine decarboxylase (ODC) during colon carcinogenesis [Abstract]. Gastroenterology 1982; 82: 1121.
176. Kingsnorth AN, King WWK, Diekema KA et al. Inhibition of ornithine decarboxylase with 2-difluoromethylornithine: reduced incidence of dimethylhydrazine-induced colon tumors in mice. Cancer Res 1983; 43: 2545–9.
177. Rozhin J, Wilson PS, Bull AW, Nigro ND. Ornithine decarboxylase activity in the rat and human colon. Cancer Res 1984; 44: 3226–30.
178. Luk GD, Baylin SB. Ornithine decarboxylase as a biologic marker in familial colonic polyposis. N Engl J Med 1984; 311: 80–3.
179. Homma Y, Kakizoe T, Samma S, Oyasu R. Inhibition of N-butyl-

N-(4-hydroxybutyl) nitrosamine-induced rat urinary bladder carcinogenesis by alpha-difluoromethylornithine. Cancer Res 1987; 47: 6176–9.

180. Bull AW, Nigro ND, Golembieski WA, Crissman JD, Marnett LJ. In vivo stimulation of DNA synthesis and induction of ornithine decarboxylase in rat colon by fatty acid hydroperoxides, autoxidation products of unsaturated fatty acids. Cancer Res 1984; 44: 4924–8.
181. Takano S, Matsushima M, Erturk E, Bryan GT. Early induction of rat colonic epithelial ornithine and S-adenosyl-L-methionine decarboxylase activities by N-methyl-N′-nitro-N-nitrosoguanidine or bile salts. Cancer 1981; 41: 624–8.
182. Weber TR, Westfall SH, Steinhardt GF et al. Malignancy associated with ureterosigmoidostomy: detection by mucosal ornithine decarboxylase. J Pediatr Surg 1988; 23: 1091–4.
183. Weber TR, Westfall SH, Steinhardt GF et al. Malignancy associated with urterosigmoidostomy: detection by mucosa ornithine decarboxylase. J Pediatr Surg 1985; 23: 1091–4.
184. Peckham JC, Experimental oncology, In: Baker HJ, Lindsey JR, Weisbroth SH (eds). The Laboratory Rat. New York: Academic Press, 1979: 119.
185. Daher N, Gautier R, Abourachid H, Decaens C, Bara J. Rat colonic carcinogenesis after ureterosigmoidostomy: pathogenesis and immunohistological study. J Urol 1988; 139: 1331–6.
186. Shands C 3rd, McDougal WS, Wright EP. Prevention of cancer at the urothelial enteric anastomotic site. J Urol 1989; 141: 178–81.
187. Strachan JR, Matthews J, Rees HC, Cooke T. Kinetic changes in experimental colonic urinary diversion. Br J Surg 1987; 74: 1046–8.
188. Kalble T, Tricker AR, Berger M et al. Tumor induction in a rat model for ureterosigmoidostomy without evidence of nitrosamine formation. J Urol 1991; 146: 862–6.
189. Gittes RE. Carcinogenesis in ureterosigmoidostomy. Urol Clin North Am 1986; 13: 201–5.
190. Spencer JR, Steckel J, May M et al. Histological and bacteriological findings in long-term ileocystoplasty and colocystoplasty in the rat. J Urol 1983; 150: 1321–5.
191. Aaronson IA, Constantinides CG, Sallie LP, Sinclair-Smith CC. Pathogenesis of adenocarcinoma complicating ureterosigmoidostomy: Experimental observations. Urology 1987; 29: 538–43.
192. Resnitzky D, Lotem J, Sachs L, Kimchi A, Oren M. Wild-type p53 induces apoptosis of myeloid leukaemic cells that is inhibited by interleukin-6. Nature 1991; 352: 345–7.
193. Herskowitz I. Functional inactivation of genes by dominant negative mutations. Nature 1987; 329: 219–22.
194. Vogelstein B, Fearon ER, Hamilton SR et al. Genetic alteration during colorectal-tumor development. N Engl J Med 1988; 319: 525–32.
195. Olumi AF, Tsai YC, Nichols PW et al. Allelic loss of chromosome 17p distinguishes high grade from low grade transitional cell carcinomas of the bladder. Cancer Res 1990; 50: 7081–3.
196. Tsai YC, Nichols PW, Hiti AL et al. Allelic losses of chromosomes 9,11, and 17 in human bladder cancer. Cancer Res 1990; 50: 44–7.
197. Fearson ER, Feinberg AP, Hamilton S, Vogelstein B. Loss of genes on the short arm of chromosome 11 in bladder cancer. Nature 1985; 318: 377–80.
198. Wu SQ, Storer BE, Bookland EA et al. Nonrandom chromosome losses in stepwise neoplastic transformation in in vitro of human uroepithelial cells. Cancer Res 1991; 51: 3323–6.
199. Magee PN, Barnes JM. The production of malignant primary hepatic tumours in the rat by feeding dimethylnitrosamine. Br J Cancer 1956; 10: 114–22.
200. Stewart M, Hill MJ, Pugh RCB, Williams JP. The role of N-nitrosamine in carcinogenesis at the ureterocolic anastomosis. Br J Urol 1981; 53: 115–18.
201. Belinsky SA, White CM, Boucheron JA et al. Accumulation and persistence of DNA adducts in respiratory tissue of rats following multiple administrations of the tobacco-specific carcinogen 4-(N-methyl-N-nitrosamino)-1-(3-pyridyl)-1-butanone. Cancer Res 1986; 46: 1280–4.
202. Lili L, Alaoui-Jamali M, EIAlami N, Castonguay A. Metabolism and DNA single strand breaks induced by 4-(N-methyl-N-nitrosamino)-1-(3-pyridyl)-1-butanone and its analogues in primary culture of rat hepatocytes. Cancer Res 1990; 50: 1810–16.
203. Druckrey H, Preussmann R, Ivankovic S, Schmahl D. Organotropic carcinogenic effects of 65 various N-nitroso-compounds on BD rats. Z Krebsforsch 1967; 69: 103–201.
204. Preussmann R, Stewart BW. N-nitroso carcinogens, In: Searle CE (ed). Chemical Carcinogens. Monograph 182. Washington DC: American Chemical Society, 1984, 643–828.
205. Brendler SY, Tompa A, Hutter KF, Preussmann, R, Pool-Zobel BL. In vivo and in vitro genotoxicity of several N-nitrosamines in extrahepatic tissues of the rat. Carcinogenesis 1992; 13: 2435–44.
206. Preussmann R, Wiessler M. The enigma of organ-specificity of carcinogenic nitrosamines. Trends Pharmacol Sci 1987; 8: 185–9.
207. Shank RC. Toxicology of N-nitroso compounds. Toxicol Appl Pharmacol 1975; 31: 361–8.
208. Hecht SS, Hoffman D. Tobacco-specific nitrosamine, an important group of carcinogens in tobacco and tobacco smoke. Carcinogenesis 1988; 9: 875–84.
209. Hoffman D, Castonguay A, Rivenson A, Hecht SS. Comparative carcinogenicity and metabolism of 4-(N-methyl-N-nitrosamino)-1-(3-pyridyl)-1-butanone and N′-nitrosonomicotine in Syrian golden hamsters. Cancer 1981; 41: 2386–93.
210. Kokkinakis DM, Subbarao V. The significance of DNA damage, its repair and cell proliferation during carcinogen treatment in the initiation of pancreatic cancer in the hamster model. Cancer Res 1993; 53: 2790–5.
211. Magee PN. The experimental basis for the role of nitrosamines in human cancer. Cancer Surv 1989; 8: 207–39.
212. Preston-Martin S, Cotrea P. Epidemiological evidence for the role of nitroso compounds in human cancer. Cancer Surv 1989; 8: 459–73.
213. Weitberg AB, Corvese D. Oxygen radicals potentiate the genetic toxicity of tobacco-specific nitrosamines. Clin Genet 1993; 43: 88–91.

214. Puisieux A, Lim S, Groopman J, Ozturk M. Selective targeting of p53 gene murational hotspots in human cancers by etiologically defined carcinogens. Cancer Res 1991; 51: 6185–9.
215. Ohshima H, Calmels S, Pignatelli B, Vincent P, Bartsch H. N-nitrosamine formation in urinary tract infections. In: Bartsch H, O'Neill I, Schulte-Hennann R (eds). Relevance of N-nitroso Compounds to Human Cancer: Exposure and Mechanisms. Lyon: IARC Scientific Publications, 1987: 384–90.
216. Tricker AR, Preussmann R. Carcinogenic N-nitrosamines in the diet: occurrence, formation, mechanisms and carcinogenic potential. Mutat Res 1991; 259: 277–89.
217. Preussmann R, Eisenbrand G. N-nitroso carcinogens in the environment, In: Searle CE (ed). Chemical Carcinogens. Washington, DC: American Chemical Society, 1984: 829–68.
218. Ellen G, Schuller PL, Bavijns E et al. Volatile nitrosamines, nitrate and nitrite in urine and saliva of healthy volunteers after administration of large amounts of nitrate. In: Bartsch H, O'Neil K, Castegnaero M, Okma M (eds). N-nitroso Compounds: Occurrence and Biological Effects. Lyon: IARC Scientific Publications; 1981; no. 41: 365–78.
219. Areiter MC, Lee L, Bruce WR. Analysis and formation of nitrosamines in the human intestine. In: Bartsch H, O'Neil K, Castegnaero M, Okma M (eds). N-nitroso Compounds: Occurrence and Biological Effects. Lyon: IARC Scientific Publications, 1981; no. 41: 357–63.
220. Wagner DA, Schultz DS, Deen WM, Young VR, Tannenbaum SR. Metabolic fate of an oral dose of 15N-labeled nitrate in humans: effect of diet supplementation with ascorbic acid. Cancer Res 1983; 43: 1921–5.
221. Preussmann R, Tricker AR. Endogenous nitrosamine formation and nitrate burden in relation to gastric cancer epidemiology. In: Reed Pl, Hill MJ (eds). Gastric Carcinogenesis. Amsterdam: Elsevier Biomedical; 1988: 147–62.
222. Saul RK, Kabir SH, Cohen Z, Bruce WR, Archer MC. Relevance of nitrate and nitrite levels in the human intestine. Cancer Res 1981; 41: 2280–3.
223. Barker HA. Amino acid degradation by anaerobic bacteria. Annu Rev Biochem 1981; 50: 23–40.
224. Padovan W, Owens C, Ferguson R. Creatinine and amino acid profiles of ileal and faecal fluids [Abstract], Clin Sci Mol Med 1975; 49: P27.
225. Ziesel SH, DeCosta K, Fox JG. Endogenous formation of dimethylamine. Biochem J 1985; 232: 403–8.
226. Tricker AR, Pfundstein B, Kalble T, Preussmann R. Secondary amine precursors to nitrosamines in human saliva, gastric juice, blood, urine and faeces. Carcinogenesis 1992; 3: 563–8.
227. Ishiwata H, Iwata R, Tanimura A. Intestinal distribution, absorption and secretion of dimethylamine and its biliary and urinary excretion in rats. Food Chem Toxicol 1984; 22: 649–53.
228. Brooks JB, Cherry WB, Thacker L, Alley CC. Analysis by gas chromatography of amines and nitrosamines produced in vivo and vitro by *Proteus mirabilis*. J Infect Dis 1972; 126: 143–53.
229. Kunicaki N, Hayashi M. Formation of N-nitroamines from secondary amines and nitrite by resting cells of *Escherichia coli*. Appl Environ Microbiol 1979; 37: 279–82.
230. Calmels S, Ohshima H, Vincent P, Gounot AM, Bartsch H. Screening of microorganisms for nitrosation catalysis at pH 7 and kinetic studies on nitrosamine formation from secondary amines by *E. coli* stains. Carcinogenesis 1985; 6: 911–15.
231. Miwa M, Stuehr DJ, Marletta MA, Wishnok JS, Tannenbaum SR. Nitrosation of amines by stimulated macrophages. Carcinogenesis 1987; 8: 955–8.
232. Dull BJ, Gittes RF, Goldman P. Nitrate production and phagocyte activation: differences among Sprague-Dawley, Wistar-Furth, and Lewis rats. Carcinogenesis 1988; 9: 625–7.
233. Kantor AF, Hartge P, Hoover RN et al. Urinary tract infection and risk of bladder cancer. Am J Epidemiol 1984; 119: 510–15.
234. Johansson SL, Anderstrom C, von Schultz L, Larsson P. Enhancement of N-[4-(5-nitro-2-furyl)-2-thiazolyl] formamide-induced carcinogenesis by urinary tract infection in rats. Cancer Res 1987; 47: 559–62.
235. Stewart M. Urinary diversion and bowel cancer. Ann R Coll Surg Engl 1986; 68: 98–102.
236. Cohen MS, Hilz ME, Davis CP, Anderson MD. Urinary carcinogen [nitrosamine] production in a rat animal model for ureterosigmoidostomy. J Urol 1987; 138: 449–52.
237. Tricker AR. Excretion of N-nitrosamines in patients with bacterial bladder infections or diversions of the urinary tract. Eur J Cancer Prevent Suppl 1996; 1: 95–9.
238. Radomski JL, Greenwald D, Hearn WL, Block NL, Woods FM. Nitrosamine formation in bladder infections and its role in the etiology of bladder cancer. J Urol 1978; 120: 48–50.
239. Hicks RM, Walters CL, Elsebai I et al. Demonstration of nitrosamines in human urine: preliminary observations on a possible etiology for bladder cancer in associarion with chronic urinary tract infections. Proc R Soc Med 1977; 70: 413–17.
240. Abdel-Tawab AR, Aboul-Azm T, Ebied SA et al. The correlation between certain tryptophan metabolites and the N-nitrosamine content in the urine of the bilharzial bladder cancer patients. J Urol 1986; 135: 826–36.
241. Stickler DJ, Chawla JC, Tricker AR, Preussmann R. N-nitrosamine generation by urinary tract infections in spine injured patients. Paraplegia 1992; 30: 855–63.
242. Creagh TA, Picramenos D, Smalley ET, Walters CL, Mundy AR. The source of urinary nitrosamines in patients with enterocystoplasties. Br J Urol 1997; 79: 28–31.
243. Groschel J, Riedasch G, Kalbe T, Tricker AR. Nitrosamine excretion in patients with continent ileal reservoirs for urinary diversion. J Urol 1992; 147: 1013–16.
244. Greenwell TJ, Woodhams SD, Smalley T, Mundy AR. Effect of antibiotics on enterocystoplasty urinary nitrosamine levels. Urology 2001; 58: 660–4.
245. Woodhams SD, Greenwell TJ, Smalley T, Mundy AR. Factors causing variation in urinary N-nitrosamine levels in enterocystoplasties. BJU Int 2001; 88: 187–91.
246. Stribling MD, Cohen MS, Fagan JD et al. The effect of ascorbic acid on urinary nitrosamines and tumor development in a rat animal model for ureterosigmoidostomy [Abstract]. J Urol 1989; 141: 304A, no. 540.

247. Weitzman SA, Weitberg AB, Clark EP, Stossel TP. Phagocytes as carcinogens: malignant transformarion produced by human neutrophils. Science 1985; 227: 1231–3.
248. Stuehr DJ, Marietta MA. Further studies on murine macrophage synthesis of nitrite and nitrate. In: Bartsch H, O'Neill IK, Schulte-Hermann R (eds). Relevance of N-Nitroso Compounds to Human Cancer: Exposures and Mechanisms. Lyon: IARC Scientific Publications, 1987: 335–9.
249. Daher N, Gautier R, Abourachid M, Decaens C, Bara J. Rat colonic carcinogenesis after ureterosigmoidostomy: pathogenesis and immuno-histochemical study. J Urol 1988; 139: 1331–6.
250. Hicks RM, Walters CL, El-Sebai I et al. Determination of nitrosamines in human urine: preliminary observations as the possible etiology for bladder cancer in association with chronic urinary tract infections. Proc R Soc Med 1976; 70: 413–16.
251. Ali MH, Satti MB, Al-Nafussi A. Multiple benign colonic polyp at the site of ureterosigmoidostomy. Cancer 1984; 53: 1006–10.
252. Lasser A, Acosta AE. Colonic neoplasms complicating ureterosigmoidostomy. Cancer 1975; 35: 1218–22.
253. Yura Y, Hayashi O, Kelly M, Oyasu R. Identification of epidermal growth factor as a component of the rat urinary bladder tumor-enhancing urinary fractions. Cancer Res 1989; 49: 1548–53.
254. Lina BAR, Woutersen RA. Effects of urinary potassium and sodium ion concentrations and pH on N-butyl-N-(4-hydroxybutyl)nitrosamine-induced urinary bladder carcinogenesis in rats. Carcinogenesis 1989; 10: 1733–6.
255. Byrne PJ, Stephens RB, Hennessy TP, West AB, Sheahan DG. Colon cancer at sites of anastomosis. Lancet 1984; i: 225.
256. Calderisi RN, Freeman HJ. Differential effects of surgical suture materials in 1,2-dimethylhydrazine-induced rat intestinal neoplasia. Cancer Res 1984; 44: 2827–30.
257. Chester JF, Gaissert HA, Ross JS, Malt RA, Weitzman SA. N-[4-(5-nitro-2-furyl)-2-thiazolyl] formamide-induced bladder cancer in mice: augmentation by sutures through the bladders. J Urol 1987; 137: 769–71.
258. Kaufman JM, Fam B, Jacobs SC et al. Bladder cancer and squamous metaplasia in spinal cord injury patients. J Urol 1977; 118: 967–71.
259. Hara I, Miyake H, Hara S et al. Increased serum carcinoembryonic antigen level in patients undergoing colon neobladder replacement compared with ileal neobladder replacement. Urology 2002; 60: 363–7.
260. Sohn M, Fuzesi L, Duetz F et al. Signet ring cell carcinoma in adenomatous polyp at site of ureterosigmoidostomy 16 years after conversion to ileal conduit. J Urol 1990; 143: 805–7.

10 Effect of enterocystoplasty on skeletal development in children

Mike Minh Nguyen and Eric A Kurzrock

Introduction

The use of bowel to reconstruct the lower urinary tract has allowed urologists to treat patients with bladder diseases at all ages. In the older patient, cancer often requires radical excision of the bladder with complete replacement with bowel segments. On the other hand, in children, congenital defects such as myelomeningocele or exstrophy are more commonly the impetus for bladder reconstruction. Enterocystoplasty has revolutionized the treatment of children with severe bladder disease, and has also highlighted the significant differences between the adult and the developing child.

As time has passed, research has elucidated a myriad of metabolic sequelae that result from the placement of bowel into the urinary tract. These include changes in acid–base balance, calcium metabolism and bone mineralization.[1] In adults, alterations in bone mineralization and homeostasis can lead to osteomalacia. In children, who are in the active phase of skeletal development, these alterations can lead to decreased growth, and in severe cases, rickets. High-risk patients are those with chronic renal insufficiency and an inability to compensate for chronic metabolic acidosis.

In children with normal renal function, the long-term skeletal consequences of enterocystoplasty remained underreported until 1992 when two retrospective studies noted that 20% of children lost 20–28 percentile height-points after enterocystoplasty.[2,3] While conceding that there existed several potential confounding factors, the authors of these reports felt that impaired growth should be added to the list of potential drawbacks to enterocystoplasty in the pediatric population. Further clinical and animal research over the past decade has added supporting, as well as conflicting, information to the debate. This chapter reviews the physiologic basis of impaired skeletal growth following enterocystoplasty and discusses the animal and clinical studies that have been performed in this subject area.

Physiology

Metabolic acidosis is a decrease in serum bicarbonate levels with a decrease in overall serum pH. This situation occurs when there is either a failure to excrete acid loads appropriately, as in renal failure, or when there is an increased load of acid, as in augmented patients. In augmented or diverted patients, metabolic acidosis is thought to result from the abnormal absorption characteristics of bowel segments interposed into the urinary tract. Unlike non-absorptive urothelium, the bowel segments used to create augments and diversions reabsorb substances excreted by the kidneys which can lead to metabolic acidosis. These substances include ammonia, ammonium, free hydrogen ions and chloride ions. Bowel segments may also excrete bicarbonate, contributing to net acidosis. Metabolic acidosis has been reported in up to 80% of patients after ureterosigmoidostomy and in 10–15% of patients after colon conduits.[1] Homeostatic mechanisms compensate for the metabolic acidosis in these patients. Increased respiratory excretion of CO_2 through hyperventilation occurs, partially and temporarily correcting the pH. In chronic metabolic acidosis however, renal compensation also occurs. Increased excretion of ammonium by the kidney effectively removes acid while creating new bicarbonate. Both mechanisms further raise the pH towards normal.

These changes occur in the time frame of several hours to days and result in 'compensated' metabolic acidosis.

However, metabolic acidosis has not been consistently found in children who have undergone enterocystoplasty or urinary diversion. In Mundy and Nurse's study, all 16 children had metabolic acidosis by arterial blood gas measurements while 6/7 myelomeningocele and 0/7 exstrophy patients were found to be acidotic when similarly tested by arterial blood gas measurements in a study by Mingin et al.[4] In studies with only serum bicarbonate measurements between 7 and 58% of patients were found to be acidotic. Mitchell and Piser found increased mean serum chloride above the normal range in 129 patients after enterocystoplasty with no difference between small and large bowel.[5] Serum bicarbonate was not significantly changed in patients with normal renal function. Children with renal insufficiency had abnormally low bicarbonate levels after surgery. In contrast, Kurzrock et al found increased bicarbonate levels in children after gastrocystoplasty.[6] This is a unique quality of stomach segments. This observation has led to composite reservoirs constructed from stomach and bowel that have been used to treat and prevent metabolic acidosis.[7]

The mechanisms behind decreased skeletal growth in patients who have undergone enterocystoplasty are not entirely clear. Currently, the prevailing theory involves mobilization of calcium carbonate from bone as a buffering response to chronic metabolic acidosis. The carbonate combines with hydrogen ions while the free calcium is then excreted in the urine.[8] Further loss of calcium stores can occur due to impairment of renal tubule calcium reabsorption. Contributions may also come from malabsorption, secondary to the removal of bowel and/or the ileocecal valve, as well as acidosis-induced changes in calcium, phosphate, and parathyroid hormone (PTH) metabolism.[1] The end result is osteomalacia or in severe cases, rickets. Subtle changes in skeletal development may occur in less severely affected children.

Animal studies

To study the physiologic effects of introducing bowel into the urinary system in a detailed, controlled fashion, several investigators have used the Wistar rat as an experimental model. Koch and McDougal performed a left ureterosigmoidostomy in 20 rats with 20 non-operated controls.[9] None of their rats had evidence of overt metabolic acidosis. Evaluation of the urine and bones demonstrated renal adaptation and changes in bone mineralization although bone length was not significantly affected by surgery.[9]

In a second study, the same group examined a group of rats in a urinary diversion model that consisted of 78 rats that were equally divided into sham-operated controls and a diverted group.[10] The diverted group underwent anastomosis of the bladder to the sigmoid colon. After surgery, this group was subdivided into those that received no water additive, sodium bicarbonate water additive, or ascorbic acid water additive. Mild metabolic acidosis was found in diverted rats when no supplemental sodium bicarbonate or ascorbic acid was given. A significant decrease in bone calcium content was also observed in this group. On the other hand, avoidance of metabolic acidosis in the other groups, through sodium bicarbonate or ascorbic acid supplementation, appeared to prevent the decrease in calcium.

Hochstetler et al examined the effects of ileal augmentation cystoplasty in Wistar rats.[11] Rats either underwent ileal augmentation cystoplasty or sham surgery, which consisted of ileal resection and primary reanastomosis. A subset of the augmentation animals received sodium bicarbonate supplementation. The authors found that an acid stress in the form of 1% ammonium chloride in the water supply was needed to demonstrate significant differences between the groups because of the rat kidney's ability to compensate for an increased acid load. When stressed in this fashion, augmented rats that did not receive sodium bicarbonate were found to have significantly decreased femur lengths, bone density, serum bicarbonate levels and serum carbon dioxide levels. Serum calcium levels were not affected. Metabolic acidosis in these animals was associated with decreased linear growth and bone density. However, when given sodium bicarbonate to correct the acidosis, these adverse changes in bone metabolism were not seen.

Recently, Gerharz et al revisited the subject in a detailed animal model of enterocystoplasty.[12] In their study, a total of 120 Wistar rats were divided into four groups: ileocystoplasty, ileocystoplasty with resection of the ileocecal segment, colocystoplasty, and a control group that underwent sagittal cystotomy and closure alone. The rats were followed for 8 months. At the end of the study, the authors found no changes in overall bone length or volume in any of the groups. Likewise, none of their groups demonstrated overt metabolic acidosis. No changes were seen in other serum markers such as calcium, PTH, vitamin D, or phosphorus. However, there were some differences in other factors in the ileocystoplasty with ileocecal segment resection group. This group alone demonstrated decreased bone mass after surgery (decreased 37.5%, $P<0.01$). This group was also unique in having statistically significant hypomagnesemia, hypocalcemia, and reduced insulin-like growth factor binding protein. They also had alterations in the cancellous compartment of their bones consistent with changes seen in osteoporosis or metabolic bone disease but not seen in osteomalacia or mineralization defects. The authors felt these changes were a result of intestinal malabsorption from the ileocecal segment resection as opposed to a direct effect of enterocystoplasty. In the other groups, no significant skeletal or metabolic changes were found.

Together, these animal studies demonstrate a negative effect on skeletal development with augmentation or diversion. When metabolic acidosis was seen, bone length decreased as was the case in Hochstetler's and Koch's study although statistical significance was reached only in the former. In McDougal's[10] study where metabolic acidosis occurred in rats which were not given

13 Patient selection criteria for orthotopic bladder replacement

Steven R Mindrup and Badrinath R Konety

Introduction

In 1888, Tizzoni and Poggi transplanted ureters into an isolated loop of ileum interposed between the ureters and the urethra in a canine that was reportedly continent and expired 30 months postoperatively after three successful pregnancies.[1] This groundbreaking work marks the origins of interest in orthotopic reconstruction of the bladder for urinary diversion after cystectomy. Lemoine first used the procedure in humans in 1913.[2] Initially, cystectomy was performed with ureteral reimplantation into the rectum. Due to complications from recurrent pyelonephritis, the rectal segment was transected and anastomosed to the urethra followed by sigmoid–anal anastomosis.

More recently, bladder substitution has revolutionized urinary diversion after cystectomy. Modern advances in orthotopic reconstruction began in 1979 with the work of Camey and Le Duc.[3] The orthotopic neobladder has since become the standard of care for urinary diversion after cystectomy; many have described the technique as the current gold standard to which other forms of diversion should be compared.[4] Consensus opinion is that urinary reconstruction to the urethra is the procedure of choice in the appropriately selected male patient with bladder cancer.[5] Quality of life after cystectomy with orthotopic neobladder creation has been compared to conduit diversion in several series. The results have been mixed with the most recent series showing a significantly higher quality of life with a neobladder.[6] Other series have shown only a marginally better quality of life in patients with neobladders compared with those with conduits.[7] However, patients with neobladders in this series were significantly younger than the cohort undergoing conduit diversion, thus leading the authors to conclude that since younger patients should have higher quality of life scores the results were further confounded and required a validated survey. While the results of these series are mixed, the trend toward improved quality of life in neobladder patients is to be expected, given their ability to resume preoperative voiding patterns without the need for a stoma or appliance. Arguably, an orthotopic neobladder may even be preferable to a cutaneous continent diversion such as the Indiana pouch since it would avoid the need for frequent catheterization.

Several bowel segments may be used for bladder substitution, including stomach, ileum, colon and, rarely, jejunum. Ileum is one of the most common segments used and will be the primary focus of this discussion. The ileal neobladder consists of an ileal pouch anastomosed to the urethra after cystectomy. There are several types of ileal neobladder currently in use, including the Melchoir, Studer and Hautmann types.[8–10] One commonly used type, the Hautmann ileal neobladder, uses a segment of small bowel arranged in an M or W shape. The Studer type neobladder uses a long segment of ileum, most of which is detubularized except for a 10–25 cm proximal segment which is left intact and into which the ureters are anastomosed. A variation of the Hautmann neobladder uses a non-detubularized proximal segment of ileum into which the ureters are anastomosed to prevent reflux as in a Studer-type neobladder. Continence rates of the Hautmann and Studer neobladders are nearly identical (Table 13.1).[11] The Kock ileal reservoir was initially used as a continent cutaneous diversion that employed intussuscepted nipple valves for both the afferent (antireflux) and efferent (continence) limbs. The procedure entailed exposed staple lines that resulted in high rates of stone formation during long-term follow-up.[20] Stein et al incorporated the serous-lined ureteral tunnel outlined by Abol-Enein and Ghoneim[21] to construct a modification of the neobladder that includes a non-refluxing ureterointestinal anastomosis called the T-pouch.[22] Other types of reservoir include the Mainz (mixed augmentation ileum and cecum) pouch and the ileocolonic (Le Bag) pouch. Like the Kock ileal reservoir, the orthotopic Mainz pouch was initially used as a continent

Table 13.1 Continence and CIC (clean intermittent catheterization) rates following neobladder diversion

Series	N	Mean follow-up (months)	Continence (%) Day	Continence (%) Night	CIC (%)	Type
Males only						
Kulkarni et al[12]	102	73	89	78	35	Multiple
Deliveliotis et al[13]	35	38	88.5	74	17	S-Pouch
Steven and Poulsen[14]	166	32	100	94	44	Kock
Females only						
Stenzl et al[15]	102	24	82	72	12	Ileal pouch
Shimogaki et al[16]	8	59.5	88	88	50	Multiple
Males and Females combined						
Lee et al[17]	130	20	67	40–47	8.3–9.5	Hautmann and Studer
Hautmann et al[18]	363	57	95.9	95	5.6	Hautmann
Parekh et al[19]	100	24	100	71	8	Multiple

catheterizable pouch, but has subsequently undergone modification to an orthotopic reservoir.[23] As the name implies, it uses both ileum and cecum with an antirefluxing anastomosis between the ureters and colonic segment. The ileocolonic (Le Bag) pouch was described by Light and Engelmann.[24] It is comprised of terminal ileum and a segment of ascending colon. Detailed discussions of the various types of neobladder are covered in other chapters of this book. It is important, however, for the surgeon to be familiar with all types as there may be situations that prompt the use of one type of neobladder over others, for example in patients with known colonic pathology, an ileal neobladder would be preferable. In patients with spinal dysraphism and concomitant neurogenic bowel, preservation of the ileocecal valve is essential for fecal continence rendering an ileal reservoir more desirable.

Indications and contraindications

The first step in the selection of the appropriate patient for orthotopic diversion involves a discussion with the patient outlining not only various forms of urinary diversion, but also the potential risks and complications of each form. Both incontinent (e.g. conduit) and continent diversion (e.g. cutaneous pouch with catheterizable stoma or orthotopic neobladder) options should be presented. Once a decision has been reached by the patient and surgeon, it should also be made clear that while a neobladder may be the optimal choice, intraoperative findings may alter the course of the diversion, and a cutaneous stoma or conduit may still be necessary. Therefore, at our institution, patients who have elected to undergo orthotopic diversion are routinely counseled in this manner and undergo abdominal marking for a conduit stoma preoperatively by a stoma nurse. In addition, stool guaiac tests are routinely done. If the colon is to be used for orthotopic diversion, some authors recommend radiologic or colonoscopic evaluation of the entire large bowel. Any patient with a heme-positive stool, past or family history of colonic polyps or colon cancer or in whom we consider using large bowel for urinary diversion will undergo preoperative colonoscopy.

Absolute contraindications for orthotopic urinary diversion include intraoperative pathologic findings within the bowel segment intended for use, including inflammatory, infectious or neoplastic disease all of which may indicate the need to use a different portion of intestine (Box 13.1). Therefore, the surgeon must be familiar with the use of different segments of bowel that could be used for orthotopic diversion. Presence of tumor at the distal urethral margin may also necessitate abandoning the orthotopic diversion in favor of a cutaneous stoma or conduit. Prior radiation therapy to the bladder may be a relative contraindication to using small bowel that may either limit options or even preclude ileal orthotopic diversion in some cases. Understanding how or when to catheterize, and the manual dexterity required for catheterization are essential prerequisites of orthotopic diversion. Mental or physical impairments interfering with these tasks can be considered absolute contraindications to orthotopic diversion as failure to comply

BOX 13.1 CONTRAINDICATIONS TO ORTHOTOPIC DIVERSION

- **Absolute**
  - Mental or physical disability
  - Unobstructed serum creatinine >2–2.5 mg/dl
  - Chronic inflammatory bowel disease
  - Intraoperative frozen sections positive for disease at urethral margin
- **Relative**
  - Bladder neck tumor
  - Pelvic irradiation
  - Recurrent urethral strictures
  - Carcinoma in situ of prostatic urethra

with a catheterization regimen, if necessary, could lead to pouch rupture with disastrous results.

Renal function is an important consideration when evaluating a patient for orthotopic diversion. Prolonged contact of urine with ileum or colon can be associated with hyperchloremic metabolic acidosis, especially in patients with altered renal function.[25] If untreated, this acidosis can result in multiple systemic manifestations including severe osteoporosis.[26] Therefore, in our opinion, patients with serum creatinine >2 mg/dl, should not undergo orthotopic bladder substitution (see Box 13.1). Some cystectomy patients present with ureteral obstruction from tumor with concomitant acute renal failure. In these patients, percutaneous drainage of the kidney to relieve the obstruction should be performed to allow renal function to return to baseline. If renal function is still borderline, creatinine clearance should be measured. Most urologists use 60 ml/min as a minimum creatinine clearance, above which orthotopic diversion can be considered.[4] It should be noted that in determining renal function during follow-up of these patients, only creatinine clearance measured under diuretic conditions correlates with renal function, and that urine concentrating ability cannot be measured accurately as osmolarity equilibrates rapidly across bowel segments.[27] With these caveats in mind, renal function can be accurately assessed both pre- and postoperatively.

Comorbid conditions and advanced patient age should not be considered absolute contraindications to orthotopic bladder substitution. Parekh et al found that patients with American Society of Anesthesiologists score of 3 or greater could undergo cystectomy with neobladder formation with morbidity and mortality rates comparable with healthier patients.[28] Continence results in men >70 years have not been significantly different from those in younger patients, provided patients are appropriately selected.[29,30] Therefore, medical comorbidities or advanced age should be taken into consideration along with the entire clinical picture of a patient, but should not be absolute contraindications to orthotopic bladder substitution. However, while results have been excellent even in older, sicker patients at high-volume centers, the same may not be applicable to all centers.[31] Hence, offering the older patient the procedure most likely to result in a successful outcome would be most advisable.

Obese patients present a unique clinical problem when deciding the route of urinary diversion. Body habitus frequently makes appliance maintenance difficult, and a thick abdominal wall can present problems for the conduit stoma or the catheterizable channel. Some workers have therefore recommended orthotopic neobladder formation as a way to circumvent these difficulties.[4] They recommend 'defatting' the mesentery to provide additional mobility when creating the reservoir as many of these patients have significant mesenteric attachments that can complicate the surgery. Obese patients may indeed be good candidates for orthotopic diversion as opposed to conduit formation or cutaneous diversion, though no specific series has been reported for this group. In such patients with a short, fatty mesentery, a longer proximal neourethra may need to be constructed to facilitate urethral anastomosis.

The management of the urethra for oncologic cases has been controversial. Historically, some authors have recommended prophylactic urethrectomy in all cases in which the bladder is removed for cancer.[32] Involvement of the prostatic urethra at cystectomy, a risk for urethral recurrence, has been quoted to be as high as 43%.[33] Incidence of carcinoma in situ or dysplasia in prophylactic urethrectomy specimens has been reported as 12.5%.[34] Urethrectomy is associated with higher rates of postoperative morbidity, anorgasmia, and erectile dysfunction.[35–37] In addition, with the current emphasis on orthotopic diversion, there is a trend towards urethral preservation in appropriate cases. Urethral recurrence rates vary from 0 to 10.6% in men and have only recently been reported in women[38] (Table 13.2). Predictors of urethral involvement include multifocality and/or presence of carcinoma in situ.[34] Prostatic urethral involvement has been extensively analyzed according to whether stromal or ductal invasion is present. Prostatic stromal invasion has shown a 30–64% urethral recurrence rate, while ductal invasion has shown a 10–25% urethral recurrence rate.[42,43] Recent series have reported that while there is an increased probability of recurrence associated with the presence of prostatic stromal invasion found on preoperative transurethral biopsy, this finding is not an absolute contraindication to orthotopic diversion as long as intraoperative frozen section is negative.[44,45] Freeman et al reported a decreased

Table 13.2 Urethral recurrence rates (URR) in oncologic urologic cases

Series	N	Median follow-up (months)	Overall URR (%)	Neobladder URR (%)
Huguet et al[39]	516	50	6.4	3.6 (men only)
Freeman et al[40]	436	72	8	4 (men only)
Deliveliotis et al[13]	35	38.2		2.8 (men only)
Stenzl et al[15]	102	26		0 (women only)
Shimogaki et al[16]	9	59.5		0 (women only)
Yossepowitch et al[41]	214	32.8	5	2 (men and women)

urethral recurrence rate when orthotopic diversion was used as opposed to cutaneous or conduit diversion.[40] This led the authors to postulate a protective effect of urine flow over the retained urethra as a cause for the reduced recurrence rates. A more plausible explanation may be better patient selection in terms of tumor biology and anatomic location. Detection of urethral recurrence can occur through routine urethral wash cytologies, or the patient may present with a bloody urethral discharge. Previous series have reported that symptomatic recurrence is associated with decreased survival.[46] In a more recent series with shorter follow-up, survival does not appear to be significantly different between recurrences detected by washings and by symptoms.[47] At our institution we continue to perform routine urethral washings for cytology with the idea that early detection may facilitate appropriate management, usually in the form of urethrectomy and cutaneous rediversion in patients with a neobladder.

Historically, neobladders were primarily used in male patients, as it was customary to remove the entire urethra in a female cystectomy to obtain adequate surgical margins. Continence was also felt to be at risk with dissection of the bladder neck and proximal urethra. In the mid 1990s, both anatomic and pathologic data were published showing oncologic safety and maintenance of preoperative continence status. Anatomic dissections outlining the neuroanatomy of the female pelvis and histologic evaluation of sphincter mechanisms have increased our understanding of the female continence mechanism and therefore facilitated orthotopic diversion in the female patient.[48,49] These studies divided the female urethra into thirds, with the proximal two-thirds containing three layers of smooth muscle and the distal third containing a transition to striated pelvic floor musculature, called the 'rhabdosphincter'. The proximal urethra is innervated by the sympathetic pelvic plexus, while the distal urethra is innervated by small branches from the pudendal nerve coursing along the pelvic floor. Therefore, preservation of the distal urethra with minimal dissection anteriorly should preserve the rhabdosphincter mechanism and subsequently preserve the female continence mechanism.

Interestingly, follow-up data have shown that instead of being incontinent, women with orthotopic reconstruction have a tendency toward retention or hypercontinence. Hautmann published results and recommendations for female neobladder based on a 10-year experience.[50] At 3 months postoperatively, 66% of the women were continent and able to void to completion without catheterization, 11% had grade I stress incontinence, and 6% had grade II stress incontinence preoperatively that was unchanged postoperatively. Seventeen percent experienced urinary retention and required clean intermittent catheterization. Further follow-up revealed that half of the women became hypercontinent and required clean intermittent catheterization.

Oncologic risk factors and safety of female neobladders have also been established. Several reports have revealed important selection criteria for female patients and demonstrated acceptable oncologic results after neobladder formation in females. Stein et al found that bladder neck involvement was a significant risk factor for urethral involvement.[51] Furthermore, in a series of 71 patients, 60% of those with bladder neck tumors had a tumor-free proximal urethra and no patient with a normal bladder neck had urethral tumor.[52] This study also underscored the importance and accuracy of intraoperative frozen sections in determining presence or absence of urethral disease, information that is critical to the choice of diversion. Similar studies have confirmed that bladder neck disease is the most important risk factor for urethral tumor involvement in women.[53]

In summary, two fundamental criteria for patient selection for orthotopic diversion have been outlined: (i) the external rhabdosphincter complex and corresponding innervation must be functionally intact to provide continence and to allow volitional voiding per urethra; and (ii) adherence to strict oncologic principles during orthotopic reconstruction with care being taken to exclude any potential residual tumor at the urethroenteric anastomosis, the retained urethra or the surgical margins.[54]

References

1. Tizzoni G, Poggi A. Die wiederherstellung der Harnblase: Experimentelle untersuchungen. Exp Untersuch Zentralbl Chir 1888; 15: 921.
2. Lemoine G. Creation d'une vessie nouvelle par un procede personnel après cystectomietotale pour cancer. J Urol Med Chir 1913; 4: 367.
3. Camey M, Le Duc A. L'enterocystoplastie avec cystoprostatectomie totale pour cancer de la vessie. Ann Urol 1979; 13: 114.
4. Stein JP, Skinner DG. Orthotopic urinary diversion. In: Walsh PC, Retik AB, Vaughan ED Jr et al (eds). Campbell's Urology, 8th edn. Philadelphia: WB Saunders, 2002; 3835–67.
5. Skinner DG, Studer UE, Okada K et al. Which patients are suitable for continent diversion or bladder substitution following cystectomy or other definitive local treatment? Int J Urol 1995; 2: 105.
6. Yoneda T, Igawa M, Shiina H et al. Postoperative morbidity, functional results, and quality of life of patients following orthotopic neobladder reconstruction. Int J Urol 2003; 10: 119–25.
7. Dutta SC, Chang SS, Coffey CS et al. Health related quality of life assessment after radical cystectomy: comparison of ileal conduit with continent orthotopic neobladder. J Urol 2002; 168: 164–7.
8. Melchior H, Spehr C, Knop-Wagemann I, Persson IM, Juenneman KP. The continent ileal bladder for urinary tract reconstruction after cystectomy: a survey of 44 patients. J Urol 1988; 139: 714–18.
9. Studer UE, Ackermann D, Casanova GA, Zingg EJ. Three years' experience with an ileal low pressure bladder substitute. Br J Urol 1989; 63: 43–52.
10. Hautmann RE, Egghart G, Frohneberg D, Miller K. The ileal neobladder. J Urol 1988; 139: 39–42.

11. Lee KS, Montie JE, Dunn RL, Lee CT. Hautmann and Studer orthotopic neobladders: a contemporary experience. J Urol 2003; 169: 2188–91.
12. Kulkarni JN, Pramesh CS, Rathi S, Pantvaidya GH. Long-term results of orthotopic neobladder construction after radical cystectomy. BJU Int 2003; 91: 485–8.
13. Deliveliotis C, Alargoff E, Skolarikos A et al. Modified ileal neobladder for continent urinary diversion: experience and results. Urology 2001; 58: 712–16.
14. Steven K, Poulsen AL. The orthotopic Kock neobladder: functional results, urodynamic features, complications and survival in 166 men. J Urol 2000; 164: 288–95.
15. Stenzl A, Jarolim L, Coloby P et al. Urethra-sparing cystectomy and orthotopic urinary diversion in women with malignant pelvic tumors. Cancer 2001; 92: 1864–71.
16. Shimogaki H, Okada H, Fujisawa M et al. Long-term experience with orthotopic reconstruction of the lower urinary tract in women. J Urol 1999; 161: 573–7.
17. Lee KS, Montie JE, Dunn RL, Lee CT. Hautmann and Studer orthotopic neobladders: a contemporary experience. J Urol 2003; 169: 2188–91.
18. Hautmann RE, De Petriconi R, Gottfried HW et al. The ileal neobladder: complications and functional results in 363 patients in 11 year follow-up. J Urol 1999; 161: 422–8.
19. Parekh DJ, Gilbert WB, Smith JA. Functional lower urinary tract voiding outcomes after cystectomy and orthotopic neobladder. J Urol 2000; 163: 56–9.
20. Stein JP, Freeman JA, Esrig D et al. Complications of the afferent antireflux valve mechanism in the Kock ileal reservoir. J Urol 1996; 155: 1579.
21. Abol-Enein H, Ghoneim MA, A novel uretero-ileal reimplantation technique: the serous lined extramural tunnel. A preliminary report. J Urol 1994; 151: 1193.
22. Stein JP, Lieskovsy G, Ginsberg DA et al. An orthotopic ileal neobladder incorporating a serosal lined ileal antireflux technique. J Urol 1998; 159: 1836–42.
23. Thuroff JW, Alken P, Riedmiller H et al. The MAINZ pouch (mixed augmentation ileum and cecum) for bladder augmentation and continent diversion. J Urol 1986; 136: 17.
24. Light JK, Engelmann UH. Le Bag: total replacement of the bladder using an ileocolonic pouch. J Urol 1986; 136: 27.
25. Mills RD, Studer UE. Metabolic complications of urinary diversion. J Urol 1999; 161: 1057–66.
26. Fujisawa M, Nakamura I, Yamanaka N et al. Changes in calcium metabolism and bone demineralization after orthotopic intestinal neobladder creation. J Urol 2000; 163: 1108–11.
27. McDougal WS, Koch MO. Accurate determination of renal function in patients with urinary diversion J Urol 1986; 135: 1175–8.
28. Parekh DJ, Clark T, O'Connor J et al. Orthotopic neobladder following radical cystectomy in patients with high perioperative risk and co-morbid medical conditions. J Urol 2002; 168: 2454–6.
29. Elmajian DA, Stein JP, Esrig D et al. The Kock ileal neobladder: updated experience in 295 patients. J Urol 1996; 156: 920.
30. Steven K, Poulsen AL. The orthotopic Kock ileal neobladder: functional results, urodynamic features, complications and survival in 166 men. J Urol 2000; 164: 288.
31. Konety BR, Inampudi L, Joslyn SA. Impact of hospital volume on outcomes from radical cystectomy: data from the Health Care Utilization Project [Abstract]. J Urol 2003; 169: 11.
32. Schellhammer PR, Whitmore WF. Transitional cell carcinoma of the urethra in men having cystectomy for bladder cancer. J Urol 1976; 115: 56–60.
33. Wood DP Jr, Montie JE, Pontes JE et al. Transitional cell carcinoma of the prostate in cystoprostatectomy specimens removed for bladder cancer. J Urol 1989; 141: 346.
34. Nixon RG, Chang SS, Lafleur BJ et al. Carcinoma in situ and tumor multifocality predict the risk prostatic urethral involvement at radical cystectomy in men with transitional cell carcinoma of the bladder. J Urol 2002; 167: 502–5.
35. Skinner DG, Stein JP, Lieskovsky G et al. 25 year experience in the management of invasive bladder cancer by radical cystectomy. Eur Urol 1993; 33 (Suppl 4): 25–6.
36. Kitamura T, Moriyama N, Shibamoto K et al. Urethrectomy is harmful for preserving potency after radical cystectomy. Urol Int 1987; 42: 375–9.
37. Tomic R, Sjodin JG. Sexual function in men after cystectomy with or without urethrectomy. Scand J Urol Nephrol 1992; 26: 127–9.
38. Jones J, Melchoir SW, Gillitzer R et al. Urethral recurrence of transitional cell carcinoma in a female patient after cystectomy and orthotopic ileal neobladder. J Urol 2000; 164: 1646.
39. Huguet J, Palou J, Serrallach M et al. Management of urethral recurrence in patients with Studer ileal neobladder. Eur Urol 2003; 43: 495–8.
40. Freeman JA, Tarter TA, Esrig D et al. Urethral recurrence in patients with orthotopic ileal neobladders. J Urol 1996; 156: 1615–19.
41. Yossepowitch O, Dalbagni G, Golijanin D et al. Orthotopic urinary diversion after cystectomy for bladder cancer: implications for cancer control and patterns of disease recurrence. J Urol 2003; 169: 177–81.
42. Levinson KA, Johnson DG, Wishnow KI. Indications for urethrectomy in an era of continent urinary diversion. J Urol 1990; 144: 73–5.
43. Hardeman SW, Soloway MS. Urethral recurrence following radical cystectomy. J Urol 1990; 144: 666–9.
44. Lebret T, Herve JM, Barre P et al. Urethral recurrence of transitional cell carcinoma of the bladder: predictive value of preoperative latero-montanal biopsies and urethral frozen sections during prostatocystectomy. Eur Urol 1998; 33: 170–4.
45. Iselin CE, Robertson CN, Webster GD et al. Does prostate transitional cell carcinoma preclude orthotopic bladder reconstruction after radical cystoprostatectomy for bladder cancer? J Urol 1997; 158: 2123–6.
46. Clark PB. Urethral carcinoma after cystectomy: the case for routine urethrectomy. J Urol 1984; 90: 173.
47. Lin DW, Herr HW, Dalbagni D. Value of urethral wash cytology in the retained male urethra after radical cystoprostatectomy. J Urol 2003; 169: 961–3.

48. Colleselli K, Stenzl A, Eder R et al. The female urethral sphincter: a morphological and topographical study. J Urol 1998; 160: 49–54.
49. Borirakchanyavat S, Aboseif SR, Carroll PR et al. Continence mechanism of the isolated female urethra: an anatomical study of the intrapelvic somatic nerves. J Urol 1997; 158: 822–6.
50. Hautmann RE. The ileal neobladder to the female urethra. Urol Clin North Am 1997; 24: 827–35.
51. Stein JP, Cote RJ, Freeman JA et al. Indications for lower urinary tract reconstruction in women after cystectomy for bladder cancer: a pathological review of female cystectomy specimens. J Urol 1995; 154: 1329–33.
52. Stein JP, Esrig D, Freeman JA et al. Prospective pathologic analysis of female cystectomy specimens: risk factors for orthotopic diversion in women. Urology 1998; 51: 951–5.
53. Stenzl A, Draxl H Posch B et al. The risk of urethral tumors in female bladder cancer: can the urethra be used for orthotopic reconstruction of the lower urinary tract? J Urol 1995; 153: 950–5.
54. Stein JP, Ginsberg DA, Skinner DG. Indications and technique of the orthotopic neobladder in women. Urol Clin North Am 2002; 29: 725–34.

14 Ileal neobladders: Camey II, Hautmann, Kock

E James Wright

Introduction

Orthotopic bladder replacement following total cystectomy developed in parallel with strategies for urethral preservation. Prior to this evolution in oncologic management, urinary diversion by ileal conduit or continent catheterizable reservoir was standard. When urethral sparing is feasible from an oncologic standpoint, orthotopic bladder replacement offers the closest approximation to normal voiding and body image. While it is not clear whether this type of reconstruction is optimal when compared to ileal conduit or catheterizable diversion,[1] many patients currently choose orthotopic bladder replacement at the time of cystectomy if it is offered as an option. For this reason, neobladder construction should be discussed will all eligible patients.

Certain features of tumor location, grade and stage can influence the suitability of orthotopic bladder construction. This is also true of some patient characteristics including renal function and medical comorbidities. Initially, neobladder construction was not favored for female patients owing to concern for the short functional urethral length and possible proximity of bladder tumors to the urogenital membrane and continence mechanism. These oncologic and functional concerns have not been shown to be contraindications to neobladder construction in women.[2] Urinary retention or 'hypercontinence' requiring self intermittent catheterization appears to be a greater risk in women with orthotopic reconstruction. Pelvic tumor recurrence rates are identical. Patient evaluation should be individualized when selecting strategies for urinary tract reconstruction. Specific selection criteria for orthotopic bladder replacement in men and women are discussed in Chapter 13.

The mechanisms for voiding and continence for orthotopic neobladders differ from those of the normal lower urinary tract. A combination of pelvic floor relaxation and increased abdominal pressure is necessary for adequate emptying. Some patients find this process difficult to master, and voiding function may be enhanced by education and counseling by nursing or physical therapy staff with expertise in pelvic floor rehabilitation.[3] Urinary continence is controlled primarily by external sphincteric function with additional factors related to neobladder configuration. Urethral sensitivity may have an important role to play in maintaining functional urinary control. Hugonnet et al observed that the sensory threshold in the proximal urethra increased following cystoprostatectomy.[4] The severity of this change influenced the ultimate continence in the patients studied. The authors concluded that relative preservation of afferent urethral function is necessary for optimal urinary control following orthotopic neobladder construction. In general, recovery of continence may continue to improve in the 3 years following orthotopic reconstruction, with roughly 90% of patients dry during the day and 70–85% dry at night.[5]

The technique of orthotopic bladder replacement evolved to fulfill two guiding principles. The first was establishment of a reservoir with adequate capacity and compliance. The second involved strategies to minimize reflux of urine into the upper urinary tract. Peristaltic activity of the bowel is an intrinsic impediment to low sustained resting reservoir pressure and may influence neobladder continence. The interplay between functional volume of an intestinal reservoir and its motor activity is variable. In spite of reconfiguration, some have observed organized motor activity to return in bowel segments.[6] Whether this is an early or late phenomenon, pressure activity can be observed in urinary reservoirs during urodynamic testing. Theoretically, a more spherical shape may have optimal pressure and volume characteristics in accordance with Laplace's law. While the idealized gains from bowel reconfiguration are never completely achieved, most evidence suggests that the contribution of increased functional volume enhances reduction in resting pressure and dissipation of peristaltic activity. In addition, intestinal reservoir capacity increases over time if filling cycles are increased. For this reason, detubularization and refolding of intestinal segments is optimal.[7]

Regarding urinary reflux and preservation of upper tract function, a multitude of ureteral–enteric reimplant techniques have been described. These make use of various tunneling or nipple valve techniques. The competing factors for each of these constructions are the balance of reflux prevention and the tendency toward obstruction. Debate continues as to the relative importance of non-refluxing ureteral implants in orthotopic reconstruction. The current consensus appears to be that preventing ureteral reflux 'may help and likely doesn't hurt'. Taken together, the principles of low pressure storage and preservation of upper tract function continue to guide the development of orthotopic neobladder construction.

This chapter discusses the development of ileal neobladders and their construction, and evaluates their merits and potential limitations for lower urinary tract reconstruction. The specific techniques addressed are the Camey II, Hautmann and hemi-Kock ileal reservoirs. These are representative of ileal reservoirs with suitable capacity and antirefluxing ureteral–enteric anastomoses. Each satisfies the requirements with a unique strategy, highlighting the creativity and characteristic innovation of urinary tract reconstruction. A more recent reservoir employing a serosal-lined tube (the T-pouch)[8,9] as an antireflux mechanism is discussed in Chapter 23. The final variant of ileal neobladder construction is the Studer reservoir, unique for its departure from traditional antirefluxing ureteral–enteric anastomoses. It relies instead on a redundant properistaltic ileal segment to protect the upper tracts. This reservoir is discussed in Chapter 15.

Principles of ileal neobladder construction

For each of the neobladders described, a segment of ileum 40–80 cm must be isolated. The distal end of this segment should be at least 15 cm proximal to the ileocecal junction. This ensures an adequate segment of terminal ileum to prevent malabsorption of bile salts and other metabolic disturbances. It is helpful to locate the ileal segment with maximal mesenteric length to ensure its mobility to the urethra for anastomosis. Stay sutures can be used to mark the margins of the ileal segment, as well as the site of any folds for reconfiguration. The ileal mesentery can be transilluminated for identification of adequate vascular branches. The ileum can support up to 15 cm lateral to a straight vessel, although more than 8 cm is rarely necessary in neobladder construction. The visceral peritoneum of the mesentery can be opened with scissors and thinned to expose crossing vessels. Once identified, these vessels are secured with hemostats, tied with 3-0 polyglycolic suture and divided. The bowel can be divided with cautery or a stapling device. Care should be taken to minimize spillage of the enteric contents during these maneuvers. The bowel continuity is re-established by ileal–ileal anastomosis. This can be done with staples or hand-sewn. The anastomosis should be constructed cephalad of the segment for neobladder construction. Closure of the mesenteric defect can be delayed until after neobladder construction, as approximation can sometimes limit mobility. The separated ileal segment should be irrigated clear with saline. Betadine solutions are unnecessary and can provoke an excessive mucous discharge during neobladder construction. For reconfiguration, the antimesenteric border of the ileum is divided with cutting current over a plastic suction tip, using coagulation current for visible crossing vessels. Ureteral implantation is undertaken following construction of the posterior reservoir wall when the LeDuc technique is used, or following reservoir completion in the case of the Kock, Studer or T-pouch neobladder. The latter make use of the Wallace, double-barrel ureteral-enteric anastomosis.

Postoperative drainage techniques for neobladders differ. Most authors advocate ureteral catheters for stenting across the ureteral-enteric anastomosis. Long 'single-J' 6 Fr or 7 Fr catheters are ideal for this purpose. As all neobladders require a urethral catheter, a useful and convenient strategy secures the ureteral catheters to a 20 Fr urethral Foley catheter leaving enough redundancy to allow access to the catheters upon Foley removal if necessary.[10] Additional drainage holes or 'fenestrations' can be cut into the distal aspect of the ureteral catheters to prevent mucous plugging or distal occlusion. This technique obviates the need for a suprapubic catheter and additional drainage apparatus despite the complex nature of neobladder construction. Dislodgment of the Foley catheter can be prevented by placing a non-absorbable suture through the catheter eye, passing it through the neobladder and body wall and securing it to the skin with a button or other pledget. In the event of balloon failure, the catheter will remain in place. This suture bridge also serves to anchor the neobladder to the body wall for future percutaneous neobladder access if necessary.

It is recommended that abdominal drains be left near the urethral-enteric and ureteral-enteric anastomoses. A single, round Jackson-Pratt suction drain #10 or larger can be looped from the left lower quadrant below the distal aspect of the neobladder and cephalad to access these two areas. The drain can be removed prior to patient discharge if the output has a creatinine value consistent with serum. The ureteral stents and Foley catheter remain in place for 14–21 days. A cystogram prior to removal confirms absence of leak.

Camey II neobladder

The original description of ileal bladder replacement by Camey and Le Duc gave impetus to develop orthotopic reconstruction more extensively.[11,12] To construct this neobladder (Camey I) a 40 cm segment of ileum is brought at its midpoint to the urethra. One ureter is implanted into each end of this segment in a unique non-refluxing fashion (Le Duc–Camey).[13] This technique requires an opening to be made in the ileum through which the ureter is advanced. A 2–3 cm mucosal incision

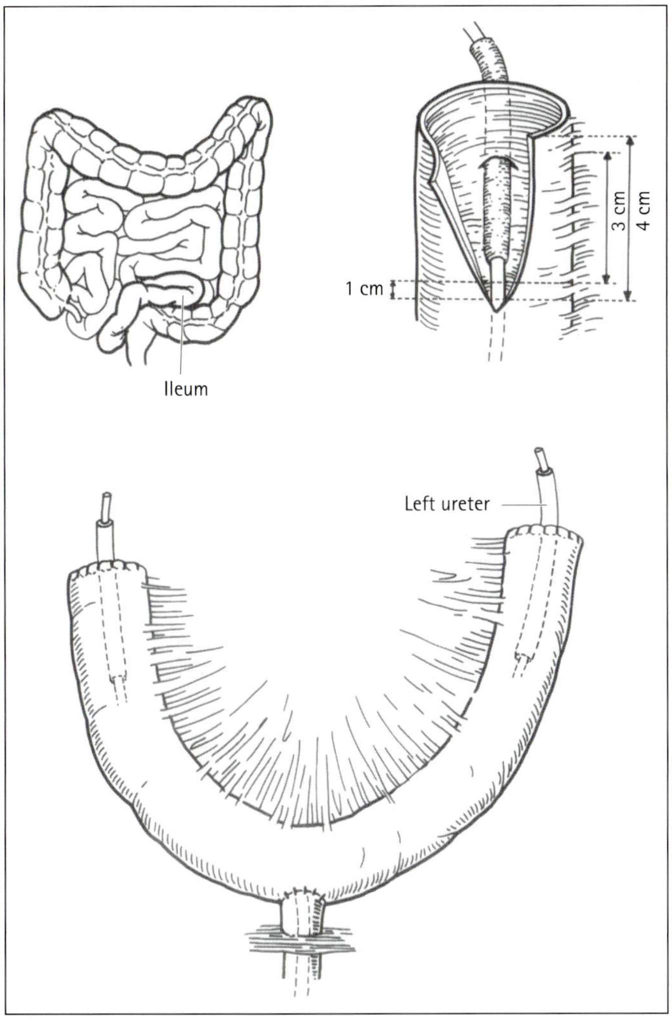

Figure 14.1 The Camey I ileal neobladder. Surgical technique showing reservoir configuration and ureteral implant method.

creates a trough to support the ureter. The distal end of the ureter is spatulated for 1 cm and fixed to the ileum with absorbable suture. The edges of the incised mucosa are similarly fixed to the lateral aspects of the ureteral segment, leaving the ureteral segment exposed inside the reservoir (Figure 14.1).

Relatively simple to construct, the Camey I is mainly of historical interest, as contemporary neobladder configurations have widely supplanted its use. Urinary continence and voiding function were problematic with the Camey I, with 20–80% of patients reporting daytime loss of control and nocturnal incontinence in 20–100%.[14] Preservation of the upper tracts followed in 95% of patients, with absence of reflux in 85%.

Camey sought to improve the functional characteristics of the original neobladder by increasing the length of ileum used to 60–70 cm. The important modification in the Camey II was detubularization and folding of the segment to allow for greater capacity and possible reduction in contraction pressure. The antimesenteric border of the ileal segment was opened and folded in a 'U' configuration. The inner edges were sewn together followed by the outer edges to complete closure. The ureteral anastomoses were again placed in the lateral limbs of the ileal reservoir in the non-refluxing fashion previously described. The most dependent midportion of the ileal segment was fixed to the urethra end-to-side (Figure 14.2). The Camey II offers advantages over the original design.[15] Daytime continence is reported to be 96%, with only 22% of patients having night wetting.[16] Continence appears to return more quickly with the detubularized reservoir. Adequate control can be seen at 4–6 months, in contrast to 8–24 months with the Camey I. Voiding, however, remains frequent. On average, patients void every 3 hours including one to three times at night. In spite of these functional differences, urodynamic comparison shows relatively similar capacity for the two reservoirs, although the maximum pressure at capacity is less with the

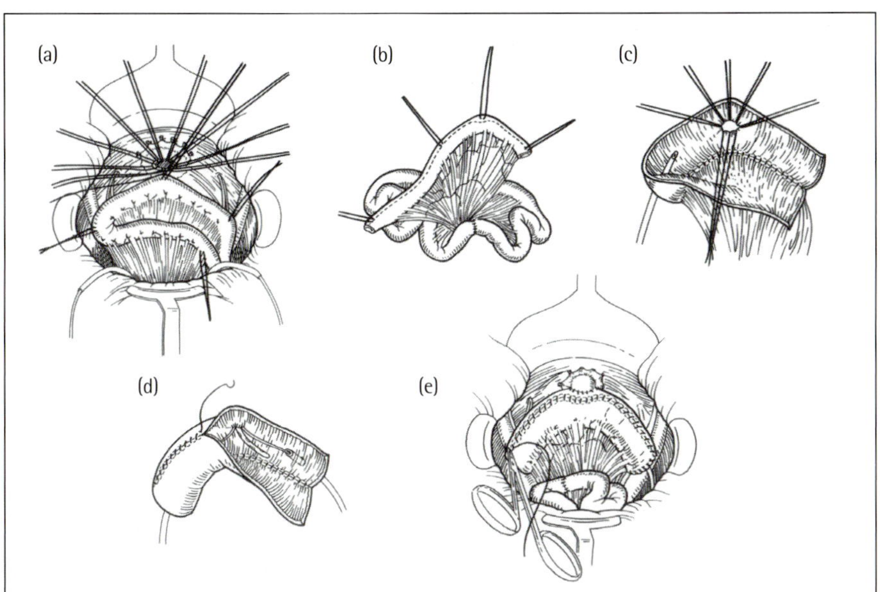

Figure 14.2 Camey II ileal neobladder construction. (a–c) A 65 cm loop of ileum is isolated and folded in a 'U' configuration. Non-refluxing ureteral implants are constructed (d) and the neobladder is fixed to the urethra at its midpoint with the lateral aspects anchored to the pelvic sidewall (e).

Camey II (32 cmH_2O vs. 43 cmH_2O). This is likely a consequence of the additional ileal length and detubularization. With regard to reflux prevention, the results are similar between the two versions.

Hautmann ileal neobladder

Hautmann attempted to create a neobladder with a more spherical reservoir than the Camey through a different folding technique: 60–80 cm of ileum is used, with detubularization along the antimesenteric border.[17] The ileum is folded into a 'W' with creation of three inner suture lines (Figure 14.3). The neobladder employs non-refluxing ureteral implants. In the original description, the ureters were placed in the posterior aspect of the medial ileal 'W' segments. This placed them between the ileal wall and mesentery. With distension of the reservoir, the ureters had a tendency to obstruct. A more recent modification of the Hautmann neobladder has the ureters implanted in the lateral ileal limbs extrinsic to the mesentery. The urethral anastomosis is placed in the right limb of the reservoir through a separate hiatus. The remainder of the outer ileal edges are approximated for complete neobladder closure.

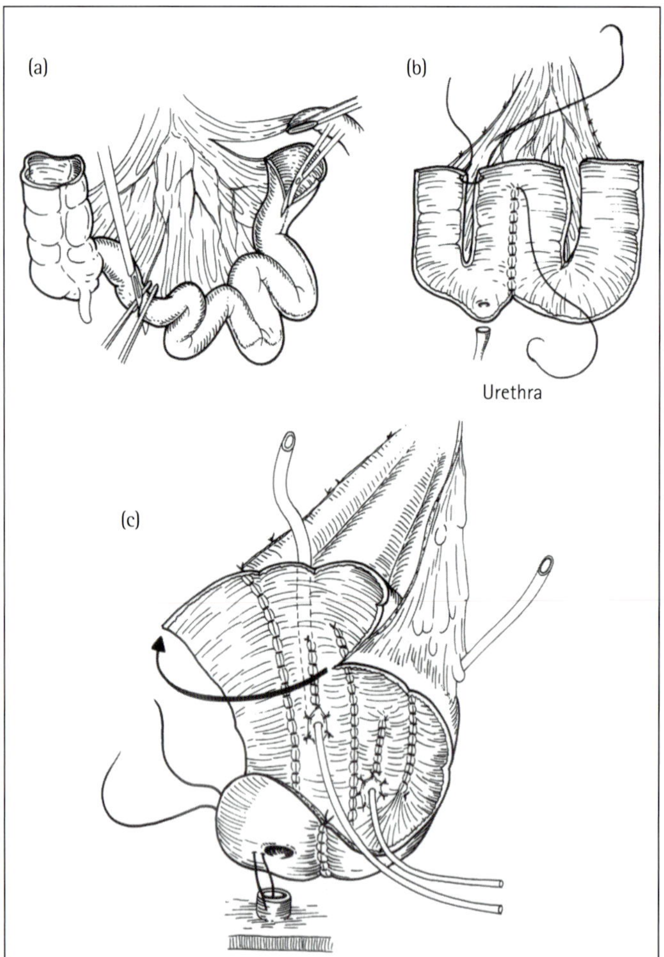

Figure 14.3 The Hautmann ileal neobladder. A 60–80 cm segment of ileum (a) is isolated for construction of a 'W' reservoir (b). The ureters are implanted in a non-refluxing manner with the dependent portion of the reservoir fixed to the urethra (c).

Hautmann et al reviewed the results in 363 men and women with neobladder construction during a follow-up of 11 years.[18] The evaluation included annual renal ultrasound, urine cytology, chest radiograph and blood analysis. An inventory of continence and voiding patterns was also recorded. The authors found a 15% rate of early neobladder-related complications including persistent urine leak (7.7%), pyelonephritis (7.4%) and obstruction of the ureteral enteric anastomosis (3%). The late complication rate was 23%. The largest number of late complications involved ureteral obstruction (9.3%); reflux was seen in 3.3% and urethral stricture in 3%. No major metabolic abnormalities were observed with respect to vitamin B_{12}, folate or acid–base balance. Notably, 48% of patients required oral bicarbonate supplementation to maintain acceptable electrolyte balance. Only three patients complained about change in stool habits following neobladder construction. This most commonly was an increase in frequency tending towards diarrhea.

Regarding voiding and continence, 96% of patients voided with relaxation of the urethral sphincter and either passive emptying or abdominal straining and 3.9% of patients required some form of intermittent catheterization to maintain an adequate emptying cycle. Stable continence during daytime and night-time hours was achieved by 5 years after neobladder construction. Good or satisfactory control (none, or <1 pad/day) was reported by 95% of the patients. This differed by day and night, with 83.7% having good daytime control and 66% with night-time continence. Patients maintained a daytime voiding frequency of 3–15/day (mean 5.2) and night-time frequency of 0–8 (mean 1.2) to achieve the stated control. Two-thirds of the patients voided once or less each night. The average neobladder volume was 433 ml (range 195–812 ml) with mean intravesical pressure of 30 cmH_2O. A mean voiding pressure of 71 cmH_2O (range 20–150 cmH_2O) was created with abdominal straining.

The authors concluded that ileal 'W' neobladder construction was highly satisfactory in terms of complication rate continence and renal preservation. A few points specific to the configuration deserve comment. While all the neobladders in their series reached the urethra, 10% required additional maneuvers to achieve this end. Greater length was established with an additional intestinal segment to bridge the gap.

Orthotopic Kock pouch

The orthotopic Kock pouch, sometimes referred to as the 'hemi-Kock', is a modification of the original continent cutaneous reservoir making use of both afferent and efferent intussuscepted nipple valves.[19,20] With anastomosis of the dependent aspect to the urethra, no efferent valve is require in the orthotopic construction. The single afferent nipple valve acts as an antireflux mechanism for protection of the upper urinary tract.

Construction of the Kock neobladder requires 60 cm of ileum (Figure 14.4) with the proximal 16 cm used for construction of the afferent nipple. The distal 44 cm are opened along the antimesenteric border and sutured along the medial aspect in a 'U' configuration. With completion of this ileal plate, construction of the nipple is undertaken. An 8 cm mesenteric window is created proximal to the junction with the ileal plate. Using two Babcock clamps, the nipple segment is grasped and intussuscepted to lie along the back wall of the ileal plate. The interior portion of the intussusception is fixed in two places with a modified (absence of the distal alignment pin to prevent ileal puncture and fistula formation) end stapling device. A third row of staples is placed to incorporate the nipple and ileal plate, fixing the nipple valve inside the neobladder. An optional absorbable mesh collar can be placed around the external portion of the nipple valve to help prevent the intussusception from expanding. With completion of the nipple valve, the distal aspect of the ileal plate is folded on itself to create a near spherical reservoir. The dependent portion of the anterior suture line is left open for final incorporation into the urethral anastomosis. The ureteral anastomosis is made with a Wallace double-barrel technique.

A recent series reviewing the functional outcome of the orthotopic Kock pouch found an early and late complication rate of 12 and 24%, respectively.[21] As with other ileal neobladders, the complications involved primarily urine leak,

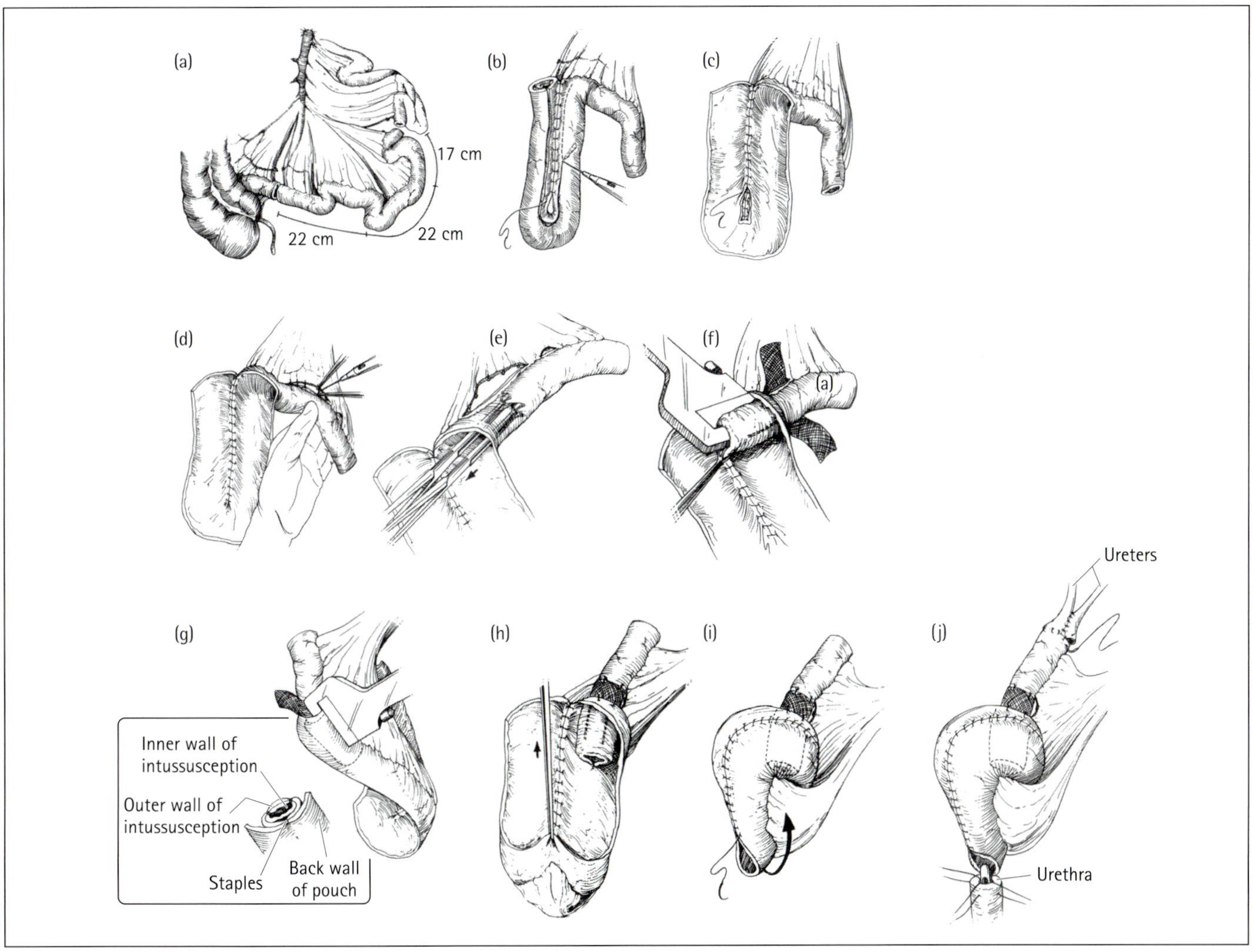

Figure 14.4 Construction of the hemi-Kock ileal neobladder. A 60 cm segment of ileum is isolated and marked as shown (a). The two long segments are folded in a 'U' configuration and ileal plate constructed (b, c). An 8 cm mesenteric window of Deaver is created at the proximal aspect of the afferent limb (d). The afferent ileal segment is intussuscepted onto the ileal plate and stapled in three locations for durable anchorage (e–g). A 1 cm Dexon mesh strip can be placed around the afferent limb for additional fixation (f). With stabilization of the afferent limb, the distal aspect of the ileal plate is folded cephalad and the reservoir closed (h). The distal aspect of the reservoir is left open for anastomosis to the urethra (i). The ureters are fixed to the proximal aspect of the afferent limb in a Wallace configuration to ensure durable patency (j). The afferent nipple valve functions as an antireflux mechanism.

pyelonephritis and urethral anastomotic stricture. Late complications in the Kock neobladder are most commonly related to the afferent nipple valve. Stenosis, thought to be due to ischemia from the intussusception or stone formation at the nipple valve staple line, is unique to this reconstruction. The rate of these secondary complications is variable, as Skinner's group found only 4.1% of 295 patients developed stones in the neobladder while 2.4% developed afferent nipple stenosis.[22] Destabilization of the nipple valve can also pose difficulties, with reflux resulting if the ileum elongates.

Continence and voiding with the Kock neobladder have a day and night variability similar to that of other ileal neobladders. Steven and Poulsen noted rates of 97 and 100% at 1 and 5 years, respectively, following surgery.[21] Night-time control varied from 75 to 94% over the same interval. This is consistent with observations of Elmajian et al[22] and Shabaan et al[23] who reported good to satisfactory daytime continence rates of 87 and 94%, respectively. Again, night-time continence was achieved in 75–86% of patients. Reflux was observed in 17% of patients in the more recent series by Shabaan et al.[23] The volume characteristics of the urethral Kock pouch in this series were consistent with other neobladders incorporating 60 cm of ileum. The capacity ranged from 225 ml to 1200 ml (mean 709 ml) with pressures less than 40 cmH_2O.

Conclusion

Ileal neobladder construction has evolved considerably in the past 20 years. Numerous modifications to reservoir configuration and ureteral enteric implant techniques offer several options for creating a 500–600 ml low pressure reservoir with acceptable urinary control and reliable preservation of upper urinary tract function.

Debate continues as to whether neobladder construction should be the 'gold' standard for lower tract reconstruction following cystectomy. As stated earlier, oncologic concerns for urethral or pelvic tumor recurrence are a potential long-term problem requiring continued surveillance. The additional time and expertise needed for neobladder construction relative to a traditional conduit diversion may also be an impediment for some surgeons. Postoperative management and education are also more intensive for patients with orthotopic bladder replacement.

Questions continually arise as to which type of ileal neobladder is the 'best'. This chapter has examined three versions employing different folding configurations and ureteral–enteric anastomosis techniques. A critical review of published series allows some comparison to be made regarding operative time for construction, early and late complications, continence and upper tract preservation. Recently, attention has also been paid to quality of life and body image issues in patients with different types of urinary tract reconstruction. It is difficult to separate the objective functional parameters of ileal neobladders relative to disease severity and comorbidity, patient self-perception and tolerance, surgeon and institutional expertise and degree of difficulty in construction. It is similarly difficult to identify a large number of patients who personally experience multiple types of urinary reconstruction in order to comment on what is best from a quality-of-life perspective.

Accepting these limitations, it is clear that each of the neobladder techniques presented can be successful. Within a reasonable margin, each satisfies the criteria of the initial guiding principles for function. Over time, there is some regression to the functional mean. Continence and upper tract preservation are nearly equivalent, and the former may have as much to do with the cystectomy technique and urethral preservation as with neobladder configuration. Potential points of separation do exist. The hemi-Kock reservoir requires specialized instrumentation (a modified stapling device) and additional experience and expertise to construct the afferent nipple valve. The mesenteric window necessary for nipple intussusception may put the ileal segment at some risk for stenosis, and the metallic anchoring staples are an ongoing nidus for possible stone formation. Regarding the Hautmann neobladder, the 'W' configuration can limit the length of the ileal mesentery, requiring additional maneuvers to allow tension-free urethral anastomosis. Finally, the Camey II may allow greater transmission of peristaltic activity with its single fold configuration.

While questions regarding optimization remain, the utility of orthotopic bladder reconstruction is certain. Ongoing study of the operative and functional issues, and impact on quality of life of these novel urinary reconstruction techniques will continue to enhance their application and evolution.

References

1. Hart S, Skinner EC, Meyerowitz BE, Boyd S, Lieskovsky G, Skinner DG. Quality of life after radical cystectomy for bladder cancer in patients with an ileal conduit, cutaneous or urethral kock pouch, J Urol 1999; 162: 77–81.
2. Stein JP, Stenzl A, Grossfeld GD et al. The use of orthotopic neobladders in women undergoing cystectomy for pelvic malignancy. World J Urol 1996; 14: 9–14.
3. Kane AM. Nursing management of neobladder surgery: the Studer pouch. Urol Nurs 2000; 20: 189–93, 197.
4. Hugonnet CL, Danuser H, Springer JP, Studer UE. Decreased sensitivity in the membranous urethra after orthotopic ileal bladder substitute. J Urol 1999; 161: 418–21.
5. Mark SD, Webster GD. Ileal reservoirs (Camey II, Hautmann, Kock, Studer). In: Webster GD, Goldwasser B (eds). Urinary diversion: scientific foundation and clinical practice. Oxford: Isis Medical Media, 1995; 140–7.
6. McDougal WS. Use of intestinal segments and urinary diversion. In: Walsh PC, Retik AB, Vaughan ED, Wein AJ (eds). Campbell's Urology, 8th edn. Philadelphia: WB Saunders, 2002; 3745–88.
7. McDougal WS. Mechanics and neurophysiology of intestinal segments as bowel substitutes. J Urol 1987; 138: 1438–9.
8. Abol-Enein H, Ghoneim MA. A novel uretero-ileal reimplanta-

tion technique: the serous lined extramural tunnel. A preliminary report. J Urol 1994; 151: 1193–7.

9. Stein JP, Lieskovsky G, Ginsberg DA, Bochner BH, Skinner DG. The T pouch: an orthotopic ileal neobladder incorporating a serosal lined ileal antireflux technique. J Urol 1998; 159: 1836–42.
10. Mark SD, Webster GD. Simplified urinary drainage following orthotopic or continent bladder replacement. J Urol 1995; 153: 334–5.
11. Camey M, Le Duc A. Le entroplasty après cystoprostatectomie total pour cancer de la vessie. Eur Urol 1979; 13: 114–23.
12. Lilien QM, Camey M. 25 year experience with replacement of the human bladder (Camey Procedure). J Urol 1984; 132: 886–91.
13. Le Duc A, Camey M, Teillac P. An original antireflux ureteroileal implantation technique: long-term follow up. J Urol 1987; 137: 1156–8.
14. Roehrborn CG, Teigland CM, Sagalowsky AI. Functional characteristics of the Camey ileal bladder. J Urol 1987; 138: 739–42.
15. Camey M, Botto H, Richard E. Complications of the Camey procedure. Urol Clin North Am. 1988; 15: 249–55.
16. Ramon J, Leandri P, Rossignol G, Botto H. Orthotopic bladder replacement using ileum: techniques and results. In Webster GD, Kirby R, King LR, Goldwasser B (eds). Reconstructive Urology. Oxford: Blackwell Scientific Publications, 1993; 445–57.
17. Hautmann RE, Egghart G, Frohneberg D, Miller K. The ileal neobladder. J Urol 1988; 139: 39–42.
18. Hautmann RE, de Petriconi R, Gottfried HW et al. The ileal neobladder: complications and functional results in 363 patients after 11 years of followup. J Urol 1999; 161: 422–7; discussion 427–8.
19. Skinner DG, Lieskovsky G, Boyd S. Continent urinary diversion. J Urol 1989; 141: 1323–7.
20. Kock NG, Ghoneim MA, Lycke KG, Mahran MR.Replacement of the bladder by the urethral Kock pouch: functional results, urodynamics and radiological features. J Urol 1989; 141: 1111–16.
21. Steven K, Poulsen AL. The orthotopic Kock ileal neobladder: functional results, urodynamic features, complications and survival in 166 men. J Urol 2000; 164: 288–95.
22. Elmajian DA, Stein JP, Esrig D et al. The Kock ileal neobladder: updated experience in 295 male patients. J Urol 1996; 156: 920–5.
23. Shaaban AA, Mosbah A, El-Bahnasawy MS, Madbouly K, Ghoneim MA. The urethral Kock pouch: long-term functional and oncological results in men. BJU Int 2003; 92: 429–35.

15 Ileal reservoir

Fiona C Burkhard, Celi Varol and Urs E Studer

Introduction

Orthotopic bladder substitutes are now the standard form of bladder replacement following cystectomy. Patient integrity remains intact, and improved cosmetic results, as well as the documented improvement in quality of life and preserved renal function are good basis for patient satisfaction. The main reason for performing the type of orthotopic bladder substitute described in this chapter is the simplicity of the surgical technique with a low complication rate and documented good long-term functional results.

Patient selection

As for any other cystectomy case preoperative assessment should exclude bone, lung and lymph node metastases and establish patient operability. Major liver, renal or bowel insufficiency, as well as incontinence due to sphincter insufficiency should be excluded. These require an alternative form of urinary diversion. In cases of bladder cancer the presence of urethral cancer in preoperative paracollicular biopsies showing tumor in the area of a future anastomotic margin are a definite contraindication. However, the most important factor determining successful outcome is the patient's willingness to comply meticulously to instructions concerning bladder function and their intellectual capacity to understand their new bladder and how it works. If these prerequisites are not met, other forms of urinary diversion should be considered since it is not the surgery itself, but the postoperative management of patients with bladder substitutes, which is the most important factor for achieving good long-term results.

Preoperative checklist

- Patient agreement for indefinite follow-up
- Adequate intellectual capacity, dexterity and mobility
- Serum creatinine ≤150 mmol/l
- Adequate liver function
- Adequate bowel function
- Continence
- No tumor in the distal urethra, paracollicular or bladder neck region

Preparation and positioning of the patient

Preoperative bowel preparation with two colonic enemas is sufficient. Subcutaneous deep venous thrombosis prophylaxis, which is commenced the evening before surgery, is injected in the upper body to prevent postoperative pelvic lymphocele formation. Patients are mobilized on the first postoperative day and wear compression stockings. Antibiotic prophylaxis with amoxicillin/clavulanic acid, aminoglucoside and metronidazole is commenced intraoperatively, aminoglucoside and metronidazole are continued for 48 hours and then stopped, amoxicillin/clavulanic acid is administered until all drains and catheters have been removed. Patients are shaved prior to surgery and placed in a slightly hyperextended supine position (Figure 15.1). The same instruments used for cystectomy and ileal conduit formation are sufficient, and no additional instrumentation is needed for the construction of the ileal bladder substitute.

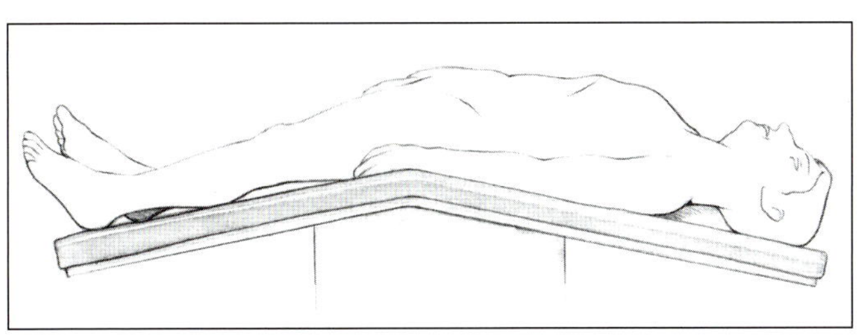

Figure 15.1 Patient supine in a slightly hyperextended position for ileal bladder replacement.

Surgical technique

Cystectomy

Pelvic lymphadenectomy and cystectomy are carried out according to standard procedures with slight modifications. For pelvic lymphadenectomy all connective and lymphatic tissues are meticulously removed from the iliac bifurcation along the external iliac vessels to the inguinal ligament. The genitofemoral nerve and the external iliac artery are the anterolateral limit. The obturator fossa is cleared completely of all tissue other than the obturator nerve. The internal iliac artery and branches, as well as the ventral aspect of the internal iliac vein is freed of all connective and lymphatic tissue. The dorsolateral pedicles, which contain the superior and inferior vesicles along the hypogastric arteries are divided, the fascia of the pelvic floor is incised and Santorini's plexus is ligated. The ureters are divided where they cross the iliac vessels allowing en bloc removal of the distal ureters and paraureteral lymphatic vessels together with the cystectomy specimen.

Nerve sparing

In men the dorsomedial pedicle is resected along the pararectal and presacral plane on the tumor-bearing side. In contrast, on the contralateral non-tumor-bearing side care is taken, whenever possible to preserve the hypogastric fibers and the plexus pelvicus situated dorsolateral to the seminal vesicle. Dissection along the dorsolateral wall is terminated at the base of the prostate. Santorini's plexus is then divided and the membranous urethra is resected as close as possible to the apex of the prostate by excavating the urethra out of the doughnut-shaped prostatic apex. The neurovascular bundles dorsolateral to the prostate are preserved on both sides.

In women the endopelvic fascia is disturbed as little as possible to minimize damage to the intrapelvic somatic fibers from the pudendal nerve, which also contributes to urethral innervation. In tumor-bearing patients the paravaginal tissue on the tumor bearing side is widely excised as far as the pararectal region to remove the lymphatics draining the bladder base (Figure 15.2a). On the non-tumor-bearing side dissection is carried out no further than the 2 o'clock or 10 o'clock position, dividing the autonomic nerve supply from the pelvic plexus passing the bladder (Figure 15.2b). This preserves the paravaginal fibers passing further dorsal to the urethra. A spongeholding forceps in the vagina facilitates dissection along the whitish vaginal wall at the height of the cervix. In patients with tumors in the trigonal area, the vaginal wall is then divided just dorsal of the portio and the anterior vaginal wall is resected en bloc with the bladder wall to the level of the bladder neck. The urethra is transsected just distal to the bladder neck. In patients without tumor in the trigone or along the bladder neck the uterus and the anterior vaginal wall can be preserved. For this the bladder is dissected from the anterior vaginal wall.

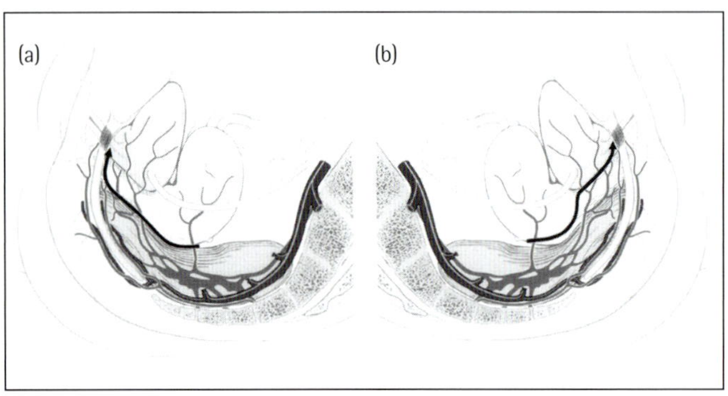

Figure 15.2 Line of dissection on the tumor-bearing (a) and the non-tumor-bearing (b) side. The line of excision is at 9 o'clock or 3 o'clock on the tumor-bearing and at 2 o'clock or 10 o'clock on the non-tumor-bearing side.

Ileal orthotopic bladder substitute

Preparing the ileal segment for the bladder substitute

For construction of the reservoir an ileal segment of approximately 54–56 cm length is isolated 25 cm proximal to the ileocecal valve (Figure 15.3). Bowel continuity is restored with a 4-0 polyglycolic acid singular seromuscular running suture. To guarantee correct measurement, the length of the ileal segment is measured with a ruler in steps of 10 or 15 cm along the border of the mesoileum without stretching the bowel. Irritation of the pelvis as well as epidural anesthesia with local anesthetics should be avoided since this can increase muscle tone and shorten the length of the bowel segment, which will result in a segment of increased length after muscle relaxation. The distal incision of the mesoileum transects the main vessels, whereas the proximal incision must be short in order to preserve the ves-

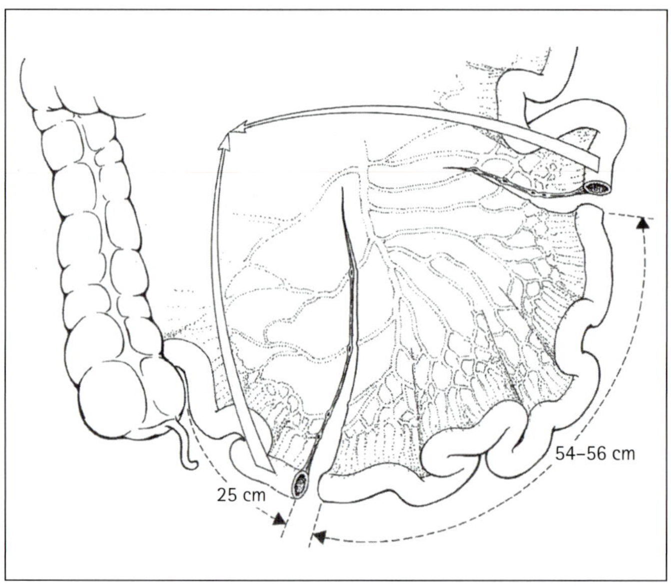

Figure 15.3 An ileal segment of 54–56 cm is isolated 25 cm proximal of the ileocecal valve. This results in a long distal incision of the mesoileum transecting the main vessels and a short proximal incision leaving the vessels intact.

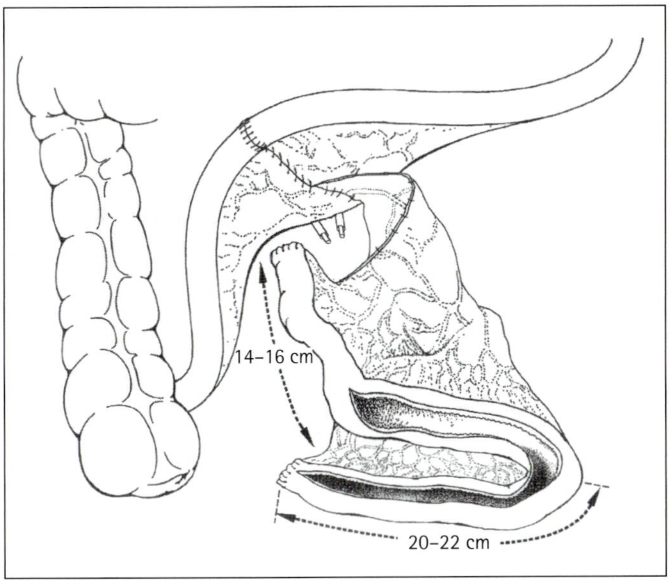

Figure 15.4 Opening of the aboral 40–44 cm of the ileal segment along the antimesenteric border.

sels perfusing the future reservoir segment (see Figure 15.3). The window in the mesoileum is closed with a 2-0 polyglycolic acid running suture in which the mesoileum of the bladder substitute is included. Care must be taken to apply the stitches superficially to preserve the blood supply to the bladder substitute. Both ends of the ileal segment are closed with seromuscular running sutures (4-0 polyglycolic acid). The distal 40–44 cm end of the ileal segment is then opened along the antimesenteric border (Figure 15.4).

The left ureter is transferred to the right side anterior to the aorta and caval vein just above the inferior mesenteric artery. Both ureters are then spatulated over a length of 1.5–2 cm. Two 1.5–2 cm long incisions are placed along the paramedian antimesenteric border at the most proximal end of the unopened part of the 14–16 cm long afferent tubular segment. The incision for the right ureter is placed approximately 1 cm distal to the incision for the left ureter. After placing a suture (4-0 polyglycolic acid) at each end of the spatulated ureter and the ileal incision, ureter and ileum are anastomosed by two running sutures using the Nesbit technique in an open end-to-side fashion (Figure 15.5). The running suture begins at the cranial/proximal end of the anastomosis. Care is taken to use as little tissue as possible at the proximal end of the suture on both sides to prevent narrowing of the ureteral lumen. Toward the distal end the amount of tissue included in the suture is gradually increased to compensate for possible pull on the ureter. A special effort should be made to always begin with the ureteral wall so that it comes to lie between mucosa and seromuscularis of the afferent tubular segment. This should prevent a fistula caused by prolapse of the mucosa and make a waterproof suture possible with a low tendency to shrink, since urine extravasation is prevented. The ureters are stented with 7–8-Fr catheters. To prevent dislocation of the stents a rapidly absorbable polyglycolic acid suture is placed through both the ureter and catheter 3–4 cm proximal to the anastomosis. This is tied loosely so as not to compromise the ureteral vasculature and allow a certain amount of movement of the catheter without resulting in pull on the ureter. Tension (on the anastomosis) is neutralized by placing sutures from the most distal periureteral tissue to the afferent ileal segment which at the same time cover the suture. The ureteral stents are passed through the wall of the most distal end of the afferent tubular segment, where they are covered by mesoileum. This provides a covered channel in the reservoir wall when removing the ureteral stents 4–7 days postoperatively.

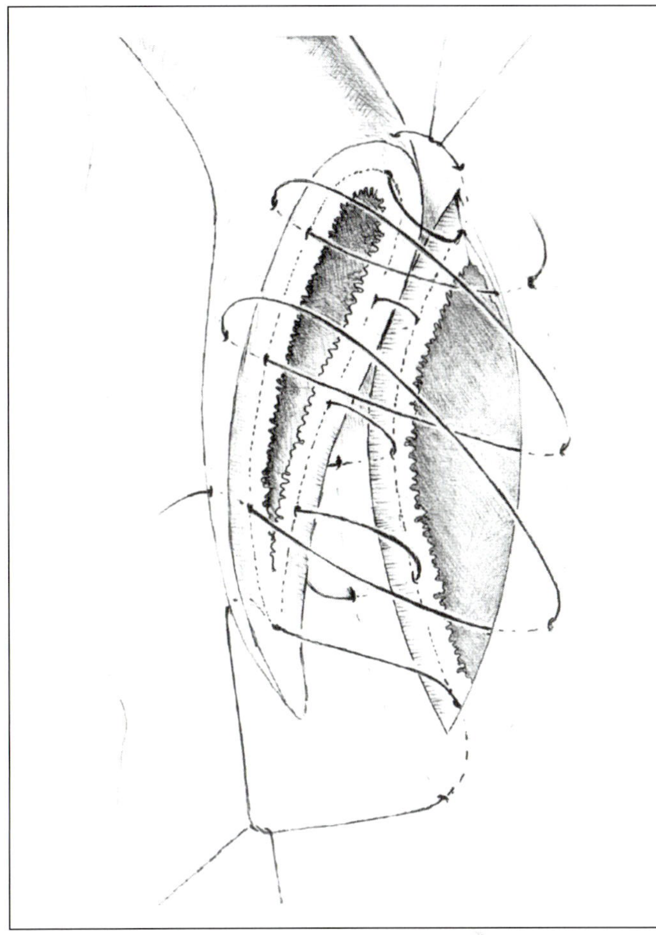

Figure 15.5 Ileoureteral anastomosis in a simple end-to-side fashion according to the Nesbit technique. Note that at the proximal end little tissue is included whereas towards the distal end increasing amount of tissue is incorporated in the suture.

Construction of the bladder substitute and anastomosis of the urethra

For construction of the reservoir the two medial borders of the open distal part of the ileal segment are folded into a U. The two medial borders are then joined by re-sewing them with a single layer seromuscular continuous polyglycolic acid suture (Figure 15.6). The bottom of the U is then folded over between

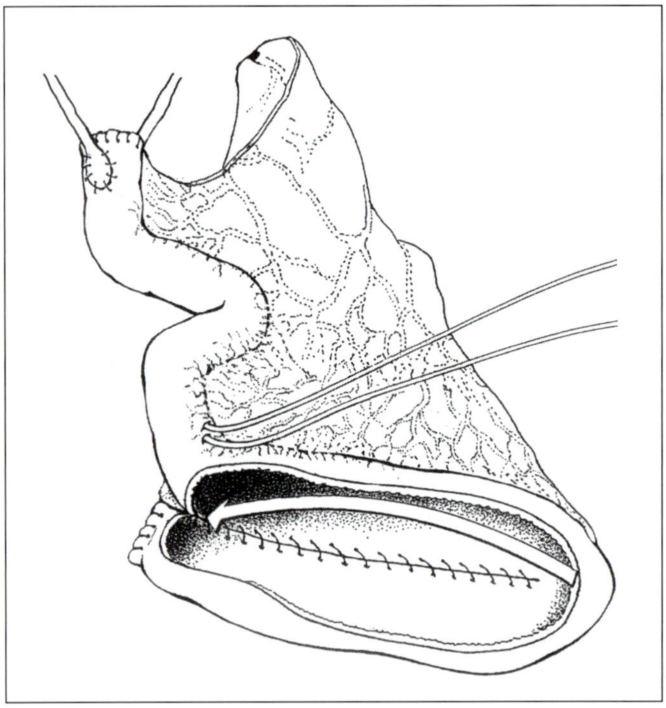

Figure 15.6 The two distal antimesenteric borders are sewn together and the opened ileum folded into a U with a continuous seromuscular suture.

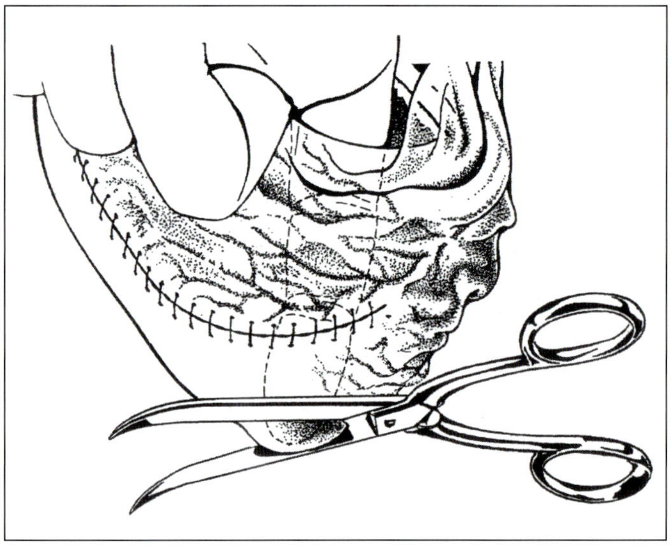

Figure 15.7 After inserting a finger into the pouch and identifying the most distal part a hole is cut.

the two ends of the U, resulting in a spherical reservoir consisting of four crossfolded ileal segments. After closure of the lower half of the anterior wall and most of the upper half the surgeon's finger is introduced through the remaining opening to determine the most caudal part of the reservoir. A hole, 8–10 mm in diameter, is cut into the pouch wall outside of the suture line, close to the mesoileum and 2–3 cm away from the edge that resulted from crossfolding the ileal segment (Figure 15.7). To achieve optimal voiding the anastomosis should not be at the end of a tunnel-shaped outlet which may kink, but should sit broadly on the pelvic floor (Figure 15.8). After placement of an 18-Fr urethral catheter, six 2-0 polyglycolic acid seromuscular sutures are placed between the hole in the reservoir wall and the membranous urethra (Figure 15.9). The two most dorsal sutures are placed at the 5 o'clock and 7 o'clock positions, followed by two sutures at the 3 o'clock and 9 o'clock positions and finally two ventral sutures are placed at the 1 o'clock and 11 o'clock positions. Care is taken to pass the two dorsal sutures through Denonvillier's fascia and the two ventral sutures through the plexus of Santorini for fixation. The sutures are tied loosely to prevent cutting or pinching of the tissue, which causes ischemia, leakage and stenosis of the sphincter apparatus. Before completely closing the pouch a 10-Fr cystostomy tube is placed into the reservoir through the fat of the mesoileum. The reservoir is flushed to remove any clots and checked for tightness (Figure 15.10).

The question of reflux prevention

To decide when reflux prevention is important in urinary diversion, it is necessary to determine under which circumstances reflux can be harmful. Clinical studies have incompletely established the pathogenesis of reflux nephropathy because it has been impossible to differentiate the effects of reflux, infection, bladder dysfunction and bladder outflow obstruction. It seems clear that generally both high-pressure reflux and urinary tract

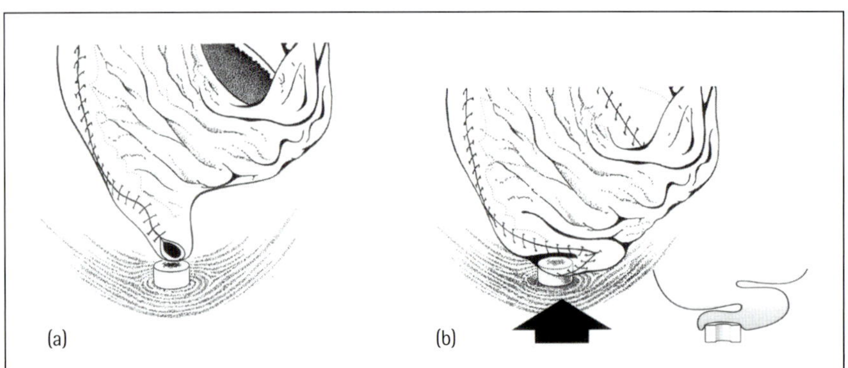

Figure 15.8 Anastomosis of the end of the suture line (a) results in kinking (b).

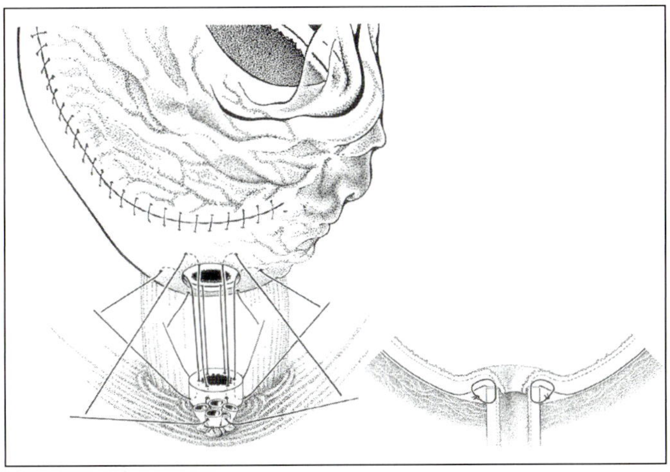

Figure 15.9 Anastomosis of the urethra to the neobladder with six seromuscular sutures. Fixation of the ventral sutures in the plexus of Santorini and the doral sutures in Denonvillier's fascia.

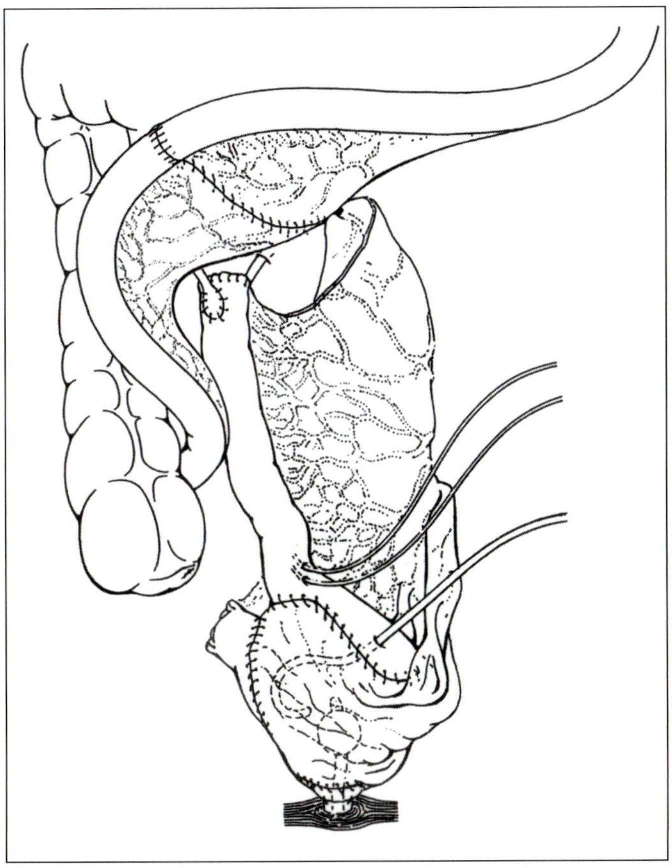

Figure 15.10 Passage of the ureteral stents and cystostomy tube before complete closure of the pouch.

infection are required for reflux nephropathy to occur, although it can occur with reflux of sterile urine over long periods or in the presence of obstruction, and as a consequence, increased bladder pressure.[1,2] The term urinary diversion implies that the normal ureterovesical junction no longer exists and that unless some form of reflux prevention is used, the ureter will experience reflux from whatever it is implanted into. However, reflux will only occur if the pressure distal to the site of implantation is higher than the peristaltic force of the ureter. Although it is not certain how damaging reflux may be, it is evident that obstruction at the entry site of the ureter into the conduit or reservoir is associated with renal damage, if this is not corrected in time. All antireflux techniques seem to have an associated risk of stenosis[3–5] and this should carefully be weighed against the risk of renal damage for uncorrected reflux. In addition, all flap valve type antireflux mechanisms portend the inherent disadvantage of intermittent functional obstruction. The valve (outlet) is compressed by the intrareservoir pressure, preventing reflux but causing outlet obstruction. In the type of ileal bladder substitute made according to Gordon's principles and described by Studer and colleagues a dynamic valve consisting of an afferent isoperistaltic tubular segment of 14–16 cm of ileum is used as the antireflux mechanism.[6] This in itself is adequate, as in this bladder substitute emptying occurs at low pressure <40 cm of H_2O by relaxation of the urethral sphincter and then by abdominal straining. As the abdominal pressure simultaneously acts on the ureters and on the renal pelvis, there is no reflux during voiding (Figure 15.11a). This in contrast to the action of a normal bladder where there is a coordinated contraction which causes an isolated rise in intravesical pressure during micturition. In addition, the urine is sterile since this is a closed system, and because the external urethral sphincter acts as a safety valve major pressure peaks in the reservoir cannot occur.

This has been confirmed in a prospective randomized study of antireflux techniques with the bladder substitute.[7] Patients were randomized to a 20-cm long afferent tubular isoperistaltic segment or one of two forms of flap valves were used. After a median follow-up of 30 months only one of the patients with the afferent tubular segment had abnormal upper tracts later than 6 months. In contrast, in the group of patients with antireflux nipples approximately 25% showed persistent, but mostly slight dilatation of the upper urinary tract more than 12 months postoperatively. In videourodynamic studies it was also shown that only when a bladder substitute was filled to its functional capacity by using elevated filling pressures was there any reflux of contrast medium toward the renal pelvis (Figure 15.11b). Even under these non-physiologic conditions of elevated pressures in the bladder substitute the peristaltic activity of the afferent tubular isoperistaltic ileal segment could actually return the contrast medium back to the reservoir.

Postoperative care

After surgery the patient leaves the operating room with an activated peridural anesthesia which remains for 5–8 days or as long as necessary. The suprapubic and transurethral catheters need to be flushed and aspirated with 0.9% saline every 6 hours

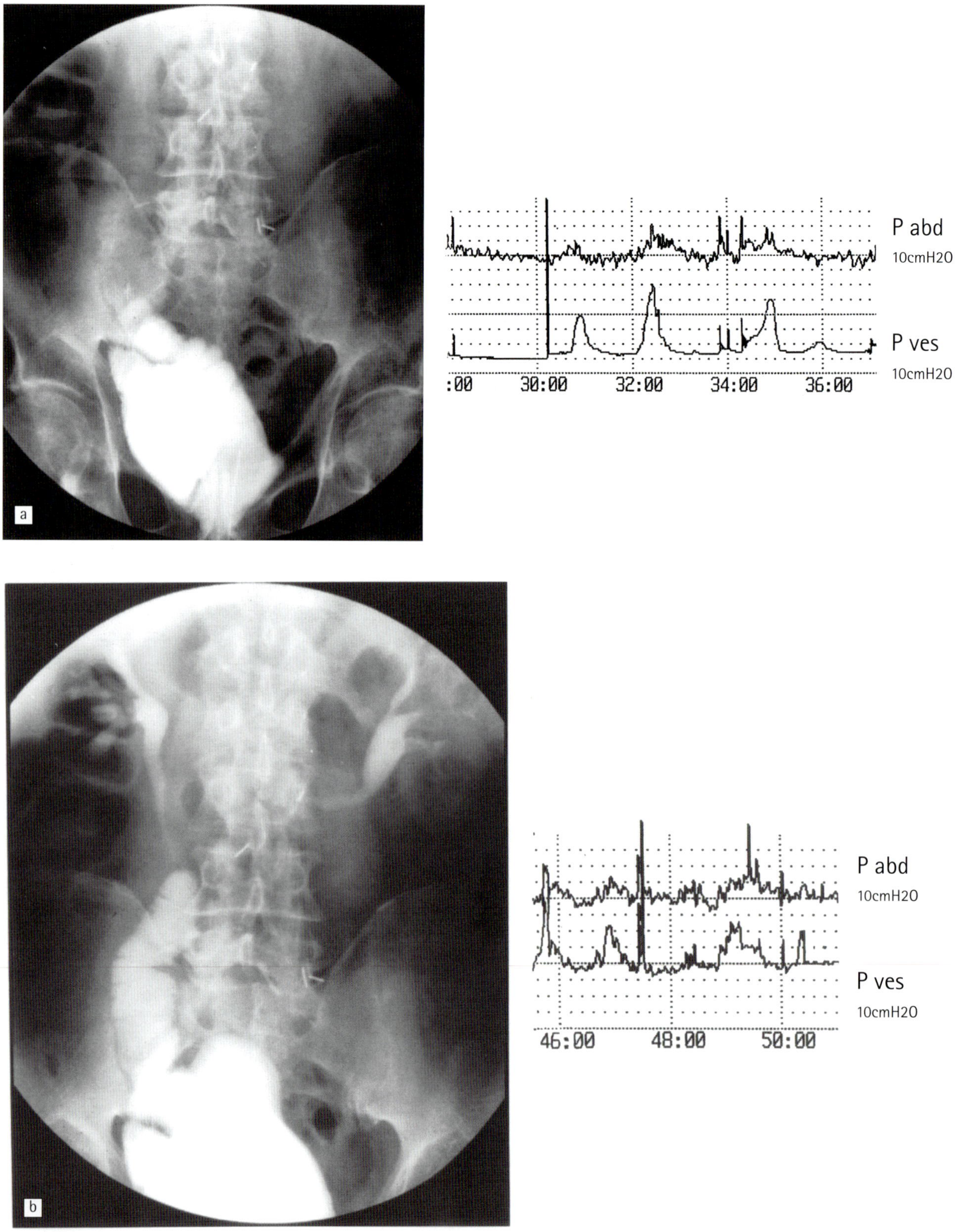

Figure 15.11 Postoperative videourodynamic studies: no reflux is seen during voiding by abdominal straining, which is documented by an increase in abdominal pressure (a). At functional capacity after retrograde filling reflux into both renal collecting systems can be observed independent of abdominal straining (b).

to prevent any catheter blockage, which may lead to rupture of the bladder substitute. This risk is most when bowel activity returns while the transurethral catheter is still in situ. The ureteral catheters must also be manually irrigated if there is a suspicion of blockage and ureteric obstruction, which should be suspected when urine output is not equal on both sides.

To prevent abdominal bloating and accelerate the return of bowel function parasympathicomimetic medication, e.g. neostigmine methylsulfate 3–6 × 0.5 mg subcutaneously, is commenced on the third postoperative day. The ureteric catheters are removed between the fifth and the eighth postoperative day. Total parenteral nutrition is commenced on the first postoperative day and stopped as soon as an oral intake is established. Between the eighth and tenth postoperative day leakage is excluded by a pouchogram and the suprapubic catheter is removed. This is followed 48 hours later by the urethral catheter allowing for the puncture site from the suprapubic catheter in the bladder substitute to seal. Following removal of the urethral catheter the patient voids initially in a sitting position every 2 hours during the day and 3-hourly with the help of an alarm clock at night.

After catheter removal in-out catheterization is done once together with an ultrasound measurement of residual urine. If ultrasound allows adequate measurement of residual urine, postvoid residual urine is then checked by ultrasound only. Any urinary tract infection due to bacteria is treated with antibiotics.

Body weight should also be routinely checked as a salt-losing syndrome by the bladder substitute can cause hypovolemia, dehydration, metabolic acidosis and a drop in body weight. If metabolic acidosis is identified (negative base excess under −4 mmol/l) then sodium bicarbonate is given orally to compensate. Patients are instructed to consume 2–3 l of fluid per day which is supplemented with an increased salt intake.

A specially trained nurse instructs and counsels patients on how to void completely. Voiding is performed by relaxation of the pelvic floor followed by slight abdominal straining. Voiding intervals are increased by 30–60 minute intervals until up to 4 hours. Patients are told not to void outside of the set time even if incontinence occurs, with the goal of increasing the bladder capacity up to 500 ml. The increase in the reservoir capacity allows the patient to achieve continence according to Laplace's law (pressure = wall tension:radius) which states that the intravesical pressure will drop with an increase in the radius of the reservoir, resulting in a low-pressure system. Postoperative time to continence depends on good counseling with daily sphincter training, surgical technique with nerve preservation to the urethra and pelvic floor as well as the patient's age.

Long-term follow-up

Meticulous lifelong follow-up is essential for optimal function of the reservoir and prevention of long-term complications. A good bladder substitute is free of infection, has no incontinence, no acidosis and no or minimal postvoid residual. Upper tract and urethral recurrences can be detected with high sensitivity by intravenous urography and lavage cytology. Postvoid residual urine needs to be evaluated, and causes such as inguinal or abdominal hernias identified and corrected, as these prevent adequate emptying. Protruding mucosa or stricture at the urethral–reservoir anastomosis may also compromise voiding and can be managed transurethrally.

References

1. Ransley PG, Risdon RA. Reflux and renal scarring. J Radiol 1978; 14 (suppl.): 1.
2. Roberts JA, Fischman NH, Thomas R. Vesicoureteral reflux in the primate IV: does reflux harm the kidney? J Urol 1982; 128: 650–2.
3. Stein JP, Freeman JA, Esrig D et al. Complications of the afferent antireflux valve mechanism in the Kock ileal reservoir. J Urol 1996; 155: 1579–84.
4. Le Duc A, Camey M, Teillac P. An original antireflux ureteroileal implantation technique: long-term followup. J Urol 1987; 137: 1156–8.
5. Steiner U, Miller K, Hautmann R. Functional results and complications of the ileal neobladder in over 200 patients. Urologe A 1994; 33: 53–7.
6. Studer UE, Ackermann D, Casanova GA, Zingg EJ. Three years' experience with an ileal low pressure bladder substitute. Br J Urol 1989; 63: 43–52.
7. Studer UE, Danuser H, Thalmann GN, Springer J, Turner H. Antireflux nipples or afferent tubular segments in 70 patients with ileal low pressure bladder substitutes: Long term results of a prospective randomized trial. J Urol 1996; 156: 1913–17.

16 Ileocolonic reservoirs: Orthotopic Mainz Pouch I, Le Bag

Joachim W Thüroff

Operative techniques for continent urinary diversion after cystectomy have greatly improved and increased in number during the last decades. The goal of orthotopic bladder substitution is to create a reservoir with an adequate capacity to store urine at low pressures. This is an essential precondition to protect the upper urinary tract and to achieve urinary continence. The procedure should not compromise cancer control.

Colonic segments are used either alone or combined with small bowel segments for orthotopic bladder substitution. The use of large bowel is associated with different advantages, which can be explained on the basis of anatomical and functional characteristics of the colonic segment.

By isolating only a short intestinal segment, a significant capacity for the continent reservoir is achieved. In this way, the total length of functionally excluded ileum is reduced, which plays an important role in the metabolism of gall bladder acids and vitamin B12.[1–3]

None of the bowel segments used for urinary diversion can compare to the physiological characteristics of the detrusor regarding distensibility and compliance. Constant distension of the bladder substitute over time leads in most cases to an increase of capacity, which may result in a largely oversized urinary reservoir. This condition can be avoided by using cecum rather than ileum due to the fact that large bowel is not as distensible as small bowel.[4] Additionally, large bowel – especially cecum and ascending colon – provides several variants for safe and effective antirefluxive ureteral implantation. Lastly, if a colonic-pouch is indicated for conversion or undiversion, an existing non-refluxive colonic-conduit may be incorporated into the pouch, avoiding ureteral reimplantation. Thus, operation time and length of bowel to be resected for creating the pouch is minimized.

However, a precondition for using large bowel for the creation of an orthotopic reservoir is the familiarity of the urologist with colonic surgery.

Utilizing large bowel-segments may also be more time consuming, since mobilization of the colon up to the right colonic flexure has to be performed, and the anastomosis to reestablish bowel continuity after exclusion of the segments for diversion is significantly larger in diameter than a small bowel anastomosis. Finally, the use of large bowel segments may also have metabolic influences.[5–8] Patients with preexisting functional intestinal disorders[9,10] may be influenced by the resection of the ileocecal valve. This may result in a faster passage of feces through the gastrointestinal tract, with consecutive disturbances.

The conclusion of these preferences and possible disadvantages – as for urinary diversion in general – is that, for the use of large bowel, no dogmas should be accepted. The applied technique and the choice of intestinal segments used for the orthotopic bladder substitution should be adapted to the patient and the pathology.

Modern concepts of intestinal urinary diversion rely profoundly on surgical versatility instead of creating 'home turfs' for one technique or the other.[11]

Indications

The indications for mixed ileocolonic orthotopic bladder substitutes do not differ in principle from the indications for other techniques of orthotopic bladder substitution. They comprise benign[12–14] and malignant disorders of the lower urinary tract at all ages[15–17] and may include simultaneous substitution cystoplasty and artificial urinary sphincter placement.[18] However, resection of the ileocecal valve may result in a faster transit of feces. This can be of importance for patients with neurogenic disorders of the sphincter mechanism. The impaired anal sphincter may not sufficiently retain the soft feces.

Another aspect to be considered regarding the indications – as in all forms of orthotopic bladder substitution – is the risk of retention requiring intermittent catheterization. Therefore, a prerequisite is motivation and cooperation as well as manual dexterity of the patient to perform transurethral self-catheterization. When applying this type of surgery to children, it must be considered that children older than nine years should be able to perform clean intermittent self-catheterization of the urethra.

Preoperative diagnosis

The patient should be in a general condition to undergo major abdominal surgery. In our series of orthotopic ileocolonic bladder substitution, the youngest patient was two-and-a-half years old, the oldest 79 years old. An important aspect is renal morphology and function. A grossly dilated upper urinary tract or impaired renal function are not drained as well by a continent urinary reservoir as by a conventional conduit, which may result in a further reduction of renal function. The intestinal urinary reservoir reabsorbs more hydrogen and chloride ions than a normal bladder. The resulting metabolic acidosis has to be compensated by respiratory mechanisms and by increased renal tubular transport mechanisms. Therefore, glomerular filtration rate should not be reduced below 50% of the normal rate in adults when a colonic orthotopic reservoir is considered. The intestinal tract should be preoperatively investigated for alterations, which may result in intra- or postoperative complications. Prior abdominal surgery or radiation can also represent a major problem for creation of ileocolonic reservoirs. Therefore, radiographic or endoscopic studies are recommended for screening the large bowel for asymptomatic diverticulosis or tumors.

Bowel preparation for reservoirs made from small/large bowel

Preoperatively

Preparation for reservoirs made from large bowel has to be more intense than for those made from small bowel. Two days prior to surgery the patient is put on liquid diet. The day before surgery the bowel can either be irrigated via orally administering 4–5 l of a hyperosmotic, non-absorbable solution or via an intestinal probe with 8–10 l of isotonic saline with a total of 50 mmol of potassium chloride added. After irrigation, serum electrolyte concentrations must be checked and, if necessary, balanced by intravenous substitution.

Intraoperatively

Small and large bowel segments that are planned to be utilized for the construction of intestinal reservoirs are flushed with saline until the irrigation fluid is clear before they are opened antimesenterically.

Perioperative antibiotics

Perioperative antibiotics should comprise broad-spectrum antibiotics including antianaerobic activity. The antibiotics are administered one hour before surgery and continued until the third to fifth postoperative day.

Technique

The patient is prone on the operation table. In the case of radical cystectomy and a planned submucosal tunnel ureter implantation into the large bowel, care should be taken to preserve as much ureter length as possible. The right colon is mobilized from the cecum to the right flexure. For tension free anastomosis with the trigonum or the urethra, and to facilitate sliding the pouch into the small pelvis this extended mobilization is essential.

The techniques of orthotopic Mainz pouch as well as the Le Bag procedure utilize the ileocecal segment.[11,24–27] Creation of the orthotopic reservoir is based on the principles of detubularization and reconfiguration of the excluded intestinal segments.[19–23]

In the Mainz pouch technique, 10–15 cm of cecum and ascending colon and two segments of terminal ileum of equal length are marked by stay sutures and isolated from bowel

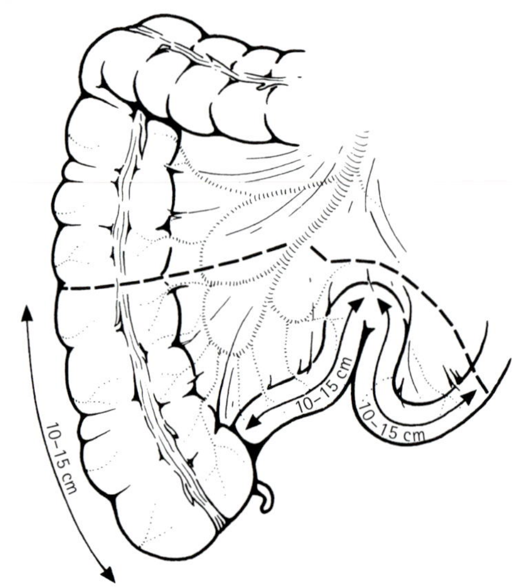

(a)

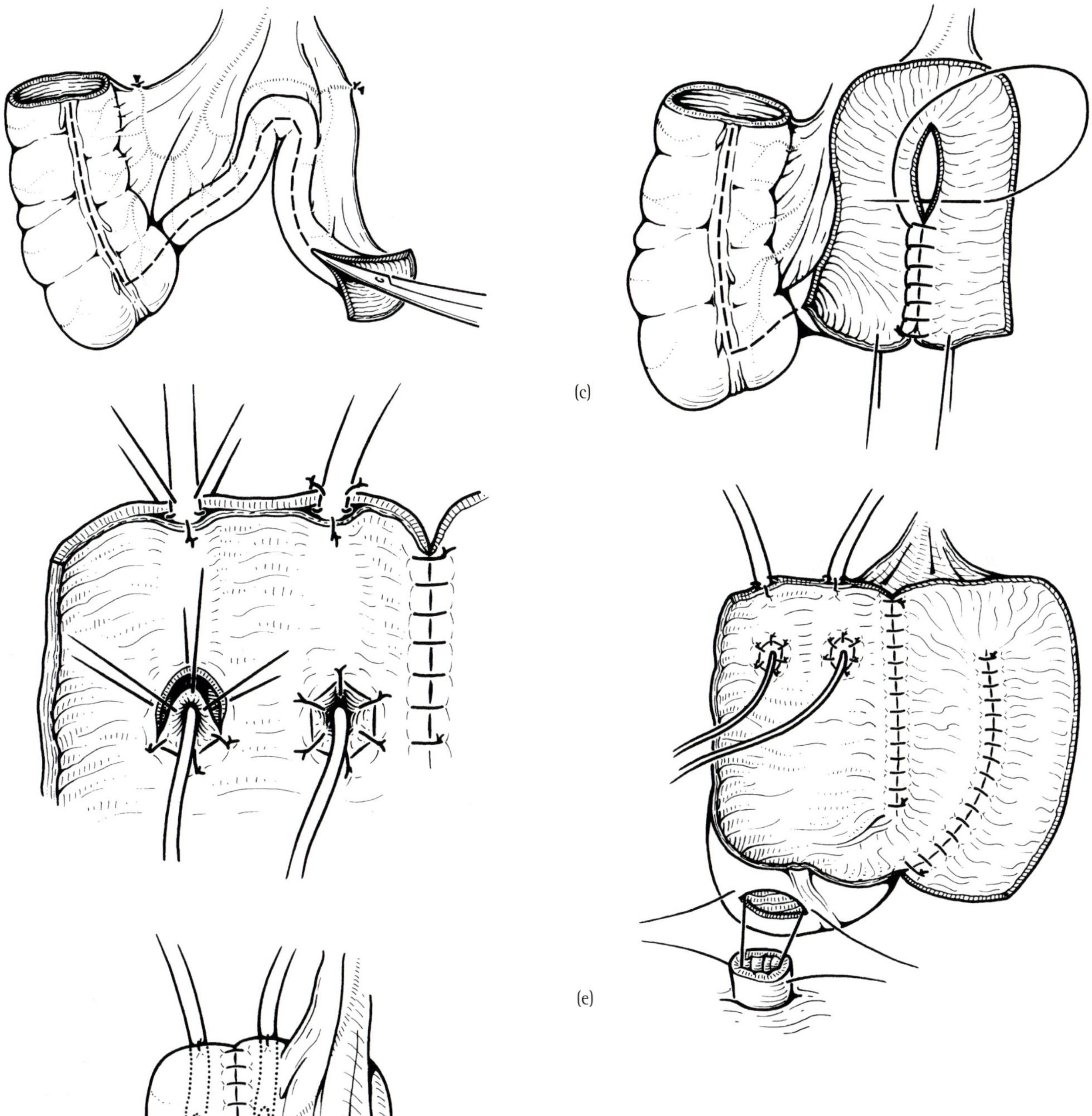

(b) (c) (d) (e)

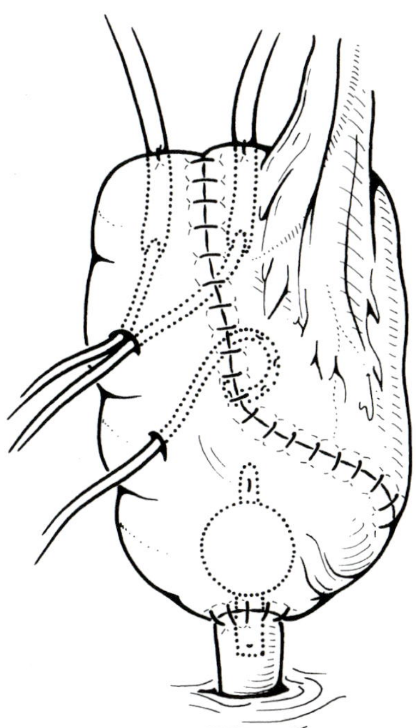

(f)

Figure 16.1 Original Mainz pouch orthotopic bladder substitution. (a) 10–15 cm of cecum and ascending colon and 20–30 cm of terminal ileum are isolated from bowel continuity. (b) The cecum and the ileum are opened at their antimesenteric borders. (c) Creation of the posterior wall of the pouch by side-to-side anastomosis of the opened segments. Subsequently cecum and ascending colon are split open and sutured the same way to the ileum. (d) Antirefluxive implantation of the ureters by means of submucosal tunnel 2–3 cm in length. (e) Anastomosis of the pouch with the membranous urethra after 20 Fr excision of the seromuscularis at the deepest point. (f) The anterior wall of the pouch is completed. Two 6–8 Fr ureteral stents and a 10 Fr pigtail cystostomy are led out through the abdominal wall. A 20 Fr transurethral Foley catheter remains indwelling for drainage and stenting of the anastomosis.

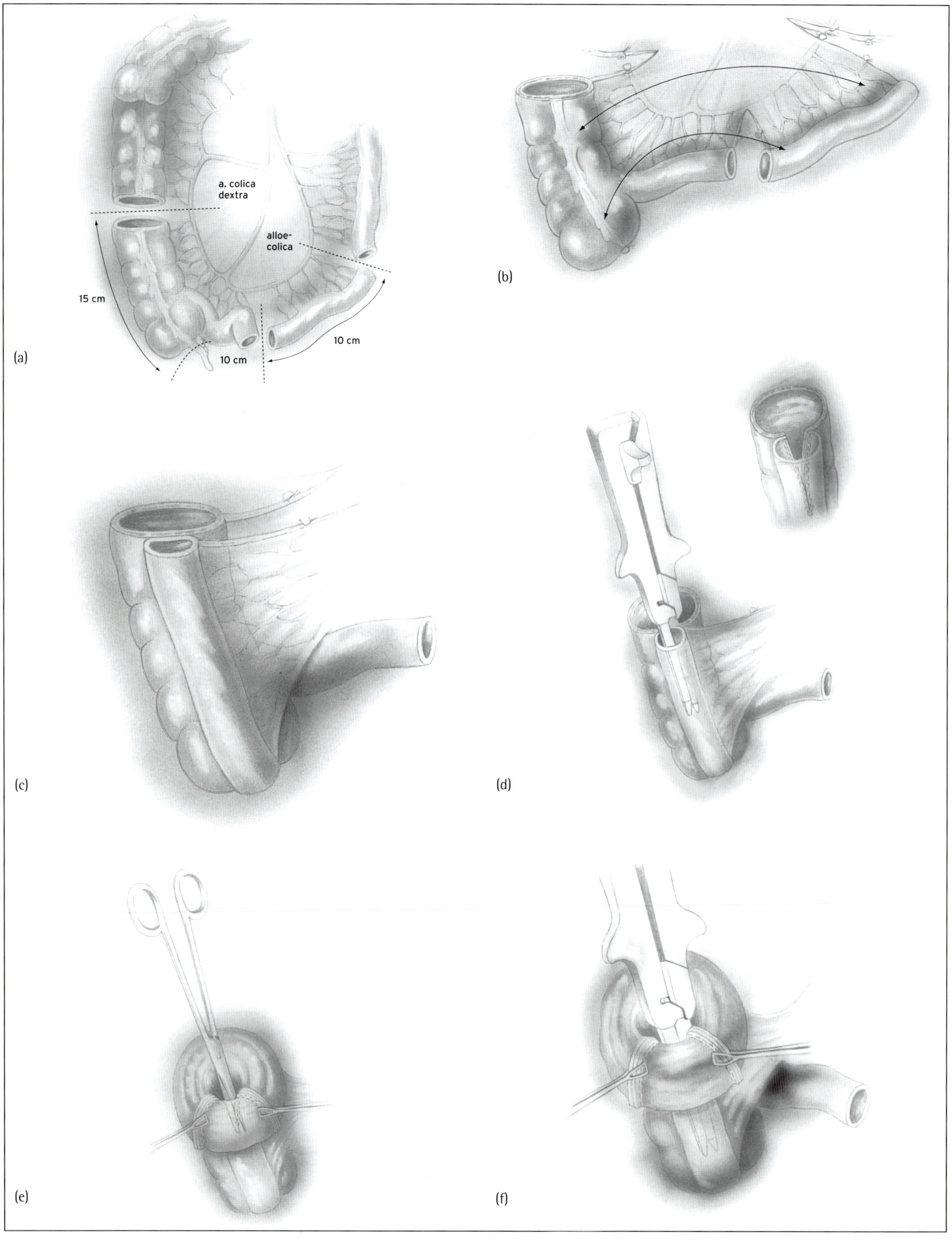

(a) (b) (c) (d) (e) (f)

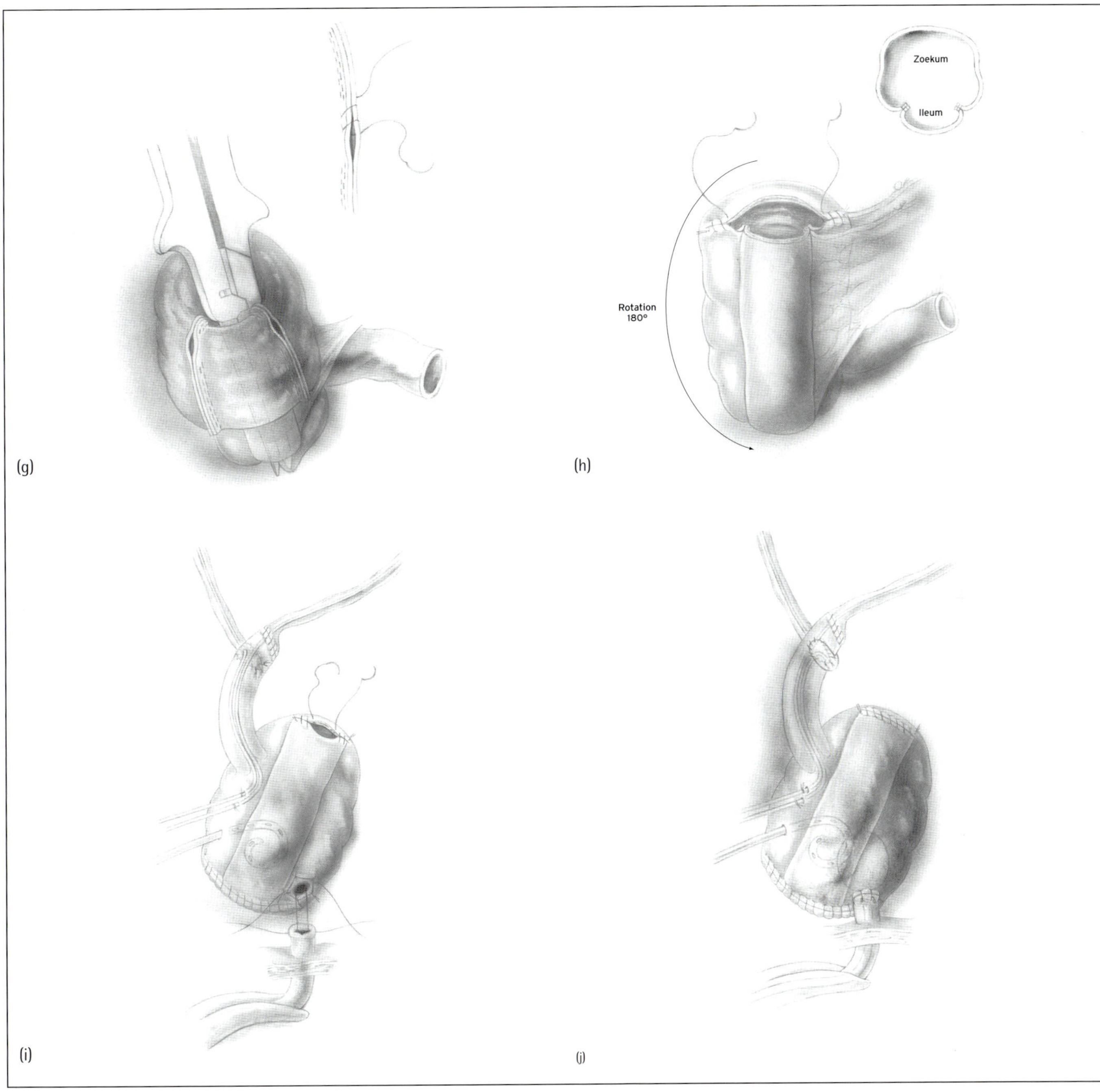

Figure 16.2 Simplified Mainz pouch orthotopic bladder substitution. (a) Isolation of ileocecal segment and separation into two parts. (b) *and* (c) Collocation of the ileal and cecal segments. (d) One-step antimesenteric opening and side-to-side anastomosis by GIA stapling technique with absorbable staples. (e) Everting and cutting open the closed end of the rows of staples. (f) Application of a second stapler. (g) Application of the final stapler and suturing the gap between the rows of staples. (h) Rotation of the pouch 180° counter-clockwise. (h) End-to-Side Nesbit implantation of the right ureter and spatulated end-to-end Wallace implantation into the prevalvular ileum. Urethral anastomosis with the pouch after mucosal eversion. (i) Completed modified orthotopic Mainz pouch.

continuity (Figure 16.1a). Ileocolostomy follows, either as sutured single row running end-to-end anastomosis after antimesenteric spatulation of the ileum for adjustment of bowel diameter or as a stapled mechanical end-to-side anastomosis of ileum to ascending colon using the EEA and TA 55 staplers. The isolated ileocecal segment is cleaned with isotonic saline. Ascending colon, cecum and both terminal ileal segments are opened at their antimesenteric borders (Figure 16.1b). The posterior wall of the pouch is created by side-to-side anastomosis of the terminal ileal loops, and of the latter with the cecum and ascending colon (Figure 16.1c). Anastomosis is performed by single-row through and through running sutures of 4/0 polyglyconate with a straight needle. After submucosal tunnel ureter implantation (Figure 16.1d), the still open pouch is slid into the small pelvis (Figure 16.1e). For bladder augmentation or subtotal substitution, the pouch is anastomosed with the posterior bladder wall using single row through-and-through sutures of 3/0 or 4/0 polyglyconate. If sliding of the pouch into the small pelvis is restricted by the length of the ileocecal artery or if implantation of the ureters into the prevalvular ileum with the ileocecal valve serving as antireflux mechanism is planned, 180° counter-clockwise rotation of the pouch for tension-free anastomosis with the urethra is performed (Figure 16.2h). For complete bladder substitution after cystoprostatectomy, a 20 Fr excision of seromuscularis is made at the lowest aspect of the cecal pole and the opened mucosa is everted with a few 5/0 absorbable stitches before anastomosis to the membranous urethra is performed by 8 interrupted sutures of 4/0 polyglecaprone (Figures 16.1ef and Figure 16.2i). Alternatively, an ileocecal pouch may be fashioned by utilizing reabsorbable staples (Figures 16.2a–g).

The isolated right colon can also be used for creating an orthotopic pouch in form of the so-called 'Le Bag' procedure. In essence, 20 cm of the ascending colon and 20 cm of the distal

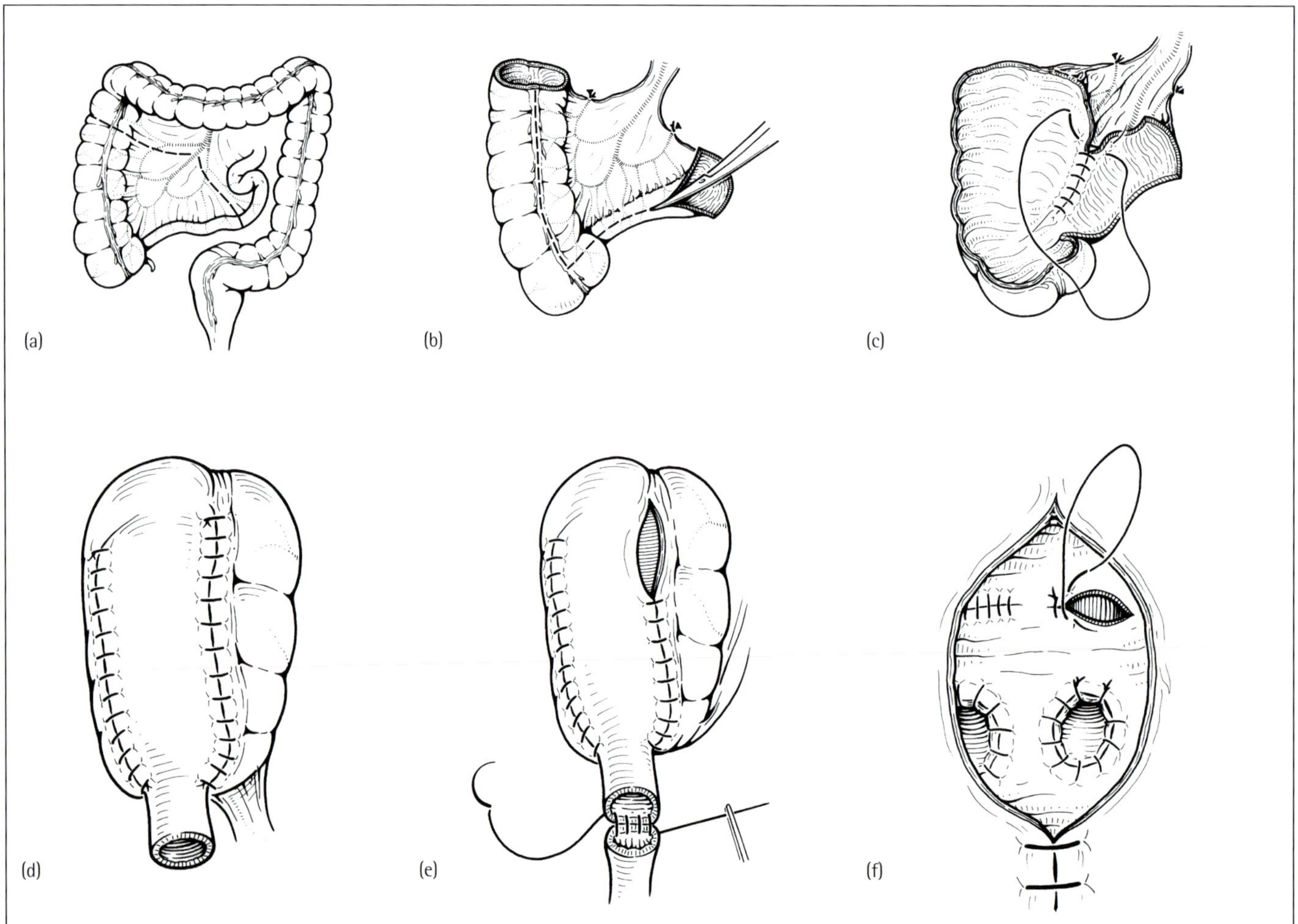

Figure 16.3 Le Bag orthotopic bladder substitution. (a) Selection of ileocolonic segment based on the ileocecal artery. (b) Incision along the antimesenteric border to create two flat sheets of bowel. (c) Suturing of ileal and colonic segments. (d) Pouch rotated 180° for urethral anastomosis. Note that for bladder substitution to the urethra, 3–5 cm of the proximal cut end of ileum are not split open for end-to-end anastomosis of ileum with the urethral stump. (e) Running suture for end-to-end anastomosis of ileum with the urethral stump. The gap in the anastomosis of the anterior pouch wall allows access to the interior of the pouch for ureteral implantation;. (f) Submucosal tunnel implantation of ureters into the colonic segment of the pouch.

ileum are isolated (Figure 16.3a). The vascular supply derives from the ileocecal artery and may include also the right colic artery. The large as well as the small bowel are opened along the antimesenteric border, thus two flat sheets are created and are in continuity only at the incised ileocecal valve (Figure 16.3b). If anastomosis of the pouch to the urethra is planned, the incision to open the small bowel segment should not be continued to the cut proximal end of ileum. This way the intact ileum end can be anastomosed to the urethral stump. The lateral border of the detubularized small bowel is anastomosed to the medial border of the colonic sheet (Figure 16.3c). The anterior wall can be reconstructed either by folding the combined bowel sheet to the bottom of the newly created pouch or by simple joining of the remaining free borders of the bowel sheets. The pouch is rotated 180° [25–27] (Figures 16.3de). The ureteral anastomosis mainly follows the principles described below (Figure 16.3f).

Implantation of the ureters

The rationale of implanting the ureters in an antirefluxive way into the orthotopic bladder substitute is to protect the upper urinary tract from pressure peaks and from ascending bacteriuria. Antirefluxive ureter implantation techniques into the intestine are derived from ureterosigmoidostomy, which meant diverting the urinary pathway into a high-pressure contaminated reservoir. The contemporary discussion about the necessity of antirefluxive ureter implantation into low-pressure reservoirs is ongoing, but still antirefluxive ureteric-intestinal reimplantation is the method of choice for colonic reservoirs.

The key point is to provide an antireflux mechanism without obstructing the ureter. The very depth of this challenge results from the number of variable conditions in the individual patients. For example, the ureters may be inflamed or dilated, bowel may have been irradiated, and one has to calculate long-term effects of the interaction between the various components of the newly created system. Thus, mechanical factors (e.g. position changes of the reservoir) or biochemical factors (e.g. effects of the urine on the adventitia of the ureter or on intestinal segments) may also play important roles. In general, it is an accepted rule of thumb that ureteral reflux is preferable to ureteral obstruction.

A variety of techniques based on different mechanisms are described. Two general principles can be distinguished. In one of them, the ureter itself becomes part of the antirefluxive mechanism while, in another, a bowel-derived antireflux mechanism is interposed between ureter and reservoir.

In any case, for implantation of the ureters into the large bowel segment, the left ureter has to be pulled into the right retroperitoneum behind the mesentery of the descending colon and through the mesentery of the ileum.

The antirefluxive implantation technique, that includes the ureter as part of the antirefluxive mechanism, relies fundamentally on the 'flap valve' mechanism. The principle is that, with an oblique entry of the ureter into the reservoir, some length of a 'tunnel' is created that allows transmission of the reservoir pressure onto the wall of the ureter, thus creating a force that occludes the ureter progressively with rising reservoir pressures. The most frequently utilized techniques of exposing the ureter to the reservoir pressure are the submucosal tunnel technique (Figures 16.1d and 16.3f) and the serosa lined extramural tunnel technique.

In the submucosal tunnel technique, both ureters are implanted into the colon with a 3–5 cm submucosal tunnel. Ureters are anchored with 6/0 polyglycolic sutures to the muscle of the bowel wall and the neo-orifices are established by 6/0 or 7/0 ureteromucosal sutures (Figure 16.1d).

In our modified technique of the orthotopic Mainz bladder substitute, the natural valve mechanism of the Bauhini valve is used as an antireflux mechanism (Figures 16.2ij). The cecal side is incorporated in the pouch, while the ureters are anastomosed in an end-to-side (Nesbit) or spatulated end-to-end (Wallace) technique to the terminal ileum. Thus, urinary flow is directed from the ureters into the pouch while reflux is prevented by the ileocecal valve.

The ureters are intubated with 6–8 F stents and a 10 F cystostomy catheter and a 20 F transurethral Foley balloon catheter are inserted into the pouch. The anastomosis of the pouch with the anterior bladder wall in bladder augmentation and subtotal substitution procedures and the anterior wall of the pouch are completed in the same way as described before. However, at the site of submucosal ureteral implantation, the pouch is closed by mucosal sutures only to prevent ureteral obstruction. A 20 F gravity drain is placed in the small pelvis and at the ureteral implantation site.

Ureter stents are removed after 10 days. The transurethral catheter is withdrawn after 3 weeks after radiographic study of the pouch. Residual urine is checked via the pouchostomy catheter when patients void spontaneously. In neurogenic cases, patients are instructed in intermittent catheterization.

Postoperative care

Non-peristaltic contractions of the bowel segments of a Mainz pouch do occur in the first months postoperatively, but subside spontaneously with increasing capacity of the pouch in most cases. For persistent incontinence due to an inadequately low compliance or persistent contractions of the pouch, anticholinergics are recommended systemically or by local instillation.

Prophylactically administered alkali is required to counteract asymptomatic postoperative acidosis demonstrated by blood gas analysis (base excess < 2.5) in about 60% of patients. In view of a maximum of 20 years of follow-up, the risk of secondary malignancies cannot be assessed ultimately at the present time. Follow-up examinations should include ultrasound of the upper urinary tract, pouchoscopy and evaluation of serum parameters such as levels of cobolamine and bile acids.

Results

Four criteria must be regarded as decisive for success or failure of orthotopic urinary diversion utilizing intestinal segments: 1) function and morphology of the upper urinary tract, 2) frequency during day and night, 3) continence and 4) ability for spontaneous micturition. Continence and capacity for spontaneous micturition, however, may be influenced significantly by the type and quality of surgery performed before orthotopic substitution itself. In this respect, related factors may be, for instance, preparation of the bladder neck and urethra,[12] sparing of the autonomous nerves,[28–31] and precautions to prevent pouch displacement.[32] Therefore, functional results rely, in fact, on myriad factors, and not only upon the segment(s) of intestine and geometrical models chosen. A ureterointestinal stricture rate of 7% is reported for ileocecal reservoirs. Continence rates for ileocecal reservoirs vary between 75% and 88% during the day and 67% during the night.[11,33]

References

1. Durrans D, Wujanto R, Carroll RN, Torrance HB. Bile acid malabsorption: a complication of conduit surgery. Br J Urol 1989; 64: 485–8.
2. Olofsson G, Fjalling M, Kilander A, Ung KA, Jonsson O. Bile acid malabsorption after continent urinary diversion with an ileal reservoir. J Urol 1998; 160: 724–7.
3. Ung KA, Olofsson G, Fae A et al. In vitro determination of active bile acid absorption in small biopsy specimens obtained endoscopically or surgically from the human intestine. Eur J Clin Invest 2002; 32: 115–21.
4. Hohenfellner M, Bürger R, Schad H et al. Reservoir characteristics of Mainz pouch studies in animal model. Urology 1993; 42: 741–746.
5. Lane TM, Shah PJ. Malabsorption after augmentation cystoplasty: the role of ileo-caecal reconstitution. BJU Int 2000; 85: 772–3.
6. Stein R, Lotz J, Andreas J et al. Long-term metabolic effects in patients with urinary diversion. World J Urol 1998; 16: 292–7.
7. Stein R, Lotz J, Fisch M et al. Vitamin metabolism in patients with a Mainz pouch I: long-term followup. J Urol 1997; 157: 44–7.
8. Stampfer D, McDougal W, McGovern F. The use of in bowel urology. Metabolic and nutritional complications. Urol Clin North Am 1997; 24: 715–22.
9. Fisch M, Wammack R, Spies F et al. Ileocecal valve reconstruction during continent urinary diversion. J Urol 1994; 151: 861–5.
10. Gillitzer R, Fisch M, Jessel D et al. Competence and function of the ileocecal valve reconstruction during uinary diversion (Mainz pouch I). J Urol 1998; 161: 66A.
11. Leissner J, Stein R, Hohenfellner R et al. Radical cystoprostatectomy combined with Mainz pouch bladder substitution to the urethra: long-term results. BJU Int 1999; 83: 964–70.
12. Linn J, Hohenfellner M, Roth S, et al. Treatment of intersitial cystitis: Comparison of subtrigonal and supratrigonal cystectomy combined with orthotopic bladder substitution. J Urol 1998; 159: 774–8.
13. Hohenfellner M, Black P, Linn J, Dahms S, Thüroff J. Surgical treatment of interstial cystitis in women. Intl. Urogynecol. J Pelvic Floor Dysfunction 2000; 11: 113–19.
14. Stein R, Fisch M, Ermert A et al. Urinary diversion and orthotopic bladder substitution in children and young adults with neurogenic bladder: a safe option for treatment? J Urol 2000; 163: 568–73.
15. Robertson C, King L. Bladder substitution in children. Urol Clin North Am 1986; 13: 333–44.
16. Riedmiller H, Thuroff J, Stockle M, Schofer O, Hohenfellner R. Continent urinary diversion and bladder augmentation in children: the Mainz pouch procedure. Pediatr Nephrol 1989; 3: 68–74.
17. Stein R, Fisch M, Beetz R et al. Urinary diversion in children and young adults using the Mainz Pouch I technique. Br J Urol 1997; 79: 354–61.
18. Miller EA, Mayo M, Kwan D, Mitchell M. Simultaneous augmentation cystoplasty and artificial urinary sphincter placement: infection rates and voiding mechanisms. J Urol 1998; 160: 750–3.
19. Giertz G, Frankson C. Construction of a substitute bladder, with preservation of urethral voiding, after subtotal and total cystectomy. Acta Chir Scand 1957; 113: 218.
20. Goodwin EW, Winter CC, Turner RD. Replacement of the ureter by small intestine: clinical application and results of the 'ileal ureter'. J Urol 1959; 81: 406–9.
21. Kock NG, Nilson AE, Nilsson LO. Urinary diversion via a continent ileal reservoir: clinical results. J Urol 1982; 128: 469–75.
22. Tasker J. Ileocystoplasty: a new technique. An experimental study with report of a case. Brit. J Urol 1953; 25: 349.
23. Hinman FJ. Selection of intestinal segments for bladder substitution: physical and physiological characteristics. J Urol 1988; 139: 519–23.
24. Thüroff JW, Alken P, Riedmiller H, Jacobi GH, Hohenfellner R. The MAINZ pouch (mixed augmentation ileum and cecum) for bladder augmentation and continent diversion. J Urol 1986; 136: 17–26.
25. Kolettis PN, Klein EA, Novick AC, Winters JC, Appell RA. The Le Bag orthotopic urinary diversion. J Urol 1996; 156: 926–30.
26. Light JK, Engelmann UH. Le Bag: total replacement of the bladder using an ileocolonic pouch. J Urol 1986; 136: 27–31.
27. Light JK, Marks JL. Total bladder replacement in the male and female using the ileocolonic segment (Le Bag). Br J Urol 1990; 65: 467–72.
28. Turner W, Danuser H, Moehrle K, Studer U. The effect of nerve sparing cystectomy technique on postoperative continence after orthotopic bladder substitution. J Urol 1997: 158; 2118–22.
29. Hugonnet C, Danuser H, Springer J, Studer U. Urethral sensitivity and the impact on urinary continence in patients with an ileal bladder substitute after cystectomy. J Urol 2001; 165: 1502–5.
30. Stenzl A, Colleselli K, Poisel S, Bartsch G. Orthotopic reconstruction of the lower urinary tract in women: Further experience and surgical refinements. J. Urol. 1996; 155: 396A.
31. Stenzl A, Colleselli K, Poisel S et al. Rationale and technique of

nerve sparing radical cystectomy before an orthotopic neobladder procedure in women. J Urol 1995; 154: 2044–9.

32. Ali-El-Din B, El-Sobky E, Hohenfellner M, Ghoneim M. Orthotopic bladder substitution in women: functional and urodynamic evaluation. J Urol 1999; 161: 1875–80.

33. Santucci R, Park C, Mayo M, Lange P. Continence and urodynamic parameters of continent urinary reservoirs: comparison of gastric, ileal, ileocolic, right colon, and sigmoid segments. Urology 1999; 54: 252–7.

17 Bladder replacement with detubularized right colon

Tamsin Greenwell, Daniela Andrich and Anthony Mundy

Introduction

The ideal bladder replacement provides a large capacity low-pressure continent storage with spontaneous volitional voiding at normal intervals with no adverse effects.

History and development

Tizzoni and Poggi described the first neobladder in a dog model in 1888,[1] whilst Verhogen reported the first cutaneous continent diversion in 1908.[2] Initial results were unsurprisingly poor given the absence of good anesthesia and antibiotics, and the technique of orthotopic neobladder did not gain popularity until the 1970s following the pioneering work of Kock.[3–6] Since this time many different techniques have been reported utilizing all segments of bowel: each of which has its own particular advantages and disadvantages. Cecal and right colonic neobladders were developed and popularized by a variety of groups in the 1980s,[7–10] and the particular benefits and pitfalls of bladder replacement with right colon will now be discussed in detail.

Indications

As with all techniques for bladder replacement the primary indications are invasive transitional cell carcinoma, aggressive superficial transitional cell carcinoma that is not controllable by more conservative means, other pelvic malignancies, congenital and acquired neurological anomalies (spinal dysraphism, cerebral palsy, multiple sclerosis, spinal cord injury), congenital urologic anomalies (vesical and cloacal exstrophy, anorectal and urogenital sinus anomaly) and chronic pelvic pain syndromes (including interstitial cystitis).[11–14]

Contraindications

The main contraindications to bladder replacement surgery can be divided into absolute and relative, physical and intellectual. Absolute physical contraindications to continent reconstruction and neobladder include inflammatory bowel disease, short bowel syndrome and significantly impaired renal function.[15] The level of renal impairment considered to be a contraindication, varies from author to author but is in the range of serum creatinine 120–250 µmol/l.[16–19] Inability to perform clean intermittent self-catheterization (CISC) secondary to poor hand function, e.g. tetraplegia, is another physical contraindication.

Absolute intellectual contraindications are refusal to perform CISC and inability to comprehend the risks and responsibilities associated with neobladder formation.[15] Advanced tumor stage is felt by many groups to be an absolute or relative contraindication[20,21] but not by all[16] as pelvic recurrence does not appear to commonly cause complications with a neobladder.[22–24] Likewise previous abdominal radiation is viewed by some as a relative contraindication as surgery is more difficult and there is a higher incidence of early and late complications for all types of reconstruction, even ileal conduit.[25–28] Likewise significant obesity, advanced age and impaired functional status are also relative contraindications.[15] An abnormal urethra is a contraindication for orthotopic urinary diversion as is a history of stress urinary incontinence[29] unless an artificial urinary sphincter is being considered.

Preoperative assessment

All patients without absolute contraindications need to be fully counseled regarding the pros and cons of each form of urinary diversion (conduit, continent pouch, orthotopic neobladder and rectal reservoir). The patient's preferences and expectations should be taken into account along with their disease characteristics, age, body mass index, physical and mental status and planned adjuvant or neoadjuvant treatment (chemotherapy and or radiotherapy). Sexual and bowel function need to be assessed preoperatively as they may be adversely affected by continent diversion surgery.

All patients should be seen prior to listing by the stoma therapist and the continent diversion nurse specialist for non-medical counseling and opinion, and if requested old patients forming a patient panel should be available to offer the patient's perspective. Patients are also seen by the continent diversion/neobladder nurse immediately prior to surgery for siting of a continent stoma site and an ileal conduit site in case of adverse findings at time of surgery precluding formation of an orthotopic neobladder.

In our unit, all patients are admitted two days prior to surgery for full bowel preparation. A rectal wash-out is performed on the day of surgery in patients with neuropathic bladders. Patients with neuropathy and severe incontinence may have a severe ammoniacal dermatitis, which may warrant a preparatory period of indwelling catheterization to allow the skin to heal. Intravenous cefuroxime and metronidazole are given at induction and for three doses postoperatively. All patients have TED stockings and subcutaneous heparin prophylactically from time of surgery until fully mobile.

Techniques

The main techniques have been described by Goldwasser, Rowland (Indiana), Mansson (Lund/Lundiana), and Lockhart (Florida).[7–10] All consist of detubularizing the right colon but vary in the length of right colon used and the method of ureteric reimplantation (Table 17.1). The issue of detubularization while held to be critical by the majority of surgeons[9,29] is not felt to be of great import in the neurologically intact patient.[30]

Ureteric reimplantation can be refluxing or non-refluxing. The main methods of ureteric reimplantation are antireflux; tunneling along the tenia from outside the urinary diversion,[31–34] or tunneling from inside the continent diversion with the ureter laid into a mucosal sulcus[35] or drawn through a submucosal tunnel (Lundiana),[36] the intussuscepted ileal nipple (Kock, Lund)[4,5,7] or the split-cuff technique.[9]

Table 17.1 Right colonic neobladder techniques

	Neobladder	Ureteric reimplantation
Goldwasser	Detubularized right colon	Goodwin
Indiana	Detubularized right colon	Tunneled in tenia
Lund	Detubularized right colon	Le Duc
Lundiana	Detubularized right colon	Le Duc
Florida	Detubularized right colon	Direct

Our technique

The right side of the colon is mobilized on the right and ileocolic vessels. The middle colic artery is transected at the level of the marginal artery to enhance mobility (Figure 17.1). The ileum and transverse colon are divided and reanastomosed with single layer seromuscular interrupted 3-0 vicryl, leaving the isolated right colon on its vascular pedicle (Figure 17.2). The right colon is detubularized by incising the midline anterior tenia (Figure 17.3). The detubularized right colon is then folded such that the superior midline of the ascending colon is sutured to the most inferior part of the divided colon. The neobladder walls are completed using continuous all-layer 3-0 vicryl (Figure 17.4). The neobladder is rotated 180° and the most dependent part opened and anastomosed to the urethra with a minimum of six 3-0 vicryl sutures (Figure 17.5). Following anastomosis the neobladder is situated orthotopically in the pelvis (Figure 17.6). The ureters are reimplanted in a direct end-to-side manner (freely refluxing) over a 6 Fr infant feeding tube as a ureteric stent with 4-0 vicryl (Figure 17.7). A 16 Fr silicone

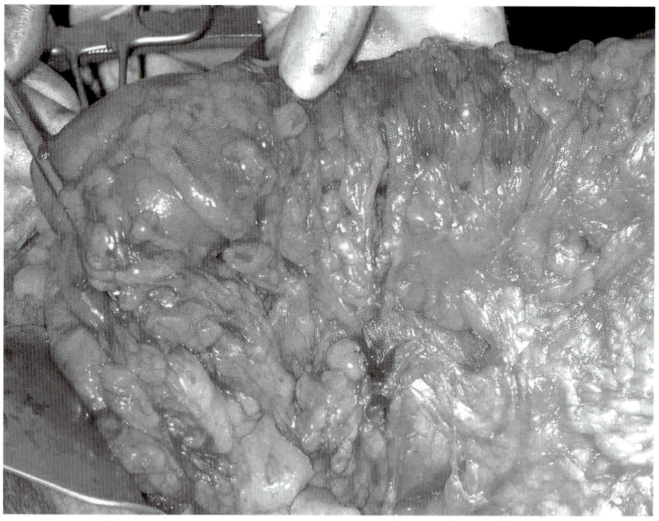

Figure 17.1 Right and transverse colon mobilized. A soft clamp is on the proximal end of the transverse colon in preparation for division of the middle colic artery and transverse colon.

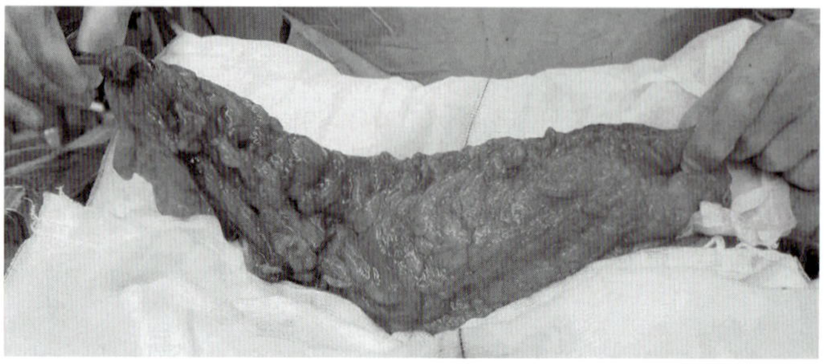

Figure 17.2 Isolated right colon on its vascular pedicle.

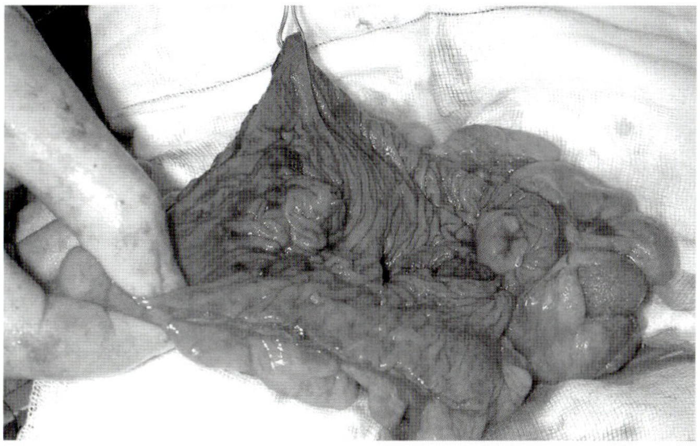

Figure 17.3 Detubularized right colon.

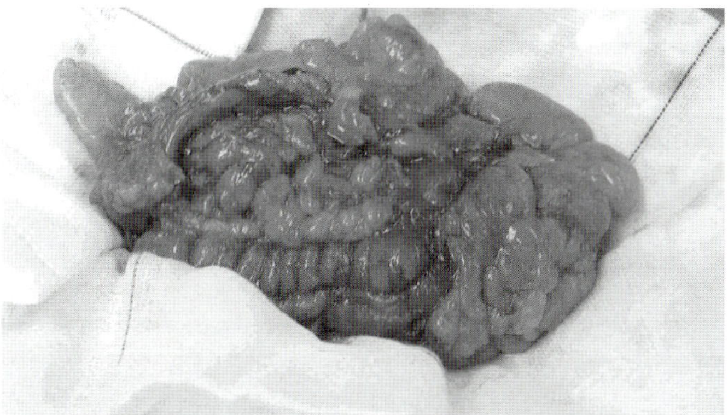

Figure 17.4 Right colonic neobladder after detubularization and suture.

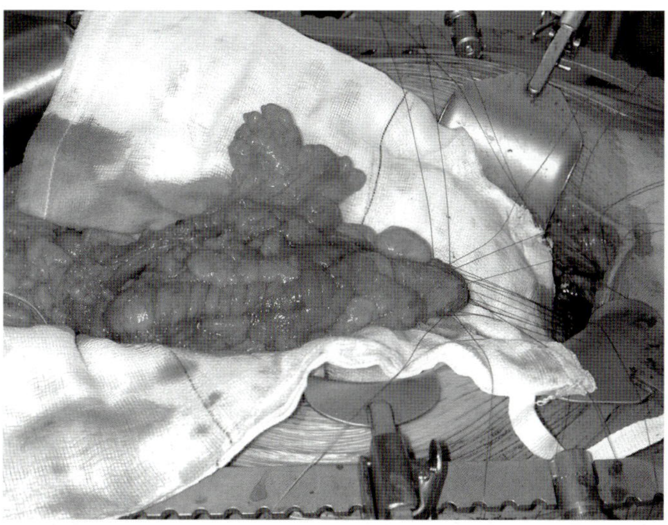

Figure 17.5 Urethro-neobladder anastomosis.

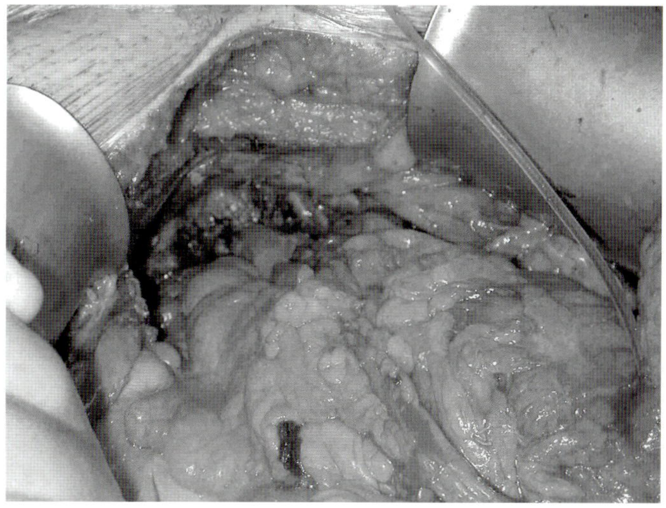

Figure 17.6 Orthotopic siting of the right colonic neobladder following completion of the urethro-neobladder anastomosis.

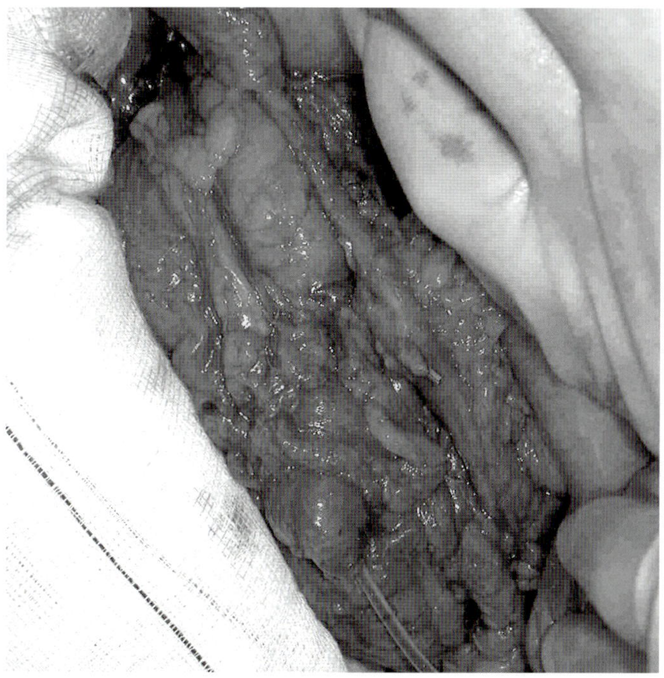

Figure 17.7 Right ureteric direct reimplantation into the neobladder.

urethral and 16 Fr silicone suprapubic catheter are sited along with a 20 Fr Robinson drain prior to closing.

Postoperative management

Many patients require a period of 6 months or so after orthotopic neobladder formation to allow their new 'bladder' to establish a new pattern of behavior. During this period many storing and voiding problems will settle down, as patients learn to use their new 'bladder' more efficiently and postoperative inflammation and irritation give way. Our patients have videourodynamics 6 months following diversion. If these reveal a good capacity, low-pressure neobladder or pouch that has a normal contour and empties well with low residual volume, they are followed up by ultrasound assessment of their upper tracts and residual volumes 6-monthly for 2 years and then annually. A plain abdominal radiograph is done biannually, or if clinically indicated, to look for stones. Children have annual measurement of their venous base excess to ensure they are not acidotic. All patients have annual isotopic measurement of their glomerular filtration rate. Those with a diversion following radical extirpative surgery for malignancy also undergo routine surveillance for recurrence depending on the underlying pathology.

Controversies

The main areas of controversy are: which segment of bowel to use; whether to perform a continent cutaneous diversion or an orthotopic neobladder in those patients who are able to have both; and whether the ureteric reimplant should be nonrefluxing or not. Current evidence supports the idea that the many different types of bowel formed into neobladders via a multitude of different folding techniques yield similar functional results, although urinary incontinence may be greater with gastric and sigmoid neobladders.[37,38]

Complications

Complications may be divided into short term (within 30 days of surgery) and long term, and are different for continent cutaneous pouches compared with neobladders.

Short-term complications

Early complications include those cardiovascular, thromboembolic, respiratory and gastrointestinal complications associated with any major abdominal procedure. Detubularized right colonic neobladder formation is reported to have a 0–3% mortality – this is impossible to divorce from the mortality associated with radical cystectomy which immediately precedes the majority of these procedures.[12,13] The deaths that have been reported have been due to pulmonary embolus, myocardial infarction, pneumonia, liver failure and acute respiratory distress syndrome.[12,13]

The short-term complications of detubularized right colonic neobladders are those due to the major abdominal nature of the procedure: bleeding, wound infection, ileus, deep vein thrombosis, pulmonary embolism, respiratory tract infections and death; and those related to the formation of the neobladder: ureteroileal leak, ureteroileal obstruction, gut leak, and neobladder-cutaneous fistula (Table 17.2).

Long-term complications

These may be broadly divided into neobladder-related and general complications. Neobladder-related complications include ureteroileal complications, metabolic acidosis, urinary tract infections, change in bowel function, stone and cancer. General complications include small bowel obstruction, deterioration in renal function, incisional hernia and abscess (Table 17.3).

Metabolic disturbances

Reabsorption of ammonia, ammonium chloride and secretion of bicarbonate by the bowel segment produces biochemically detectable acid–base and electrolyte disturbances in virtually all patients but this is clinically significant in very few.[39–41] The amount of electrolyte exchange across a colonic segment depends upon the area of the colonic segment and the time

Table 17.2 Short-term neobladder-related complications

Complication	Rate (%)
Local	
Neobladder leak	0
Entero-neobladder fistulas	0–1.5
Ureteroenteric obstruction	0
Ureteroenteric reflux	0
Urethral anastomotic stricture	0
Urinary incontinence	0
ISC	0
Acute pyelonephritis	0
Other	0–4.2
General	
Superficial infection	0
Deep infection	0–5.9
Prolonged ileus	0–8.4
Small bowel obstruction	0–3.0
Respiratory tract infection	0
Deep vein thrombosis	0
Pulmonary embolism (PE)	0–1.5
Other	0–8.4
Death (liver failure, PE, pneumonia, femoral embolism)	0–4.8

Table 17.3 Long-term neobladder-related complications

Complication	Rate (%)
Local	
Urinary incontinence due to neobladder	0-7.5
Urethral anastomotic stricture	0-4.8
Stress urinary incontinence	0-4.2
Daytime incontinence	7.1-64.2
Nighttime incontinence	33.3-79.1
ISC	0-34.3
Rupture	0-1.5
Neobladder stones	0-11.9
Upper tract stones	0-1.5
Ureteroenteric obstruction	0-4.5
Ureteroenteric reflux	0
Acute pyelonephritis	0-1.5
Hyperchloremic metabolic acidosis	0-16.7
Change of bowel habit	0-55
Asymptomatic bacteriuria	74
Enteroneobladder fistula	0-5.9
General	
Wound infection	0
Wound hernia	0-1.5
Abscess	0
Bowel obstruction	0-4.2
Renal deterioration	0-4.8
Other	0

period for which it is in contact with urine.[42] Chronic metabolic acidosis causes mobilization of calcium carbonate from bone as a buffer. The carbonate combines with hydrogen and the calcium is excreted in the urine.[43] The acidosis is also buffered using protein from bone matrix.[44] This buffering can cause reduction in growth potential in children and an increased number of orthopedic problems.[39,45] Colocystoplasty is also occasionally associated with hypokalemia as a result of secretion of potassium into the urine by the colon patch.[39]

Vitamin B_{12} deficiency

This occurs very rarely although there is a tendency for low normal vitamin B_{12} levels consequent to reduced absorption if terminal ileum is resected.[46]

Changes in the sensorium

These may occur secondary to magnesium deficiency, ammonia excess secondary to failure of hepatic clearance of the increased portal ammoniacal load, enhanced drug reabsortipon and failure of drug excretion – especially for those drugs undergoing obligatory renal excretion such as theophylline.[47]

Renal function

Deterioration of renal function has been reported in 0–4.8% of patients with continent intestinal reservoirs and neobladders.[48,49] The presence or absence of deterioration following detubularized right colonic neobladder appears to be related to baseline renal function, and formation is not recommended in patients with glomerular filtration rate (GFR) <55 ml/min[48,50] as this appears to be the critical level of renal function required to successfully deal with the excess chronic endogenous acid load after urinary diversion. At 10 years post-reconstruction GFR is slightly to moderately reduced in all patients. This reduction occurs in ileal and colonic conduit patients as well as those with right colonic reservoir.[51]

CISC in neobladders

Spontaneous voiding is a fine balance between an adequate fall in outlet resistance and an adequate increase in intra-neobladder pressure. The former can only happen if the native sphincter system is functional or by use of an artificial urinary sphincter (AUS). Emptying of the neobladder is not based on the coordinated contraction of the urinary reservoir because the neobladder cannot contract volitionally. Spontaneous voiding is achieved, if it is achieved, by abdominal straining to increase abdominal pressure with simultaneous relaxation of the pelvic floor.[52] As there is no reliable way to predict preoperatively if a patient will be able to void spontaneously or not, all patients must learn how to perform CISC before surgery. CISC is required in 50% of women and 4–8% of men with right colonic neobladder.[12,13,53–55]

Mucus

Mucus production can be a problem in patients using CISC and in the immediate postoperative period.[48] Elimination of mucus production is not easy and may indeed be inadvisable as it may protect the bowel mucosa against urinary carcinogens and other substances.[56] Mucus accumulation can predispose to urinary tract infection, stone formation, bladder outlet obstruction and bladder perforation.[57,58]

Bacteriuria

Although asymptomatic bacteriuria with mixed organisms occurs in 50–100% of neobladders[59] the incidence of significant urinary tract infection has been reported to be lower (4–43%).[60,61] Although secretion of immunoglobulin A by the bowel segment may be beneficial,[62] large residuals, presence of mucus and the need to perform CISC are predisposing factors to clinically relevant urinary tract infections. Infection while performing CISC is harmless in the normal urinary tract except in the presence of high-grade reflux[63,64] and the same is probably true for neobladders. While bacteriuria is implicated in stone formation[65] and the development of malignancy[66] it is currently unclear whether its elimination is desirable or possible.

Stones

Urinary tract stones, especially bladder stones, form in 1–13% of neobladders.[12,13,65] Stones occur in only 2% of patients who void spontaneously and efficiently. However, they occur in 10% of patients who need to perform CISC – implicating stasis as an important factor in pathogenesis.[67] Stones are usually triple phosphate, implying that bacteriuria with urease-producing bacteria (*Proteus*, *Providencia* and *Klebsiella*) may be a causative factor.[68] Other risk factors are the presence of intravesical foreign bodies, mucus[65] and hypocitraturia.[69] Stones may be prevented by ensuring complete emptying, performing regular wash-outs to eliminate mucus build up and pharmacotherapy with citrate supplementation, thiazide diuretic or acetohydroxamic acid.[70]

When stones are detected they must be removed because they represent a nidus for infection and have a tendency to enlarge if left in situ. The majority of stones can be removed endoscopically as long as they can be removed completely without leaving fragments behind. Large or multiple stones require open removal.[12,67]

Vesico ureteric reflux

This is not thought to be of significance in practice as it has not been associated with deterioration in renal function[70–72] – however, reflux has been associated with renal parenchymal damage secondary to pyelonephritis in animal models.[73] Conversely in practice renal damage consequent to obstruction has been a far greater problem in those ureters reimplanted in an antireflux manner (13.2% vs. 4.2%).[74]

Rupture

Neobladder rupture is a rare but life-threatening complication occurring in up to 1% with a reported mortality of 23–25%.[12,75–77] It is generally traumatic in etiology related to ISC, overdistension and/or external trauma.[75] The diagnosis is often delayed due to lack of awareness of this condition, the often unimpressive clinical findings on examination and negative radiological investigation.[78] Diagnostic delay is especially problematic in patients with neuropathy, who have altered sensory pathways and develop peritonitis and intra-abdominal abscesses without significant signs and symptoms. Perforation is more common in neuropathy, in those with competent bladder outlets (including those with AUS, in individuals with recurrent urinary tract infections and in those performing CISC.[77,79] The usual site of perforation is the suture line. The rupture may be explained by local ischemia of this area.[80]

Alternatively, bladder overdistension or high intravesical pressures can cause transient localized microvascular occlusion – creating a weak point which can easily rupture after an abrupt intrinsic or extrinsic pressure rise.[81] Because most patients with colonic neobladders (especially those who do CISC) have infected urine, conservative treatment with catheter drainage and antibiotics is inadequate. If the clinical picture is that of bladder rupture, exploration of the abdomen must be performed even if contrast cystography has been negative as the diagnosis is made preoperatively in only 43–75%[75,77,82,83] and most perforations are intra-abdominal.[75]

Carcinoma

The appearance of a new malignancy in a right colonic neobladder is very rare, although local recurrence occurs in 4–10% of patients having neobladder formation for malignancy.[19–22] In general there is a long latent period of 10 years or more between urinary reservoir construction and malignancy in those treated for benign disease. Malignancy may be associated with chronic inflammation, urine stasis and recurrent urinary tract infection[66,84,85] or may be related to field change in the colonic mucosa.

Pathogenesis may be related to chronic reservoir inflammation and bacteriuria. This allows for the reduction of urinary nitrates to nitrites by colonic bacteria, which in turn react with urinary secondary amines to form *N*-nitrosamines.[86] It is these *N*-nitrosamines that are implicated in the pathogenesis of the cancers that develop in ureterosigmoidostomies.[87]

Bowel disturbance

The natural role of the ileum is the absorption of water and electrolytes, vitamin B_{12}, bile acids and fats from the small bowel lumen. Bowel disturbances, in particular, intractable diarrhea have been reported in up to 50% of patients having right colonic neobladders.[12,13,88] Colonization of distal ileum by colonic commensals following resection of the ileocecal valve,[89] combined with an increased bile acid and fat load on the colon consequent to distal ileal resection both increase the total load of water and electrolytes reaching the colon and result in secretion of salt and water by the colon.[90,91] The colon cannot adequately reabsorb this extra load. The increased bile acid load also produces an increase in gut motility that compounds the problem.[92]

This post-neobladder bowel disturbance can be extremely troublesome especially for patients with neuropathic bladder and bowel dysfunction – whose fecal continence is generally dependent upon chronic constipation. The preoperative preparation and the relative starvation of the postoperative period also disturb this.[93,94]

Incontinence

When it comes to an evaluation of urinary continence following orthotopic neobladder diversion there is a wide variation in the definition of continence. This varies from 'dry without the need of any pads' through to 'loss of a few drops of urine or less on the majority of days and nights'.[15,95,96]

Incontinence can be a significant problem after detubularized right colonic neobladder formation, particularly at night and particularly in the elderly.[97] Bedwetting is attributed to a reduction in urethral closing pressure, relaxation of the pelvic floor muscles, increased urine output and failure of the sphincter to increase in tone in response to contractions from the bowel patch during sleep, individually or in combination and occurs in 15–63% of patients.[12,97–101] Daytime incontinence in patients with orthotopic neobladders is thought to be consequent to loss of the sacral reflex arc, incomplete neobladder detubularization and/or sphincter damage[98,99] and occurs in 0–37% of women and 2–64% of men.[12,53,54,98,99]

The AUS is the outlet procedure that theoretically at least offers the maximum chance of spontaneous voiding for those patients who are incontinent secondary to sphincter incompetence post orthotopic neobladder. The use of the AUS has been reported in 0–5% of patients following detubularized right colonic orthotopic neobladder.[12,13,97]

To prevent sphincter incompetence following orthotopic neobladder formation a meticulous apical dissection during cystoprostatectomy is required along with full control of the dorsal venous plexus of Santorini,[102] urethral tears should be avoided, as should bleeding or prolonged urine leak as this will result in fibrosis with distraction and a consequent loss of elasticity in the region of the urethral anastomosis. Optimal detubularization and refashioning of the right colonic segment are also required.

Investigation of urinary incontinence following neobladder formation requires endoscopy, post-void residual assessment and videourodynamic assessment of the neobladder and the sphincter mechanism. Urethral profilometry is advocated by some but we have not found this to be of benefit.

Incontinence is managed according to cause with voiding retraining, pads, pharmacotherapy, ISC, AUS and neobladder manipulation.

Quality of life

Improved quality of life is the main reason cited for offering patients bladder replacement as opposed to incontinent diversion; however this is a rather ephemeral concept. There is no set definition of 'quality of life' and no set and hence repeatable means of measurement. Assessment of quality of life is multifactorial and depends upon the individual, their circumstances as well as their disease. There have been many studies comparing quality of life in patients with continent diversions or neobladders and those with ileal conduits.[103–105] In general these have shown no significant benefit in favor of neobladder or continent diversion with the exception of the studies by McGuire et al[106] and Hobisch et al[107] who reported a better quality of life in those with continent diversion or neobladder.

Conclusion

Patients with congenital and acquired problems of urinary storage and voiding remain a therapeutic challenge. Treatment may be considered to be a success if a large volume low-pressure continent reservoir that empties completely can be constructed. This prevents upper tract deterioration, avoids significant urinary tract infection, helps in the maintenance of continence and provides optimal personal and social acceptance. The detubularized right colonic neobladder provides an attractive versatile alternative with acceptable morbidity and minimal mortality.

References

1. Tizzoni G, Foggi A. Die Wiederherstellung der Harnblase. Centralbl Chir 1888; 15: 921–4.
2. Verhogen J. Neostomie uretero-cecale. Formation d'une nouvelle poche vesicale et d'un nouval uretre. Assoc Franc d'Urol 1908; 12: 352–65
3. Kock NG. Intraabdominal 'reservoir' in patients with permanent ileostomy. Preliminary observations on a procedure resulting in fecal 'continence' in five ileostomy patients. Arch Surg 1969; 99: 223–31.
4. Kock NG, Nilson AE, Norlen L, Sundin T, Trasti H. Urinary diversion via a continent ileum reservoir: clinical experience. Scand J Urol Nephrol 1978; Suppl 49: 23.
5. Kock NG, Nilson AE, Nilsson LO, Norlen LJ, Philipson BM. Urinary diversion via a continent ileal reservoir: clinical results in 12 patients. J Urol 1982; 128: 469–75.
6. Lieskovsky G, Boyd SD, Skinner DG. Management of late complications of the Kock pouch form of urinary diversion. J Urol 1987; 137: 1146–50.
7. Mansson W, Collen S, Sundin T. Continent caecal reservoir in urinary diversion. Br J Urol 1984; 56: 359–65.
8. Rowland RG, Mitchell MR, Birhrle R. The cecoileal continent urinary reservoir. World J Urol 1985; 3: 185–9.
9. Goldwasser B, Barrett DM, Benson RC Jr. Bladder replacement with use of detubularised right colon segment. Preliminary report of a new technique. Mayo Clin Proc 1986; 61: 615–21.
10. Lockhart JL. Remodelled right colon: an alternative urinary reservoir. J Urol 1987; 138: 730–4.
11. Whitmore WF, Gittes RF. Reconstruction of the urinary tract by cecal and ileocecal cystoplasty: review of a 15-year experience. J Urol 1983; 129: 494–8.
12. Mansson W, Davidsson T, Konyves J et al. Continent urinary tract reconstruction; the Lund experience. BJU Int 2003; 92: 271–6.
13. Levy OM, Phillips MH, Algen A, Kivart AM. Bladder replacement after radical cystectomy using detubularised right colonic segment. Urology 1988; 32: 492–7.
14. Kirsch AJ, Olsson CA, Heisle JW. Pediatric continent reservoirs and colocystoplasty with absorbable staples. J Urol 1996; 156(Suppl): 611–14.
15. Elmajnan DA, Stein JP, Esrig D et al. The Kock ileal neobladder: updates experience in 295 male patients. J Urol 1996; 156: 920–5.

16. Hautmann RE. Complications and results after cystectomy in male and female patients with locally invasive bladder cancer. Eur Urol 1998; 33(Suppl 4): 23–4.
17. Hohenfellner M, Dahms S, Pfitzenmaier J, Thuroff JW. Orthotopic bladder augmentation and substitution. Curr Opin Urol 1999; 9: 309–14.
18. Studer UE, Zingg EJ. Ileal orthotopic bladder substitutes. What we have learned from 12 years experience with 200 patients. Urol Clin North Am 1997; 24: 781–93.
19. Lebret T, Herve JM, Yonneau L et al. After cystectomy is it justified to perform a bladder replacement for patients with lymph node positive bladder cancer? Eur Urol 2002; 42: 344–9.
20. Hautmann RE, Simon J. Ileal neobladder and local recurrence of bladder cancer; patterns of failure and impact on function in men. J Urol 1999; 162: 1963–6.
21. Ward AM, Olencki T, Peerbook D, Klein EA. Should continent diversion be performed in patients with locally advanced bladder cancer? Urology 1998; 51: 232–6.
22. Tefilli MV, Gheiler EL, Tiguert R et al. Urinary diversion related outcome in patients with pelvic recurrence after radical cystectomy for bladder cancer. Urology 1999; 53: 999–1004.
23. Yossepowitch O, Dalbagni G, Golijanin D et al. Orthotopic urinary diversion after cystectomy for bladder cancer: implications for cancer control and patterns of disease recurrence. J Urol 2003; 169: 177–81.
24. Mansson W, Collen S, Stigsson L. Four method of uretero-intestinal anastomosis in urinary conduit diversion. A comparative study of early and late complications and the influence of radiotherapy. Scand J Urol Nephrol 1979; 13: 191–9.
25. Wammock R, Wricke C, Hohenfellner R. Long term results of ileocecal continent diversion in patients treated with and without previous pelvic irradiation. J Urol 2002; 167: 2058–62.
26. Ahlering TE, Kennello S, Boyd SD, Lieskovsky G, Skinner DG, Bernstein L. A comparative study of preoperative complications with Kock pouch urinary diversion in highly irradiated versus non-irradiated patients. J Urol 1988; 139: 1202–4.
27. Gschwend JE, May F, Paiss T, Gottfried HW, Hautmann RE. High dose pelvic irradiation followed by ileal neobladder urinary diversion: complications and long term results. Br J Urol 1996; 77: 680–3.
28. Aboseif SR, Borirakchanyavat S, Lue TF, Carroll PR. Continence mechanism of the ileal neobladder: a urodynamic study in women. World J Urol 1998; 16: 400–4.
29. Cheng C, Hendry WF, Kirby RS et al. Detubularisation in cystoplasty: clinical review. Br J Urol 1991; 67: 303–7.
30. Nurse DE, McRae P, Stephenson TP, Mundy AR. The problems of substitution cystoplasty. Br J Urol 1988; 61: 423–6.
31. Politano VA, Leadbetter WF. An operative technique for the correction of vesicoureteric reflux. J Urol 1958; 79: 932–41.
32. Leadbetter WG, Clark BG. Five years experience with ureteroenterostomy by the 'combined' technique. J Urol 1955; 73: 67–9.
33. Coffey RC. Physiologic implantation of the severed ureter or common bile duct into the intestine. JAMA 1911; 156: 397–8.
34. Barry JM. Unstented extravesical ureteroneocystotomy in kidney transplantation. J Urol 1983; 129: 918–19.
35. Camey N, Le Duc 1979. L'entero-cystoplastie apres cystoprostatectomie totale pour cancer de vessie. Indications, technique operatoire, surveillance et resultants sur quatre-vin sept cas. Ann Urol 1979; 13: 114–17.
36. Goodwin WE, Winter CC, Barker WF. 'Cup-patch' technique of ileocystoplasty for bladder enlargement or partial substitution. Surg Gynecol Obstet 1959; 108: 180–240.
37. Parekh DJ, Gilbert WB, Smith JA Jr. Functional lower urinary tract voiding outcomes after cystectomy and orthotopic neobladder. J Urol 2000; 163: 56–8.
38. Santucci RA, Park CH, Mayo ME, Lange PH. Continence and urodynamic parameters of continent urinary reservoirs: comparison of gastric, ileal, ileocolic, right colon and sigmoid segments. Urology 1999; 54: 252–7.
39. Wagstaff KE, Woodhouse CRJ, Rose GA et al. Blood and urine analysis in patients with intestinal bladders. Br J Urol 1991; 68: 311–16.
40. Nurse DE, Mundy AR. Metabolic complications of cystoplasty. Br J Urol 1989; 63: 165–70.
41. McDougal WS. Metabolic complications of urinary intestinal diversion. J Urol 1992; 147: 1199–208.
42. Koch MO, McDougal WS. The pathophysiology of hyperchloraemic metabolic acidosis after urinary diversion through intestinal segments. Surgery 1985; 98: 561–70.
43. Lemann J Jr, Litzow R, Lennon EJ. The effect of chronic acid loads in normal man: further evidence for the participation of bone mineral in the defence against chronic metabolic acidosis. J Clin Invest 1966; 45: 1608–14.
44. McDougal WS, Koch MO, Shands G 3rd et al. Bony demineralisation following urinary intestinal diversion. J Urol 1988; 140: 853–5.
45. Mundy AR, Nurse DE. Calcium balance, growth and skeletal mineralisation in patients with cystoplasties. Br J Urol 1992; 69: 257–9.
46. Terai A, Okado Y, Shichiri Y et al. Vitamin B12 deficiency in patients with urinary intestinal diversion. Int J Urol 1997; 4: 21–5.
47. Ekman I, Mansson W, Nyberg L. Absorption of drugs from continent caecal reservoir. Br J Urol 1989; 64: 412–16.
48. Fontaine E, Leaver R, Woodhouse CR. The effect of intestinal urinary reservoirs on renal function: a 10 year follow-up. BJU Int 2000; 86: 195–8.
49. Jonsson O, Olafsson G, Lindholm E, Tornquist H. Long term experience with the Kock ileal reservoir for continent urinary diversion. Eur Urol 2002; 40: 632–40.
50. Kristjansson A, Davisson T, Mansson W. Metabolic alterations at different levels of renal function following continent urinary diversion through colonic segments. J Urol 1997; 157: 2099–103.
51. Mansson W, Ahlgren G, White T. Glomerular filtration rate up to 10 years after urinary diversion of different types. A comparative study of ileal and colonic conduit, refluxing and non-refluxing anastomosis and continent caecal reservoir. Scand J Urol Nephrol 1989; 23: 195–200.
52. Strawbridge LR, Kramer SA, Castillo O et al. Augmentation cystoplasty and the genitourinary sphincter. J Urol 1989; 142: 297–301.

53. Ali El Dein B, el-Sobky E, Hohenfellner M, Ghoneim MA. Orthotopic bladder substitution in women: functional evaluation. J Urol 1999; 161: 1875–80.
54. Jarolim L, Babjuk M, Grim M et al. Reconstruction of the lower urinary tract in women after cystectomy. Cas Lek Cesk 1999; 138: 716–18.
55. Shimogaki H, Okada H, Fujisawa M et al. Longterm experience with orthotopic reconstruction of the lower urinary tract in women. J Urol 1999; 161: 573–7.
56. Iannoni C, Marcheggiano A, Pallone F et al. Abnormal patterns of colorectal mucin secretion after urinary diversions of different types. Hum Pathol 1986; 17: 834–40.
57. Rushton HG, Woodard JR, Parrott TS et al. Delayed bladder rupture after enterocystoplasty. J Urol 1988; 140: 344–6.
58. Khoury AE, Salomon M, Doche R et al. Stone formation after augmentation cystoplasty: the role of intestinal mucus. J Urol 1997; 158: 1133–7.
59. Lockhart JL, Davies R, Persky L, Figuroa TE, Ramirez G. Acid-base changes following urinary tract reconstruction for continent diversion and orthotopic bladder replacement. J Urol 1994; 152(2 Pt 1): 338–42.
60. Mitchell ME, Kulb TB, Backes DJ. Intestinoplasty in combination with clean intermittent catheterization in the management of vesical dysfunction. J Urol 1986; 136: 288–91.
61. Khoury JM, Timmons SL, Corbel L et al. Complications of enterocystoplasty. Urology 1992; 40: 9–14.
62. Murray K, Nurse DE, Mundy AR. Secreto-motor function of intestinal segments used in lower urinary tract reconstruction. Br J Urol 1987; 60: 532–5.
63. Lapides J, Diokno AC, Silber SJ et al. Clean intermittent self-catheterisation in the treatment of urinary tract. J Urol 1972; 107: 458–61.
64. Kass EJ, Koff SA, Diokno AC et al. The significance of bacilluria in children on long term intermittent catheterisation. J Urol 1981; 126: 223–5.
65. Blyth B, Ewalt DH, Duckett JW et al. Lithogenic properties of enterocystoplasty. J Urol 1992; 148: 575–7.
66. Golomb L, Klutke CG, Lewin KJ et al. Bladder neoplasms associated with augmentation cystoplasty: report of 2 cases and a literature review. J Urol 1989; 142: 377–80.
67. Nurse DE, McInerney PD, Thomas PJ et al. Stones in enterocystoplasties. Br J Urol 1996; 77: 684–7.
68. Griffith DP, Musher DM, Itin C. Urease. The primary cause of infection-induced urinary stones. Invest Urol 1976; 13: 346–50.
69. Terai A, Arai Y, Kawakita M, Okada Y, Yoshida O. Effect of urinary intestinal diversion on urinary risk factors for urolithiasis. J Urol 1995; 153: 37–41.
70. Pantuck AJ, Han K, Perotti M, Weiss RE, Cummings KB. Ureterointestinal implantation and complications of refluxing versus non-refluxing techniques. J Urol 1999; 161(Suppl): 237.
71. Pantuck AJ, Hank R, Perrotti M et al. Ureteroenteric anastomosis in continent urinary diversion: long-term results and complications of direct versus nonrefluxing techniques. J Urol 2000; 173: 450–5.
72. Kristjansson A, Mansson W. Refluxing or non-refluxing anastomosis. BJU Int 1999; 84: 905–10.
73. Richie JP, Skinner DG, Wassman J. The effect of reflux on the development of pyelonephritis in urinary diversion: an experimental study. J Surg Res 1974; 16: 256–61.
74. Lockhart JL, Pow-Sang JM, Persky L, Stanford E, Helal M. Results, complications and surgical indications of the Florida pouch. Surg Gynecol Obstet 1991; 173: 289–96.
75. Mansson W, Bakke A, Bergman B et al. Perforation of continent urinary reservoirs. Scandinavian experience. Scand J Urol Nephrol 1997; 31: 529–32.
76. Elder JS, Snyder HM, Hulbert WC et al. Perforation of the augmented bladder in patients undergoing clean intermittent catheterization. J Urol 1988; 140: 1159–62.
77. Couillard DR, Vapnec JM, Rentzepis MJ et al. Fatal perforation of an augmentation cystoplasty in an adult. Urology 1993; 42: 585–8.
78. Bauer SB, Hendren WH, Kozakewich H et al. Perforation of the augmented bladder. J Urol 1992; 148: 699–703.
79. Crane JM, Scherz HS, Billman GF et al. Ischemic necrosis: a hypothesis to explain the pathogenesis of spontaneously ruptured enterocystoplasty. J Urol 1991; 146: 141–4.
80. Essig KA, Sheldon CA, Brandt MT et al. Elevated intravesical pressure causes hypoperfusion in canine colocystoplasty: a fluorometric assay. J Urol 1991; 146: 551–3.
81. Slaton JW, Kropp KA. Conservative management of suspected bladder rupture after augmentation enterocystoplasty. J Urol 1994; 152: 713–15.
82. Braverman RM, Lebowitz RL. Perforation of the augmented urinary bladder in nine children and adolescents: importance of cystography. AJR Am J Roentgenol 1991; 157: 1059–63.
83. Sheiner JR, Kaplan GW. Spontaneous bladder rupture following enterocystoplasty. J Urol 1988; 140: 1157–8.
84. Kirby RS, Lloyd-Davies RW. Adenocarcinoma occurring within a caecocystoplasty. Br J Urol 1985; 57: 357–8.
85. Filmer RB, Spencer JR. Malignancies in bladder augmentations and intestinal conduits. J Urol 1990; 143: 671–7.
86. Hill M. Nitrates and bacteriology: are these important etiological factors in gastric carcinogenesis? Adv Biosci 1986; 32: 35–45.
87. Stewart M. Urinary diversion and bowel cancer. Ann R Coll Surg Eng 1986; 68: 98–102.
88. Ben Chaim J, Shenfield O, Goldwasser B, Shemesh E. Does the use of the ileocaecal region in reconstructive urology cause persistent diarrhoea? Eur Urol 1995; 27: 315–17.
89. Fromm D. Ileal resection or disease and the blind loop syndrome: current concepts and pathophysiology. Surgery 1973; 73: 639–48.
90. Debongnie JC, Phillips SF. Capacity of human colon to absorb fluid. Gastroenterology 1978; 74: 698–703.
91. Cummings JH, James WP, Wiggins HS. Role of colon in ileal resection diarrhoea. Lancet 1973; i: 344–7.
92. Jacobsen M, Hojgaard L, Hylander Moller E et al. Effect of enterocoated cholestyramine on bowel habit after resection: a double blind cross over study. BMJ 1985; 290: 1315–18.
93. Singh G, Thomas DG. Bowel problems after enterocystoplasty. Br J Urol 1997; 79: 328–32.

94. Soong CS, Thompson JB, Poley JR et al. Hydroxy fatty acids in human diarrhoea. Gastroenterology 1972; 63: 748–57.
95. Chen L, Allen TD. Continence in the myelodysplastic patient following enterocystoplasty. J Urol 1993; 149: 1103–6.
96. Iwakiri J, Gill H, Anderson M, Freiha F. Functional and urodynamic characteristics of an ileal neobladder. J Urol 1993; 149: 1072–6.
97. Goldwasser B, Mansson W, Davidsson T et al. Cystourethrometric findings in patients with detubularised right colonic segment for bladder replacement. J Urol 1991; 145: 538–41.
98. Stein JP, Grossfeld GD, Freeman JA et al. Orthotopic lower urinary tract reconstruction in women using the Kock ileal neobladder: updated experience in 34 patients. J Urol 1997; 158: 400–5.
99. Steven 1K, Poulson AL. The orthotopic Kock ileal neobladder: functional results, urodynamic features, complications and survival in 166 men. J Urol 2000; 164: 288–98.
100. Jakobsen H, Steven K, Stigsby B et al. Pathogenesis of nocturnal urinary incontinence after ileocaecal bladder replacement: continuous measurement of urethral closure pressure during sleep. Br J Urol 1987; 59: 148–52.
101. Akerlund S, Berglund B, Kock NG et al. Voiding pattern, urinary volume, composition and bacterial contamination in patients with urinary diversion via a continent ileal reservoir. Br J Urol 1989; 63: 619–23.
102. Koraitim MM, Atta MA, Foda MK. Impact of prostatic apex on continence and urinary flow in patients with intestinal neobladders. Br J Urol 1996; 78: 534–6.
103. Kitamura H, Miyao N, Yanase M et al. Quality of life in patients having an ileal conduit, continent reservoir or orthotopic neobladder after cystectomy for bladder carcinoma. Int J Urol 1999; 6: 393–9.
104. Hart S, Skinner EC, Meyerowitz BE et al. Quality of life after radical cystectomy for bladder cancer in patients with an ileal conduit, or a cutaneous urethral Kock pouch. J Urol 1999; 162: 77–81.
105. Mansson A, Davidsson T, Hunt S, Mansson W. The quality of life in men after radical cystectomy with a continent cutaneous diversion or orthotopic bladder substitution; is there a difference. BJU Int 2002; 90: 386–90.
106. McGuire MS, Grimaldi G, Grotas J, Russo P. The type of urinary diversion after radical cystectomy significantly impacts on the patients' quality of life. Ann Surg Oncol 2000; 7: 4–8.
107. Hobisch A, Tosin K, Kinzl J et al. Patients' assessment of life after cystectomy and orthotopic neobladder versus ileal conduit. J Urol 1999; 161(Suppl 90): 344.

18 Sigmoid neobladder

Jerilyn M Latini

Introduction

Every segment of the gastrointestinal system has been used for urinary diversion, bladder replacement or urinary tract reconstruction. The ideal bladder substitute has yet to be determined. Continent urinary diversions have traditionally been classified according to their efferent continence mechanism. Continent urinary diversions that anastomose to the urethra, using the native urethral sphincter as the continence mechanism, are termed bladder replacements, orthotopic bladder substitutes or neobladders. The ideal neobladder should allow (i) normal urethral voiding, (ii) low-pressure urine storage, (iii) preservation of renal function, (iv) socially acceptable continence, (v) no significant metabolic/nutritional disturbances and (vi) maintenance of quality of life.

Orthotopic bladder substitution was first popularized by Camey.[1] Following experience with the non-detubularized Camey ileal neobladder, various techniques for orthotopic bladder replacement using the urethral sphincter as the continence mechanism have been described. Virtually all gastrointestinal segments alone and in combination have been used. When removing the native urinary bladder, the urethral sphincter mechanism must be preserved, as the neobladder will ultimately be anastomosed to the urethral sphincter as the efferent continence mechanism.

These urinary diversions are attractive because they have no abdominal stoma. Almost all patients void per urethra by increasing the abdominal pressure (by the Valsalva maneuver) with simultaneous urethral sphincter relaxation. Urine elimination occurs most often by voiding, less commonly by intermittent catheterization. Urine will be potentially sterile at all times, if no foreign bodies, such as indwelling or intermittent catheters, are inserted into the neobladder. The main drawback associated with neobladders is possible chronic nocturnal enuresis. Having the patient void once or twice during the night can minimize this. Patients must also be prepared that it may take 1–3 months to achieve continence postoperatively.

The sigmoid neobladder was initially described in 1987 by Reddy.[2–4] Minor technical modifications have been described since this initial experience.[5–8] The sigmoid neobladder is an orthotopic bladder substitute that is low-pressure, highly compliant and non-refluxing. Daytime and nighttime continence is ideally achievable, with the ability to void volitionally at socially acceptable intervals. Diurnal continence is possible in most cases of bladder substitution, given available detubularization techniques. The sigmoid neobladder is performed similar to the procedure popularized by Reddy,[9,10] Parra et al,[8] Chen et al,[6] Da Pozzo et al[5] and Libertino.[7]

Indications

The indications for urinary diversion include both malignant and non-malignant conditions: congenital problems (posterior urethral valves, epispadias complex, bladder exstrophy), neurogenic bladder, inflammatory conditions, interstitial cystitis, infection (tuberculosis, schistosomiasis), radiation, chemical cystitis, fistula, trauma, iatrogenic causes, undiversion, and idiopathic conditions.

Patient selection

In the past, a minimum level of renal function was required before urinary diversion would be performed. The intestinal segment interposed into the urinary tract may absorb and excrete urinary electrolytes and metabolites, causing significant metabolic disturbances. Patients with compromised renal function were much less able to compensate for these metabolic derangements, leading to severe morbidity and potential mortality, if untreated. Experience with modern techniques for urinary diversion demonstrates that severe metabolic abnormalities are uncommon, even in patients with compromised renal function. Currently, there is no cut-off minimum level of renal function below which urinary diversion is absolutely contraindicated.

There are other requirements that must be met prior to continent urinary diversion using the urethral sphincter. Occult bowel disease (carcinoma, polyps, dysplasia, severe diverticular disease) must be ruled out by colonoscopy or barium enema. Following neobladder creation, adequate length of healthy bowel must remain to minimize gastrointestinal compromise.

Those with benign functional urinary tract pathology may require urodynamic study of the urethral sphincter. Those with malignant disease should have no residual urethral or pelvic floor tumor involvement following cystectomy and/or exenteration. Relative contraindications include multifocal carcinoma in situ in the bladder or tumor near the bladder neck. Absolute contraindications include tumor into the prostatic urethra, or tumor involving the bladder neck/urethral margin in both sexes. Those with positive intraoperative frozen sections or positive preoperative urethral or bladder neck biopsies are not offered neobladders. In recent years, increasing numbers of neobladders have been performed in females following anterior exenteration, given the oncologic criteria discussed above.

Patient motivation is crucial. The patient must be physically and psychologically capable of clean intermittent self-catheterization, should this become necessary at any point, on a temporary or chronic basis. Some patients with neurogenic bladder dysfunction, selected patients with exstrophy, and those who have undergone prior surgery resulting in incontinence are not suitable candidates, as a functioning external urinary sphincter is critical for a functional, continent neobladder.

Preoperative patient preparation

Mechanical and antibiotic bowel preparation is required prior to urinary diversion using small or large bowel. In addition to oral antibiotics administered following cathartic, mechanical bowel preparation, intravenous perioperative antibiotics are used. Anti-embolism stockings and sequential compression devices are used to prevent thrombotic complications during and following surgery.

Prior to any urinary diversion, the patient must be evaluated and marked by the enterostomal therapist in conjunction with the operating surgeon. The optimal stoma position varies depending on the patient and the type of diversion planned. Even in patients in whom continent urinary diversion utilizing the urethral or anal sphincter is planned must be evaluated for alternative stoma position(s), in the event that the planned surgical procedure cannot be performed for technical, anatomic or other unanticipated intraoperative reasons.

Anatomy

Branches of the superior and inferior mesenteric arteries supply the small intestine and colon. The inferior mesenteric artery (IMA) divides into the left colic artery and sigmoid artery, which gives rise to the superior rectal artery and two or three left inferior colic arteries. These branches anastomose with the left colic artery as the marginal artery near the mesenteric colonic border (Figure 18.1). When ligating the lateral vascular bladder pedicles during radical cystectomy, care must be taken to preserve the internal iliac arteries. This maneuver protects the middle and inferior rectal (hemorrhoidal) arteries, minimizing the risk of distal rectal ischemia and the potential for intestinal leakage at the colorectal anastomosis.

Surgical technique

In the supine position with the lower extremities in a slightly abducted position, a lower midline transperitoneal or paraumbilical incision is made from just above the umbilicus to the pubic symphysis to expose the entire sigmoid colon. If greater exposure is necessary, the incision can be extended cephalad, allowing the descending colon to be taken down from the splenic flexure, to better achieve a tension-free descending colonic anastomosis. An appendectomy should not be performed at this time, as appendix may be needed as a cutaneous conduit in the future.

An abdominal retractor is placed, packing the small intestine into the upper abdomen to gain necessary exposure. If cystectomy is performed, the left internal iliac artery must be preserved. Excessive dissection of the pelvic floor and urethra is to be avoided, as the integrity of both is vital for maintaining continence. Attention should be given to preserving the urethra for anastomosis to the neobladder. In men, the prostatic apex is transected as during radical prostatectomy. Preservation of prostatic tissue/capsule to enhance continence is not necessary and may compromise the oncologic operation. In women, the posterior bladder wall is dissected off of the anterior vagina to the vaginocervical junction, preserving the autonomic sympathetic nerve fibers running laterally. Urethral margin frozen sections should be obtained to confirm the absence of residual prostatic tissue in men, and to rule out carcinoma, carcinoma in situ or dysplasia in all patients.

The colon is freed from the retroperitoneum by incising the entire white line of Toldt to ensure adequate visualization and mobilization. The mesenteric vascular supply to the sigmoid/descending colon should then be backlit and examined, specifically following the sigmoid artery and its branches from the IMA. A 35–40-cm segment of sigmoid on a broad, mobile mesentery is then selected. The proximal and distal ends of the selected length are marked with silk stay sutures. The proximal end of the sigmoid segment is then gently guided into the deep pelvis to be sure that it reaches for tension-free urethral anastomosis. Only if the sigmoid colon mesentery has sufficient length, allowing the sigmoid to reach the pelvis and urethra, will neobladder creation be possible. Once it has been decided to continue with neobladder creation, the mesentery is isolated and divided. Incising too deeply into the mesentery should be avoided, as important collateral blood supply comes from the middle colic and superior hemorrhoidal arteries. A tension-free colon–colon anastomosis is performed between the proximal end of the transected left colon and the distal sigmoid to re-establish intestinal continuity. Our preference is to use a stapling technique. Alternatively, one may use various suture techniques.

The descending colon is carefully placed anterior to the isolated sigmoid segment. Mesenteric length should be checked again, and, if necessary, the splenic flexure can be released to allow for adequate mobility to the deep pelvis and urethral stump on no tension. The mesocolon is closed with interrupted 3-0 silk sutures, incorporating only the peritoneum and taking care to not traumatize the mesenteric vessels. The isolated sigmoid segment lies lateral to the reanastomosed sigmoid colon.

The sigmoid segment is then flushed with antibiotic irrigation until clear. The isolated sigmoid segment is folded into a U-shape with the most dependent portion (the midpoint towards the pelvis) marked, identifying the optimal site for urethral anastomosis (Figure 18.2a). The segment is detubularized by incising the sigmoid using the Bovie on coagulation current along the posteromedial teniae, near the mesenteric border. The medial edges of the detubularized limbs of the U are aligned and the posterior neobladder wall is closed using two layers of continuous 2-0 synthetic absorbable suture (SAS; we prefer Vicryl). The first layer approximates the serosa and muscularis, followed by the second approximating the mucosal edges.

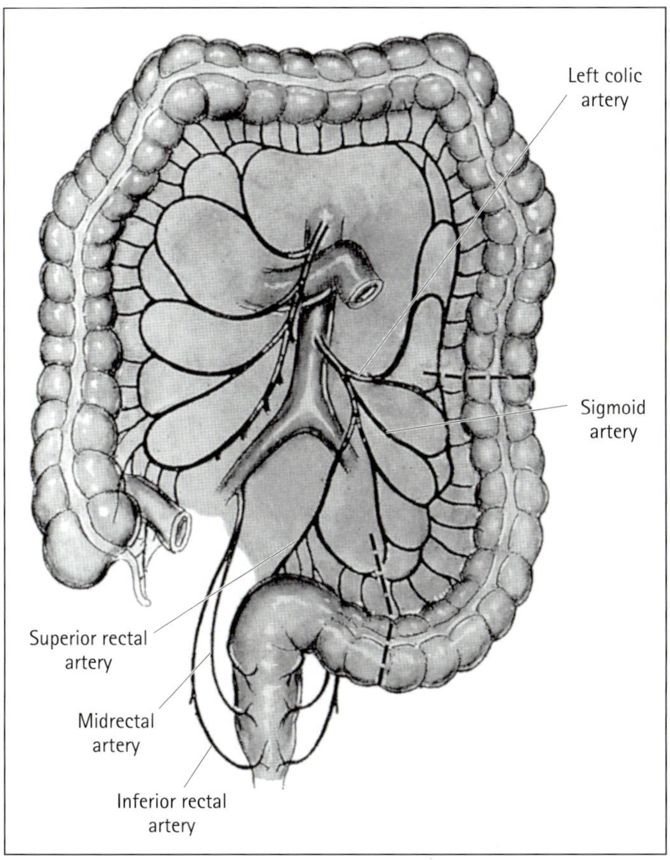

Figure 18.1 Technique to reconstruct detubularized sigmoid neobladder. The sigmoid colon is isolated on a broad mesenteric pedicle. (Reprinted with permission of the Lahey Clinic, Burlington, MA, USA and adapted from Reddy PK. J Urol 1991; 145: 51 with permission from Lippincott Williams & Wilkins.)

The ureterointestinal anastomoses are performed in an antirefluxing manner. The ureters are implanted through the posterolateral (omental) teniae of each limb of the U from within the neobladder using the submucosal transcolonic technique using 4-0 SAS suture (Figure 18.2b). Saline is injected submucosally to create the submucosal tunnels. Using a right angle clamp, the ureters are brought through the submucosal tunnels in the posterior neobladder wall and into the neobladder 'lumen'. Alternatively, the ureterointestinal anastomoses may be performed from outside the neobladder, prior to detubularization, using the seromuscular technique. Here, the ureters are brought anteriorly and implanted into the posterolateral tenia of each limb of the U using the Leadbetter technique. For either technique, each ureterointestinal anastomosis is stented with a 7-Fr 90-cm single-J ureteral stent. Each ureteral stent is secured to the neobladder with 4-0 chromic catgut suture to the colon.

Closure of the anterior neobladder wall is begun, in a similar manner to the posterior wall, but the cephalad-most portion is not completed, to allow for visualization during urethral anastomosis. A 24-Fr Malecot catheter is inserted into the neobladder through the open cephalad portion and brought out of the neobladder through a counter-incision in a convenient location. The Malecot catheter is secured to the neobladder using a 3-0 SAS pursestring suture. The ureteral stents are eventually brought out through the anterior wall of the neobladder through a similar counter-incision as the Malecot catheter.

The urethral anastomosis is performed by first redetermining the most dependent portion of the completed neobladder and optimal location for the urethral anastomosis. This may or may not be in the exact location that was marked earlier. A 1-cm (30-Fr) opening in the serosa muscularis is made at the most dependent portion, with a smaller opening created in the mucosa. Six interrupted 2-0 SAS (Monocryl or Vicryl) sutures are used to anastomose the neobladder to the urethra. Our preference is to pre-place the urethrointestinal anastomotic sutures with a urethral suture guide in place. Once the six anastomotic sutures are placed circumferentially and tagged, the suture guide is removed and a 20-Fr Council catheter is placed under direct vision and the urethral catheter balloon inflated. The six anastomotic sutures are then tied on no tension, completing the urethrointestinal anastomosis.

The remaining half of the anterior neobladder wall and cephalad opening of the neobladder are folded and approximated using continuous 2-0 SAS suture in a two-layer watertight closure (Figure 18.2c). Once the neobladder is completed and the Malecot and stents are secured, the neobladder is filled through the Malecot and tested for leakage. Additional reinforcing 2-0 SAS sutures are placed if needed, ensuring that the neobladder is watertight.

Two closed suction drains are then placed, one in the deep pelvis near the urethrointestinal anastomosis and a second near the ureterointestinal anastomoses. The neobladder is covered

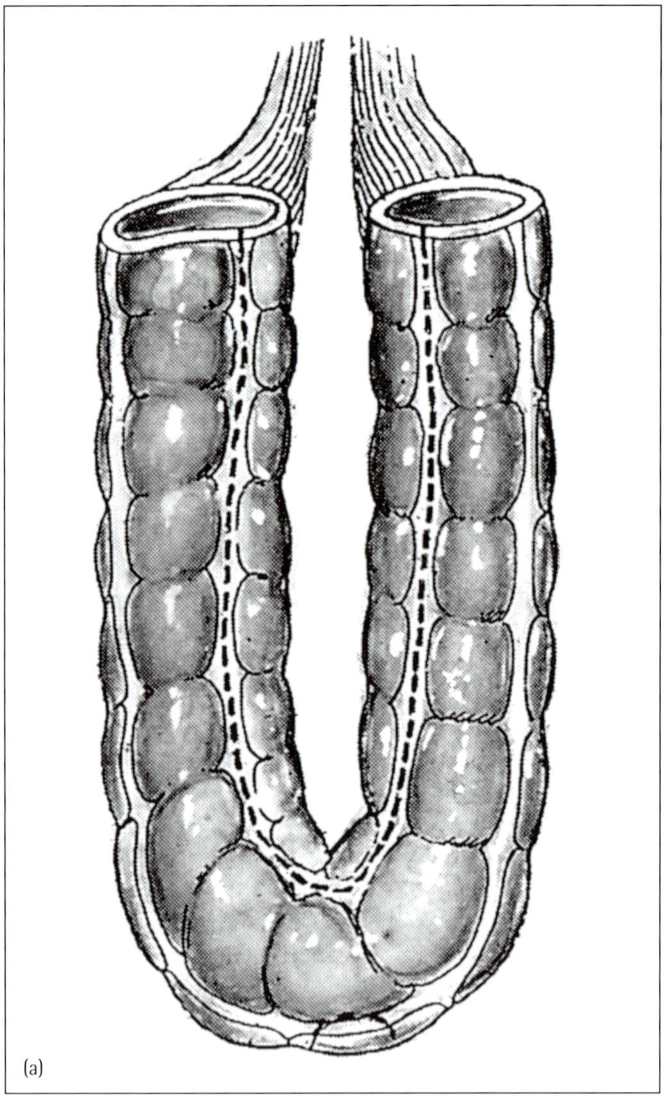

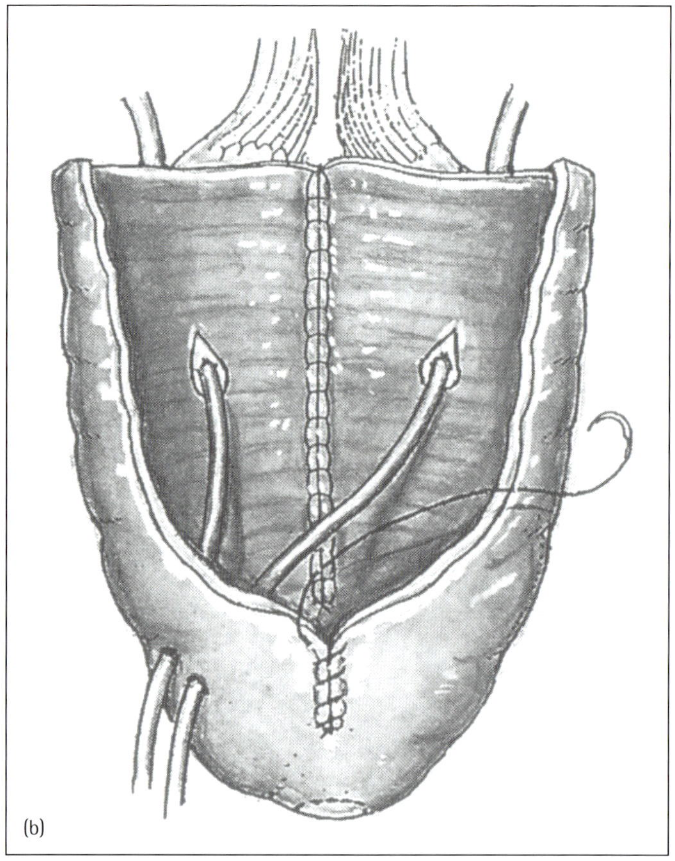

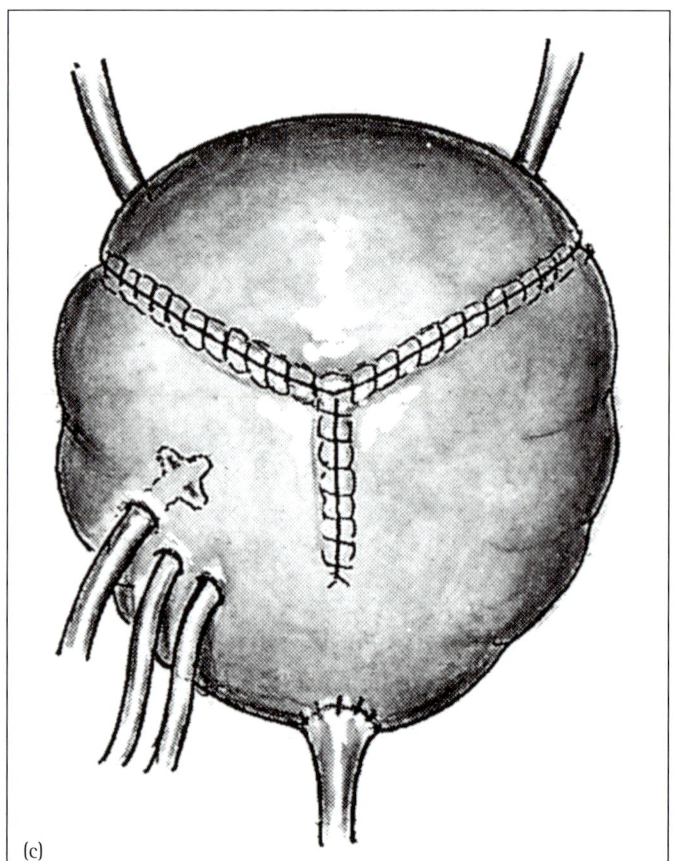

Figure 18.2 Sigmoid colon neobladder: technical procedure. (a) Tract of sigmoid colon 35–40-cm long is isolated and positioned in U shape at bladder site. It is completely detubularized along the medial tenia. (b) The posterior edges are realigned and ureters are reimplanted in the posterior layer. (c) The anterior layer is sutured in a Y shape. (Reprinted with permission from the Lahey Clinic, Burlington, MA.[12])

with omentum. The abdominal incision is closed in standard fashion, after bringing the Malecot cystostomy catheter and ureteral stents out via counter-incisions in the anterior abdominal wall. The two drains are brought out on the contralateral abdominal wall. All catheters, stents and drains are secured externally using non-absorbable drain sutures.

Postoperative care

The Malecot cystostomy catheter and urethral catheter are irrigated every 6 hours and as needed to prevent mucous plugging. The ureteral stents are irrigated as needed. The pelvic drains are removed once their output falls and it is determined that the creatinine of the drained fluid is consistent with serum. The stents are removed at 14 days. At 3 weeks, the urethral catheter is removed if gravity cystogram shows no extravasation. The Malecot is then clamped and the patient instructed in cycling the neobladder and a trial of urethral voiding. Postvoid residuals are measured via the Malecot for 1–2 weeks. The patient should continue to irrigate the neobladder via the Malecot periodically. Neobladder capacity will stretch to accommodate 250–800 ml.[5,6,9,10,13–15] Once progress and success is achieved with urethral voiding, the Malecot is removed. All patients are taught Kegel exercises to better achieve urinary continence.

Six weeks postoperatively, a baseline excretory intravenous pyelogram (or renal ultrasound or radionuclide renal scan, if there is allergy to intravenous contrast) is obtained to assess the upper tracts and rule out silent hydroureteronephrosis. Long-term routine oncologic evaluation is as indicated. In addition, postvoid residual urine volumes and serum electrolytes are monitored in neobladder patients initially every 3 months for the first year, then every 6 months thereafter. Urine cytology, intravenous pyelography and urethroscopy/pouchoscopy are performed annually.

Urodynamic studies

Reddy and colleagues reported the results of urodynamic studies for 27 men with sigmoid neobladders following radical cystoprostatectomy for transitional cell carcinoma of the bladder.[2–4] Mean maximum capacity ranged from 450 ml at 3 months follow-up to 600 ml at 12 months. Filling pressures and maximum pressure at capacity decreased from 3 to 12 months, as residual urine volumes increased slightly (Table 18.1). With time, neobladders will become more capacious and compliant with lower reservoir pressures.

Chen and colleagues reported outcomes for six men with sigmoid neobladders with follow-up of 8–20 months (mean 14.6).[6] All six were continent during the day within 1 month after beginning to void per urethra. Of the four who were continent at night, two had to awaken twice each night to remain dry. The two who were not continent at night did not try to awaken to void and used one to two pads per night. Neobladder capacity was reported to be 310 ml on average. Mean maximal filling pressures were 16.7 ± 6.2 cmH_2O (range 14–28) and mean maximal intravesical pressure was 49.0 ± 9.7 cmH_2O (range 26–60). Compliance was not specifically reported. No patient had pressure spikes documented at urodynamics.

Da Pozzo reported outcomes for 24 sigmoid neobladders with follow-up of 7–70 months (mean 38.3).[5] Twenty of the 21 (95.2%) patients evaluated at 9 months with urodynamics were continent during the day, with 16 of the 17 (94.1%) patients evaluated at 18 months stating the same. The mean neobladder capacity was 414 ml (range 310–800) at 9 months, 492 ml (range 360–800) at 18 months and 465 ml (range 450–560) at 26–39 months. Mean endoluminal pressure at maximum capacity was reported to be 31 cmH_2O (range 16–42), 29 cmH_2O (range 14–42) and 28 cmH_2O (range 19–39) at 9, 18 and 26–39 months, respectively. Mean residual urine volumes were 35 ml (range 0–300), 42 ml (range 0–300) and 27 ml (range 15–40) at 9, 18 and 26–39 months, respectively. Nocturnal continence, defined as total involuntary enuresis of no more than two awakenings per night, was present in 12 of 21 (57.2%) and 12 of 17 (70.6%) patients evaluated at 12 and 18 months, respectively. The pathogenesis of nocturnal incontinence is probably related to a reduced level of consciousness, making it impossible to consciously increase external urethral sphincter tone during contractions of the intestinal neobladder. Loss of recruitment through spinal reflex pathways of the external sphincter to bladder filling also plays a role.[16]

Santucci et al reported the continence and urodynamic parameters of four sigmoid neobladders in a series of 40 patients who had undergone various types of gastrointestinal urinary diversions (Tables 18.2 and 18.3).[15] Continence was defined as

Table 18.1 Detubularized sigmoid neobladder: urodynamic data

Follow-up (months)	Maximum capacity in ml (range)	Filling pressure in cmH_2O (range)	Pressure at capacity in cmH_2O (range)	Residual urine in ml (range)
3	450 (230–720)	25 (15–40)	40 (20–70)	26 (0–110)
6	580 (360–800)	15 (10–22)	19 (12–30)	35 (5–75)
12	600 (380–780)	12 (10–16)	16 (10–22)	40 (4–80)

From Reddy PK. Urol Clin North Am 1991; 18: 609–14 with permission from Elsevier.[10]

Table 18.2 Continence by pouch type

Diversion	Continence Day (%)	Continence Night (%)
Stomal urinary reservoirs		
Ileocecal (Mainz)	10/11 (91)	10/11 (91)
Right colon (Indiana)	6/6 (100)	6/6 (100)
Neobladders		
Gastric	2/6 (33)	2/6 (33)
Sigmoid	2/4 (50)	2/4 (50)
Ileocecal (Mainz)	6[a]/8 (75)	6/8 (75)
Ileum (Hautmann)	4[a]/5 (80)	5/5 (100)

[a]Mild incontinence.
From Santucci RA et al. Urology 1999; 54: 252–7 with permission from Elsevier.[15]

complete dryness or wearing one pad per day for 'safety', given that the pad was dry at the day's end. Continence rates were lower in sigmoid neobladder patients (50%) compared with the ileal (80%) and ileocecal (75%) neobladders in this series, but were better than with gastric neobladders (33%, 2 of 6). Nighttime and daytime incontinence rates were almost the same in all patients. All four sigmoid neobladder patients were able to void spontaneously, compared with four of the eight ileocecal neobladder patients who required clean intermittent catheterization. Capacity was not significantly different between the ileal, ileocecal and sigmoid neobladders (402–600 ml) but was significantly greater than gastric neobladders (311 ml). Compliance was also significantly lower in the gastric neobladders (31 cm/ml) compared with all other types of intestinal neobladders studied (46–88 cm/ml). Sigmoid neobladders had the highest average pressures at capacity (40 cmH_2O) compared with gastric (23 cmH_2O), right colon (21 cmH_2O), ileocecal and ileal (4–10 cmH_2O) segments. Okada et al compared the operative time, blood loss and reservoir capacity of three types of neobladder using colon segments (right colon, ileocecal and sigmoid) and found no significant differences between them.[17]

Fujisawa et al evaluated 11 women who underwent modified sigmoid neobladder following nerve- and urethral support-sparing cystectomy for transitional cell carcinoma of the bladder.[13] All but one woman achieved acceptable continence during the day. Eight had mild stress incontinence. Eight of the 11 were continent at night with or without arising to void regularly. All 11 women voided volitionally, but one required clean intermittent catheterization to empty high postvoid residuals, due to excessive neobladder capacity. Eight of the 11 women underwent urodynamic study, revealing mean intrareservoir filling pressures at maximal filling of 20.3 ± 7.9 cmH_2O (range 10–31) and mean reservoir compliance of 21.0 ± 10.2 ml/cmH_2O (range 12–43.7). Capacity ranged from 236 ml to 450 ml.

This group later compared voiding and urodynamic parameters in 14 men and nine women with sigmoid neobladders.[14] Mean intrareservoir filling pressures at maximal filling were 21.9 ± 12.7 cmH_2O (range 10–40) in men and 24.2 ± 14.0 cmH_2O (range 10–56) in women. Mean reservoir compliance was 25.3 ± 14.1 ml/cmH_2O (range 9.5–51.1) in men and 19.3 ± 10.8 ml/cmH_2O (range 12–43.7) in women. Mean residual urine volumes were 57.0 ± 35.1 ml (range 4–110) in men and 21.3 ± 15.1 ml (range 7–50) in women, when notably one woman with a residual urine volume of 600 ml was excluded.

The urodynamic findings were used to determine factors important for a functional neobladder. In females compared with males, outlet angulation, neobladder morphology and location influenced voiding more than intrareservoir pressure. Women voided with much lower intrareservoir pressures than men (due to lower urethral resistance), but this was not a major factor. The distance between the neobladder outlet (ideally at the most dependent portion of the neobladder) and coccyx was

Table 18.3 Urodynamic data by pouch type[a]

Diversion	N	Capacity (ml)	Compliance (ml/cmH_2O)	Pressure spike at capacity (%)	Patients with pressure spikes at capacity (%)	Maximum flow rate (ml/sec)	Postvoid residual (ml)
Stomal urinary reservoirs							
Ileocecal (Mainz)	11	543 ± 71	88 ± 73	10 ± 10	55	NA	NA
Right colon (Indiana)	6	535 ± 101	61 ± 33	21 ± 24	50	NA	NA
Neobladders							
Gastric	7	311 ± 97	31 ± 35	23 ± 15	83	13 ± 8	19 ± 28
Sigmoid	4	402 ± 139	46 ± 43	40 ± 22	100	17 ± 11	6 ± 7
Ileocecal (Mainz)	8	585 ± 112	65 ± 42	7 ± 13	25	9 ± 13	544 ± 581
Ileocecal (Hautmann)	6	600 ± 0	62 ± 35	4 ± 9	33	22 ± 7	18 ± 21

[a]All values are mean ± SD.
From Santucci RA et al. Urology 1999; 54: 252–7 with permission from Elsevier.[15]

greater in females, which is not unexpected, but the wider pelvis allows the neobladder to descend towards the bottom of the pelvis, falling backwards, creating a narrow neocysto-urethral angle and the potential for voiding dysfunction. Further, if the pelvic floor is weak and the neobladder cannot be effectively compressed by abdominal straining, it may be displaced deeper into the pelvis, creating greater outlet angulation. In their description, Fujisawa refers to the 'pouchocele' that may result in these women with postoperative voiding dysfunction. The neocystourethral angle, as well as pelvic floor support, were found to be the crucial factors in effective neobladder emptying in women compared with men.

A timely study of bladder cancer patients with ileal (24) and colon neobladders (18 sigmoid and 10 right colon) comparing health-related quality of life (QOL) and urinary continence has recently been reported.[18] No significant difference was documented between patients with either type of neobladder and all were overall satisfied with their health-related and disease-specific QOL. Given the impact that urinary diversion has from physical, psychological, functional, social, and economic standpoints, this type of study is invaluable.

Conclusions

The sigmoid colon can be used in those patients with adequate mobility in the left colon mesentery and IMA. It is especially useful in patients with diseased or irradiated small bowel and/or ileocecum. Advantages of sigmoid are that it is expendable in the sense that there is essentially very low risk for malabsorption (Vitamin B_{12}, folic acid, bile salts) and diarrhea.[1] In fact, published sigmoid neobladder series report no metabolic acidosis, malabsorption or diarrhea.[2–6,13] The small bowel is left intact and not compromised. The sigmoid is ideally situated for orthotopic neobladder creation and ureteral anastomosis, given the central location of the sigmoid colon in the pelvis. It almost always reaches down into the pelvis on no tension, unlike other intestinal segments.

The sigmoid colon provides a capacious reservoir once detubularized.[20] Significant urinary retention due to an overcapacious neobladder has not been reported with over 5 years of follow-up.[5] Good neobladder capacity is achieved at 12–18 months and does not appear to increase over time, as may be the case with ileal and ileocolic neobladders. The teniae provide reliable antireflux mechanisms for ureteral implantation.

Sigmoid neobladders provide excellent functional results with no significant metabolic consequences. The surgical technique is straightforward and not time-consuming. The basic surgical principles do not vary significantly from other types of neobladders, reservoirs and urinary diversions. Patient satisfaction is high. Volitional voiding through the urethra, urinary continence, low residual urine volumes and preservation of renal function provide the neobladder patient with a high level of physical, psychological and social satisfaction. Some may experience chronic nighttime enuresis, which is often manageable through conservative maneuvers such as behavioral modification and/or condom catheters, or much less commonly by placement of an artificial urinary sphincter. Neobladders are arguably the optimal form of urinary diversion in the appropriate, motivated patient.

References

1. Lilien OM, Camey M. 25-year experience with replacement of the human bladder (Camey procedure). J Urol 1984; 132: 886–91.
2. Reddy PK. Detubularized sigmoid reservoir for bladder replacement after cystoprostatectomy: preliminary report of new configuration. Urology 1987; 29: 625–8.
3. Reddy PK, Lange PH. Bladder replacement with sigmoid colon after radical cystoprostatectomy. Urology 1987; 29: 368–71.
4. Reddy PK, Lange PH, Fraley EE. Bladder replacement after cystoprostatectomy: efforts to achieve total continence. J Urol 1987; 138: 495–9.
5. Da Pozzo LF, Colombo R, Pompa P et al. Detubularized sigmoid colon for bladder replacement after radical cystectomy. J Urol 1994; 152: 1409–12.
6. Chen K-K, Chang LS, Chen M-T. Neobladder construction using completely detubularized sigmoid colon after radical cystoprostatectomy. J Urol 1991; 146: 311–15.
7. Libertino JA. Sigmoid colon neobladder. Use of intestine in urologic surgery. Atlas Urol Clin North Am 1995; 3: 65–8.
8. Parra RO, Cummings JM, Boullier JA. Simple detubularization technique for construction of continent colonic urinary reservoirs. Urology 1994; 44: 35–7.
9. Reddy PK, Lange PH, Fraley EE. Total bladder replacement using detubularized sigmoid colon: technique and results. J Urol 1991; 145: 51–5.
10. Reddy PK. The colonic neobladder. Urol Clin North Am 1991; 18: 609–14.
11. Reddy PK. Total bladder replacement. J Urol 1991; 145: 51.
12. Libertino JA. Sigmoid colon neobladder. Use of intestine in urologic surgery. Atlas Urol Clin N Am 1995; 3: 65–8.
13. Fujisawa M, Gotoh A, Miyazaki S et al. Sigmoid neobladder in women after radical cystectomy. J Urol 2000; 163: 1505–9.
14. Fujisawa M, Gotoh A, Nakamura I et al. Long-term assessment of serum B(12) concentrations in patients with various types of orthotopic intestinal neobladder. Urology 2000; 56: 236–40.
15. Santucci RA, Park CH, Mayo ME, Lange PH. Continence and urodynamic parameters of continent urinary reservoirs: comparison of gastric, ileal, ileocolic, right colon, and sigmoid segments. Urology 1999; 54: 252–7.
16. Jakobsen H, Steven K, Stigsby B, Klarskov P, Haldt T. Pathogenesis of nocturnal urinary incontinence after ileocaecal bladder replacement. Continuous measurement of urethral closure pressure during sleep. Br J Urol 1987; 59: 148–52.
17. Okada H, Yamanaka N, Oh-Öka H et al. Construction and voiding functions of three types of orthotopic neobladders using colonic segments: the Kobe University experience. Int J Urol 1998; 5: 22–9.

18. Miyake H, Nakamura I, Eto H et al. An evaluation of quality of life in patients who underwent orthotopic bladder replacement after cystectomy: comparison of ileal neobladder versus colon neobladder. Urol Int 2002; 69: 195–9.
19. Koch MO, McDougal WS, Reddy PK, Lange PH. Metabolic alterations following continent urinary diversion through colonic segments. J Urol 1991; 145: 270–3.
20. Hinman F Jr. Selection of intestinal segments for bladder substitution: physical and physiological characteristics. J Urol 1988; 139: 519–23.

19 The gastric continent urinary reservoir

Pasquale Casale, Mark Horowitz and Michael E Mitchell

Introduction

The notion of bladder emptying by means of intermittent catheterization has gained universal acceptance by both patients and physicians. This has led to an enormous expansion in the use of continent urinary reservoirs for patients without bladders. Leg bags and stomal appliances play only a small role in the surgical armamentarium of urinary diversion. Since 1950 when Gilchrist et al[1] described a technique for construction of a continent urinary reservoir (CUR) many techniques have been described. The CUR has to fit certain criteria, hold large volumes at low pressures, prevent reflux, be continent and allow for complete emptying. Most of the described reservoirs such as the Indiana Pouch,[2] the Kock Pouch,[3] and the Mainz Pouch[4] use varying lengths of ileum and/or cecum to meet these objectives. Neobladders have also been constructed from ileum and sigmoid colon. In 1989, Bihrle et al[5] described a technique for creating continent reservoir using transverse colon with tubularized segment of stomach implanted beneath the tinea as a catheterizable stoma. Each bowel segment has its own advantages and disadvantages and certainly a surgeon must feel comfortable with the segment used. Many times, however, particularly in pediatric patients, the clinical situation dictates unique reservoir composition.

In the broadest sense, the continent reservoir is designated by (i) the structure of the reservoir, (ii) the mechanism of antireflux and (iii) the mechanism of emptying. For example, the Indiana pouch is a cecal reservoir (or cecal composite with large or small bowel), ureters tunneled into the tenia, and continence based on the ileocecal valve with tapered terminal ileum a catheterizable channel. However, if continence is based on the normal urethral mechanism, even if the bladder consists totally of bowel, this is technically a bladder replacement, not a CUR. On the other hand, if a patient preferably uses a catheterizable channel other than the urethra for continence, such as an appendix tunneled into the reservoir (Mitrofanoff procedure),[6] this is a CUR. What is even more confusing is the nomenclature of a reconstruction which uses a bladder augmented with bowel in which the urethra is tunneled into the bladder base.[7] Is this simply a bladder augmentation in a patient dependent on intermittent catheterization or a CUR variation? In reality, these differences make little impact on this discussion. The term 'gastric CUR' will be used in its purest sense, a reservoir constructed totally of stomach tissue emptied through a catheterizable channel other than the native urethra. The principles, however, can be applied to composite reservoirs (stomach and bladder, stomach and small bowel, etc.) and bladder augmentation with stomach as well.

The major reason that alternative forms of CUR construction come from the pediatric literature is that pediatric urologists are often confronted with unique anatomic problems that are uncommon in the adult patient population. These include patients with severe cloacal malformations, exstrophy and cloacal exstrophy patients. In 1980, Mitrofanoff described using the appendix as a means of catheterizing the bladder in neurogenic bladder patients.[6] The appendix is tunneled in a submucosal manner into the bladder and the other end is brought out through the abdominal wall usually to the umbilicus. If appendix is not available, other tubes may be used. We have employed ureters, tapered small bowel, fallopian tubes and tubes of stomach. Techniques to create a continent cutaneous stoma which is cosmetically pleasing has made it possible for young patients to catheterize a hidden stoma without difficulty or pain. We recently reviewed our unpublished experience with the creation of a Mitrofanoff catheterizable channel in 33 patients. Eleven patients have the ability to catheterize either their Mitrofanoff or urethra. All 11 patients choose to catheterize their Mitrofanoff in preference to urethral catheterization. The reasons for this include easier access to the stoma (abdominal wall vs perineum), less discomfort and less time involved. The advantage of the gastric reservoir is that most catheterizable tubes can be easily tunneled into the gastric wall for continence.

The gastric reservoir

Sinaiko[8] in 1956 first described the use of stomach in reconstruction of the urinary tract. His experiments initially centered on the creation of a gastric reservoir in dogs. He later applied these techniques to humans. Leong and Ong[9] used the antrum for bladder replacement in adults undergoing cystectomy for cancer and for augmentation. Both groups observed that gastric mucosa washed with urine maintained its acid secretory activity. In the dog model we demonstrated a clear net chloride flux into the urine in bladders augmented with stomach.[10] Herein lies one of the major differences between a reservoir of stomach and large or small bowel. A gastric reservoir is basically a secretory organ with minimal net water loss, but significant hydronium, chloride and sodium ions flux into the urine. Large and small bowel on the other hand have resorptive mucosa which results in net flux of hydronium and chloride ions and ammonia from the urine back into the serum (Figure 19.1). In a healthy adult with good renal function, the flux of ions should have no major impact. In young patients, particularly with altered renal or hepatic function, resorption of hydronium and chloride ions may lead to chronic clinical (or subclinical) metabolic acidosis. Worsening metabolic acidosis is seen in young patients who demonstrate acidosis prior to urinary reconstruction with small bowel.[11] Because ammonium chloride is one of the significant buffer systems in the urine (see Figure 19.1), resorption of chloride ultimately potentiates the resorption of ammonia which has little consequence except in patients with altered hepatic function. Gastric secretory function, however, stabilizes this ammonium chloride buffer system. Ion flux, particularly with resorptive epithelium, is accentuated in intestinal reservoir patients presumably because of the increased contact time with urine. This situation is analogous to the ureterosigmoidostomy patients who have long been known to have potential for hyperchloremic acidosis. Therefore, hyperchloremic acidosis can be anticipated in patients with large or small bowel reservoirs. Conversely, alkalosis with low serum, sodium, potassium and chloride is observed in some patients with gastric reservoir.

Stomach and the large and small bowel all have potential for mucus production. The character of the mucus, however, varies. Usually the gastric reservoirs secrete mucus which provides little change in the viscosity of urine and tends to be more gelatinous than particulate so the urine has a clear appearance, in contrast to the more flocculate, viscous and stringy mucus of distal small bowel and colon. Urine specimens from gastric reservoirs have fewer 'mucus' cells and smaller mucus pellets with centrifugation. This may be of significance in patients who require catheterization with small catheters in whom significant increase in urine viscosity can reduce flow rate to the point of catheter obstruction. Reduced urine viscosity after gastric urinary reconstruction is beneficial in patients who are voiding spontaneously or using the artificial sphincter.

Blyth et al reported the incidence of stone formation in different bowel segments following augmentation enterocystoplasty.[12] Stones formed in all segments used except for gastric

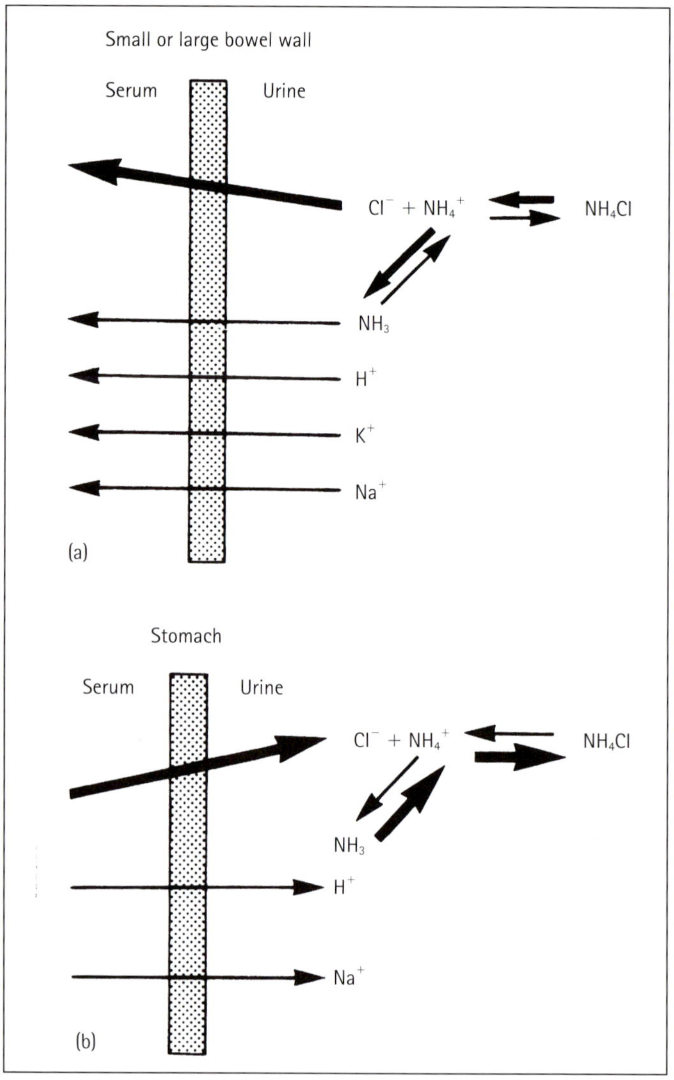

Figure 19.1 Net ion flux differs for (a) small and large bowel and (b) stomach. The net flux of chloride with large and small, net ion bowel is from the urine to the serum. This reduces the chloride ion activity in the urine and shifts the equilibrium of the ammonium chloride buffer releasing ammonia which also has a net flux to the serum. The situation is exactly the reverse for stomach as chloride and hydronium ions are actively secreted into the urine. This forces the equilibrium to stabilize or increase ammonium chloride concentration in the urine.

augmentation. No stones were reported in a study of 73 gastrocystoplasties.[13] Theoretically, stones which commonly form in acid media, such as uric acid stones, would potentially form in gastric reservoirs, but this has been a problem in only one patient to date.[14] Random urine pH in animal models and in human studies demonstrates a remarkable ability of normal urine to buffer acid production of the gastric flap. However, close monitoring of urine pH will show variation during the day, usually related to anticipated dietary shifts. The pH of the urine rarely goes below 5 in patients with gastric reservoirs except patients with significant chronic elevations in serum gastrin or in patients with reduced salt excretion or renal concentration defects.

There are two characteristics of the gastric flap which make it technically favorable for reconstruction: rich blood supply with a single pedicle and excellent potential for submucosal tunneling. The unique pedicle of the gastric wedge flap makes it very easy to construct a reservoir deep in the pelvis or in any location. The rich blood supply also facilitates the construction of gastric tubes and reservoir simultaneously. Submucosal tunnels can be constructed either from the mucosal or serosal side, analogous to the bladder. Furthermore, because of the muscle backing, a relatively short tunnel can secure continence or antireflux. We have used appendix, ureter, tapered ileum, fallopian tube and gastric tube for this purpose. In addition to these characteristics, the dynamics of stomach seem to be favorable for construction of a reservoir. Although it takes, relative to small and large bowel, longer for a gastric augmentation or neobladder to distend with time (6–8 months), most patients expand far beyond the size of the original flap. Bladders augmented with stomach and gastric neobladders also, either because of the geometry or because of the nature of the elastic character of the flap, tend to empty well with minimal residual volumes. For example, in 18 patients with artificial sphincter and gastrocystoplasty, 11 (61%) were completely dry and emptied without catheterization.[15] Goselblez et al reported a 90% success rate in 30 consecutive patients who underwent gastrocystoplasty or construction of a continent urinary reservoir with stomach.[16] Nine of the patients received a CUR and 90% of this group was dry for greater than 3 hours, had normal electrolytes, normal acid–base balance and preservation or improvement of renal function.

Availability, nevertheless, makes stomach a very important consideration for reconstruction in certain patient groups. These include: cloacal exstrophy patients; some patients with severe cloaca malformation; patients with bowel that is either severely deficient or not suitable for use in reconstruction (as in patients who have had extensive abdominal radiation therapy or multiple previous attempts at reconstruction). Furthermore, stomach neurogenic bladder patients may be a strong consideration where resection of the ileocecal valve may not be appropriate because of the potential for creating a problem with diarrhea.[17]

The downside for using stomach relates primarily to the secretory nature of the epithelium. Patients with gastric reservoir who have no bladder tissue or urethral tissue in the reconstruction do not have a problem with pain secondary to acid production from the flap. However, these patients may occasionally have very mild hematuria. Approximately 36% of patients with either gastrocystoplasty or gastric reservoir will have either hematuria, bladder spasm or dysuria.[18] A metabolic alkalosis (hyponatremic, hypokalemic) can also result from acid and salt loss in the urine in some patients with stomach in the lower urinary tract. The patients most subject to this phenomenon are those with a tendency to salt loss; (i) short bowel syndrome, (ii) salt-losing nephropathy or (iii) vomiting and diarrhea. If it is known that salt balance is a problem in a patient, gastric augmentation or reservoir may be contraindicated and a flap with resorptive mucosa should be considered. The gastric flap has been removed in several patients with severe salt loss and alkalosis. Chronic elevation of serum gastrin may relate to the pathophysiology in these patients and may reflect excessive resection of acid-producing tissue resulting in gastrin production from the gastric antrum. Unfortunately, treatment with Omeprazole (Merck Colner Westpoint, PA), which blocks H^+, K^+ exchange, will potentially make this situation worse by increasing serum gastrin. The treatment strategy in such patients should be to increase acid intake (carbonated soft drinks or vitamin C) particularly with meals. Renal patients compromised with anuria or very dilute urine may also have problems with excessive irritation or hematuria relating to the reduced buffering capacity of the urine. Such patients will need to be placed on H_2-blockers and bladder or reservoir buffer irrigations until transplantation. After transplantation, these patients do well. Patients who have normal renal function rarely have problems with salt loss.

A loss of one-third to one-half total stomach volume has not, to this point, created a major problem with either a 'small stomach' or with resorption problems (loss of intrinsic factor). Most patients will have early satiety for the first month or so after resection. In over 130 gastrocystoplasties we have not observed permanent reduction in dietary capacity; in fact general growth and development after gastric urinary reconstruction has been accelerated.

Technique

A large wedge of the mid-portion of the stomach body is taken with its blood supply which can either be based on the right or the left gastroepiploic artery. In most patients, the right gastroepiploic is the more constant. This is true for all patients except for patients with cloacal exstrophy. Most patients are placed on a liquid diet for 48 hours preoperatively and given a bottle of magnesium citrate 24 hours before surgery. Mechanical and antibiotic bowel preparation are not necessary except in the patients with history of chronic and severe constipation.

A vertical incision is made in the midline to the left of the umbilicus (if the umbilicus is to be the site of a continent stoma) from the symphysis pubis to the xiphoid process. In the case of creating a gastric reservoir, a large segment is necessary. A wedge-shaped flap is taken from the mid-portion of the body of the stomach (Figure 19.2). Length along the greater curvature should be approximately 15–17 cm depending on the size of the patient. The usual length of the two sides of the wedge is 7–10 cm and, therefore, 90-mm gastrointestinal stapler is required. Any shorter instrument requires several applications, which can be very awkward. Staples reduce potential for peritoneal spill. The greater omentum is incised parallel to and several centimeters inferior to the greater curvature of the gastroepiploic vessels (see Figure 19.2). The omental vessels are

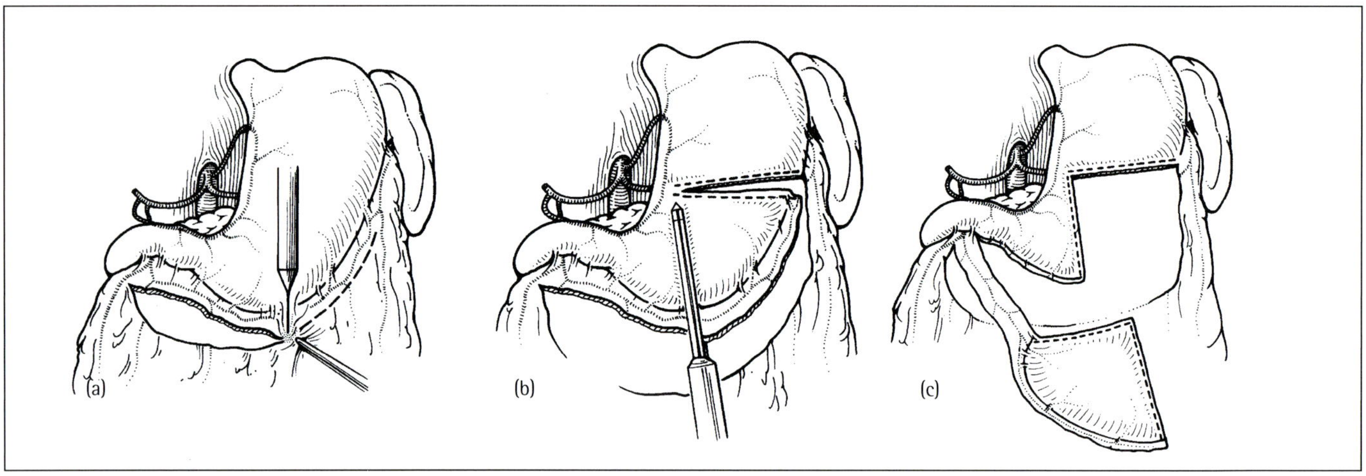

Figure 19.2 (a) The technique of harvesting a gastric flap includes first the incision of the omentum 2 cm inferior to the gastroepiploic artery then selecting the wedge and dividing the short vessels between the future pedicle and the greater curvature. (b,c) The wedge is taken with a GIA 90 stapler and the staples are removed from the anterior gastric wall and the stomach is closed in two layers.

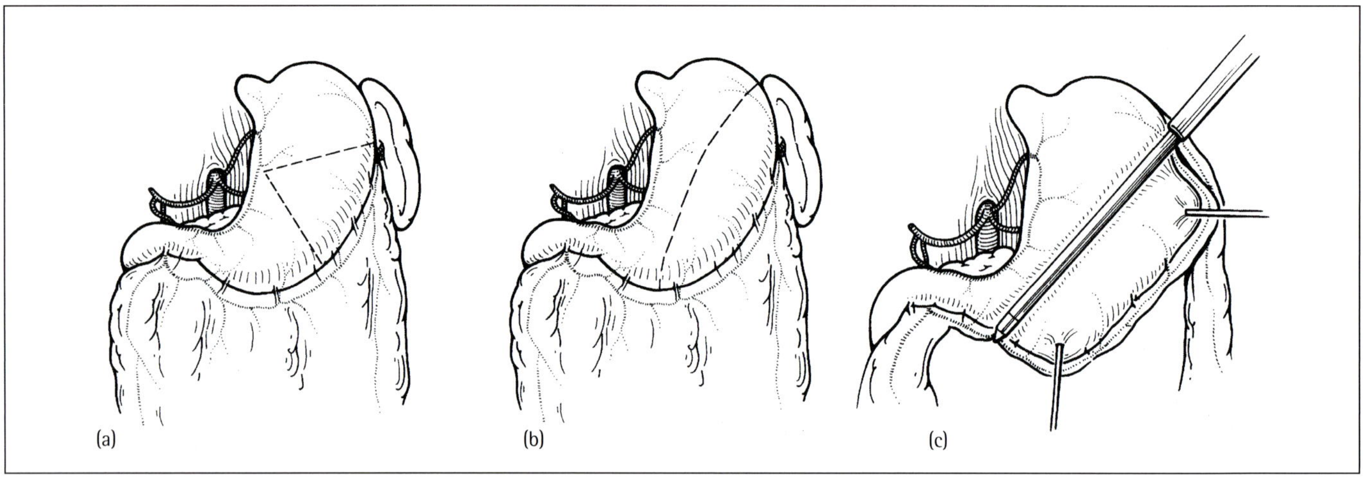

Figure 19.3 An alternative oblique or transverse incision which may obviate the need for gastric closure. (a) Wedge flap. (b,c) Oblique flap; note the shorter pedicle. (Reproduced from Ehrlich et al. J Urol 1993; 150: 713–15[19] with permission from Lippincott Williams & Wilkins.)

ligated with 3-0 or 4-0 silk ties. The appropriate gastroepiploic artery is then selected for the pedicle. The short communicating vessels between the stomach and proximal portion of the gastroepiploic artery are then tied in place with 4-0 silk and divided. During the development of the pedicle to the flap, we apply papaverine solution to the artery to prevent spasm. Once the pedicle is defined, the stapling device is used to resect the wedge of the stomach. In this process, great care is taken to make sure that the posterior aspect of the stomach and structures such as the pancreas are avoided. The apex of the wedge is not extended to the lesser curvature. Depending on the shape of the stomach, it is sometimes possible to make a very oblique wedge almost going straight across the greater curvature (Figure 19.3), but this maneuver is only effective in those stomachs which tend to 'hang down' and tends to shorten the pedicle length (but obviates the need for gastric closure).[19] The staples are then removed from the anterior wall and the stomach is closed in two layers: an inner layer of running locking 3-0 resorbable suture and an outer seromuscular layer of interrupted 3-0 silk. The staples are left in the gastric wedge while the stomach is repaired. Protect the wedge and pedicle with a moist lap pad placed over the flap to avoid any possibility of injury. After the stomach is repaired, a nasogastric tube is passed and placed beyond the anastomosis and secured by the anesthesiologist. The wedge flap is then brought through an opening in the transverse mesocolon and usually through the small bowel mesentery into the pelvis. The final position, of course, depends on the particular needs of the patient (Figure 19.4). It is important to remember that this wedge is potentially producing acid during the procedure, therefore H_2-blockers are given prior to and during surgery.

After the wedge has been brought to the appropriate position and the bowel and abdominal contents properly protected it can be opened and irrigated with saline and antibiotic solu-

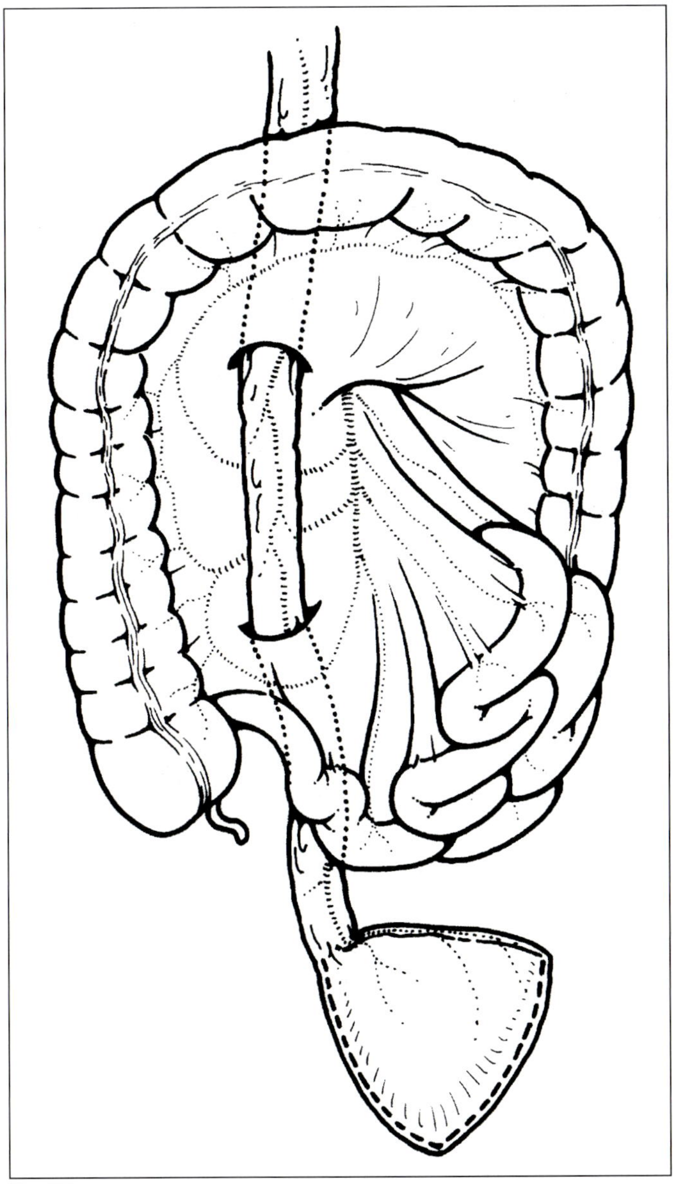

Figure 19.4 Bringing the flap into the pelvis through the mesocolon and omentum of the small bowel (arrows). Because of the length of the pedicle the gastric reservoir can be placed in any location within the abdomen.

tion. All the staples are removed. Usually, ureteral reimplantation is performed with the reservoir open. This is done in a manner analogous to ureteral reimplantation into the bladder. It is usually easier to tunnel under the gastric mucosa than to open the mucosa. A small nipple is made at the end of the ureter to prevent stenosis of the ureteral orifice (Figure 19.5). Ureters can also be reimplanted into the intact reservoir with standard extravesical techniques. Construction of a continence mechanism can be done before or after closure of the reservoir. Tunnel technique (ureter, appendix, gastric tube, or tapered bowel) can be used as with ureteral reimplantation. However, a contiguous gastric tube with proximal nipple may be constructed (similar to a continent gastrostomy) (Figure 19.6). The continent stoma is constructed after closure of the reservoir and proper abdominal positioning. The gastric reservoir is closed in two layers: a 3-0 chromic inner mucosa and submucosal layer and an outer running simple 3-0 Vicryl or Monocryl suture.

It is possible to augment a gastric reservoir with a segment of large or small bowel or bladder. If a composite reservoir is constructed, the Malencott tube is usually brought through the gastric wedge. The reservoir adjacent to the tube is sutured to the anterior abdominal wall and matured just as a gastrostomy tube would be matured to make sure that there is no potential leak from the reservoir upon removal of the tube. This gastric reservoir drainage tube will remain in place for at least 3 weeks and possibly longer depending on the ability of the patient to empty.

Clinical experience

We have performed the construction of a total gastric CUR in seven patients, five with cloacal exstrophy, one with cloaca and one with classic exstrophy (two patients with cloacal exstrophy and bladder remnants had these converted into neovaginas due to absence of vaginal tissue). The ureters were reimplanted with long submucosal tunnels into the gastric reservoir in four patients and combined with contralateral trans-ureteroureterostomies in three. Continence was achieved with the intussusception of a contiguous gastric tube in two patients. Continent Mitrofanoff stoma using ureter was performed in two patients. Two patients had a tapered ileal segment and one patient had an artificial urinary sphincter placed on a gastric tube. The continent stomas were placed in the perineum of all patients.

Our mean follow-up is approximately 7 years. The renal function has remained stable in six patients. One patient had transient worsening in renal function due to obstruction of a ureter at the bladder which was subsequently corrected. Six patients are dry in the day and in the night on intermittent catheterization every 3–4 hours and require no anticholinergics. One patient voids to completion by Valsalva. Our total gastric CUR constructions have decreased mainly because our overall rate of augmentation in this unique group of exstrophy patients has diminished. The time when we implemented early primary closure of both the classic and cloacal exstrophy patients correlates with a decreased augmentation rate in this group.

Case examples

Case 1

MG, aged 4 years, was born with cloacal exstrophy and had abdominal closure and end colostomy as a newborn. She had a small contracted bladder, bilateral vesicoureteral reflux, total urinary incontinence and no vagina. She had chronic perineal

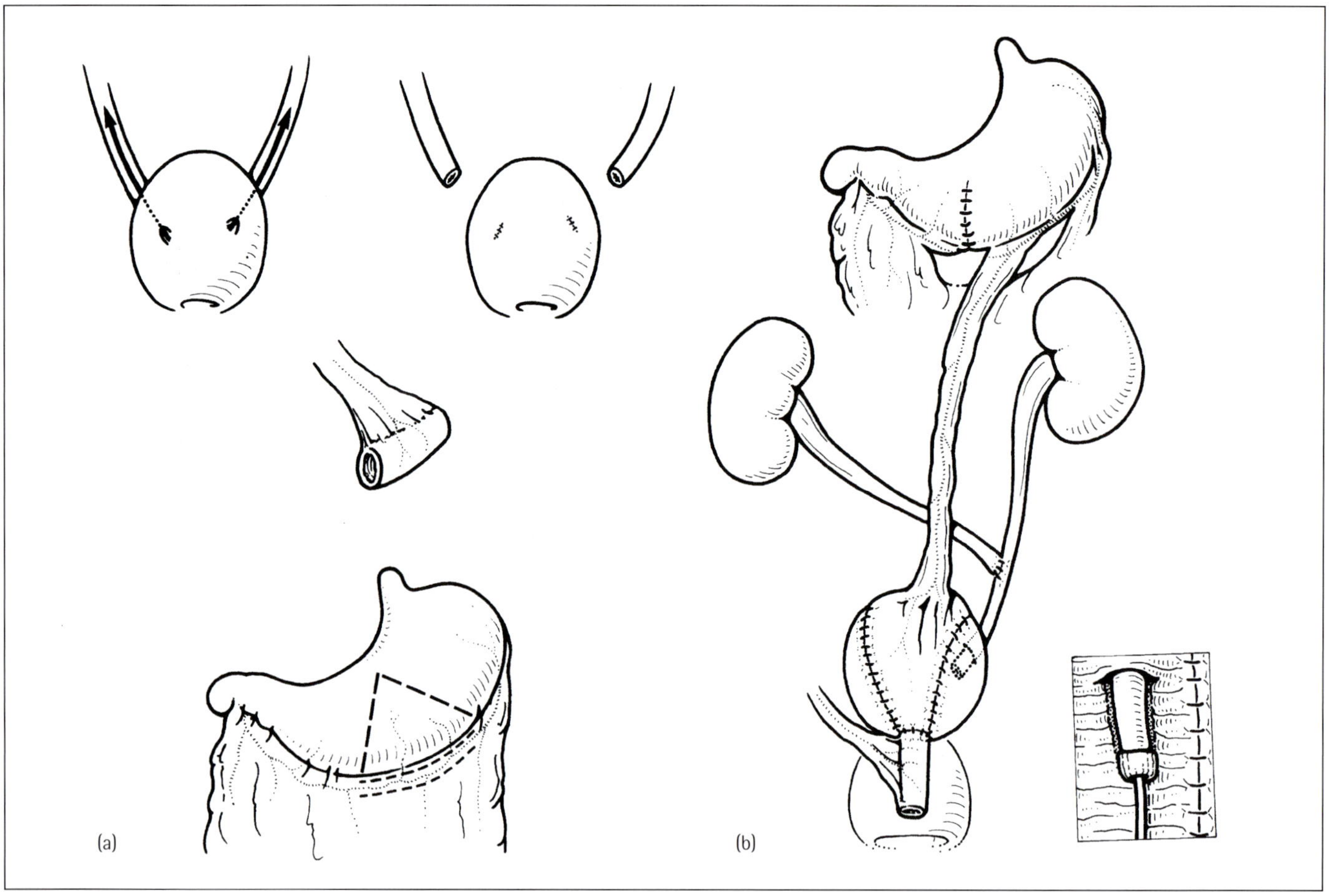

Figure 19.5 Patient MG. (a) Preoperative small bladder with no compliance and massive reflux. (b) Reconstruction utilizing gastric reservoir and distal right ureter versus orthotopic catheterizable channel.

breakdown because of the incontinence. She also had a short bowel syndrome without any excess bowel available for urinary reconstruction (see Figure 19.5a). After bowel preparation, extensive reconstruction was undertaken in which a reservoir was constructed from a wedge-shaped gastric flap. A distal third of the right ureter was brought into the perineum distally, the proximal end being tunneled into the gastric reservoir which was placed in the pelvis. The distal end of the proximal two-thirds of the ureter was then anastomosed to the left ureter as a trans-ureteroureterostomy, the distal left ureter was tunneled in the gastric reservoir. The bladder, which was quite small and contracted, was moved posteriorly to construct a vagina (see Figure 19.5b).

The patient initially had some problem with fungal infections of the reservoir. This now is only a rare problem. She does intermittent catheterization, is dry by day and night, has stable serum chemistries, and stable upper tracts by ultrasound.

Note: This young girl is a good example of a child whose reconstruction was facilitated by the gastric reservoir. She literally had no other tissue which could have been used for urinary reservoir. Her bladder was small and not expansile, but we felt would probably form an adequate vagina. Use of a distal ureter for an orthotopic catheterizable stoma is applicable primarily in the exstrophy patients because of the nature of the pelvis and a very constant blood supply to the distal third of the ureter from the internal iliac artery.

Case 2

D.H. is a 16-year-old girl, born with cloacal exstrophy and total urinary incontinence. At birth, she had excision of her ectopic bladder. The dilated ureters were brought to the perineum as end cutaneous ureterostomies. She also had the construction of an end ileostomy. A very large abdominal defect was closed with non-resorbable mesh, but subsequently this was removed because of multiple enterocutaneous fistulas and infection. Prior to her referral she had had 30 operations, but because of her chronic wetting she was referred for reconstruction.

At surgery, an orthotopic gastric CUR was constructed based on the left gastroepiploic artery. A catheterizable and continent orthotopic urethra was constructed from a short segment of small bowel which was tapered with the GIA stapler. The proximal end of this segment was tunneled into the gastric reservoir and the distal end was brought out to the perineum.

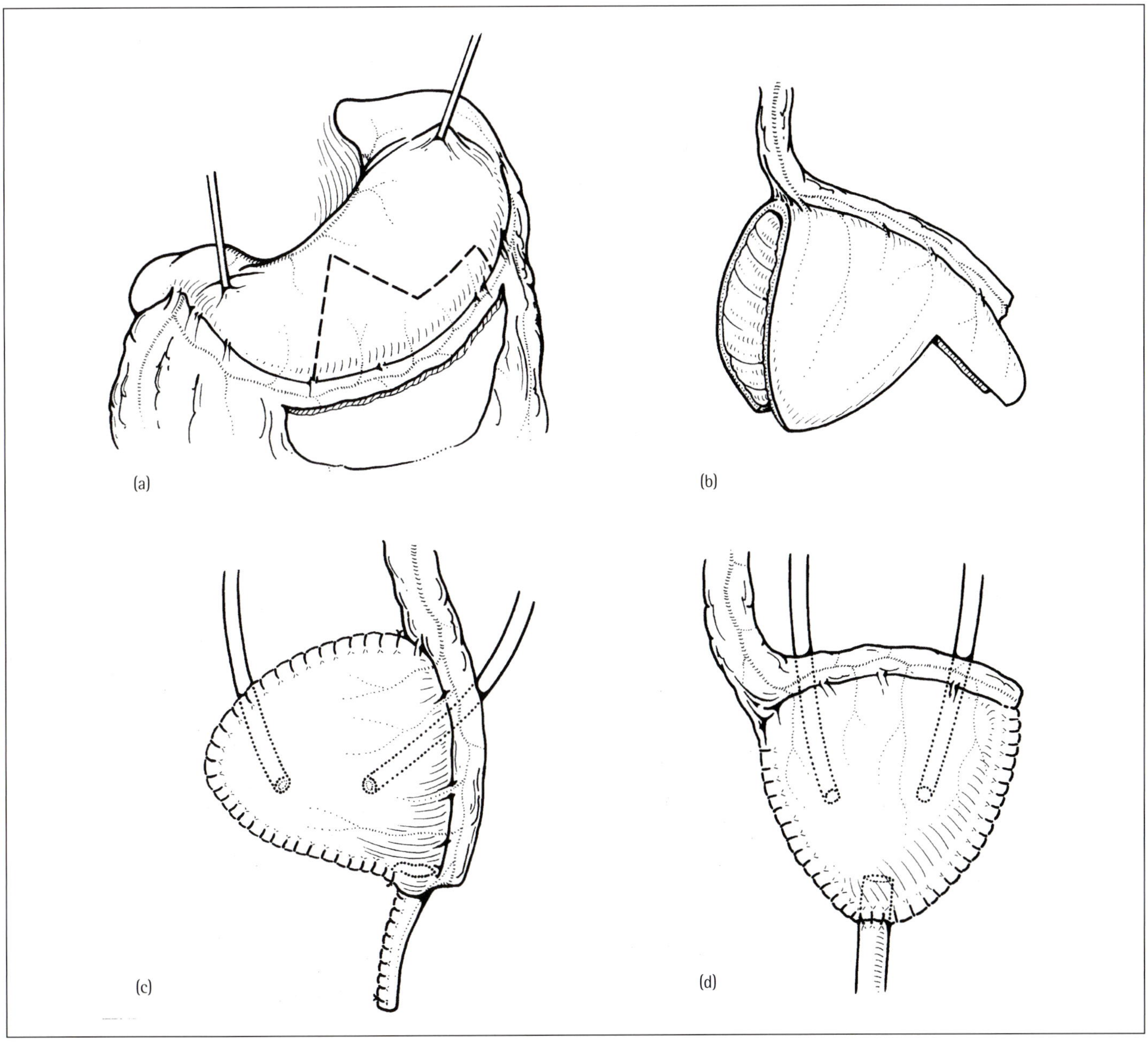

Figure 19.6 (a–c) The technique of reservoir construction using the contiguous gastric tube. (D) Tunnel technique.

The ureters were massively dilated and the distal right ureter was so dilated that it was opened and folded on itself and brought into the perineum as a vagina (Figure 19.7). The left ureter, which was also massively dilated, was tapered and tunneled into the reservoir. The proximal right ureter was anastomosed to the side of the left ureter forming a right to left trans-ureteroureterostomy. Due to the massive abdominal wall defect the abdomen was closed with polypropylene mesh. Although the patient healed and did well initially, at 3.5 weeks after surgery she developed bowel obstruction secondary to adhesions and after exploration developed a small bowel fistula which was subsequently closed.

She currently does intermittent catheterization through a continent stoma and is dry; renal function is stable. She has had to have one operation to straighten the catheterizable channel because of an episode of difficulty with catheterization.

Note: This patient represents the advantage of having tissue not involved with the primary pathophysiology. She had a significant deficiency of bowel and problem with nutrition because of short bowel syndrome. We were fortunate to be able

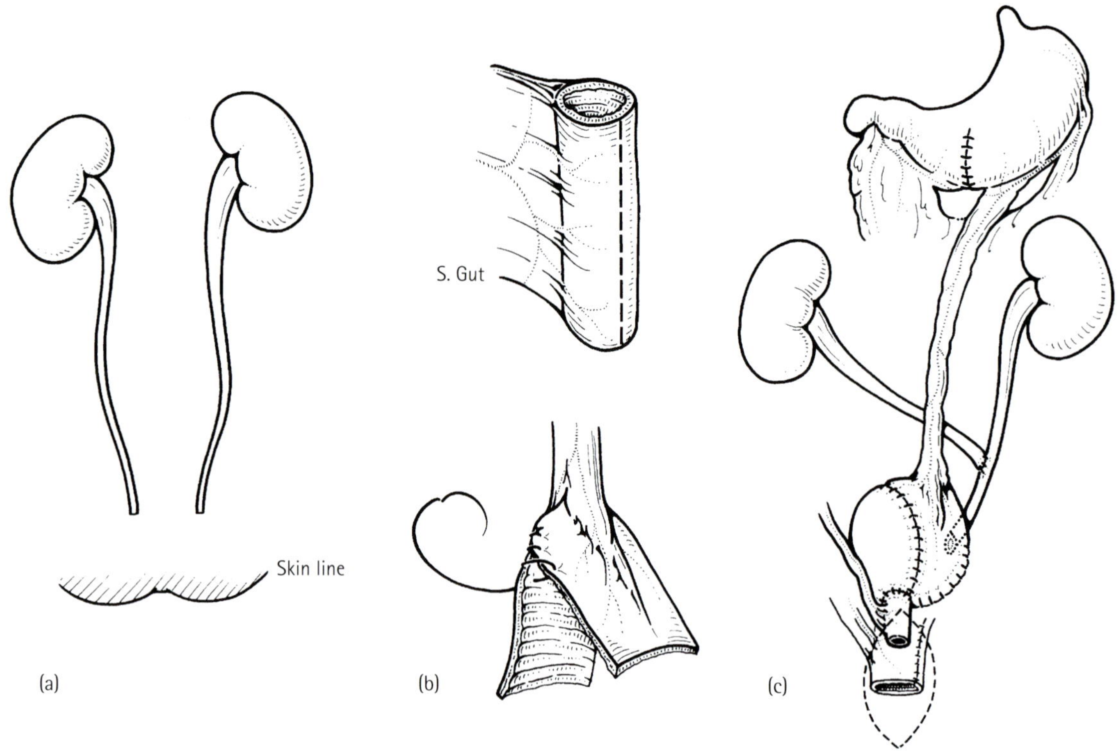

Figure 19.7 (a) Preoperative anatomy of patient DH. Bilateral hydroureteronephrosis, perineal urethrostomies, no vagina. (b) Distal right ureter folded and used to construct a vagina. (c) Reconstruction utilizing a gastric reservoir and tunneled segment ileum for continence.

to use a dilated ureter to form a vagina which has held up well and, in fact, calibrates to an 18-Fr Hagar dilator. In general, we have not been as happy with small bowel tapered to form a catheterizable channel. The incidence of complications seems to be higher with this form of Mitrofanoff construction.

Conclusion

The gastric CUR is one of many reconstructive procedures that should be in the armamentarium of the reconstructive surgeon. The use of stomach to form a complete reservoir is limited to a specialized patient group as demonstrated in the discussion above. However, stomach can be used in combination with large and small bowel to form composite reservoirs and augmentations. The advantage is that this gastric tissue provides excellent potential for tunnel formation to secure continence and antireflux. The secretory function may be balanced with resorption function of large or small bowel.

Ideally, transitional epithelium should be used for all urinary reconstructions. In our laboratory, as in several other centers of the USA, we are experimenting with techniques for bladder reconstruction using seromuscular flaps and transitional epithelial grafts to alleviate the downside of secretory and resorptive epithelium. The day is not far away when we will have true bladder reconstruction.

References

1. Gilchrist RK, Merricks JW, Hamlin HW et al. Construction of a substitute bladder and urethra. Surg Gynecol Obstet 1950; 90: 752–60.
2. Roland RG, Mitchell ME, Bihrle R. The cecoileal continent reservoir. World J Urol 1985; 3: 185–90.
3. Koch NG, Ghoneim NA, Lycke KG et al. Replacement of bladder by the urethral Kock pouch: functional results, urodynamic and radiologic features. J Urol 1989; 141: 1111–16.
4. Thüroff JW, Alken P, Reed Miller H et al. The Mainz pouch (mixed augmentation ileum and cecum) for bladder augmentation and continent diversion. J Urol 1986; 136: 17–26.
5. Bihrle R, Foster RS, Steidle CP et al. Creation of a transverse colon gastric composite reservoir: a new technique. J Urol 1989; 141: 1217–20.
6. Mitrofanoff P. Cystostomie continent trans-appendiculare dans le traitement des vessie neurologiques. Chir Pediatr 1980; 21: 297–305.
7. Kropp KA, Angwafo FF. Uretheral lengthening and reimplanta-

tion for neurogenic incontinence in children. J Urol 1986; 135: 534–6.

8. Sinaiko ES. Artificial bladder from segment of stomach and study of the affect of urine on gastric secretion. Surg Gynecol Obstet 1953; 102: 433–8.
9. Leong CH, Ong GB. Gastrocystoplasty. Br J Urol 1972; 47: 236.
10. Piser JA, Mitchell ME, Kulb TB et al. (1987) Gastrocystoplasty and colocystoplasty in canines: the metabolic consequences of acute saline and acid loading. J Urol 1987; 138: 1009–13.
11. Mitchell ME, Piser JA. Intestinocystoplasty and total bladder replacement in children and young adults: follow-up in 129 cases. J Urol 1987; 138: 579–84.
12. Blyth B, Ewalt DH, Duckett JW, Snyer HM. Lithogenic properties of enterocystoplasty. J. Urol 1992; 148: 575–7.
13. Ganesan GS, Mitchell ME et al. Bladder reconstruction using stomach: 73 patients in six years later [Abstract]. American Urologic Association Annual Meeting, Washington, DC, 1991. J Urol 1991; 147: 253A.
14. Walker RD. Uric acid stone in a patient with gastrocystoplasty. (Personal communication.)
15. Ganesan GS, Nguyen DH, Adams MC et al. Lower urinary tract reconstruction using stomach and the artificial sphincter. J Urol 1993; 149: 1107–9.
16. Goselblez R, Woodard JR et al. The use of stomach in pediatric reconstruction. J Urol 1993; 150: 438–40.
17. Nguyen DH, Ganesan GS and Mitchell ME. Lower urinary tract reconstruction using stomach tissue in children and young adults. World J Urol 1992; 10: 76–9.
18. Nguyen DH, Bain MA, Samuelson KL. et al. The syndrome of dysuria and hematuria in pediatric urinary reconstruction with stomach. J Urol 1993; 150: 707–9.
19. Ehrlich RM, Babiarz JW and Payne CK. Gastrocystoplasty without opening the stomach. J Urol 1993; 150: 713–15.

20 Orthotopic bladder replacement in women

Cheryl T Lee and James E Montie

Introduction

In 2004, bladder cancer will be diagnosed in 60 240 people in the USA, 44 640 men and 15 600 women; 12 710 will die from disease, 8780 men and 3930 women.[1] Thus, women account for 26% of the cases and 31% of the deaths, which demonstrates the need for early and aggressive treatment. Radical cystectomy is the most effective means of cancer control of non-metastatic high-risk transitional cell carcinoma (TCC) of the bladder.[2] An appropriate choice for urinary diversion must then be made. Orthotopic substitution in women may pose technical challenges and has previously been approached with reluctance due to concerns of urethral recurrence and urinary incontinence. Moreover, neobladder performance in women was uncertain, but now it is clear that good long-term results are achievable.[3–7] Consequently, orthotopic diversion has increasingly been done in female patients. It is therefore important periodically to examine the techniques, outcome and general standard under which orthotopic substitution is done. Attention to issues of body image, fertility and functional preservation of sexual organs is critical to achieving an acceptable functional result to accompany the excellent local control that cystectomy provides in the treatment of primary bladder cancers.[2]

Clinical considerations

Urethral recurrence

The field of urinary diversion has grown tremendously in the past decade with successful use of the orthotopic diversion. Intense scrutiny has focused on proper patient selection to avoid anastomosis of a urinary reservoir to a high-risk urethra resulting in urethral recurrence and the need for a second major reconstructive procedure. In women, the incidence of urethral involvement of the bladder in TCC ranges between 2% and 13%.[8,9] As demonstrated by Stein et al in a review of 67 female cystectomy patients, the primary risk factor for urethral involvement is tumor presence at the bladder neck.[9] This finding was confirmed by Stenzl and colleagues in a population of 356 women with bladder cancer followed for a mean of 5.5 years.[10] Secondary urethral tumors were associated with bladder tumors at the trigone ($P = 0.035$) and the bladder neck ($P < 0.001$).[10] Other series have demonstrated similar associations with tumor at the bladder neck.[11] Essentially all female patients found to have urethral tumor have disease at the bladder neck. Intraoperative frozen section of the bladder neck has been shown to correlate well with pathologic evaluation of the bladder neck and urethra.[12] After orthotopic diversion, one can anticipate a 2–4% rate of urethral recurrence, which is less than the rate for patients undergoing cutaneous diversion.[3,13,14]

Non-traditional candidates

Indications for orthotopic diversion in men continue to expand, permitting this procedure in traditionally poor-risk patients such as the elderly, those previously treated with radiation, those with locally advanced disease, and those with pelvic malignancies requiring neoadjuvant chemotherapy and radical exenterative procedures.[15–18] A relaxation of certain relative contraindications is therefore only natural in females. Relative and absolute contradictions of female orthotopic substitution are outlined in Box 20.1. It is clear that favorable tumor characteristics and patient selection are critical to maximize the benefits of orthotopic diversion.

However, urologists will encounter highly motivated patients who have had advanced disease requiring pretreatment but who strongly desire a natural voiding pattern. These patients should be considered for orthotopic diversion when possible.

Female orthotopic diversion in the setting of advanced local disease or previous radiotherapy for pelvic malignancy must be approached carefully, as the prior treatment or subsequent cystectomy resection may undermine the integrity of the pelvic anatomy resulting in postoperative incontinence. Although technically challenging at times, orthotopic diversion after neoadjuvant treatment or post-radiation salvage cystectomy is feasible in male patients and is associated with

BOX 20.1 RELATIVE AND ABSOLUTE CONTRAINDICATIONS FOR ORTHOTOPIC NEOBLADDER DIVERSION IN WOMEN

Relative
- Significant stress urinary incontinence
- Bulky tumor involvement of the trigone
- Multifocal CIS (carcinoma in situ)

Absolute
- Positive frozen section urethral margin
- Gross tumor involvement of the urethra
- Patient refuses or is unable to perform intermittent self catheterization
- Poor performance status

moderate complete day and nighttime continence rates of 67% and 56%, respectively.[16] Two women, aged 69 and 51 years, who underwent cystectomy and orthotopic diversion 2 and 3 months after radiotherapy were included in this series by Bochner et al.[16] Both had good continence and did not require use of pads or intermittent self-catheterization (ISC). This result also reflects our initial experience in two women treated with preoperative radiotherapy who are fully continent after orthotopic substitution without the need for ISC.[19] Although consideration must be given to the benefit that may or may not be realized in patients with a high risk of treatment failure and uncertain long-term survival, we believe that the benefits of orthotopic diversion do not hamper or impede subsequent treatment and may offer improved quality of life. For similar reasons we have not allowed age alone to be a deterrent for orthotopic substitution.

Surgical considerations

Management of reproductive organs

Cystectomy in women may pose technical challenges. Although the female pelvis is larger and can offer better exposure, many urologists are unfamiliar with female pelvic anatomy. Commonly, anterior pelvic exenteration is required because of high volume disease or involvement at the trigone or posterior wall necessitating removal of neighboring pelvic structures that are at risk for direct extension. The surgeon must be prepared to proceed with total abdominal hysterectomy and anterior vaginectomy with subsequent vaginal reconstruction. Vaginal reconstruction can be complex, occasionally requiring tissue flaps to maximize organ function in younger women. Bilateral salpingo-oophorectomy is generally performed, as well, unless the patient is premenopausal and has grossly benign ovaries. Certainly, the age, child-bearing status and sexual function of the patient must be considered when planning such radical extirpative procedures (Table 20.1).

If the extent of disease is felt to be organ-confined and located favorably, it is reasonable in young women with child-bearing potential to spare the reproductive organs since it is increasingly clear that most female organs are not involved by primary bladder cancer and that local recurrence is uncommon.[20,21] When orthotopic diversion is planned in the sexually active postmenopausal woman with a tumor site away from the trigone or bladder neck, the anterior vagina should be preserved. The plane between the anterior vaginal wall and posterior aspect of the bladder is developed (Figure 20.1). This dissection must hug the anterior vaginal wall so as not to compromise the cancer surgery and also to avoid the considerable bleeding that can be encountered when the dissection is in the wrong plane. An advantage of this approach is avoidance of the rich vascularity of the vagina appreciated when the entire anterior vaginal wall is resected.

Total cystectomy and total abdominal hysterectomy would include removal of the bladder, uterus and cervix, with or without the fallopian tubes and ovaries. The anterior vaginal wall and urethra are preserved and the fornix of the vagina is closed (see Figure 20.3 later). This strategy maintains the natural vaginal architecture and provides the greatest potential for timely return to prior sexual activity. Moreover, the risk of neo-vesicovaginal fistula is essentially negligible as the surgeon avoids opposing vaginal and neo-vesicourethral anastomotic suture lines. Another reconstructive strategy is total cystectomy and orthotopic reconstruction with removal of the bladder and preservation of the uterus and ovaries, anterior vaginal wall and urethra. This is an optimal choice for the sexually active female with

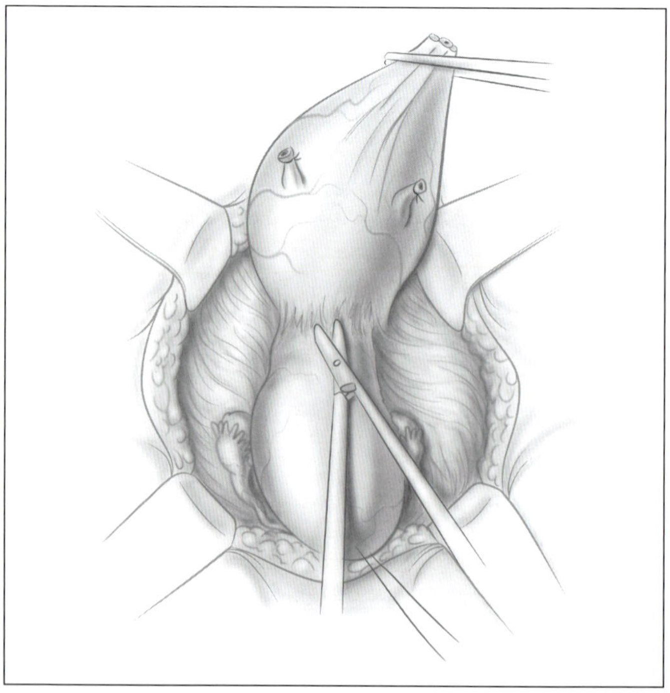

Figure 20.1 Preservation of the anterior vagina. The bladder is dissected away from the anterior vaginal wall.

Table 20.1 Indications for surgical extent of radical cystectomy in women

Type	Extent	Indication
I	Cystectomy, alone Preserve reproductive organs/vagina/urethra (for neobladder)	≤ T2 Child-bearing potential desired Potentially sexually active
II	Cystectomy plus TAH/BSO (if uterus and ovaries are present) Preserve vagina/urethra (for neobladder)	≤ T2, Post child-bearing Post-menopausal Potentially sexually active
IIa	Cystectomy plus TAH (if organs present) Preserve vagina/urethra (for neobladder)	≤ T2, Post child-bearing Pre-menopausal; grossly normal ovaries Potentially sexually active
III	Cystectomy plus TAH/BSO (if organs present) plus anterior vaginectomy Preserve urethra for neobladder	T2 or T3 Posterior wall tumor away from bladder neck
IIIa	Cystectomy plus TAH (if organs present) plus anterior vaginectomy Preserve urethra for neobladder	T2 or T3 Posterior wall tumor away from bladder neck Premenopausal; grossly normal ovaries
IV	Cystectomy plus TAH/BSO (if present) plus anterior vaginectomy and urethrectomy	T2 or T3 Tumor at bladder neck or urethra
IVa	Cystectomy plus TAH (if present) plus anterior vaginectomy and urethrectomy	T2 or T3 Tumor at bladder neck or urethra Premenopausal; grossly normal ovaries

TAH, total abdominal hysterectomy; BSO, bilateral salpingo-oophorectomy.

low-volume or early-stage disease who has concerns about future fertility.

Continence and urethral preservation

An understanding of the continence mechanism in women is critical prior to creation of an orthotopic neobladder. There are at least two continence mechanisms in women.[22,23] One is in the proximal urethra, which is innervated via autonomic nerves that travel via an intrapelvic course from the pelvic plexus coursing adjacent to the bladder neck and vagina. These nerves often are transected during a radical cystectomy. In the mid to lower third of the urethra there is an intermingling of smooth and striated muscle fibers called the rhabdosphincter muscle that is innervated via somatic fibers from the sacral spinal cord, believed to travel via an extrapelvic course, reaching the urethra through the pudendal nerves. The rhabdosphincter muscle, the second mechanism, appears to be critical for continence in women. Since the rhabdosphincter is present in the mid to lower urethra, the entire bladder and bladder neck can be resected in a woman without compromising eventual continence.

A third intrapelvic pathway of somatic fibers derived from the S2–S4 sacral roots, distinct from the peripheral pudendal nerve, may also supply the urethral sphincter.[23] These fibers travel beneath the endopelvic fascia in close relation to the inferior vascular pedicle of the bladder and are susceptible to injury during radical cystectomy.

When planning orthotopic diversion, it is important to maintain the integrity of the endopelvic fascia and pubo-urethral ligaments and thus preserve the support of the external sphincter. Dissection of the lateral wall of the vagina should also be avoided to prevent injury to the urethral innervation described above. Moreover, the bladder neck must be removed entirely to minimize the risk of local tumor recurrence in remaining urothelium and postoperative urinary retention (hypercontinence). The urethra is amputated sharply at the junction with the bladder neck, avoiding distal mobilization or dissection of the urethra (Figure 20.2). After the bladder has been removed a sample of the urethra is circumferentially excised from the specimen or the urethral stump (if necessary) and sent for frozen section to ensure a negative urethral margin. Exposure (Figure 20.3) is often ideal for the placement of urethral

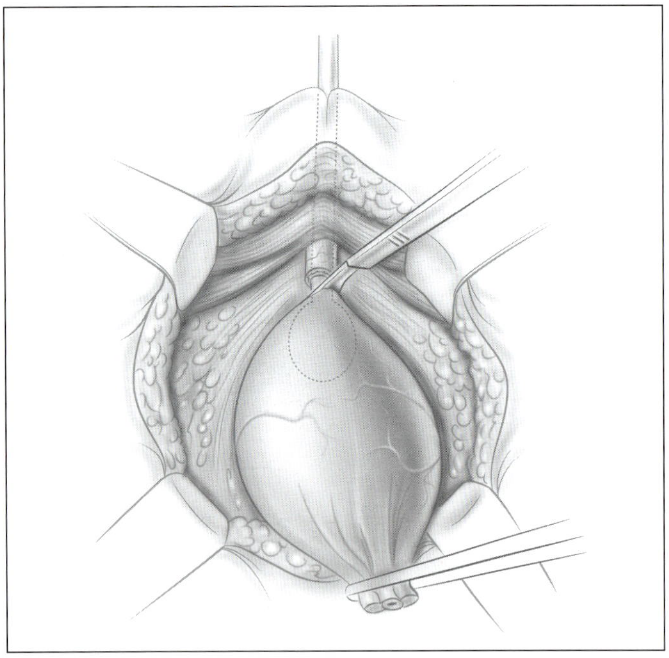

Figure 20.2 In preparation for orthotopic diversion, neither the endopelvic fascia nor the anterior venous plexus is disturbed. An incision is made in the anterior urethra just distal to the junction with the bladder neck. The urethra is divided completely, and the dissection of the bladder off the anterior vaginal wall can be done in either an antegrade or a retrograde fashion.

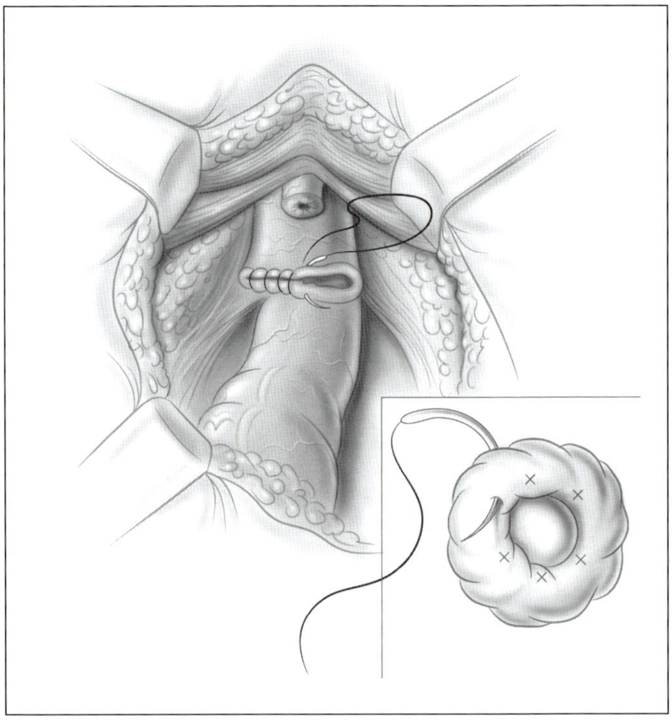

Figure 20.3 The anterior vaginal wall and urethra have been preserved in preparation for orthotopic diversion. The fornix of the vagina has been closed. (Inset) Fine absorbable urethral sutures are placed.

sutures after confirmation of a negative margin. The authors prefer six to ten fine absorbable sutures using 2-0 to 3-0 Monocryl taking small bites on the urethra (see Figure 20.3 inset).

In the initial experience with orthotopic diversion, the concern for stress incontinence was such that anterior urethral fixation sutures were placed to prevent hypermobility of the urethra. This maneuver is not only unnecessary (unless documented stress incontinence from hypermobility is evident preoperatively) but is counterproductive since it contributes to increased urinary retention. A possible additional mechanism for postoperative urinary retention may be exacerbation of a pre-existing but previously insignificant cystocele. After the cystectomy, the urethra is fixed anteriorly, and the patient voids by Valsalva maneuver after relaxing the external sphincter. The increased abdominal pressure needed for voiding across the fixed urethra and bladder neck could be blunted by the cystocele, if present.

Orthotopic diversion

A discussion of the pros and cons of the various types of bowel segment that can be used as orthotopic reservoirs is beyond the scope of this chapter and is covered in detail elsewhere in this book. Suffice it to say that the increasing popularity of the orthotopic neobladder in the 1990s led to substantial research on both orthotopic neobladders and continent cutaneous reservoirs, which resulted in the identification of two basic surgical principles.[24–27] First, it is necessary to detubularize the bowel segment to minimize peristaltic contractions. Secondly, it is also necessary to re-form the reservoir to a spherical shape as much as possible, to provide ideal volume–pressure characteristics. A more spherical reservoir results in a larger capacity neobladder with lower functional pressures. There is a multitude of technical descriptions for creation of an orthotopic neobladder. The differences between the types of reservoir are often minor; thus, broad categories of reservoirs have been described.[28] The authors currently utilize the technique popularized by Hautmann, but have used the techniques popularized by Studer prior to this.[29] Both of these orthotopic reservoirs offer similar advantages to women.

The reservoir is constructed from a 40–60 cm segment of terminal ileum and/or large intestine (Figure 20.4). The loop is divided at its antimesenteric border (see Figure 20.4 inset) and fashioned in a spherical shape specific to the given orthotopic technique. We currently utilize a W-shaped sphere (Figure 20.5). The ureteroenteric anastomosis is performed using a variety of refluxing and non-refluxing techniques. The neourethra is created at a dependent portion of the pouch, which will generally have no difficulty in reaching down to the urethral stump, particularly in women; however, a tension-free urethral anastomosis may be difficult in short, obese patients with thick mesenteries. Preplaced sutures in the urethral stump (see Figure 20.3 inset) are placed in appropriately

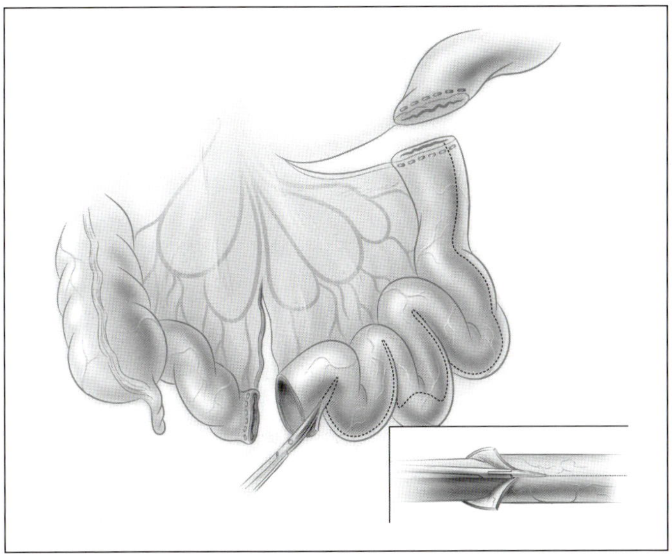

Figure 20.4 Isolation of the desired bowel segment with close attention to maximal preservation of the mesenteric blood supply. (Inset) Bowel loop is divided at the antimesenteric border.

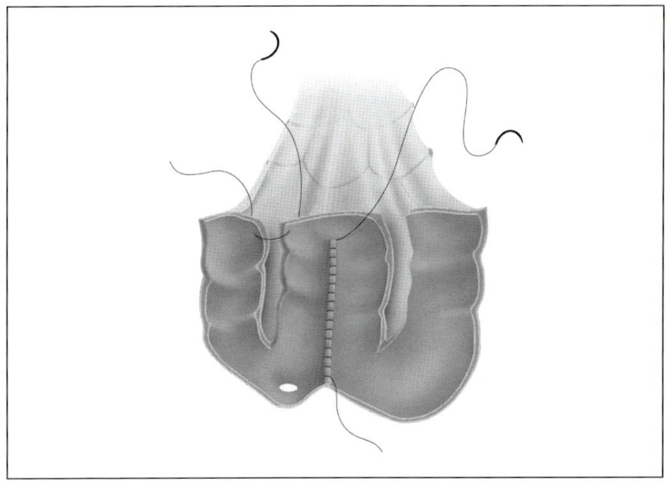

Figure 20.5 Fashioning the reservoir. Reservoir characteristics, provided by both detubularized ileal and ileocecal pouches include adequate capacity, absence of contractions, sperical shape and favorable compliance. The neourethra is created at a dependent portion of the reservoir.

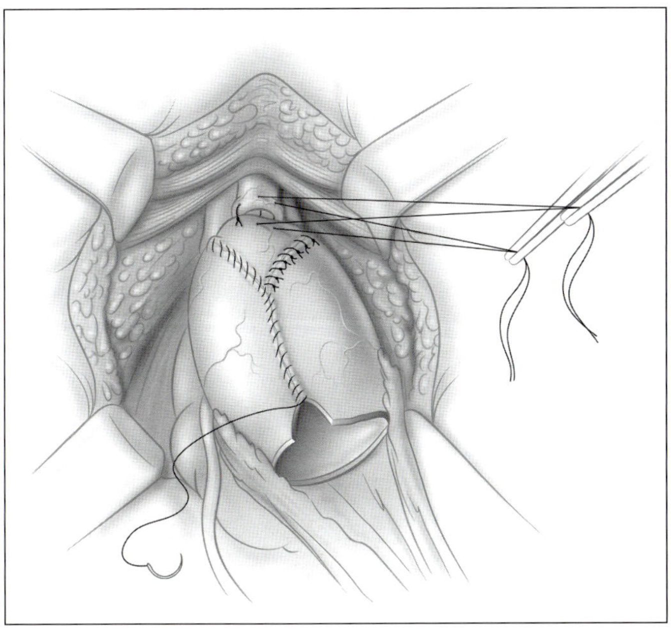

Figure 20.6 Completion of the urethroenteric anastomosis.

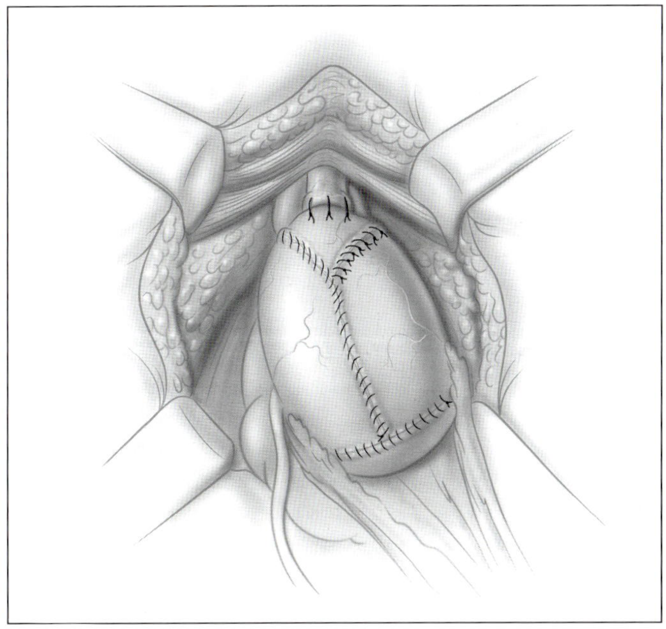

Figure 20.7 Closure of the neobladder.

corresponding locations around the neourethra over an 18–20 Fr Foley catheter (Figure 20.6). The urethral anastomosis is accomplished by tying down the sutures. The remainder of the neobladder is closed and then irrigated using the indwelling Foley catheter (Figure 20.7). If anterior vaginectomy has been performed, the surgeon must be vigilant about excluding the urethral anatomosis from the vaginal reconstructive anastomotic line. This can be readily accomplished by securing omentum between the two lines. A pelvic drain is placed.

Postsurgical considerations

Chapter 22 specifically reviews voiding function and continence following orthotopic diversion, though there are two concerns of particular importance to female patients.

Urinary retention

Despite careful intraoperative attention to anatomic structures, 10–20% of women will have chronic urinary retention or hypercontinence.[30] The etiology is not completely clear, but is felt to be mechanical, as distinguished by Ali-El-Dein and colleagues.[30] This group reviewed their series of 100 women who underwent cystectomy and orthotopic diversion primarily using a W-shaped ileal technique and found that 16 women had chronic urinary retention. They thoroughly evaluated these women using videourodynamics, pelvic floor electromyography, magnetic resonance imaging of the pelvis and cystourethroscopy. Medical therapy using doxazosin was ineffective at improving evacuation, despite previous reports.[31] Ultimately there was evidence that retention resulted from an altered positioning of the pouch in the pelvic cavity, caused by acute angulation of the posterior pouch–urethral junction. Herniation of the pouch wall through the prolapsed vaginal stump was also observed in most cases. When vaginal wall descent was mechanically corrected by a pessary, there was significant improvement in evacuation. This group has advocated intraoperative technique to suspend the vaginal stump and urinary pouch.

Chronic urinary tract infection

Female patients undergoing orthotopic diversion may be at an increased risk of urinary tract infection (UTI). Wood and colleagues[32] examined the rate of bacteriuria, positive urinalysis, positive urine culture and actual urosepsis in 66 patients (58 men and 8 women) who had orthotopic neobladders. At a mean followup of 30 months, 55 patients voided normally and 11 required ISC. Normal voiders experienced a rate of 78% positive urinalysis, 36% UTI (sypmtomatic low level bacteriuria or $>10^5$ bacteriuria with or without symptoms), and 13% urosepsis. At 5 years, the rates of UTI and urosepsis rose to 58% and 18%, respectively. Those requiring ISC experienced a rate of 100% positive urinalysis, 55% UTI and 9% urosepsis. There were no apparent statistical differences between the normal voiders and those on ISC in this small series. However, on multivariate analysis, female sex was a predictor of UTI, but not urosepsis; women were nearly three times more likely than men to suffer from UTI. ISC was not related to UTI or urosepsis. This study demonstrated the high incidence of positive urinalysis and a comparatively low but substantial rate of urosepsis, particularly in those with recurrent UTIs. These patients, particularly females, may benefit from prophylactic antibiotic therapy.

Contemporary outcomes at the University of Michigan

From 1 September 1995 to 6 February 2003, 105 women required radical cystectomy. Of these women, 53 (mean age 62 years, range 35–86) underwent orthotopic bladder substitution with mean follow-up of 32 months. For the entire group, mean operative time, estimated blood loss and length of hospital stay were reasonable at 6.2 hours, 1.1 l and 8.2 days, respectively. There were no perioperative deaths. Forty-two patients (79%) are disease free, two are alive with disease, and eight died (six from bladder cancer and two from other causes). Tumor was organ-confined in 38 (73%) and non-organ-confined in 14 (27%) cancer patients. Hautmann and Studer neobladder diversions were performed in 33 and 20 patients, respectively. Complete daytime or nighttime continence was reported by 46 (87%) and 45 (85%) patients, respectively. A total of 42 women (79%) void to completion, while 11 (21%) require intermittent catheterization.

A subset ($n = 22$) of patients were considered non-traditional because of preoperative clinicopathologic or functional characteristics. This subset included women over 70 years ($n = 12$), with a history of prior pelvic radiation/pelvic malignancy ($n = 2$), neoadjuvant chemotherapy for locally advanced disease ($n = 6$), or previous stress urinary incontinence ($n = 2$). When compared to the traditional group, the non-traditional patients were older (mean age 68 years; $P = 0.0003$) and had more comorbidities with a mean American Society of Anesthesiologists (ASA) class of 2.3 ($P = 0.01$); differences could not be detected in other parameters, including pathologic stage, complication rate or continence in this small series. Highly encouraging complete daytime and nighttime continence in the non-traditional group was reported in 19 (86%) and 20 (91%), respectively; 4 (18%) require ISC.

Conclusions

Orthotopic neobladder formation provides a desired alternative to incontinent or continent stomal diversion and has acceptable rates of morbidity and functional outcome. Patients can maintain their body image and ultimately achieve natural voiding patterns with a similar or improved quality of life over incontinent reservoirs.[15,33] The application of this technique to female patients has increased substantially in the recent past. Unfortunately, many women who choose orthotopic diversion are not considered desirable or traditional candidates for the procedure because of advanced disease, age, prior incontinence, or prior pelvic surgery or radiotherapy. The biggest concern in non-traditional women is often the potential risk of associated incontinence and local tumor recurrence. Our philosophy has been to broadly recommend orthotopic diversion to traditional candidates and to carefully select interested and appropriate non-traditional candidates. We have had very favorable initial results using this approach.

Although a neobladder is not a panacea for patients with bladder cancer, and difficult treatment decisions remain, it does provide a more tolerable alternative to an ileal conduit and makes the concept of early cystectomy more palatable to the patient. A bladder preservation strategy using multimodality treatment (aggressive transurethral resection, chemotherapy and radiation therapy) is still worthy of continued investigation, but as cystectomy remains the most effective local treatment for high-risk bladder cancer, orthotopic substitution can provide a safe and functional option for women.

References

1. Jemal A, Tiwari RC, Murray T et al. Cancer statistics, 2004. CA Cancer J Clin 2004; 54: 8–29.
2. Stein JP, Lieskovsky G, Cote R et al. Radical cystectomy in the treatment of invasive bladder cancer: long-term results in 1054 patients. J Clin Oncol 2001; 9: 666–75.
3. Abol-Enein H. Ghoneim MA. Functional results of orthotopic ileal neobladder with serous-lined extramural ureteral reimplantation: experience with 450 patients. J Urol 2001; 165: 1427–32.
4. Studer UE, Zingg EJ. Ileal orthotopic bladder substitutes: What we have learned from 12 years' experience with 200 patients. Urol Clin North Am 1997; 24: 781.
5. Mills RD, Studer UE. Female orthotopic bladder substitution: A good operation in the right circumstances. J Urol 2000; 163: 1501–4.
6. Hautmann RE, Petriconi RD, Gottrried H-W. The ileal neobladder: complications and functional results in 363 patients after 11 years of followup. J Urol 1999; 161: 422–8.
7. Madersbacher S, Mohrle K, Burkhard F, Studer UE. Long-term voiding pattern of patients with ileal orthotopic bladder substitutes. J Urol 2002; 167: 2052–7.
8. Stenzl A, Bartsch G, Rogatsch H. The remnant urothelium after reconstructive bladder surgery. Euro Urol 2002; 41: 124–31.
9. Stein JP, Cote RJ, Freeman JA et al. Indications for lower urinary tract reconstruction in women after cystectomy for bladder cancer: A pathological review of female cystectomy specimens. J Urol 1995; 154: 1329–33.
10. Stenzl A, Draxl H, Posch B et al. The risk of urethral tumors in female bladder cancer: can the urethra be used for orthotopic reconstruction of the lower urinary tract? J Urol 1995; 153: 950–5.
11. Stein JP, Esrig D, Freeman JA et al. Prospective pathologic analysis of female cystectomy specimens: Risk factors for orthotopic diversion in women. Urology 1998; 51: 951.
12. Lebret T, Herve J-M, Barre P et al. Urethral recurrence of transitional cell carcinoma of the bladder: Predictive value of preoperative later-montanal biopsies and urethral frozen sections during prostatocystectomy. Eur Urol 1998; 33: 170–4.
13. Yossepowitch O, Dalbagni G, Golijanin D et al. Orthotopic urinary diversion after cystectomy for bladder cancer: implications for cancer control and patterns of disease recurrence. J Urol 2003; 169: 177–81.
14. Freeman JA, Tarter TA, Esrig D et al. Urethral recurrence in patients with orthotopic ileal neobladders. J Urol 1996; 156: 1615–19.
15. McGuire MS, Grimaldi G, Grotas J, Russo P. The type of urinary diversion after radical cystectomy significantly impacts on the patient's quality of life. Ann Surg Oncol 2000; 7: 4–8.
16. Bochner BH, Figueroa AJ, Skinner EC et al. Salvage radical cystoprostatectomy and orthotopic urinary diversion following radiation failure. J Urol 1998; 160: 29–33.
17. Saika T, Suyama B, Murata T et al. Orthotopic neobladder reconstruction in elderly bladder cancer patients. Int J Urol 2001; 8: 533–8.
18. Ward AM, Olencki T, Peerboom D, Klein EA. Should continent diversion be performed in patients with locally advanced bladder cancer? Urology 1998; 51: 232–6.
19. Lee CT, Hafez K, Sheffield JH, Joshi DP, Montie JE. Orthotopic bladder substitution in women: nontraditional applications. J Urol 2004; 171: 1585–8.
20. Chen ME, Pisters LL, Malpica A, Pettaway CA, Dinney CP. Risk of urethral, vaginal and cervical involvement in patients undergoing radical cystectomy for bladder cancer: results of a contemporary cystectomy series from MD Anderson Cancer Center. J Urol 1997; 157: 2120–3.
21. Chang SS, Cole E, Cookson MS, Peterson M, Smith JA Jr. Preservation of the anterior vaginal wall during female radical cystectomy with orthotopic urinary diversion: technique and results. J Urol 2002; 168: 1442–5.
22. Studer UE, Hautmann H, Hohenfellner K et al. Indications for continent diversion following cystectomy and factors affecting long term results. Fifth International Consensus Meeting on Bladder Cancer. 1997. Toyko, Japan.
23. Borirakchanyavat S, Aboseif SR, Carroll PR, Tanagho EA, Lue TF. Continence mechanism of the isolated female urethra: an anatomical study of the intrapelvic somatic nerves. J Urol 1997; 158: 822–6.
24. Turner WH, Bitton A, Studer UE. Reconstruction of the urinary tract after radical cystectomy: the case for continent urinary diversion. Urology 1997; 49: 663.
25. Studer UE, Danuser H, Merz VW et al. Experience in 100 patients with an ileal low pressure bladder substitute combined with an afferent tubular isoperistaltic segment. J Urol 1995; 154: 49.
26. Hautmann RE, Miller K, Steiner U et al. The ileal neobladder: 6 years of experience with more than 200 patients. J Urol 1993; 150: 40.
27. Skinner DG, Boyd SD, Lieskovsky G et al. Lower urinary tract reconstruction following cystectomy: experience and results in 126 patients using the Kock ileal reservoir with bilateral ureteroileal urethrostomy. J Urol 1991; 146: 756.
28. Bachor R, Hautmann R. Options in urinary diversion: a review and critical assessment. Semin Urol 1993; 11: 235–50.
29. Lee KS, Montie JE, Dunn RL, Lee CT. Hautmann and Studer orthotopic neobladders: the Michigan experience. J Urol 2003; 169: 2188–91.
30. Ali-El-Dein B, Gomha M, Ghoneim MA. Critical evaluation of the problem of chronic urinary retention after orthotopic bladder substitution in women. J Urol 2002; 168: 587–92.
31. Jarolim L, Babjuk M, Pecher SM et al. Causes and treatment of residual urine volume after orthotopic bladder replacement in women. Euro Urol 2000; 38: 748–52.
32. Wood DP Jr, Bianco FJ Jr, Pontes JE, Heath MA, DaJusta D. Incidence and significance of positive urine cultures in patients with an orthotopic neobladder. J Urol 2003; 169: 2196–9.
33. Hara I, Miyake H, Hara S et al. Health-related quality of life after radical cystectomy for bladder cancer: a comparison of ileal conduit and orthotopic bladder replacement. BJU Int 2002; 89: 10–13.

21 Bowel and bladder replacement after total pelvic exenteration

Anne K Schuckman, John Stein and Donald G Skinner

Introduction

Total Pelvic Exenteration (TPE) is an important surgical technique in the management of advanced pelvic malignancies. Since the first report of pelvic exenteration by Bruschwig[1] in 1948, the majority of exenterations have been performed for gynecologic malignancies. However, exenteration may also be appropriate therapy for advanced prostate, bladder and rectosigmoid carcinomas and pelvic sarcomas. Pelvic exenterations may be required in the surgical management of complications from radiation therapy including rectovesical fistulas and persistent bleeding from radiation proctitis, as well as in the salvage setting following incomplete tumor resection or locally recurrent disease. Exenteration offers a solution for patients who require palliation from urinary or bowel obstruction from bulky pelvic masses and palliation from pelvic pain. Exenteration may also offer a chance for long-term survival in patients with extensive disease.

Total pelvic exenteration is an aggressive operation used as salvage or palliation following previous surgery, chemotherapy or radiation, and carries the potential for significant morbidity and mortality. Surgeons and potential candidates for exenteration must understand the potential complications and post operative recovery before proceeding with the operation. With a traditional abdominal and perineal approach to exenteration, requiring creation of both urinary and fecal stomas for external diversion, the morbidity of TPE is high.[2] Sources of morbidity include: local complications from the perineal and abdominal wounds, complications related to the abdominal stomas including stenosis, prolapse or parastomal herniation, and the need for external appliances. Additionally, because many patients undergoing this extensive operation have received preoperative radiation, they are at significantly higher risk for fistula formation and suture line breakdown. Finally, the empty pelvis predisposes the patient to abscess formation, perineal herniation, and small bowel obstruction from pelvic adhesions.[2]

The expectations of both surgeon and patient should be clear and realistic prior to undergoing TPE. The possibility of undergoing a tumor resection without the creation of dual stomas or the need for permanent external appliances greatly enhances patient acceptance for this operation.[3] Additionally, concurrent reconstruction of the vagina in female patients may aid in their psychological recovery following radical surgery.[4] The development of reconstruction techniques has been important including: orthotopic urinary diversion in the male and female, anal sparing colorectal surgery with preservation of normal bowel function (thereby avoiding a permanent colostomy), and concurrent vaginal reconstruction. These surgical improvements have allowed us to provide a more aggressive surgical approach in the management of extensive and recurrent pelvic malignancies.

Since 1986, the Urology Department at University of Southern California (USC) has offered male patients the option of lower urinary tract reconstruction by means of an orthotopic substitute using an ileal reservoir. Currently, 90% of male patients are able to undergo orthotopic urinary diversion at the time of radical cystoprostatectomy.[5] Since 1992, in appropriately selected women, we have employed the orthotopic ileal neobladder for urinary reconstruction in female patients as well.[6] Prior to 1996, the Kock reservoir was used as the orthotopic reservoir for urinary diversion, and subsequently we have applied the 'T-pouch' ileal reservoir in men and women as the primary neobladder.[7]

Complete surgical removal with wide surgical margins remains the cornerstone for long-term cure of patients with extensive pelvic disease. We believe the TPE, with simultaneous bowel and urinary reconstruction, accomplishes this goal without the undesirable psychological sequelae of a permanent colostomy and an external urinary diversion.

Candidates for TPE with simultaneous bowel and urinary reconstruction

Any candidate for TPE with simultaneous reconstruction of the fecal and urinary systems should have a disease process confined to the pelvis without involvement of the membranous urethra, anus, or urogenital diaphragm. Patients with locally advanced bladder, prostate and rectal carcinomas and pelvic sarcomas may be candidates for exenterative procedures. Patients with recurrent prostate carcinoma following seed or external beam radiation therapy or incomplete primary resection may also be candidates for exenterative procedures. Those suffering complications from radiation therapy such as debilitating fistulas or experiencing symptoms of bowel obstruction or renal failure due to large compressing pelvic masses may be candidates for TPE and simultaneous reconstruction. In our experience, prior radiation and chemotherapy has not been an absolute contraindication for orthotopic urinary and bowel reconstruction.

Many pelvic sarcomas present as a large mass involving the prostate or bladder, and may also be adherent to the anterior rectal wall. In general, our policy for the treatment of pelvic sarcomas has been pre-operative chemotherapy, with or without radiation therapy, followed by an exenterative procedure and reconstruction. Anterior exenteration or radical cystoprostatectomy, while sparing the rectum, increases the chances of rectal laceration, positive surgical margins, and local recurrence. Following neo-adjuvant chemotherapy or radiation, tissue planes may be obliterated and the distinction between scar and tumor impossible. An exenterative procedure may be the operation of choice to safely resect all disease.

Preoperative evaluation of the patient should be geared towards defining whether the disease process is confined to the pelvis. In cases of malignancy, patients should have no obvious clinical evidence of pelvic side-wall tumor extension, tumor fixation, or gross lymphadenopathy. Metastatic workup should included chest X-ray, liver function tests and an alkaline phosphatase. If the alkaline phosphatase is elevated, a bone scan should be performed. CT scans should be ordered to assess pelvic adenopathy and potential pelvic side-wall or adjacent organ involvement. A final, critical component of the clinical evaluation is a bimanual examination performed under anesthesia. Additionally, patients should be counseled preoperatively regarding the possibility of cutaneous urinary and fecal diversion and evaluated for abdominal stoma placement by an enterostomal therapist.

Surgical technique

After induction of general anesthesia, a bimanual exam is performed with the patient in the lithotomy position. This examination provides information on the resectability of the mass and on its adherence to the anterior rectal wall. In addition, it helps the surgeon to determine if enough anus can be preserved above the sphincter mechanism to perform a low rectal/anal anastamosis and maintain fecal continence. For heavily irradiated patients or those with bulky pelvic masses, the operation may be initiated perineally using the exaggerated lithotomy position with the perineum parallel to the floor (Figure 21.1). It is important to adequately position the shoulder supports so that there are no pressure points and to prevent overextension or the arms, which may result in brachial plexus injury. A curved 180° anterior incision around the anus allows dissection of the distal rectum within the ischiorectal fossa and dissection of the distal prostate or bladder off the anterior rectal wall. If simultaneous urethrectomy is performed, then the incision is extended vertically over the bulbar urethra and the entire urethra is removed en bloc. This incision also allows for an inferior pubectomy if deemed necessary to ensure clean margins. A long (7.5–10.0 cm) GIA stapling device can be used to divide the rectum proximal to the anal sphincter via the perineal incision. The perineal wound is closed by re-approximating the perineal body.

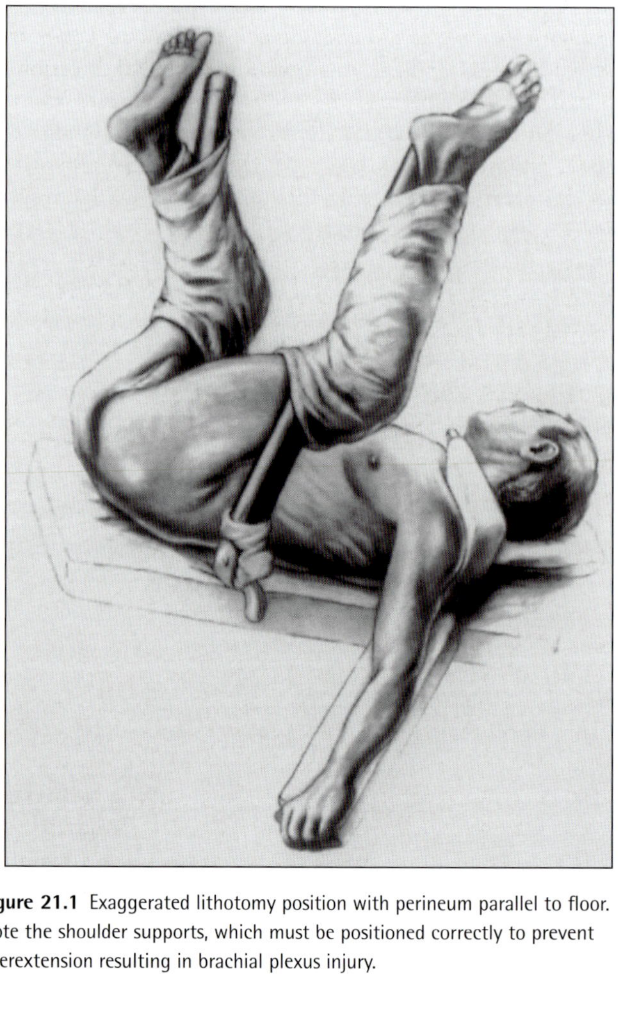

Figure 21.1 Exaggerated lithotomy position with perineum parallel to floor. Note the shoulder supports, which must be positioned correctly to prevent overextension resulting in brachial plexus injury.

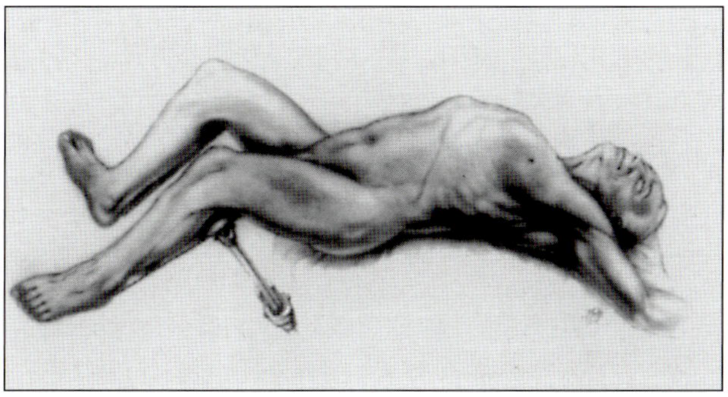

Figure 21.2 Hyperextended frog-leg position with legs supported by Krauss adjustable arm supports. This position allows free access to the perineum and anus for bowel reconstruction. (Reproduced from Skinner and Sherrod. J Urol 1990; 144: 1433–9[17] with permission from Lippincott Williams & Wilkins.)

The patient is then repositioned supine with the legs supported by Krauss adjustable arm supports according the method of Lange and Reddy.[8] The table is hyperextended and the foot of the table is lowered to provide free access to the perineum and anus (Figure 21.2).

The abdomen and retroperitoneum are thoroughly explored through a midline incision extending from the pubis to the epigastrium to determine the presence of distant metastatic disease and to assess the extent and resectability of the primary tumor. The cecum, ascending colon, terminal ileum, and small-bowel mesentery are mobilized in a cephalad direction to the point at which the duodenum crosses the midline. The sigmoid colon and its mesentery are freed off the sacral promontory and divided at an appropriate level approximately 10 cm above the peritoneal reflection. The ureters are then divided at or just distal to the common iliac arteries. These initial maneuvers gives the specimen early mobility and facilitate subsequent posterior dissection. The bowel is then packed as in a routine cystectomy leaving the divided sigmoid colon accessible in the field.

An extended pelvic iliac lymph node dissection is begun at the level of the inferior mesenteric artery and continued distally to the node of Cloquet and laterally to the genitofemoral nerve. Following division of the lateral and posterior pedicles, including the cardinal ligaments in the female, the rectum is completely freed from the hollow sweep of the deep pelvis. In the male, the prostatic dorsovenous complex is controlled. In the female the urethropelvic ligaments are left intact and the rhabdosphincter preserved to aid in postoperative continence. The urethra is prepared similarly as for a radial cystectomy with lower urinary tract reconstruction or a radical prostatectomy. (Figure 21.3). Eight 2-0 Vicryl (polyglycolic acid) sutures are placed circumferentially in the urethra as it is divided. A frozen section is sent from the proximal bladder margin. If a negative margin cannot be obtained, an orthotopic diversion is not appropriate and an alternate form of urinary diversion performed (as discussed with the patient preoperatively).

The rectourethralis muscle is divided and the distal prostate or vagina is mobilized off the anterior rectal wall for several centimeters. This provides the appropriate and necessary length proximal to the anal sphincter to complete the coloanal anastamosis. The rectum is then isolated, stapled shut and divided using a PI-55 automatic stapler (Figure 21.4). The entire specimen may then be removed en bloc.

The greater omentum is then mobilized off the transverse colon and prepared as a vascularized pedicle graft based on the left gastro-epiploic vessels in the manner of Turner-Warwick[9] (Figure 21.5). The rectal J-sigmoid pouch is constructed according to the manner of Wheeless[10] (Figure 21.6). To provide adequate colonic mobility and ensure a tension free anastamosis, the inferior mesenteric artery may need to be divided and the splenic flexure of the colon mobilized. The anvil of the EEA stapling device is then inserted into the dependant portion of the J-Pouch and secured with a pursestring suture. A large caliber EEA device is then inserted through the anus with the opened screw end puncturing the rectal staple line (Figure 21.7) After firing the EEA device, the surgeon should confirm there are two complete rings of tissue removed from the anastamosis, confirming two complete circular suture lines and limiting the chance of anastamotic leak.

Reconstruction of the urinary tract is accomplished by means of an orthotopic antirefluxing ileal reservoir. Since November 1996, we have employed the 'T-Pouch' as previously described by Stein et al.[5] If a urethrectomy is performed, a continent cutaneous diversion is constructed using a 'Double T' technique (see Chapter 23 for technique description), or other catheterizable continent reservoir.

Female patients may require primary vaginal reconstruction at the time of total pelvic exenteration using a detubularized cylinder of ileum, a rectus myocutaneous flap, a peritoneal flap, or an omental flap. The specific technique used is based on surgeon preference, available tissues and technical feasibility. The rectus myocutaneous flap is our preferred method, as it provides additional vascularized tissue to fill the pelvis and eliminates the problem of mucous drainage from the ileal neovagina.

Finally, the previously prepared omental pedicle graft is secured to the levators in the deep pelvis anterior to the J-sigmoid pouch to separate the fecal and urinary streams. In the female, it is important to place a split omentum between a neovagina and urinary stream as well. A closed suction drain is placed posterior to the omental graft in the hollow of the sacrum and removed on approximately the fifth postoperative day if there is no drainage. A penrose drain is placed near the urethral anastamosis and the afferent limb of the ileal reservoir. Ureteral stents (8F feeding tubes) are left through the ureteroileal anastamoses and secured to the urethral catheter or suprapubic tube. A temporary loop colostomy is performed in those patients who had prior heavy irradiation or in any patient in whom there is any question regarding the sigmoid-anal anastamosis. A gastrostomy tube is placed for post-operative decompression.[11] Figure 21.8 schematically demonstrates the completed reconstruction in a male.

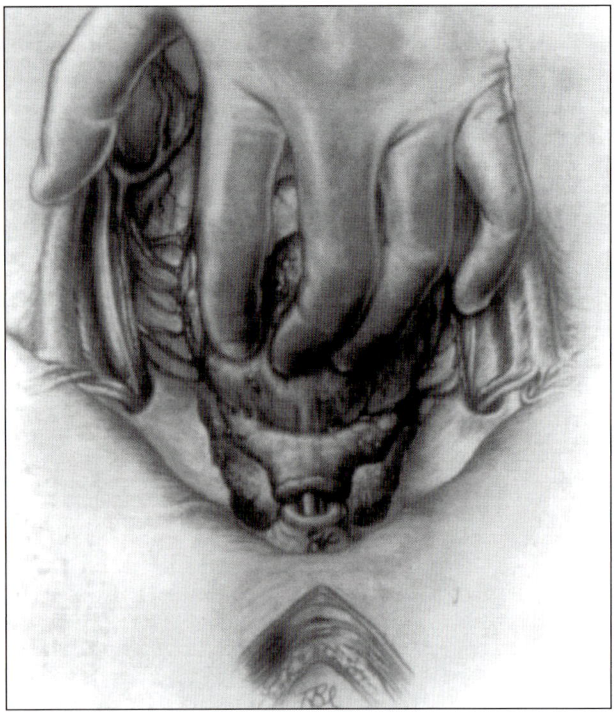

Figure 21.3 Preparation of the membranous urethra as for radical cystectomy with orthotopic reconstruction. Eight 2-0 poly-glycolic (Vicryl) sutures are placed circumferentially in the urethra as it is divided. (Reproduced from Skinner and Sherrod. J Urol 1990; 144: 1433–9[17] with permission from Lippincott Williams & Wilkins.)

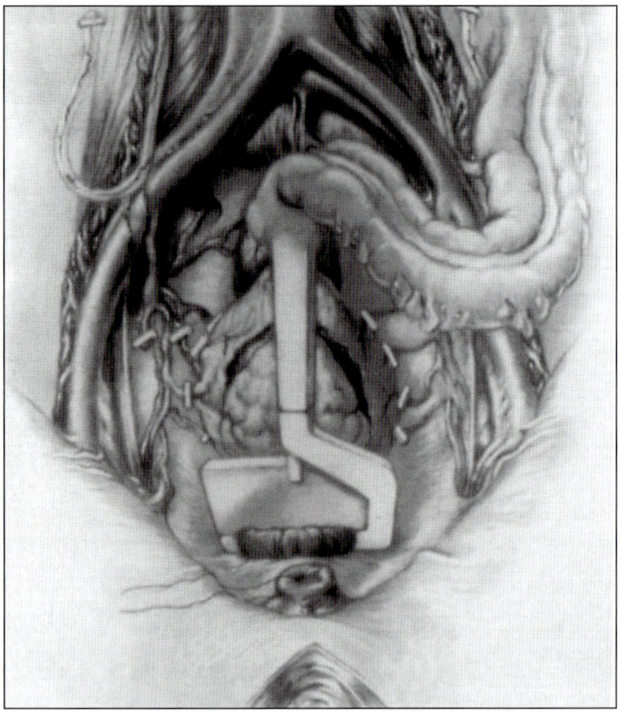

Figure 21.4 Rectum is isolated and stapled above the urogenital diaphragm using a PI-55 stapling device. The rectum is divided cephalad to the stapler to complete the en-bloc exenteration. (Reproduced from Skinner and Sherrod. J Urol 1990; 144: 1433–9[17] with permission from Lippincott Williams & Wilkins.)

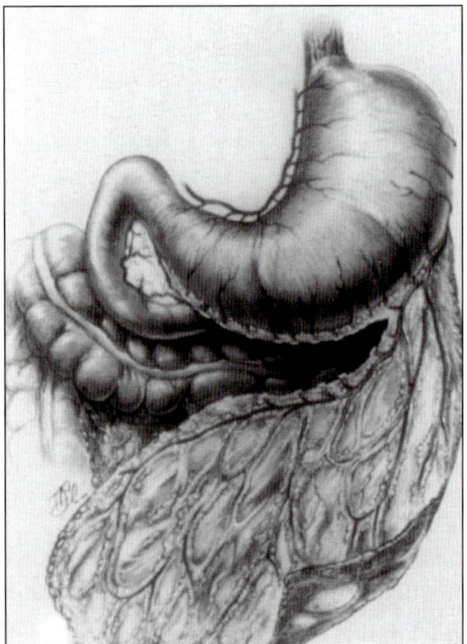

Figure 21.5 The omentum prepared as a vascularized pedicle graft based on the left gastroepiploic artery in the manner or Turner-Warwick.[9] (Reproduced from Skinner and Sherrod. J Urol 1990; 144: 1433–9[17] with permission from Lippincott Williams & Wilkins.)

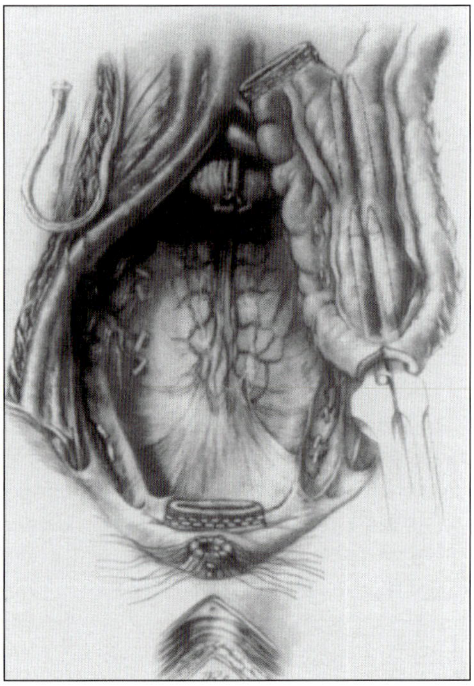

Figure 21.6 The rectal J-Sigmoid pouch is constructed with two applications of the GIA stapler. To allow the sigmoid pouch to reach the anus without tension, the inferior mesenteric artery may be divided and the splenic flexure mobilized. Note the stapled anus and pre-placed sutures in the membranous urethra. (Reproduced from Skinner and Sherrod. J Urol 1990; 144: 1433–9[17] with permission from Lippincott Williams & Wilkins.)

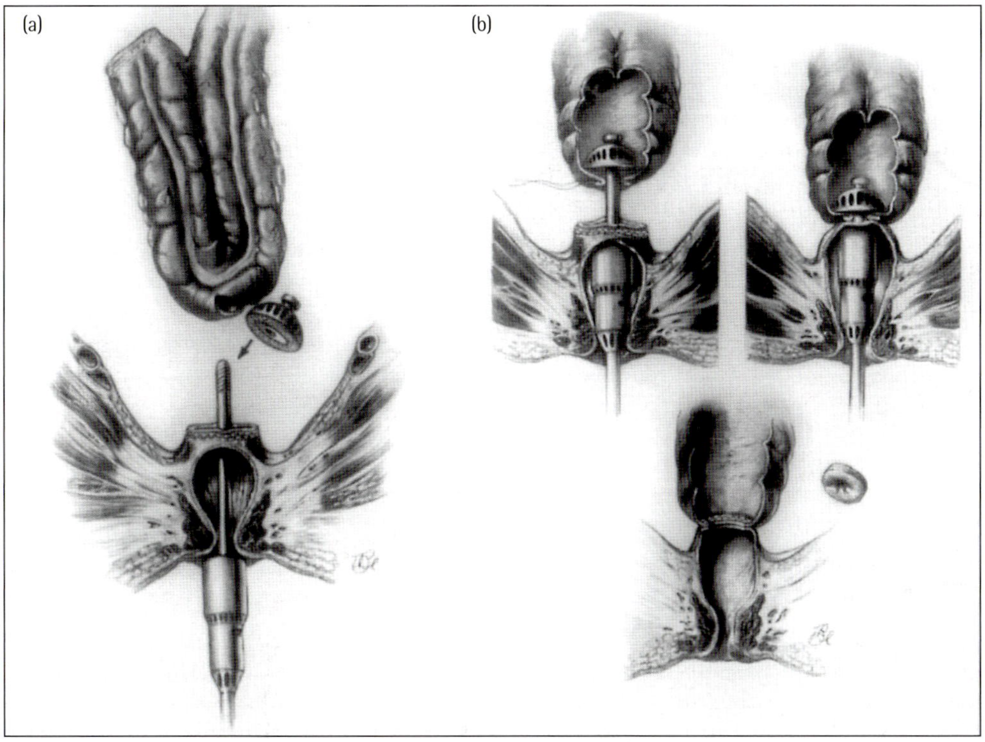

Figure 21.7 Bowel reconstruction using J-sigmoid pound and colo-anal anastamosis. (a) EEA device inserted through the anus with the open screw puncturing the anal staple line. (b) Anvil of the stapler inserted in the dependant portion of the J-sigmoid pouch and secured with pursestring suture. Complete anastamosis produced two full rings of excised tissue. (Reproduced from Skinner and Sherrod. J Urol 1990; 144: 1433–9[17] with permission from Lippincott Williams & Wilkins.)

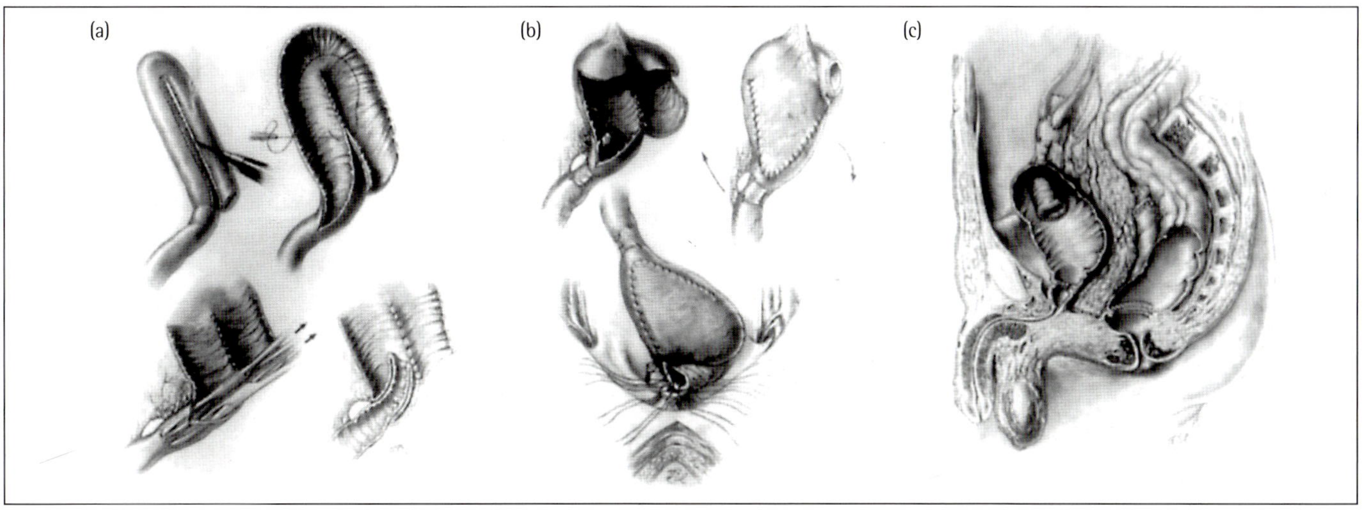

Figure 21.8 Schematic of completed urinary and fecal reconstruction. Note the omental interposition separating the suture lines. (Reproduced from Skinner and Sherrod. J Urol 1990; 144: 1433–9[17] with permission from Lippincott Williams & Wilkins.)

Post-operative follow up

The usual hospital stay following exenteration is 10–12 days including one to two days in the intensive care unit. Patients are discharged home with the urethral catheter and Penrose drain left in place for a total of three weeks. At the three-week postoperative mark, a gravity cystogram of the ileal reservoir may be obtained and, if no leak is demonstrated, the catheter and attached ureteral stents (as well as Penrose drain) are removed. The patient is discharged home on antibiotics for several days. Patients are monitored annually with cystograms.

Discussion

Over 40 years have now passed since the original description of total pelvic exenteration by Bruschwig.[1] Surgical and anesthetic techniques have clearly improved and allow physicians to offer a broader spectrum of surgical choices to even their sickest patients. A surgeon may realistically counsel a patient on recovery, free of external urinary or fecal appliances and without compromising oncologic principles.[12] In fact, simultaneous reconstruction of the bowel, bladder and vagina may offer not only psychological benefits to a patient, but also limit local complications secondary to an empty pelvis. Therefore, reconstruction of the lower urinary tract combined with re-establishment of bowel continuity has become the goal in the appropriate patient with extensive disease confined to the pelvis.

Morbidity following the traditional pelvic exenteration is high, with major complication rates reported to be 50%.[2] In contrast, the peri-operative complication rate following TPE with simultaneous urinary and bowel reconstruction is similar to that reported for radical cystectomy and orthotopic neobladder construction.[13] This can be attributed to the viability of the tissue that fills the pelvis following TPE. Reconstruction with an ileal reservoir and sigmoid J-pouch with an interposed omental flap leaves well-vascularized tissue within the operative bed and reduces the excess space for herniation or obstruction. In females, reconstruction of the vagina can be performed with a rectus myocutaneous flap, ileum or a rectus-peritoneal flap based on the inferior epigastic artery, all of which additionally fill the pelvis and promote healing. Hatch et al[14] demonstrated a lower complication rate in patients undergoing TPE with a low rectal anastamosis and improved healing in patients in which an omental wrap was utilized.

Many patients with extensive pelvic malignancy have received high dose preoperative radiation and neoadjuvant chemotherapy resulting in compromised pelvic tissues. Success of the colo-anal anastamosis depends both on the vascularity of the bowel segments and on creating a tension free anastamosis. Harris and Wheeless[15] recommend a diverting colostomy in all irradiated patients with a low rectal anastamosis. We have followed this recommendation, and create a temporary diverting loop colostomy in our heavily irradiated patients. The colostomy is generally reversed 3–4 months postoperatively.[16] Additionally, we attempt to create a tension-free anastamosis through complete mobilization of colon to the splenic flexure and division of the IMA when necessary. However, no report conclusively demonstrates an improved rate of rectal anastamotic healing in non-radiated patients utilizing a diverting colostomy. We therefore do not routinely perform a colostomy on patients with no prior radiotherapy unless the surgeon is not satisfied with some aspect of the colo-anal anastamosis.

The end-to-end circular stapling device has greatly assisted the surgeon in performing the low rectal anastamosis. The stapling device allows for the use of a shorter rectal stump than is needed for a hand-sewn anastamosis. Reconstruction of the bowel using the J-sigmoid reservoir anastamosed to the anus reduces the tenesmus and diarrhea associated with end-to-end descending coloproctostomy. Rectal continence has been excellent with the low J-sigmoid pouch with a return to control within 3–4 weeks in patients not previously radiated, including patients who have undergone a combined perineal and abdominal exploration.

Conclusions

Effective management of extensive pelvic malignancy requires complete excision with wide surgical margins. Frequently this can only be accomplished with total pelvic exenteration. Advances in continent orthotopic urinary diversion, anus-sparing surgery and vaginal reconstruction allow the surgeon to perform exenterative surgery without the psychological disturbance of multiple stomas. Patients can return to urethral voiding, sexual function and bowel control in a reasonable period of time following surgery. The complication rate following TPE with bowel and urinary reconstruction is comparable to radical cystectomy with continent diversion. The lower complication rate of simultaneous bowel and urinary reconstruction with TPE makes this procedure a clear improvement over traditional exenteration.

References

1. Bruschwig A. Complete excision of the pelvic viscera for advanced carcinoma. Cancer 1948; 1: 177–83.
2. Jackwatz JG, Porudominsky D, Riihimaki DU et al. Complications of pelvic exenteration. Arch Surg 1985; 120: 1261–5.
3. Boyd SD, Feinberg SM, Skinner DG et al. Quality of life survey of urinary diversion patients: comparison of ileal conduits versus continent Kock reservoirs. J Urol 1987; 138: 1386–9.
4. Mirashemi R, Averette HE, Lambrou N et al. Vaginal reconstruction at the time of pelvic exenteration: a surgical and psychosexual analysis of techniques. Gynecol. Oncol 2002; 87: 39–45.
5. Skinner DG, Boyd SD, Lieskovsky G et al. Lower urinary tract reconstruction following cystectomy: experience and results in 126 patients using the Kock ileal reservoir with bilateral ureteroileal urethrostomy. J Urol 1991; 146: 756–60.
6. Stein, JP, Strenzl, A, Esrig D et al. Lower Urinary Tract Reconstruction following cystectomy in the female using the Kock ileal reservoir with bilateral ureteroileal urethrostomy: initial experience. J Urol 1994; 152: 1404–8.
7. Stein JP, Lieskovsky G, Ginsberg DA, Bochner BH, Skinner DG. T-Pouch: an orthotopic ileal neobladder incorporating a serosal lined antireflux technique. J Urol 1998; 159: 1836–42.
8. Lange PH, Reddy PK. Technical nuances and surgical results of radical retropubic prostatectomy in 150 patients. J Urol 1987; 138: 348–52
9. Turner-Warwick R. The use of the omental pedicle graft in urinary tract reconstruction. J Urol 1976; 116: 341–7.
10. Wheeless CR Jr. Rectal reservoir colonic pouch. In: Atlas of Pelvic Surgery, 2nd edition. Wheeless CR Jr (ed.) Philadelphia: Lea & Febiger, 1988.

11. Buscarini M, Stein JP, Lawrence MA, Lieskovsky G. Tube gastrostomy after radical cystectomy and urinary diversion: surgical technique and experience in 709 patients. Urology 2000; 56: 150–2.
12. Morley GW, Hopkins MP, Lindenauer MS et al. Pelvic exenteration, University of Michigan: 100 patients at 5 years. Obst Gynec 1989; 74: 934–43.
13. Skinner DG, Lieskovsky G (eds). Diagnosis and Management of Genitourinary Cancer, Philadelphia: WB Saunders, 1988, 295–312.
14. Hatch KD, Gelder MS, Soong S. Pelvic exenteration with low rectal anastamosis: survival, complications and prognostic factors. Gynecol Oncol 1990; 38: 462–7.
15. Harris WJ, Wheeless CR Jr. Use of the end-to-end anastamosis stapling device in low colorectal anastamosis associated with radical gynecologic surgery. Gynecol Oncol 1986; 23: 350–7.
16. Skinner DG. Urinary diversion after total pelvic exenteration for rectal cancer, Annals of Surg Oncol 1999; 6: 717–18.
17. Skinner DG, Sherrod A. Total pelvic exenteration with simultaneous bowel and urinary reconstruction. J Urol 1990; 144: 1433–9.

22 Voiding function and continence following orthotopic diversion

Kilian Walsh

Introduction

Since Tizzoni and Foggi anastamosed an ileal loop to the bladder neck of a dog in 1888 many forms of orthotopic bladder have been described.[1] Voiding through the urethra is a natural desire for most patients, however, this must be balanced against the recognized difficulties in creating a new bladder from a section of bowel. While orthotopic bladder was originally introduced and popularized in men, the technique is now offered routinely to women .

An alteration of voiding function is inevitable in each case. By careful follow-up of the patients who have undergone different procedures, our knowledge of what dysfunction patients can expect after a procedure has increased dramatically in recent years. It is essential that this knowledge be imparted to patients so that they can make an informed choice on the advantages and disadvantages orthotopic bladder substitution can offer. It is only when a technique is reproducible and of value to those in whom it is employed that it can be called a success.

Voiding function and continence are key concerns to anyone contemplating an orthotopic bladder. This chapter attempts to illustrate the variety of techniques available as well as the underlying mechanisms that give rise to voiding problems and their reported results, so the surgeon and patient can have a knowledgeable discussion prior to therapy and should dysfunction arise treat it appropriately.

Orthotopic neobladder is a generic term and the multiplicity of surgical procedures makes comparison difficult. The outcome measures used in reported series are also variable and single institutions reporting on a particular technique may have some inherent bias.

Historical perspective

Knowledge of the historical development of the orthotopic bladder helps to compare the value of different techniques. The initial reports of the Camey I (see Figure 14.2) highlighted the important continence problems with orthotopic bladder, daytime urinary frequency varied between 8 and 15 times a day and nocturnal incontinence was reported in over 50% of patients.[2]

Although significant changes in the design of orthotopic bladders have improved the situation these problems are still reported and remain the key concerns for patients both pre- and postoperatively.

The construction technique of 40 cm of ileum arranged as a 'U' shape was felt to have contributed to the incontinence, and with the Camey II (Figure 14.2) the ileum was detubularized therefore increasing the radius and capacity of the continent reservoir. This modification helped improve the interval of daytime continence to 3 hours and episodes of nocturnal continence. However 28% of patients still required the use of pads or a convene catheter overnight.[3] The Hautmann bladder detubularizes 60–80 cm ileum but it is reconstructed as a 'W' plate, which leads to an increased bladder capacity. In a review of 211 patients, the urodynamic studies estimated a mean bladder volume of 775 ml as opposed to the mean 520 ml for the Camey II. Patients were reported to void 5.1 times a day and an average of 1.6 times at night. However 3.6% of patients required clean intermittent catheterization.[4]

The orthotopic Kock pouch is also constructed from ileum and incorporates an antireflux nipple. Reported series have suggested that 92% of patients were continent by day and 73% by night. The construction of a nipple within the reservoir has led to stone formation and for this reason the technique has somewhat fallen out of favor. In a urodynamic evaluation the average maximum reservoir capacity was 709 ml (range 225–1200 ml), maximum pressure at capacity was

<40 cmH_2O (range 10–40 cmH_2O).[5] A combination of large and small bowel with the ileocecal segment for the construction of an orthotopic bladder may have potential benefits over the use of ileum alone. The wide lumen of the cecum allows for ease of creation of a spherical reservoir. The cecum rarely has diverticular disease and the ileocecal vessels are remarkably constant and long enough to allow the pouch to be mobilized into a small pelvis for anastamosis.

The Mainz pouch was first introduced in 1983 and constructed in the form of a spherical pouch with 10–15 cm of detubularized cecum and ascending colon and two ileal loops of the same length. A daytime incontinence rate of 5.3% and nighttime incontinence of 21% with a mean bladder capacity of 426 ± 34 ml and a mean residual of 37 ± 8.2 ml have been reported, at least 1 year after surgery.[6] Light and Engelman in 1985 also isolated an ileocolic segment for use as an orthotopic bladder: 20 cm of ascending colon and a corresponding segment of terminal ileum are used. A full-length incision along the ileocecal remnant is made 2 cm distal to the cut end of ileum continuing through the ileocecal valve and into the anterior tenia of the ascending colon. A horizontal mattress forming a large pouch joins the outermost layers. The technique was called Le Bag (see Figure 16.3). However, in an early series of 11 patients only five out of nine were continent and one required an artificial sphincter suggesting some problems with voiding and storage.[7] More contemporary series have shown continence rates of up to 80%.[8]

With a concern about the effectiveness of vitamin B_{12} and bile acid resorption when incorporating the distal ileum into a neobladder, detubularized right colon for use as a reservoir was described and investigated. The distal part of the colonic bowel segment is folded over to close the neobladder with running 3-0 sutures. In a reported series of 41 patients, two required placement of an artificial urinary sphincter for severe day and night incontinence. Two-thirds of the patients were dry at night if they awoke every 2–3 hours to void.[9] The sigmoid neobladder can provide a low-pressure, high-volume reservoir from 30 cm to 35 cm of large bowel. It has been popularized by Reddy and he published urodynamic data of 27 patients who had undergone total bladder replacement using detubularized sigmoid colon. He claimed that all patients were continent during the day and 67% were continent at night, the remainder using pads or a condom catheter at night. The average bladder capacity was 600 ml with low pressures during filling and at capacity.[10]

The stomach was initially used in dogs for the reconstruction of the urinary tract. There are inherent advantages in the use of stomach wall. It characteristically stores under low pressure and empties on an intermittent basis similarly to the bladder. It produces a smaller amount of mucus, it does not absorb electrolytes, and hydrochloric acid has a bactericidal action. However the potential for hematuria, bladder spasm and dysuria has decreased the popularity of the procedure. While the stomach has often been used in augmentation (see Figure 19.6) its assessment in orthotopic bladder replacement has been limited and small series have been reported. In a study in which a 4-year follow up was done the urodynamic parameters and incontinence rates (8–23%) were less favorable in those with a gastric orthotopic neobladder compared with those who had an ileocecal bladder with incontinence reported in up to 63% of patients.[11]

Hence multiple case series using different sections of bowel, of differing lengths configured in a different manner and resulting in variable capacities have reported fairly similar problems with orthotopic bladder. Daytime continence in the majority of cases is good; around 10% of patients will require intermittent catheterization. However, nighttime continence is a universal problem often requiring the use of catheters, pads and even insertion of a sphincter. The problem with the array of small case series with limited follow-up describing a variety of techniques is that it is difficult to determine the advantages and disadvantages of each technique. Common scientific and surgical principles, however, underlie the reason for the voiding characteristics of orthotopic bladders. The management of voiding dysfunction following orthotopic bladder, should it arise, involves an understanding of these principles and accurate recognition and classification of the underlying disorder. Videourodynamics help to identify the primary problem, classify it accordingly and allow the appropriate management depending on the findings.

Surgical and scientific principles underlying voiding dysfunction

The advantage of a surgeon adopting one technique is that they become familiar with the technical aspects of the procedure and a greater reliability can be expected based on their previous experience. It does, however, make a valid comparison of different procedures more difficult. Where this has been attempted there has been a suggestion, but the case has in no way been proved that ileal or ileocecal configurations may achieve slightly better continence rates than gastric and sigmoid reconstructions,[12] or that the Studer bladder has slightly better nighttime continence than the Hautmann bladder.[13] Continence is dependent upon suitable storage of urine and appropriately timed voiding. These in turn, are dependent on an adequate volume low-pressure storage system and the generation of voiding contraction of sufficient length and amplitude that is coordinated with appropriate relaxation of component sphincter mechanisms.

The storage characteristics depend on the choice of bowel segment, its length and its new configuration. The sphincter mechanism is related to sex and age of the patient and the effect of pelvic surgery on the vascular and neurological control of the sphincter. The relationship between sphincter control and bladder contraction is altered dramatically by the introduction of an orthotopic bladder.

In essence it is difficult to judge how these components will relate to each other postoperatively, however there are scientific and surgical principles on the basis of which we can make some predictions. It is the understanding of these principles that allows us direct appropriate therapy.

Detubularization

It has been argued that detubularization is essential to allow adequate capacity for an orthotopic bladder. It is achieved by opening the bowel along the antimesenteric border and creating a reservoir. Certainly on mathematical principles the volume of a cylinder is dependent on its length and radius. However, it is not possible to fashion the bowel into a perfect cylinder and therefore the final configuration of the bowel will also influence its volume. It has been shown based on calculations the desired shape is that of a spherical reservoir. An optimal number of sections for each length of bowel will be required to produce a spherical shape. A 'W' pouch requires shorter lengths of segments to produce a given volume than an 'S' pouch and an 'S' requires shorter lengths than a 'U'. In order to create the greatest volume reservoir for a given length of bowel it should be spherical in shape with a relationship of 1 between the length and diameter but in practical terms an ovoid reservoir with a length:diameter ratio of between 1 and 2 will give adequate volume.[14] The pressure within any new reservoir is important in a number of contexts:

- It should be kept low during filling to preserve potential upper tract deterioration and help continence.
- There should be no spontaneous unconscious episodes of contraction increasing the bladder reservoir pressure.
- During timed voiding the bladder pressure generated should be of an amplitude sufficient to overcome sphincter mechanisms and of a duration sufficient to allow complete emptying.

Laplace' law relates the pressure difference across a thin curved membrane. It states that pressure is related to the tension in the wall of the bladder and the radius. During normal bladder filling because of the compliant nature of the detrusor wall the relationship between tension and radius is kept constant allowing low pressure filling. When the pressure–volume relationship for a tubular reservoir was compared with a detubularized spherical reservoir in neobladders constructed from 40 cm of ileum with a diameter of 3.2 cm, the tubular reservoir has been shown to have a substantially smaller capacity and a larger pressure for a given volume than the detubularized bowel.[15]

Bladder contractility

Spontaneous contractions of bowel are physiological, whereas in the bladder they are considered pathological. A concern is that if they are of large enough amplitude they can overcome the sphincter mechanism and produce incontinence.

When bowel contracts it will produce an increase in muscle tone but because the volume of the reservoir constructed from detubularized bowel is about twice that of tubularized bowel and the pressure range is half, this reduces the amplitude of pressure rises caused by partial contractions.[14] This helps decrease spontaneous leakage at normal bladder volumes.

With overdistension, however, the pressure rise produced by partial contractions is further reduced, perhaps decreasing the efficiency of complete voiding which means the voiding characteristics may change over time and could be a contributing factor in the development of orthotopic bladder retention.

Another point of view is that the extrapolation of mathematical principles that apply rigidly to geometric principles is misleading in the human context. The argument is that the intestine is asymmetrical in its caliber and that even with the correct detubularization technique the observed increase in capacity can fall to as low as a 40% of the expected increase and not double as calculated by mathematical principles. Gut mobility is also severely restricted by detubularization and this may offset any geometrical advantage. In a comparative study of the effects of detubularization on outcome in substitution cystoplasty it was acknowledged that detubularization shifts the detrusor pressure curve of a urodynamic study to the right but does not abolish contractility and that mechanisms other than detubularization may be important in determining the functional outcome. It was also observed that those patients with better continence had a greater capacity and lower contractility. The behavior of the sphincter could influence the orthotopic bladder characteristics over time rather like the development of low pressure chronic retention observed in patients with bladder outflow obstruction.[16] An appreciation by both patient and surgeon that the relationship between sphincter and bladder can alter helps in choosing the most appropriate non-surgical methods of treatment for voiding dysfunction when warranted. Traditionally detubularization has been carried out at the antimesenteric border but in an interesting technical alteration a perimesenteric incision of the ileal segment has been shown to improve compliance and increase capacity of the neobladder[17] suggesting that surgical technique can influence the characteristics of the neobladder. While detubularization is a theoretical advantage for orthotopic bladder construction, in practice the gain may not be as great as predicted and could lead to an increased likelihood of retention.

Bladder–urethral anastamosis

Reports from the pediatric literature demonstrating that tubularizing the bladder at the level of the trigone can improve continence in children with spina bifida, such as with the Kropp or Young–Dees–Leadbetter[18] procedure led to the concept of tubularizing the lower end of the bowel segment prior to its anastamosis on to the remnant urethra. Somewhat surprisingly this led to more complications and did not help in terms of continence. In fact the use of a tube led to a kink arising between the orthotopic bladder and the urethra resulting in retention. After this was recognized and the tubularized lower segment was resected continence improved, demonstrating an important principle that the anastamosis onto the urethra should be to the most dependent portion of the orthotopic bladder.[19] It is not only the site of the urethral anastamosis which is important but also the functional urethral length that has an effect on day time continence in both orthotopic bladder and radical prostatectomy. Those with a short urethral length have demonstrated an increased risk of dribbling when walking with a full bladder.[20]

Structural changes in orthotopic bladder

The structure and organization of detrusor muscle is designed to produce efficient storage and bladder emptying, obviously bowel wall is quite different and designed to give peristalsis which is a propulsive motor pattern orchestrated by neuronal excitation and inhibition in cooperation with intrinsic muscular control mechanisms. The interstial cells of Cajal form a network of cells in which electrical slow waves originate and then propagate into the musculature initiating rhythmic contractile activity upon excitation by enteric nerves. Interstitial cells of Cajal (Figure 22.1) have now been isolated and their intrinsic properties reveal the presence of rhythmic inward currents not found in smooth muscle cells. These cells act as pacemaker cells in the gut and are located in two specific areas. One population is located between longitudinal and circular muscle layers and is related to the myenteric plexus. It is important for normal peristalsis. The second population is located between the innermost circular layer and outermost subdivisions of the circular muscle in association with the deep muscular (enteric) plexus. Changes have been observed when bowel has been used as an orthotopic bladder. In detubularized segments from ileal bladders of more than 1 year, interstitial cells of Cajal were rare in the myenteric plexus and absent in the deep enteric plexus, and the innermost circular muscle layer and deep enteric plexus nerve fibers could not be identified. Within tubular segments normal features were maintained up to 3 years post surgery.

An association between the presence of a normal interstitial cell population in relation to the myenteric plexus and the maintenance of pressure waves has been suggested. Segments with intact interstitial cells of Cajal related to the deep enteric plexus had a contractile response to distension thus producing a better functional outcome. These structural changes may influence the characteristics of orthotopic bladder behavior over time.[21]

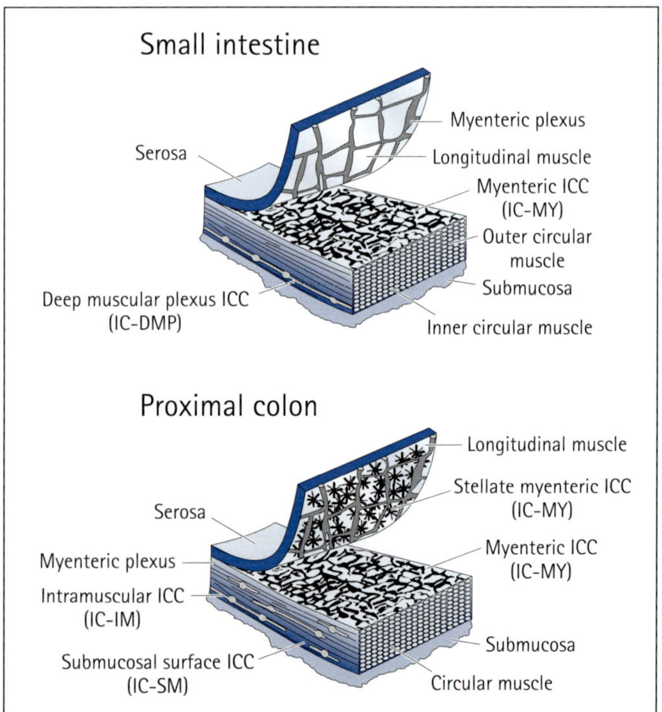

Figure 22.1 Interstitial cells of Cajal (ICC) of the small intestine and colon. (Reproduced with permission of Dr Kenton Sanders, University of Nevada.)

Pharmacological response

A change has been observed in the contractile responses to pharmacological stimulants of the α-adrenergic and purinergic systems from ileal segments incorporated in an ileocystoplasty and studied as muscle strips. The strips display a response more suggestive of detrusor than bowel activity suggesting that an alteration in its structure has led to a change in function.[22] Evidence from cecal urinary reservoirs where the effect of muscarinc receptor blockade, stimulation and smooth muscle relaxation was studied demonstrated that responses to agents such as atropine, bethenacol and glucagons were greatly altered after detubularization, and that reconfigured bowel may alter its pharmacologic response which in turn will have a significant effect on voiding function and pattern.[23]

Response to changes in pressure and fluid constituents

A lively debate exists as to whether small or large bowel is preferential in the construction of a neobladder. A model has been developed using the Mainz pouch that enables the assessment of the structural properties of both small and large bowel and their changes during filling and alterations in intraluminal pressure. It was noted that the most distensible layer was the circular ileal layer, which could be advantageous for urinary storage. Also, altering the osmolality of the instilling solution could influence the characteristics of intracavity pressure waves, with a hyperosmotic solution resulting in the greatest amplitude. Given the fact that nocturnal urine tends to be of greater concentration it was postulated that this may have an effect on nocturnal continence.[24]

Urethral sphincter control

Although the characteristics of the neobladder will be defined by the nature of bowel incorporated, it is the relationship between bowel and sphincter that determines continence. The dissection required in a cystectomy can certainly affect the anatomy of the external urethral sphincter (EUS). The sphincter itself is described as a striated muscle extending from the bladder base to the urogenital diaphragm.[25] Most investigators have suggested that the EUS is a horseshoe-shaped sphincter that loops around the urethra so that on contraction it can produce a kinking. The EUS is derived from the puborectalis muscle, and the two contract simultaneously upon stimulation of the latter with a concentric needle electromyographic electrode. The perineal branch of the pudendal nerve innervates the EUS. It is formed predominantly of skeletal fibers, however, it contains smooth muscle which receives noradrenergic innervation.[26] Lack of knowledge of the precise anatomical relation of the somatic nerve termination to the sphincters renders these nerve branches susceptible to injury during pelvic surgery.[27] The intrapelvic somatic pathway derived from the S2, S3, and S4 sacral roots and distinct from the peripheral pudendal nerve, supplies somatic innervation to the levator ani and the striated urethral sphincter. Nerve fibers can be identified throughout the loose areolar tissue planes dissected during cystectomy (Figure 22.2). Injury to the somatic innervation may potentially impact on urinary continence.

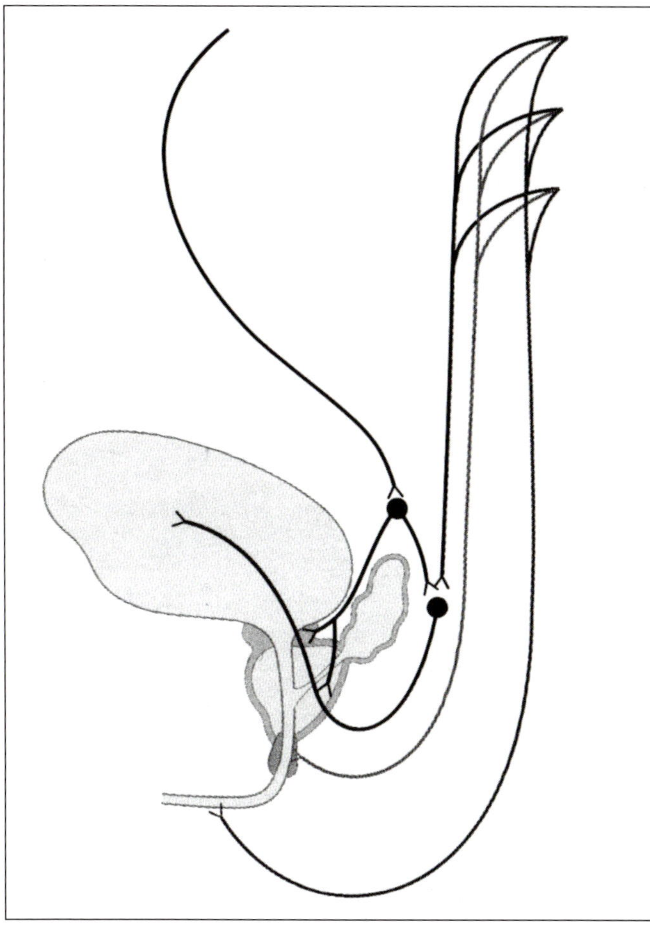

Figure 22.2 Four components of innervation of the lower urinary tract (sympathetic, parasympathetic, somatic, pudendal nerve). (Reproduced from Gosling JA et al.[28]).

Voiding dysfunction: unable to store

How do these principles relate to voiding dysfunction? Different rates of daytime incontinence have been reported in different series, due to a variety of definitions. However, in a recent review it was estimated that daytime incontinence in patients undergoing orthotopic bladder replacement developed in a mean of 13.3%.[20] Factors such as advancing age and lack of nerve-sparing techniques have been shown to contribute to this as well as the relationship between the new bladder and existing sphincter.[29] Aging is an extremely important factor and it has been reported that continence rates can decrease 5–10 years after surgery due to changes within the orthotopic bladder and aging of the urethral sphincter.[30] While these factors are of extreme importance in daytime continence, it is perceived that it is nighttime incontinence which is of most concern. The decrease in urethral strength following dissection and a noted decrease in urethral tone during sleep result in the urethra being unable to resist changes in bladder pressure at night resulting in incontinence. Increased urine output at night leads to a greater need for nocturnal capacity. However, the use of an alarm clock and regular timed voiding until the patient has learnt to recognize the nocturnal sensation of bladder fullness has been proved to help significantly in nighttime incontinence.[31] Stress incontinence can be treated with moderate success with periurethral bulking agents and if required an artificial urinary sphincter. In a recent small series this was found to be well tolerated and reliable with a positive impact on the patient's quality of life.[32] A history of stress incontinence in women preoperatively appears to be an important predictive factor for sphincteric weakness postoperatively. This should be fully assessed prior to orthotopic replacement and patients warned about its potential to remain postoperatively.[33]

Voiding dysfunction: unable to empty

Much has been made of the fact that with time an orthotopic bladder will increase its functional capacity. This is a physiological event and related to structural changes discussed earlier. However, this tendency has been claimed by some authors to be advantageous in so far as it improved daytime and nighttime continence. It is perhaps therefore an opportune moment to suggest that the term 'hypercontinence', which has been used by some authors is misleading. It is simply retention of residual urine and should be classified as such and treated accordingly.

The treatment is clean intermittent catheterization and the reported incidence of the introduction of such therapy has again varied in different series between 0 and 53%.[34] The keys to avoiding retention would seem to be clear instruction on pelvic floor relaxation, regular voiding to prevent overdistension and regular follow-up.[35]

Urinary incontinence: the evidence base

As has been previously mentioned, the difficulty in drawing conclusions from a variety of reported case series is that there is an inherent bias. Within the past decade in medical education an emphasis has been placed upon evidence-based practice. In some circles this has been considered a minor revolution with the traditional surgical apprenticeship being replaced by a more broad-based view of treatment outcomes. The desire is to select and standardize appropriate treatments for specific conditions. Inevitably those treatments that have been in practice for the longest period of time, and are widely used with the greatest number of reports are probably the easiest to study. With orthotopic neobladder being a relatively new technique, performed predominantly in specialized centers that have incorporated their own modifications it is has been more difficult to build a consensus. The Cochrane review process has been instrumental in helping create a body of reference literature. Recently the Cochrane Collaboration has reported on the use of intestinal segments for intractable incontinence or following cystectomy. The goal was to determine the best way of improving or replacing the function of the lower urinary tract using intestinal segments when the bladder has to be removed. Only randomized or quasi-randomized controlled trials of surgery were selected as these represent the most robust evidence. The trials were analyzed with appropriate statistical methodology for categorical outcomes and a relation between the numbers reporting an outcome to the numbers at risk in each group was used to derive a relative risk. For continuous variables means and standard deviations were used to derive a weighted mean difference with 95% confidence intervals. The intention was to undertake a meta-analysis using a fixed effects model and explore differences between trials. The types of outcome measure that were assessed were general measures of health status, disease-specific measures of quality of life and other measures of patient satisfaction (including sexual function). The number of participants in high-quality studies that were deemed suitable for inclusion in the review of urinary incontinence was 140. The relative risk for both daytime and nighttime incontinence was 1 (Figure 22.3) suggesting no difference in incontinence between a variety of orthotopic techniques. However, the confidence intervals were wide suggesting that a clinical difference could exist but that it could not be demonstrated statistically.[36] The problem in using an evidence base as a guide to practice is that the criteria for selection are so robust that sample sizes are small and it can be difficult to show differences. But it is a sobering thought that

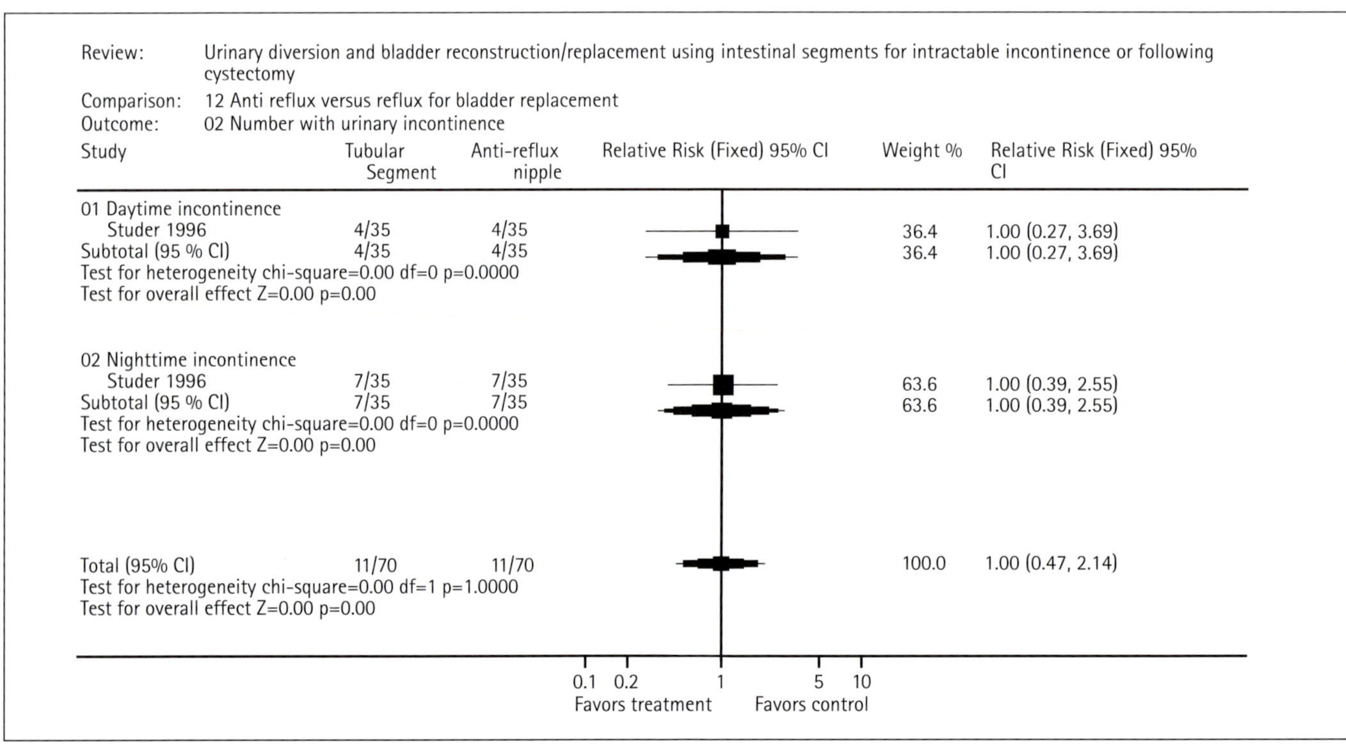

Figure 22.3 Relative risk of urinary incontinence following urinary diversion. (Reproduced from Yong SM et al. Cochrane Library. Issue 1, 2003.[36] © Cochrane Library. Reproduced with permission.)

evidence-based analysis has been unable to show a difference in quality of life terms between ileal conduit and orthotopic bladder.[36]

Future directions

Because gastrointestinal segments can lead to the complications of metabolic disturbances, urolithiasis, increased mucus and the potential for malignancy, recent experimental work has tried to produce tissue-engineering techniques to create functional new bladder segments. Donor tissue is dissociated into individual cells, which are implanted directly into the host or expanded in culture, attached to a support matrix and reimplanted after expansion. The implanted tissue can be heterologous, allogenic or autologous.[37] The supporting matrix is composed of biodegradable artificial or natural polymers that can allow cell survival by diffusion of nutrients across short distances, once the cell-support matrix is implanted. The cell-support matrix becomes vascularized in concert with expansion of the cell mass after implantation. A system of urothelial cell harvest where cells are expanded until the desired numbers are obtained is employed. Using this method it is possible to expand a urothelial strain from a single specimen which initially covers a surface area of 1 cm to one covering a surface area of 4202 m within 8 weeks.[38] The urothelial and muscle cells can be expanded in vitro, seeded onto the polymer scaffold and allowed to attach and form sheets of cells. The cell polymer scaffold can then be implanted in vivo. To address the function of tissue-engineered bladders, an animal model has been designed which requires a subtotal cystectomy and subsequent replacement with a tissue-engineered organ. In a trial, 14 beagle dogs underwent trigone-sparing cystectomy: the animals were randomly assigned to one of three groups. Urodynamics were undertaken serially before and after surgery, and animals killed at 1, 2, 3, 4, 6 and 11 months after surgery and gross, histologic and immunocytochemical analyses were done. In dogs in whom a bladder was reconstructed the mean bladder capacity retained 95% of its original volume and showed no difference in compliance Histologic differentiation was maintained and immunostaining indicated the presence of neural structures. Within the bladder, the results indicated that it is possible to tissue-engineer bladders which are anatomically and functionally normal.[39] It is hoped engineered bladder tissues will prove safe and effective; clinical trials are in progress and although exciting it will be some time before the long-term clinical validity of these techniques can been assessed.

Summary

By studying the historical development of orthotopic bladder and understanding the underlying scientific principles, patients can be counseled preoperatively about the expected outcomes from such a procedure. When problems do arise, videourodynamics help classify the underlying problem as predominantly bladder contraction or retention, or sphincter-related or a combination of both and will help direct appropriate the secondary therapy – be it educational, pharmacologic, surgical or catheterization.

References

1. Tizzoni G, Poggi A. Die Widerherstellung der Harnblase. Experimentale Untersuchungen. Zentrabl Chir 1888; 15: 921–4.
2. Camey M, Le Duc A. Le enteroplasty après cystoprostattectomie total pour cancer de la vesi. Eur Urol 1979; 13: 114–23.
3. Camey M, Richard F, Botto H. Ileal replacement of bladder In: King LR, Stone AR, Webster GD (eds). Bladder Reconstruction and Continent Urinary Diversion, 2nd edn. Chicago: Mosby Yearbook, 1991: 398–410.
4. Hautmann RE, Miller K, Steiner U, Wenderoth U. The ileal neobladder: six years of experience with more than 200 patients. J Urol 1993; 150: 40–5.
5. Ghoneim MA, Shaban AA, Mahran MR, Kock NG. Further experience with the urethral Kock pouch. J Urol 1992; 147: 361–5.
6. Beduk Y, Turkolmez K, Baltaci S, Gogus C. Comparison of clinical and urodynamic outcome in orthotopic ileocaecal and ileal neobladder. Eur Urol 2003; 43: 258–62.
7. Light JK, Marks JL. Total bladder replacement in the male and female using the ileo-colonic segment (Le Bag). Br J Urol 1990; 65: 467–72.
8. Kolettis PN, Klein EA, Novick AC, Winters JC, Appell RA. The Le Bag orthotopic urinary diversion. J Urol 1996; 156: 926–30.
9. Goldwasser B. Bladder replacement. In: Glenn JF, and Graham SD (eds.) Urologic Surgery, 4th edn. Philadelphia: JB Lipincott, 1991: 1059–67.
10. Reddy PK. The colonic neobladder. Urol Clin North Am 1991; 18: 4.
11. Lin DW, Santucci RA, Mayo ME, Lange PH, Mitchell ME. Urodynamic evaluation and long term results of the orthotopic gastric neobladder in men. J Urol 2000; 164: 356–9.
12. Santucci RA, Park CH, Mayo ME, Lange PH. Continence and urodynamic parameters of continent urinary reservoirs: comparison of gastric, ileal, ileocolic, right colon and sigmoid segments. Urology 1999; 54: 252–7.
13. Lee KS, Montie JE, Dunn RL, Lee CT. Hautmann and Studer orthotopic neobladders: a contempary experience. J Urol 2003: 169: 2188–91.
14. Colding-Jorgensen M, Poulsen AL, Steven K. Mechanical characteristics of tubular and detubularised bowel for bladder substitution: theory, urodynamics and clinical results. Br J Urol 1993: 72: 586–93.
15. Colding-Jorgensen M, Nordling J and Steven K. A model for the plasticity of soft tissues. In: Mosekilde E (ed.) Proceedings of First Copenhagen Symposium on Computer Simulation in Biology, Ecology and Medicine. Copenhagen, 1993; 153–7.

16. PJ Thomas, NM De Souza, AR Mundy. The effects of detubularisation and outflow competence in substitution cystoplasty. Br J Urol 1996; 78: 681–5.
17. Nikolaev VV. Perimesenteric detubularisation of ileum for ileocystoplasty improves compliance and increases capacity. BJU Int 2001; 88: 577–80.
18. Mouriquand PD, Sheard R, Phillips N et al. The Kropp-onlay procedure (Pippi Salle procedure): a simplification of the technique of urethral lengthening. Preliminary results in eight patients. Br J Urol 1995; 75: 656–62.
19. Studer UE, Gerber E, Springer J, Zing EJ. Bladder reconstruction with bowel after radical cystectomy. World J Urol 1992; 10: 11–19.
20. Steers WD. Voiding dysfunction in the orthotopic neobladder. World J Urol 2000; 18: 330–7.
21. Faussone-Pellegrini MS, Seni S, Carini M. Distribution of ICC and motor response characteristics in urinary bladders reconstructed from human ileum. Am J Physiol 1997; 273: 147–57.
22. Batra AK, Hanno PM, Ruggieri MR. Detubularization-induced contractile response change of the ileum following ileocystoplasty. J Urol 1992; 148: 195–9.
23. Tammela TL, Kiiholma PJ, Chancellor MB. Effects of atropine, glucagons and bethanechol on urodynamics of continent cecal urinary resevoir before and after complete, partial and sham detubularizations in dog. Neurol Urodyn 1993; 12: 81–9.
24. Hohenfellner M, Burger R, Schad H et al. Resevoir characteristics of Mainz pouch studied in animal model. Osmolality of filling solution and effect of oxybutynin. Urology 1993; 42: 741–6.
25. Strasser H, Kilma G, Poisel S et al. Anatomy and innervation of the rhabdosphincter of the male urethra. Prostate 1996; 28: 24–31.
26. Katazaki H, Koyangi T, Kars M. Sympathetic innervation of the female feline urethra rhabdosphincter. Neurosci Lett 1991; 129: 165–7.
27. Borirakchanyavat S, Aboseif SR, Carroll PR et al. Continence mechanism of the isolated female urethra: an anatomical study of the intrapelvic somatic nerves. J Urol 1997; 158: 827–9.
28. Gosling JA, Dixon JS, Humphreys JR. The Functional Anatomy of the Lower Urinary Tract. Edinburgh: Churchill Livingstone, 1983.
29. Park JM, Montie JE. Mechanisms of incontinence and retention after orthotopic neobladder diversion. Urology 1998; 51: 601–9.
30. Madersbacher S, Mohrloe K, Burkhard F, Studer UE. Long term voiding pattern of patients with ileal orthotopic bladder substitutes. J Urol 2002; 157: 2052–7.
31. Studer UE, Zingg EJ. Ileal orthotopic bladder substitute. What have we learned from 12 years experience with 200 patients. Urol Clin North Am 1997; 24: 781–800.
32. O'Connor RC, Kuznetsov DD, Patel RV et al. Artificial urinary sphincter placement in men after cystectomy with orthotopic ileal neobladder: continence, complications and quality of life. Urology 2002; 59: 542–5.
33. Aboseif SR, Borirakchanyavat S, Lue TF, Carroll PR. Continence mechanism of the ileal neobladder in women: a urodynamics study. World J Urol 1998; 16: 400–4.
34. Hautmann RE, Paiss T, De Petriconi R. The ileal neobladder in women: 9 years experience with 18 patients. J Urol 1996; 155: 76–81.
35. Mills RD, Studer UE. Female orthotopic bladder substitution: a good operation in the right circumstances. J Urol 2000; 163: 1501-4.
36. Yong SM, Dublin N, Pickard R et al. Urinary diversion and bladder reconstruction/replacement using intestinal segments for intractable incontinence or following cystectomy. Cochrane Library, Issue 1, Oxford, 2003.
37. Atala A. Tissue engineering in the genitourinary system. In Atala A, Mooney D (eds), Tissue Engineering. Boston: Birkhauser Press, 1997: 149.
38. Cliento BG, Freeman MR, Schneck FX, Retik AB, Atala A. Phenotypic and cytogenetic characterization of human bladder urothelial expanded in vitro. J Urol 1994; 152: 665–70.
39. Oberpenning FO, Meng J, Yoo J Atala A. De novo reconstitution of a functional urinary bladder by tissue engineering. Nature 1999; 17: 149–55.

23 The continent Kock and T-pouch reservoirs: crossover techniques

John P Stein and Donald G Skinner

Introduction

Over the past 25 years, dedicated efforts have been made continually to improve upon lower urinary tract reconstruction in patients requiring urinary diversion following removal of their bladder. The goals of urinary diversion have evolved from simply diverting the urine and protecting the upper urinary tracts. Contemporary objectives of urinary diversion should provide a continent means to store and eliminate urine in an effort to provide a socially improved quality of life. Currently, there are four potential options regarding lower urinary tract reconstruction:

- Incontinent cutaneous diversion – including the ileal or colon conduit
- continent cutaneous reservoir – requiring catheterization of a cutaneous abdominal wall stoma
- continent rectal reservoir – with elimination of urine via the rectum
- orthotopic bladder substitute – with reconstruction to the native intact urethra.

In 1950, Bricker's introduction of the ileal conduit established a simple and reliable form of urinary diversion.[1] This form of urinary diversion remained, even until the early 1990s, the 'gold standard' with which other forms of urinary diversion were compared. Concurrent with Bricker's establishment of the ileal conduit, Gilchrist et al independently reported on the concept of a continent cutaneous form of urinary reconstruction.[2] This urinary diversion utilized the ileocecal valve as the continence mechanism, and the distal ileum as a catheterizable stoma. While technical reasons prevented the popularization of Gilchrist's ileocecal reservoir, the simpler Bricker ileal conduit became the urinary diversion of choice for the next several decades.

The concept of a continent cutaneous urinary diversion was eventually popularized in the 1980s at several large academic institutions.[3–5] These experiences revolutionized lower urinary tract reconstruction from a wet stoma, such as the ileal conduit, to a continent cutaneous form of urinary diversion. Patients were relieved from the issues of an external collection device, however catheterization of an abdominal wall stoma was still required. Although these continent cutaneous urinary diversions were technically a more challenging form of urinary reconstruction, they were considered an improvement upon the standard ileal conduit.

A natural progression of the continent cutaneous urinary diversion was the orthotopic bladder substitute – anastomosed directly to the native intact urethra.[6–11] The orthotopic neobladder most closely resembles the original bladder in both location and function. This form of lower urinary tract reconstruction now eliminated the need for a cutaneous abdominal wall stoma and a cutaneous collection device. Orthotopic bladder substitution relies on the patient's intact rhabdosphincter continence mechanism (external striated sphincter muscle). It eliminates the need for intermittent catheterization and the often plagued efferent continence mechanism of most continent cutaneous reservoirs. Voiding is therefore accomplished by concomitantly increasing intra-abdominal pressure (Valsalva) with relaxation of the pelvic floor musculature. The majority of male and female patients undergoing orthotopic reconstruction are continent and void to completion without the need for intermittent catheterization.[11,12]

Two important criteria must be fulfilled when considering patients for orthotopic urinary diversion. First, if an exenteration is performed for a pelvic malignancy, the cancer operation must not be compromised by the reconstruction at the urethroenteric anastomosis, retained urethra or surgical margins. Second, the rhabdosphincter mechanism should be competent and remain intact following surgery to provide a continent means of storing urine. If these criteria can safely be maintained, both male and female patients may be considered appropriate candidates for orthotopic urinary diversion. From an oncologic perspective, it has been our practice to perform intraoperative frozen-section analysis of the proximal urethra just distal to the prostate apex in men and distal to the bladder neck in women. If no tumor or high-grade dysplasia are demonstrated pathologically at this time orthotopic reconstruction can be performed safely with a low risk of a urethral recurrence in most patients.[6]

Evolution of the intussuscepted Kock nipple and T-mechanism

Over the past 25 years, an important component in the evolution of urinary diversion has been the development of a reliable and durable means to provide continence (via a catheterizable stoma) and prevent the reflux of the urinary constituents, in order to protect the upper urinary tract. The intussuscepted nipple valve was one technique that satisfied these goals.[12] With a growing body of experience and longer follow-up, it became clear that complications existed with this technique and improvements upon the intussuscepted nipple valve were needed.[13–17] The widespread application of the intussuscepted nipple was therefore, limited primarily to academic institutions with large clinical experience in lower urinary tract reconstruction. In 1993, Abol-Enein and Ghoneim reported their experimental[18] and subsequent early clinical experience on a novel concept employing an extramural serous-lined tunnel for reflux prevention.[19,20] Based upon this concept and the success of the serous-lined extramural tunnel, the notion of the T-mechanism was developed at the University of Southern California (USC).[21]

The theory of an intussuscepted nipple valve mechanism to provide continence at the skin level, and to prevent reflux of urine dates back to the pioneering work of Perl in 1949.[22] He described an intussuscepted jejunal nipple to provide jejunostomy feedings with an inserted catheter while preventing the associated skin maceration with so-called incontinent jejunostomies. Perl also recognized the importance of an intraluminal valve location that would maintain continence with increasing intraluminal pressures by concomitantly increasing coaptation of the walls of the intussuscepted intraluminal nipple valve.

Basso's experimental work with the intussuscepted valve in 1951 resulted in the clinical application of this nipple to prevent ascending cholangitis following duodenal or pancreatic resections in which the sphincter of Oddi was sacrificed.[23] Furthermore, he performed the initial experimental work demonstrating urologic application of the intussuscepted nipple for reflux prevention in a ureteroileosigmoidostomy. This concept of ureteral intussusception was subsequently applied directly to the ureter by Mathisen[24] in 1953, and confirmed by Grey and associates in 1957.[25] During this same time period, tunneled antireflux techniques gained popularity and the enthusiasm for the intussuscepted ureter dissipated.

The application of the intussuscepted ileum for continence in a cutaneous urinary diversion was first reported by Smith and Hinman in 1955.[26] Elegant experimental studies were performed comparing various cutaneous continence mechanisms including an antiperistaltic ileal segment, the ileocecal valve, and an intussuscepted ileal nipple valve. It was demonstrated that the ileocecal valve and the ileal intussusception techniques successfully provided appropriate continence. These procedures were then applied to pediatric patients with neurogenic bladders requiring catheterization of the continent stoma.

The most recognizable pioneer in the development and clinical application of the intussuscepted nipple valve was Dr Nils Kock. In 1973, Kock successfully reported on 37 patients with inflammatory or neoplastic diseases of the colon who had undergone creation of a continent detubularized ileostomy reservoir employing the intussuscepted nipple valve as the catheterizable limb.[27] The concept of detubularization of the bowel to provide a low-pressure urinary reservoir, without peristaltic pressure waves was subsequently validated urodynamically.[28] This landmark experience paved the way for the continent Kock ileal urinary diversion.

In 1982, Kock subsequently published the initial results of the continent ileal reservoir (Kock pouch) with the intussuscepted nipple mechanism in 12 patients for a cutaneous urinary diversion.[3] Importantly, this was the first report in which the concepts of modern day continent urinary diversion were applied: detubularization and folding of the bowel into a sphere to provide a low-pressure, large capacity reservoir with an antireflux mechanism to protect the upper urinary tracts and a continent catheterizable stoma.

Beginning in 1982, the continent Kock ileal reservoir became the primary form of urinary diversion at our institution.[5,29] The continence and antireflux mechanism in this ileal reservoir required construction of intussuscepted nipple valves as described by Kock. The evolution of the orthotopic neobladder was a direct result of the success of the continent cutaneous reservoir, as well as a need to eliminate the need to catheterize an abdominal stoma. In 1986, the orthotopic Kock ileal neobladder became the procedure of choice in selected male[7] patients undergoing cystectomy and subsequently, in 1990 was successfully applied to women[30] with excellent functional results.

Throughout this period, significant technical advances and improvements in lower urinary tract reconstruction have been made. We have been committed to the concept of the Kock ileal reservoir and reflux prevention in all patients with continent urinary diversions. Although the principles of the continent Kock ileal reservoir (cutaneous and orthotopic form) are sound, complications can occur.[13–17] Most complications associated with the Kock ileal reservoir involve the intussuscepted nipple (valve): either the antirefluxing (afferent limb) nipple or the continent catheterizable (efferent limb) nipple.

An extensive review of the Kock ileal reservoir at USC demonstrated a 10% complication rate associated with the intussuscepted antireflux nipple in over 800 patients (undergoing either a continent cutaneous or orthotopic Kock ileal reservoir).[17] The most common complications associated with the intussuscepted afferent nipple included: (i) the formation of pouch calculi (usually on exposed staples that secure the afferent nipple valve) in 5%, (ii) afferent nipple stenosis (thought to be caused by ischemic changes resulting from the mesenteric stripping required to maintain the intussuscepted limb) in 4% and (iii) extussusception (prolapse of the afferent limb) in 1% of patients.[17] Although the majority of these afferent nipple valve complications (60%) can be managed with endoscopic techniques, they nonetheless result in some morbidity. In fact, approximately 3% of all patients undergoing a continent Kock ileal reservoir will require an open surgical revision to repair an afferent nipple-associated complication.[17]

The need to improve upon the intussuscepted nipple valve was obvious. Based on reports from Abol-Enein and Ghoneim[18–20] employing a ureteral extramural serous-lined tunnel, as well as our own experience with the Mitrofanoff appendiceal extramural serous-lined technique,[31] we subsequently developed and described a novel extramural, serous-lined ileal flap valve method called the T-mechanism.[21,32] This flap valve T-mechanism can be applied as a continence, as well as an antireflux technique. This technique was first successfully incorporated into an afferent antireflux limb of an orthotopic reservoir (T-pouch)[21] and subsequently into an afferent antireflux and efferent continence limb of a cutaneous reservoir (double-T-pouch).[32] The application of the flap valve T-mechanism should help eliminate the complications associated with the intussuscepted nipple valve while maintaining an effective antireflux or continence mechanism.

The concepts and principles of the continent Kock ileal reservoir are logical and ultimately paved the way for the development of the T-mechanism. The implementation of the T-mechanism in continent urinary diversion may represent a small step forward in the evolution of lower urinary tract reconstruction. It would be beneficial for surgeons dedicated to lower urinary tract reconstruction to be familiar with both techniques (intussuscepted nipple and T-mechanism) as they have considerable crossover. The continent cutaneous Kock ileal reservoir, the orthotopic Kock ileal reservoir, the orthotopic T-pouch and the continent cutaneous double-T-pouch will be described in this chapter.

Preoperative preparation

Patients undergoing radical cystectomy are admitted the morning prior to surgery for a mechanical and antibacterial bowel preparation, intravenous hydration, and to be evaluated and counseled by the enterostomal therapy nurse. A clear liquid diet may be consumed until midnight, at which time the patient takes nil by mouth. A standard modified Nichols bowel prep[33] is initiated the morning of admission: 120 ml of Neoloid orally at 9:00 am; 1 g of neomycin orally at 10:00 am, 11:00 am, 12:00 pm, 1:00 pm, 4:00 pm, 8:00 pm and 12:00 am; and 1 g of erythromycin base orally at 12:00 pm, 4:00 pm, 8:00 pm and 12:00 am. This regimen is well tolerated, obviates the need for enemas, and maintains nutritional and hydrational support. Intravenous crystalloid fluid hydration is begun in the evening prior to surgery, and maintained to ensure an adequate circulating volume as the patient enters the operating room. In addition, intravenous broad-spectrum antibiotics are administered en route to the operating room, providing adequate tissue and circulating levels at the time of incision.

Preoperative evaluation and counseling by the enterostomal therapy nurse is a critical component of the successful care of all patients undergoing cystectomy and urinary diversion. Patients determined to be appropriate candidates for orthotopic reconstruction are instructed how to catheterize per urethra should it be necessary postoperatively. Regardless, all patients are site marked for a cutaneous stoma, instructed in the care of a cutaneous diversion (continent or incontinent form), and instructed in proper catheterization techniques should medical or technical factors preclude orthotopic reconstruction. The ideal cutaneous stoma site is determined only after the patient is examined in the supine, sitting and standing position. Proper stoma site selection is important for patient acceptance, and to the technical success of lower urinary tract reconstruction should a cutaneous form of diversion be necessary. In general, incontinent stoma sites are best located higher on the abdominal wall, while stoma sites for continent diversions can be positioned lower on the abdomen (hidden below the belt line) since they do not require an external collecting device. Furthermore, the umbilicus is also an ideal catheterizable stoma site which is cosmetically very pleasing.

Continent cutaneous Kock ileal reservoir

Most patients undergoing continent urinary diversion have bladder cancer and undergo the cystectomy portion of the procedure initially. Identification of the appropriate segment of ileum for the pouch begins by identifying the avascular plane of Treves between the terminal branches of the superior mesenteric artery and the ileocolic artery. The mesentery is divided deep into the base which allows adequate mobility for the reservoir. This is an important step in both the continent cutaneous and the orthotopic reconstruction when incorporating ileum to construct the pouch to allow for proper mobility. The segments of ileum utilized for the specific components of the reservoir are then measured and marked with silk sutures for the cutaneous Kock ileal reservoir: 17 cm for the efferent nipple, two 22-cm segments for the reservoir portion, and a second proximal 17-cm segment for the afferent antireflux nipple. A more proximal 5-cm segment of ileum is discarded with a wedge of mesentery to provide mobility to the reservoir and for the small bowel anastomosis. Note, the proximal mesenteric division is very shallow, maintaining the blood supply to the reservoir (Figure 23.1).

The proximal end of the ileum (afferent limb) is then closed with a running Parker-Kerr suture (3-0 chromic) and a third layer of imbricating seromuscular layer (3-0 silk). The small-bowel anastomosis is then completed, and the mesenteric window closed anterior and cephalad to the ileum isolated for the reservoir.

The reservoir portion (two 22-cm segments) is then laid out in a 'U' fashion, with the apex directed in a caudal direction. The serosal walls of the 22-cm segments are reapproximated to each other with 3-0 polyglycolic acid (PGA) sutures (Figure 23.2). The bowel is then opened adjacent to the suture line, and for an additional 1–2 cm proximally and 3 cm distally along the nipple valve limbs to facilitate the intussusception later on. This posterior mucosal incision is then oversewn in two layers with a continuous 3-0 PGA suture. This suture line forms the posterior wall of the reservoir.

The intussuscepted nipples are then constructed in similar fashion. The mesentery of the wings of ileum proximal and distal to the pouch are divided for about 5 cm and 7–8 cm (windows of Deaver), respectively (Figure 23.3). This maneuver reduces the amount of mesenteric fat adhering to the bowel wall which facilitates the intussusception of the limbs and helps reduce issues of extussusception of the nipples later on. Two or three vascular arcades are spared and a separate small window of Deaver is developed in the mesentery to allow passage of a 2–3-cm strip of tetracycline-soaked PGA mesh. This mesh will serve as an anchoring collar at the base of both nipple valves.

The nipple valves are then intussuscepted into the reservoir by passing two Allis clamps approximately two-thirds of the way into the lumen of the ileal limb toward the PGA mesh. The mucosa is grasped with the clamps and then drawn toward the reservoir. A third Allis clamp on the cut edge of the ileum facilitates the intussusception (Figure 23.4). The nipples are then secured with three parallel rows of permanent staples. This can be done with a standard TA55 stapler, or with a custom-made non-cutting GIA device (no knife). Two rows of staples should be placed in the anterior 180° of the nipple (Figure 23.5). Care should be taken to use the full length of the stapler to obtain appropriate nipple length. If a standard GIA device is used, two rows of staples should be manually removed in addition to the six staples from the base of the cartridge before use. This provides for two rows of staples at the base of the nipple with no staples at the tip. We prefer the GIA over the TA55 stapling device because the TA55 requires a pin for proper staple alignment which may result in a fistula at the base of the intussusception. The third row secures the nipple to the back wall of the pouch, and is best applied from the outside the reservoir using a full cartridge. The tip of the nipple is then anchored and further secured to the back wall of the pouch (Figure 23.6).

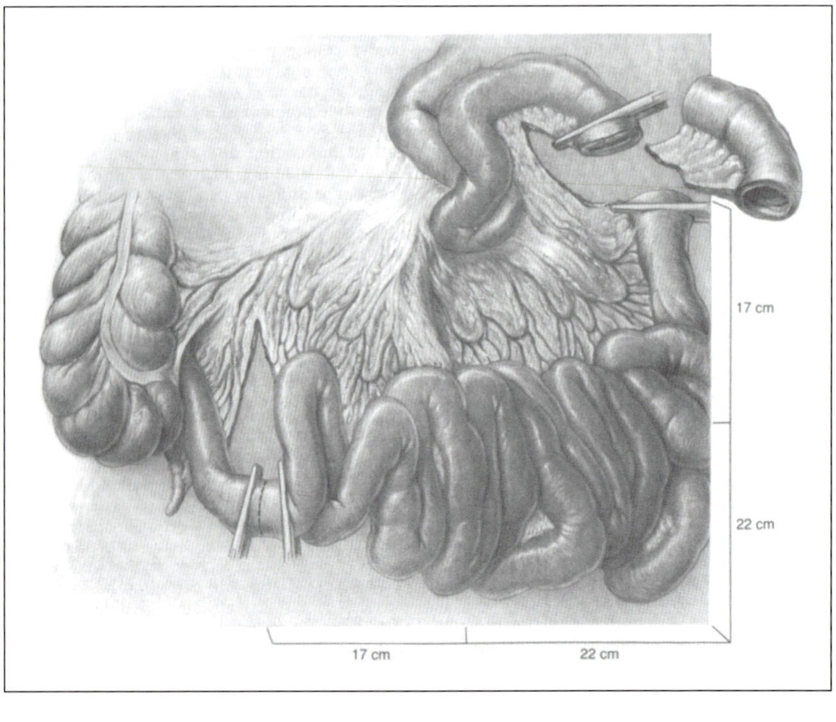

Figure 23.1 The bowel is divided distally in the avascular plane between the terminal branches of the superior mesenteric artery and the ileocolic artery. The segments for the cutaneous Kock ileal reservoir are identified: 17 cm for the efferent nipple (distal segment), two 22-cm segments for the reservoir (middle segment), and another 17-cm segment for the antireflux nipple (proximal segment). Note that a 5-cm segment that is most proximal is discarded with a portion of the mesentery to provide mobility to the reservoir and allow for the small-bowel anastomosis.

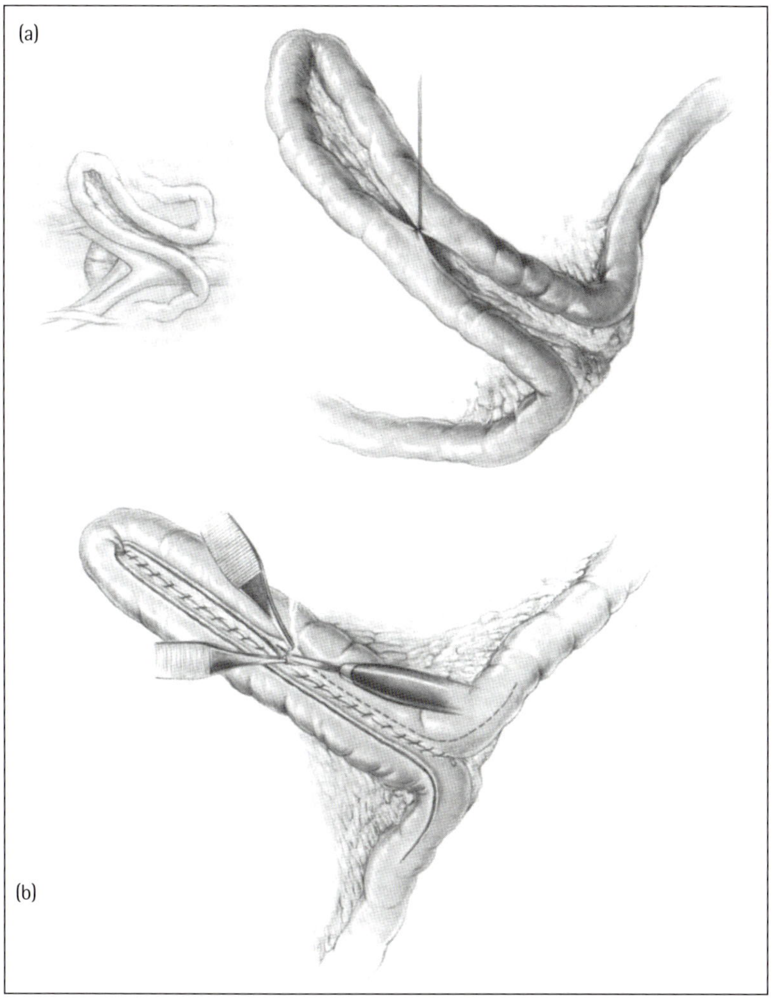

Figure 23.2 (a,b) The cutaneous Kock ileal reservoir is placed in a 'U' shape and the serosal walls of the 22-cm segments reapproximated 1 cm away from the mesenteric attachment to the bowel. The bowel is opened adjacent to this suture line and sutured in two layers to provide a watertight closure of the back wall.

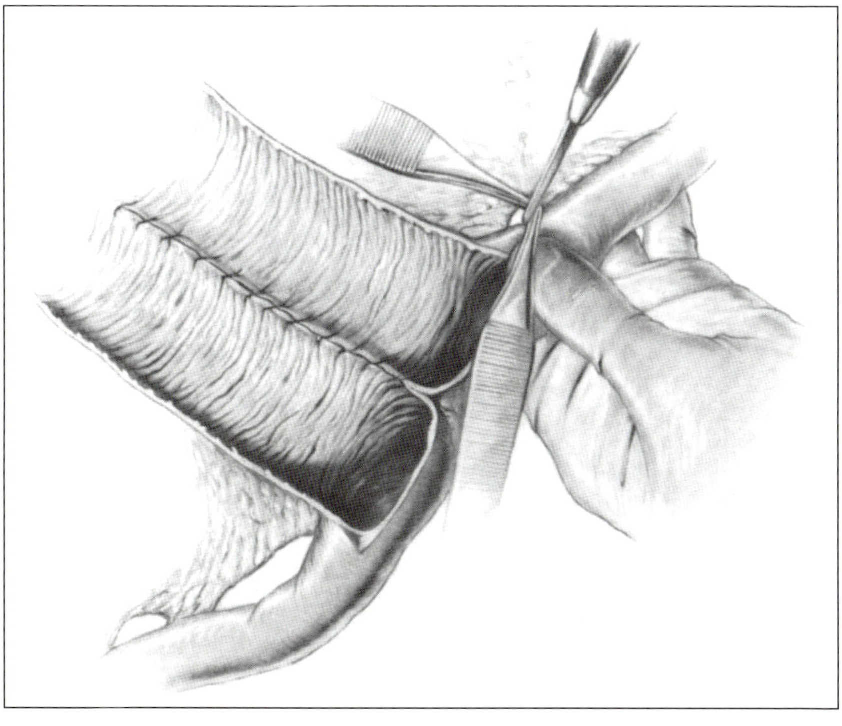

Figure 23.3 The windows of Deaver are developed by dividing the mesentery of the ileum proximal and distal to the pouch for 7–8 cm of the efferent nipple and slightly shorter (5–6 cm) for the afferent nipple. After two or three vascular arcades are spared, another small mesenteric opening is made to accommodate the PGA mesh that acts as an anchoring collar at the base of the nipple valves.

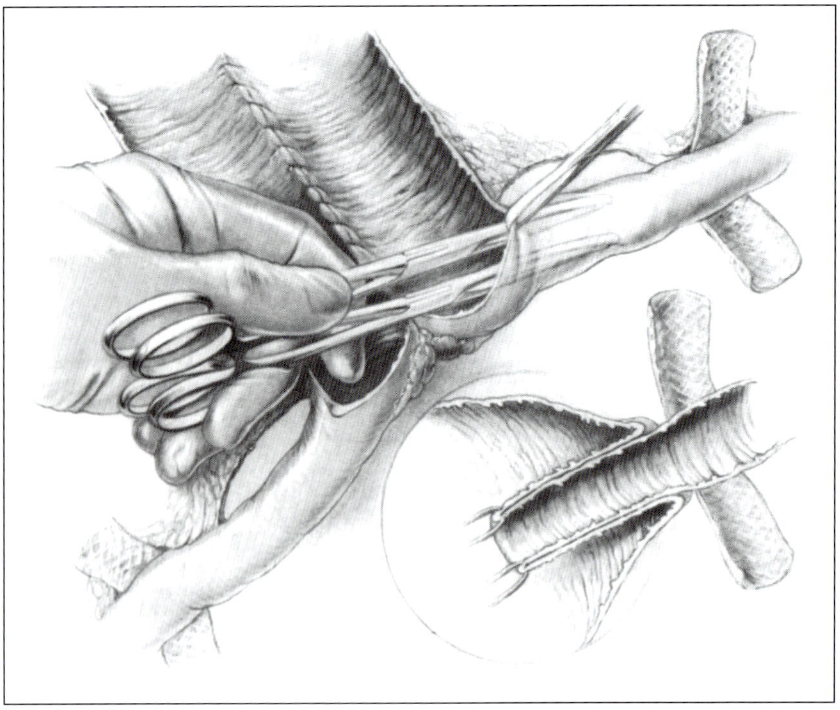

Figure 23.4 The nipple valves are intussuscepted into the reservoir lumen with Allis clamps. A third Allis clamp on the cut edge of the ileum will provide counter traction and facilitate the intussusception.

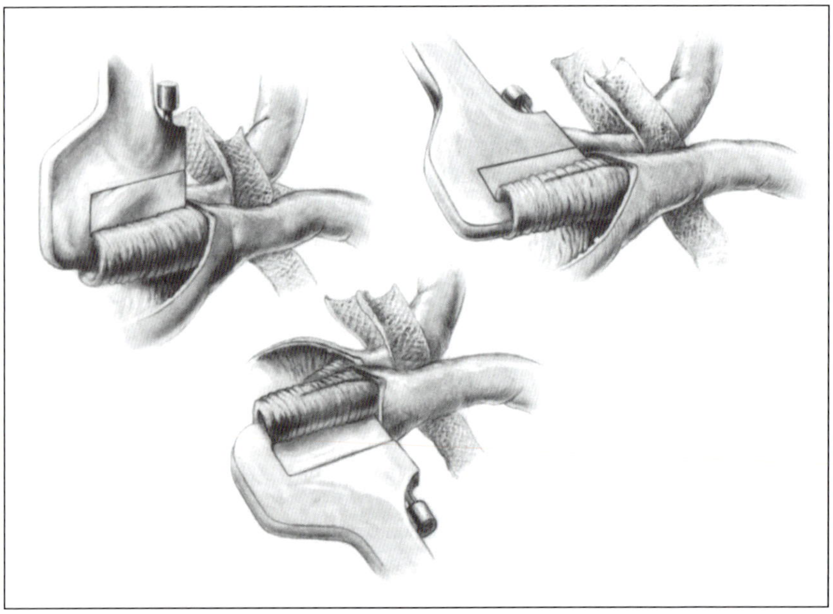

Figure 23.5 Two rows of staples are placed in the anterior 180° of the nipple lying in the lumen of the reservoir. Note the entire length of the nipple should be secured with the staple line. The custom made non-cutting GIA stapler (no knife) or a TA55 device can be used (as illustrated).

The final step in nipple fixation is suturing the PGA mesh collars circumferentially to the serosal base of the nipple (Figure 23.7). A 30-Fr Medina tube is passed up the nipple to act as a template and prevent the circumferential interrupted sutures from being placed too tightly. The excess mesh is excised, and the remaining mesh secured to the bowel serosa of both the reservoir and the ileal wing with 2-0 chromic sutures. Importantly, the mesh on the efferent limb will be integral in the later fixation of the catheterizable limb to the abdominal fascia.

After the nipples are constructed and secured, the anterior wall of the reservoir is closed. The cephalad portion of the 'U' is folded up and sutured to the free mucosal edge midway between the base of the nipples. This creates a spherical urinary reservoir allowing for large volumes under low pressure. A running 3-0 PGA suture is used to close the anterior wall in two

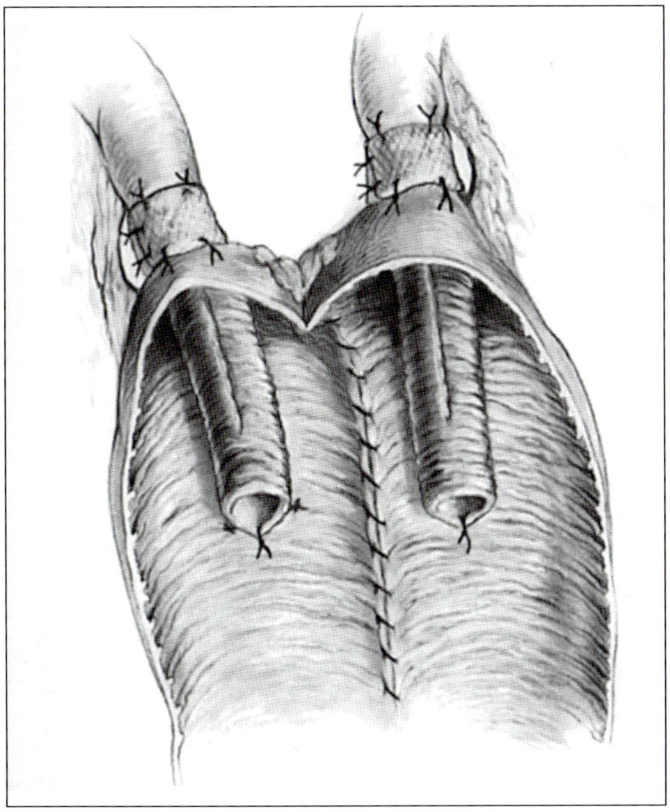

Figure 23.6 The intussuscepted nipples are further secured to the reservoir wall with a suture at the tip of the nipple to the pouch.

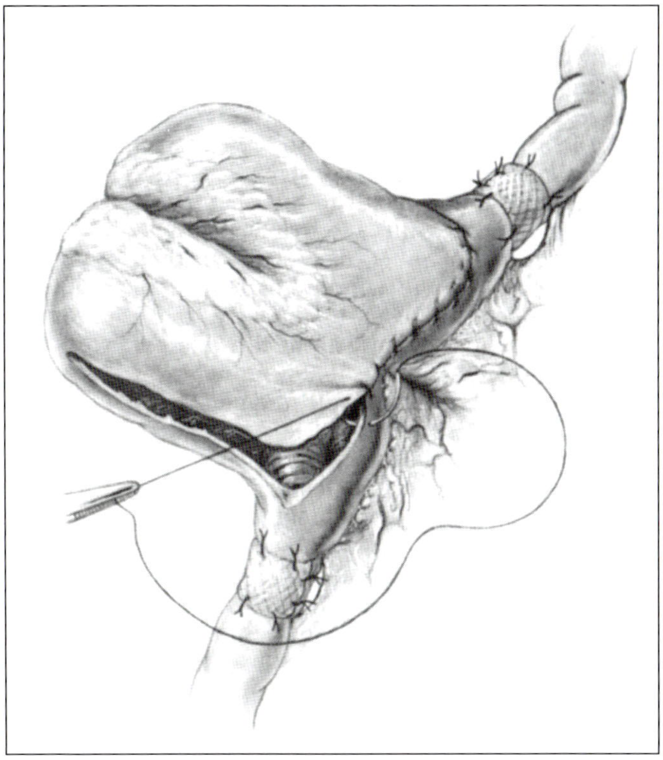

Figure 23.8 The reservoir is closed and rotated (a) so the afferent limb is orientated posteriorly toward the sacral promontory for the ureteral anastomoses and the efferent limb oriented anteriorly for the cutaneous stoma (b).

layers. Once the anterior wall is closed, the reservoir is rotated so the afferent limb points toward the sacral promontory for the ureteral anastomoses and the efferent limb rotates anteriorly for the cutaneous stoma (Figure 23.8).

The ureters are spatulated and anastomosed to the proximal portion of the afferent limb in an end-to-side fashion with 4-0 PGA sutures. The ureteroileal anastomoses are stented with no. 8 infant feeding tubes.

Attention is then directed to the cutaneous stoma. This portion of the procedure is most crucial to the patient on a day-to-day basis. Attention to surgical detail is important. A small skin plug is excised using the flat end of a 10 ml syringe plunger as a template. The anterior rectus fascia is incised vertically for 2–3 cm, and the rectus muscle split. The posterior rectus fascia is then incised in a similar manner. Three no. 1 PGA horizontal mattress sutures are placed through the anterior rectus fascia

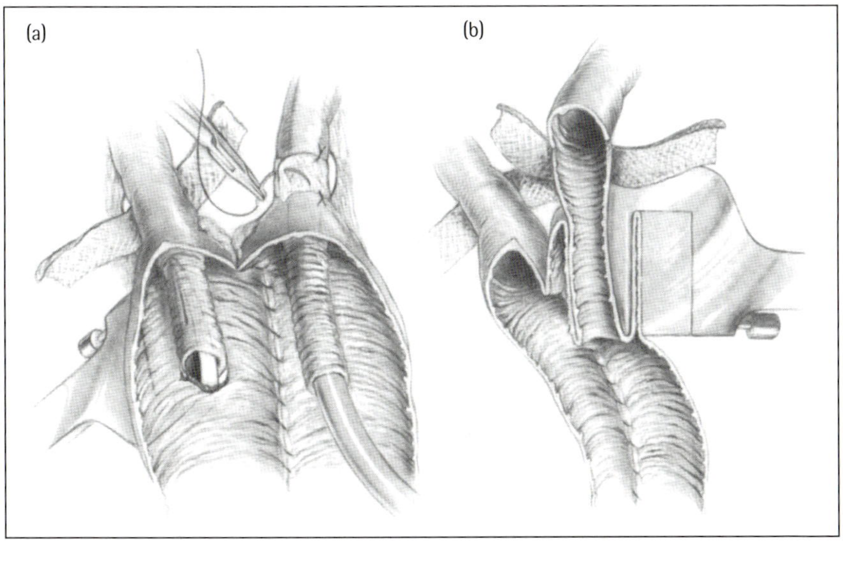

Figure 23.7 The back wall of the reservoir is anchored to the nipple incorporating either two (b) or three (a) layers of the bowel wall. This can be done with a non-cutting GIA (no knife) with the two-layered technique, or with the TA55 device as shown. Note, care must be taken to close enterotomies and pinholes to prevent fistula formation.

on the lateral, inferior and medial portions of the incision and affixed in their corresponding site on the PGA collar of the efferent limb (Figure 23.9). Care must be taken to assure that the sutures do not become crossed when passing them through the abdominal wall and securing them to the collar. The distal end of the efferent ileal limb is then brought through the stomal opening. The PGA sutures are tied down, which then secures the reservoir to the abdominal wall. Any excess ileum at the skin level is excised and a flush stoma is matured with circumferential 3-0 interrupted PGA sutures.

A 30-Fr Medina tube is then passed through the stoma into the reservoir and sutured in place at the skin level. This should irrigate freely without resistance. A Penrose drain is placed through a separate stab wound and positioned in a dependent portion of the abdomen and pelvis. The catheters and drain are kept in place for approximately 3 weeks.

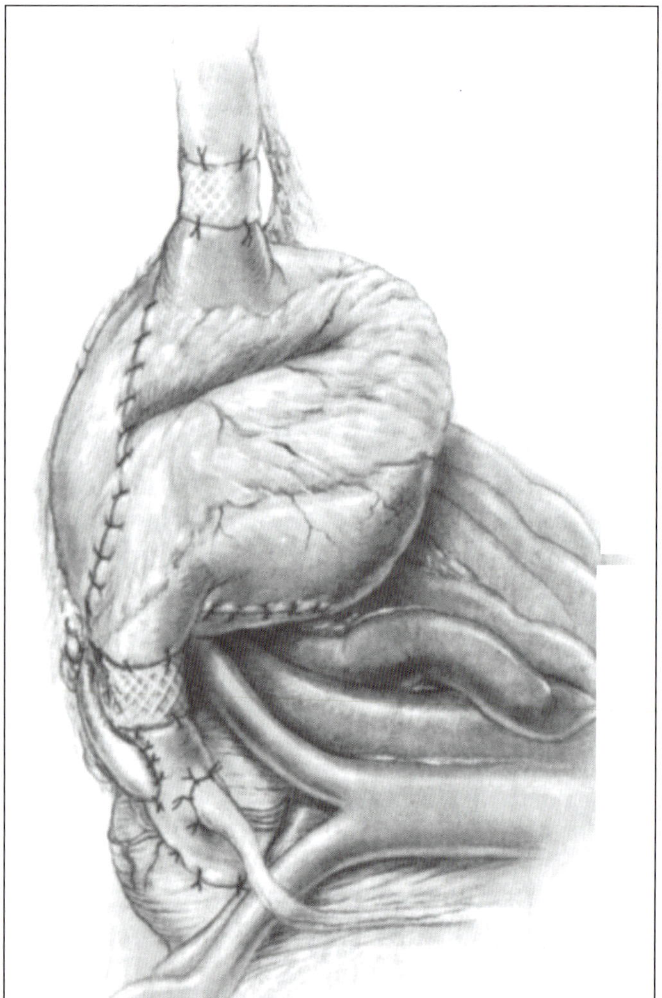

Figure 23.9 Fixation of the efferent limb for the cutaneous stoma. Note, the lateral and medial sutures (no. 1 PGA), and the PGA collar of the efferent limb to anchor these sutures. A Marlex strut (optional) can be used to further anchor the limb and help prevent mesenteric herniation.

Orthotopic Kock ileal reservoir

The orthotopic Kock ileal neobladder is constructed from approximately a 61-cm segment of terminal ileum (Figure 23.10). The reservoir portion of the neobladder is constructed from two 22-cm segments of distal ileum, and a single 17-cm segment of more proximal ileum is used to form the antireflux afferent nipple valve. The distal mesenteric division of the terminal ileum is performed along the avascular plane of Treves, between the ileocolic artery and the terminal ileal branches of the superior mesenteric artery, extending to the base of the small bowel mesentery. The proximal mesenteric division is short to ensure a broad vascular supply to the proximal ileal segment. A 5-cm portion of proximal ileum is discarded proximal to the overall segment in order to ensure adequate mobility of the pouch and the small bowel anastomosis. The proximal end of the isolated ileal segment is closed with a running Parker-Kerr suture (3-0 chromic) and imbricated with a layer of 3-0 silk sutures. The small bowel continuity is reestablished with a standard small bowel anastomosis and the mesenteric trap closed.

The two isolated 22-cm ileal segments are positioned adjacent to one another in a 'U' fashion with the apex again directed caudally (Figure 23.11a). The 22-cm ileal segments are again sewn together along the serosa (side-to-side) approximately 1 cm from the mesentery with a 3-0 PGA running suture. The ileum is opened just lateral to this serosal basting suture. The incised mucosa is approximated and over sewn the entire length with a 3-0 PGA suture in two layers (Figure11b). This suture line forms the posterior wall of the orthotopic reservoir.

Attention is then directed toward the proximal 17-cm ileal segment and construction of the intussuscepted afferent nipple valve. A windows of Deaver is developed along the afferent limb mesentery adjacent to the serosa of this proximal 17-cm segment. The mesentery is divided away from the pouch, extending for 5–6 cm. This is best performed with electrocautery. This helps prevent future prolapse or extussusception of the afferent nipple valve. One additional window of Deaver is created beyond the previously stripped mesentery, while preserving at least one vascular arcade in between. A 2.5-cm strip, tetracycline soaked, piece of doubled PGA mesh is then brought through this smaller window. This mesh will serve as an anchoring collar at the base of the nipple valve.

The intussuscepted antireflux afferent nipple valve is then created similarly described for the cutaneous Kock ileal reservoir (Figure 11c). The afferent nipple is intussuscepted by passing two Allis clamps toward the anchoring collar, grasping the mucosa, and inverting the ileum into the pouch. This positions the mesh adjacent to the wall of the pouch at the base of the intussuscepted nipple. Next, two single rows of parallel 4.8-mm non-hemostatic staples (applied with a custom no-knife GIA50 stapler), with the proximal four staples removed from each row, are applied to the medial and anterior aspect of the nipple. A third parallel staple line is applied from outside the pouch between the posterior wall of the pouch along the mesenteric border and one layer of the intussuscepted nipple (applied with

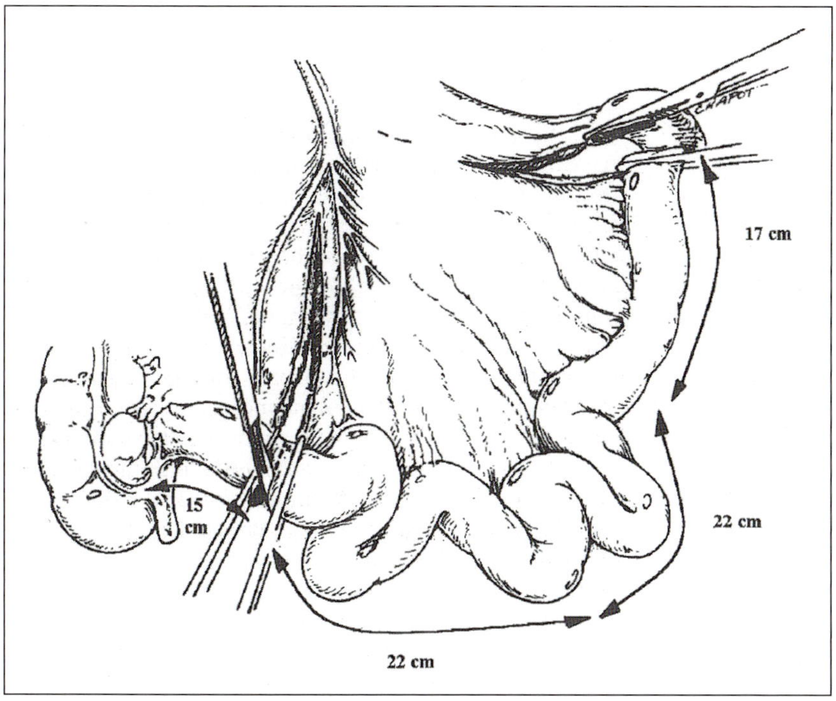

Figure 23.10 The ileal segment used to construct the orthotopic Kock ileal reservoir. A total of 61 cm of ileum is required in the construction including: two 22-cm segments for the reservoir portion of the pouch and a proximal 17-cm segment for the intussuscepted afferent nipple valve.

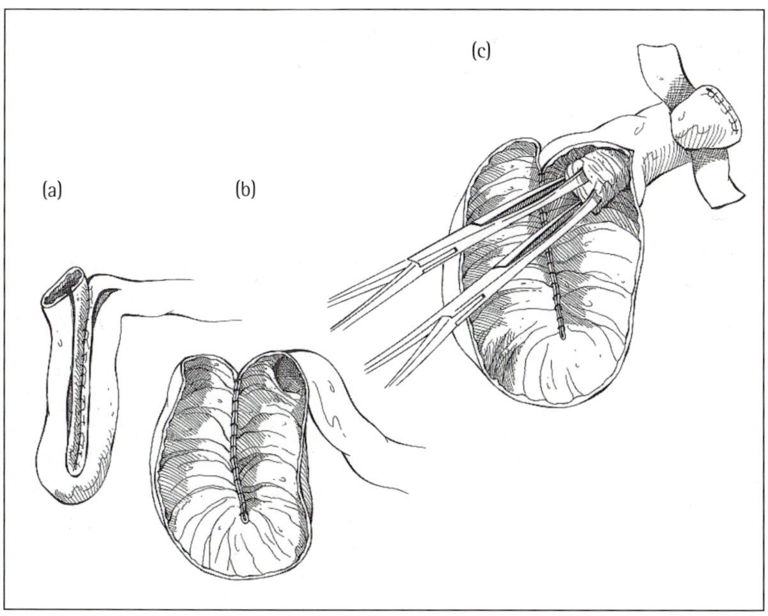

Figure 23.11 Creation of the orthotopic Kock ileal reservoir. (a) The two 22-cm segments are approximated in a 'U' formation with a serosal basting suture 1 cm from the mesentery. The ileum is opened with electrocautery adjacent to this basting suture line. (b) The posterior wall of the reservoir is sutured in two layers. (c) A 5–7-cm antireflux nipple valve is created by intussusception of the afferent limb with Allis clamps.

a TA55 stapling device). The pinhole created by the TA55 is over sewn from within the pouch to prevent formation of a fistula. This maneuver effectively fixes the afferent nipple valve to the posterior wall of the reservoir. The anchoring PGA mesh collar is fixed to the base of the afferent nipple valve and reservoir. The mesh is circumferentially sutured (over a 30-Fr catheter) to the serosa at the base of the nipple with 2-0 chromic suture. This helps prevent prolapse of the nipple valve.

The reservoir is closed by folding the ileum in the opposite direction back onto itself, creating a totally detubularized reservoir. The anterior aspect of the pouch is closed in two layers with 3-0 PGA sutures in a watertight fashion. It should be noted that the anterior suture line is stopped just prior to reaching the end of the right side, allowing easy entry of one finger into the neourethra (Figure 23.12). This is the most mobile and dependent portion of the reservoir and will be the portion of the reservoir anastomosed to the native urethra.

The ureteroileal anastomosis is then completed, end-to-side, with interrupted 4-0 PGA sutures. The ureters are again stented with no. 8 pediatric feeding tubes. In the orthotopic

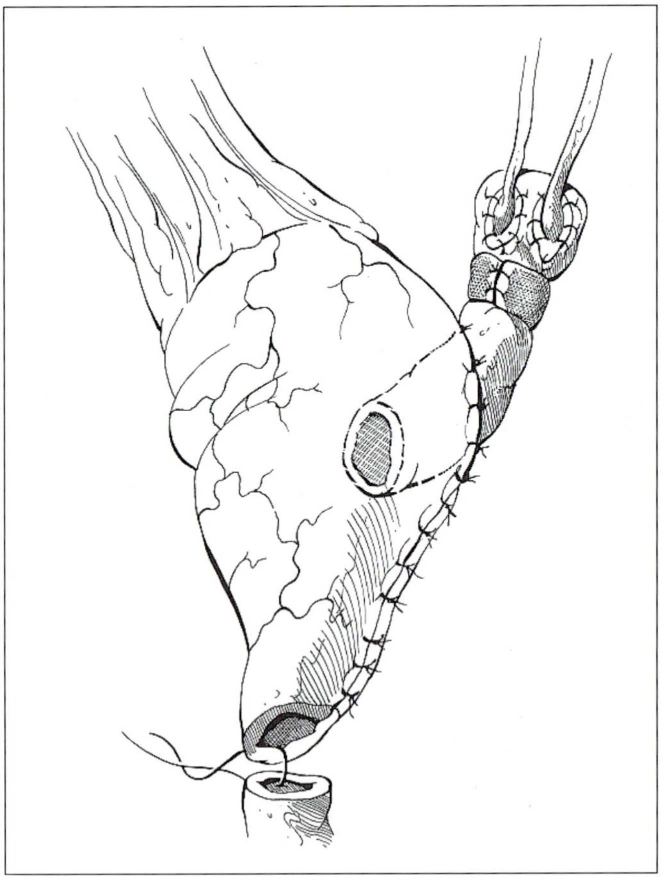

Figure 23.12 After the afferent valve is constructed the reservoir is completed by folding the ileum upon itself in an opposite direction to which it was opened. The most dependent portion is left open for the urethral anastomosis. Note the ureteroileal anastomosis is completed prior to the urethral anastomosis.

Kock ileal reservoir, these feeding tubes will be sutured to a 24-Fr hematuria catheter which is passed per urethra and positioned into the pouch. The urethral sutures (placed at the time of cystectomy) are placed into the neobladder and tied down to form a tension-free, mucosa-to-mucosa, urethroileal anastomosis. The pelvis is drained by a one-inch Penrose drain for 3 weeks and removed along with the urethral catheter and stents at that time.

Orthotopic T-pouch ileal neobladder

The terminal portion of the ileum is used to construct the orthotopic T-pouch ileal neobladder (Figure 23.13). Similarly as in the Kock ileal reservoir, the distal mesenteric division is made along the avascular plane of Treves between the ileocolic artery and terminal branches of the superior mesenteric artery. This division should extend deep into the avascular portion of the mesentery, essential for adequate mobility of the reservoir. The proximal mesenteric division, however, is short and provides a broad vascular blood supply to the reservoir. In addition, a small window of mesentery and 3–5 cm portion of small bowel proximal to the overall ileal segment are discarded, ensuring mobility to the pouch and small bowel anastomosis.

The T-pouch is created from a 44-cm segment of distal ileum placed in an inverted 'U' configuration – each limb of the 'U' measuring 22 cm. A more proximal 8–10-cm segment of ileum (afferent limb) used to form the afferent antireflux mechanism. Note, if ureteral length is short or compromised a longer afferent ileal segment (proximal ileum) may be harvested.

The ileum is divided between the afferent ileal segment and the 44-cm segment that will form the reservoir. The mesentery between these segments is carefully incised for 2–3 cm with preservation of all major vascular arcades. The afferent ileal segment will ultimately be advanced in the serosal-lined ileal trough formed by the base of the two adjacent 22-cm segments of ileum. The proximal end of the isolated afferent ileal seg-

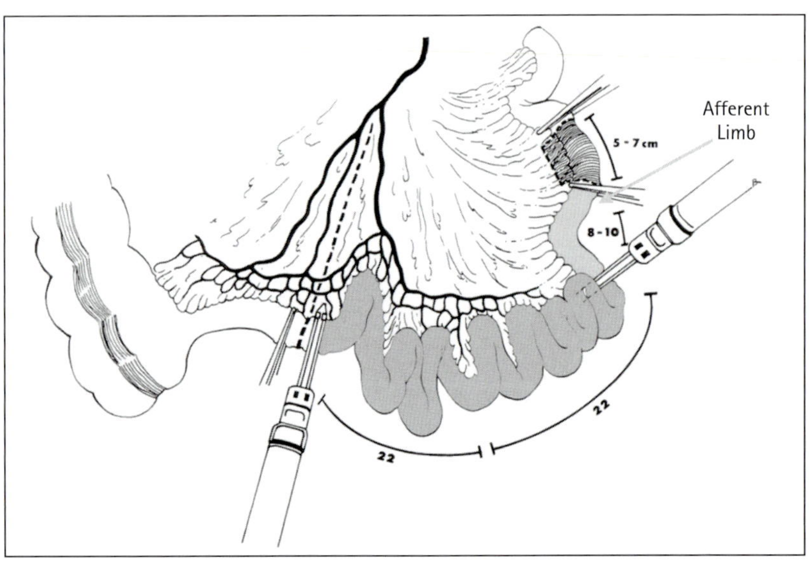

Figure 23.13 Designated segments of terminal ileum for construction of the orthotopic T-pouch ileal neobladder. Note that the distal mesenteric division is made between the ileocolic and terminal branches of the superior mesenteric artery extending deep into the avascular plane of the mesentery. A small window of mesentery and a 3–5-cm segment of proximal small bowel is discarded to allow mobility to the pouch and small bowel anastomosis.

ment is closed with a running Parker-Kerr suture of 3-0 chromic, and a third layer of interrupted 3-0 silk sutures. A standard small-bowel anastomosis is made to re-establish bowel continuity, and the mesenteric trap closed.

The isolated 44-cm ileal segment is then laid out in an inverted 'U' configuration with the apex of the 'U' directed inferiorly (caudal) and with a suture marking a point between the two 22-cm adjacent segments of ileum (Figure 23.14). The opened end (base) of the 'U' is directed superiorly (cephalad).

The antireflux mechanism is then created by anchoring the distal 4 cm of the afferent ileal segment into the serosal-lined ileal trough formed by the base of the two adjacent 22-cm ileal

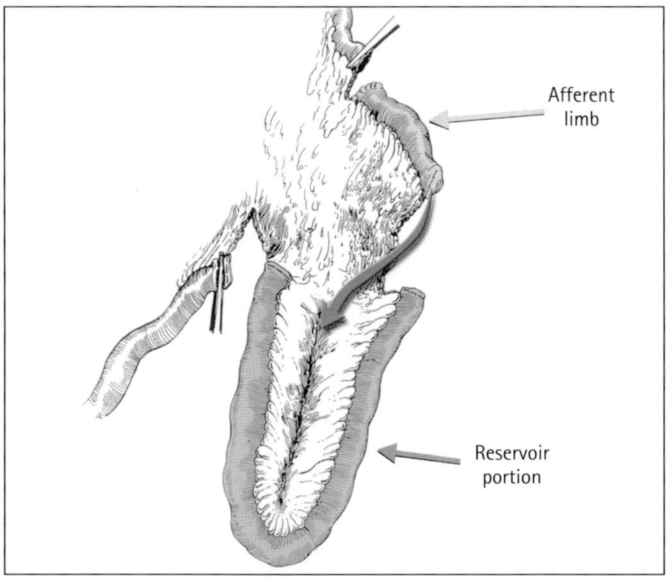

Figure 23.14 The T-pouch is constructed from an isolated 44-cm ileal segment (laid out in an inverted 'U' configuration) which forms the reservoir portion of the pouch, and a proximal 8–10-cm segment of ileum to form the afferent antireflux limb. Note, the mesentery between the afferent ileal segment and the proximal portion of the 44-cm ileal segment is carefully incised (1–2 cm) with preservation of the major vascular arcades.

segments. First, mesenteric windows of Deaver are opened between the vascular arcades (carefully excising mesenteric fat adjacent to the serosa of the ileum) for 3–4 cm proximal to the distal most portion of the isolated afferent ileal segment (Figure 23.15). Preserving these arcades maintains a vascularized afferent limb, and allows for the permanent fixation of this limb into the serous-lined ileal trough with complete preservation of the mesentery and blood supply.

A series of 3-0 silk sutures are then used to approximate the serosa of the two adjacent 22-cm ileal segments at the base of the 'U' with the sutures being passed through the previously opened windows of Deaver. Specifically, a silk suture is placed in the serosa (adjacent to the mesentery) at the base (most cephalad portion of the 'U') of one of the 22-cm ileal segments (Figure 23.16a). The suture is then passed through the most proximal window of Deaver opened in the afferent limb and placed in a corresponding site of the serosa (next to mesentery) of the adjacent 22 cm ileal segment. The suture is then brought back through the same window of Deaver and tied down (Figure 23.16b). Generally, two silk sutures are placed within each window of Deaver to ensure that the back wall of the reservoir does not separate. This process is repeated through each individual window of Deaver until the distal 4 cm of the afferent segment is permanently fixed in the serosal-lined ileal trough. The placement of small (¼ inch) Penrose drains through each window of Deaver provides traction and facilitates passage of the silk suture back and forth through the mesentery without difficulty. The Penrose drains are systematically removed as the afferent limb is fixed within the serosal-lined ileal trough.

Next, the previously anchored portion of the afferent ileal segment (distal 4 cm) is tapered on the antimesenteric (anterior) border over a 30-Fr catheter (Figure 23.17). This portion of the afferent ileal segment can be tapered with a stapler or simply with a running suture. Regardless of the technique, this maneuver reduces the bulk and lumen of the afferent limb, and facilitates later coverage of the anchored afferent limb with ileal flaps. This tapering of the afferent limb will also increase

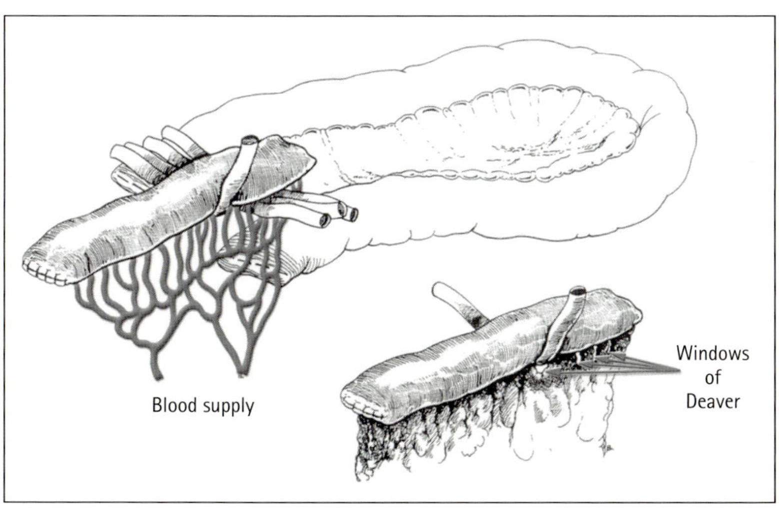

Figure 23.15 Creation of the antireflux T-mechanism. First, three to four mesenteric windows of Deaver are opened (adjacent to the serosa of the ileum) 4 cm distal of the isolated afferent ileal segment. Placement of small Penrose drains through each mesenteric window helps identify and facilitates passage of suture through each (see insert with arrows). The distal 4 cm of the afferent segment will be anchored into the serous-lined ileal trough formed by the base of the two adjacent 22-cm ileal segments.

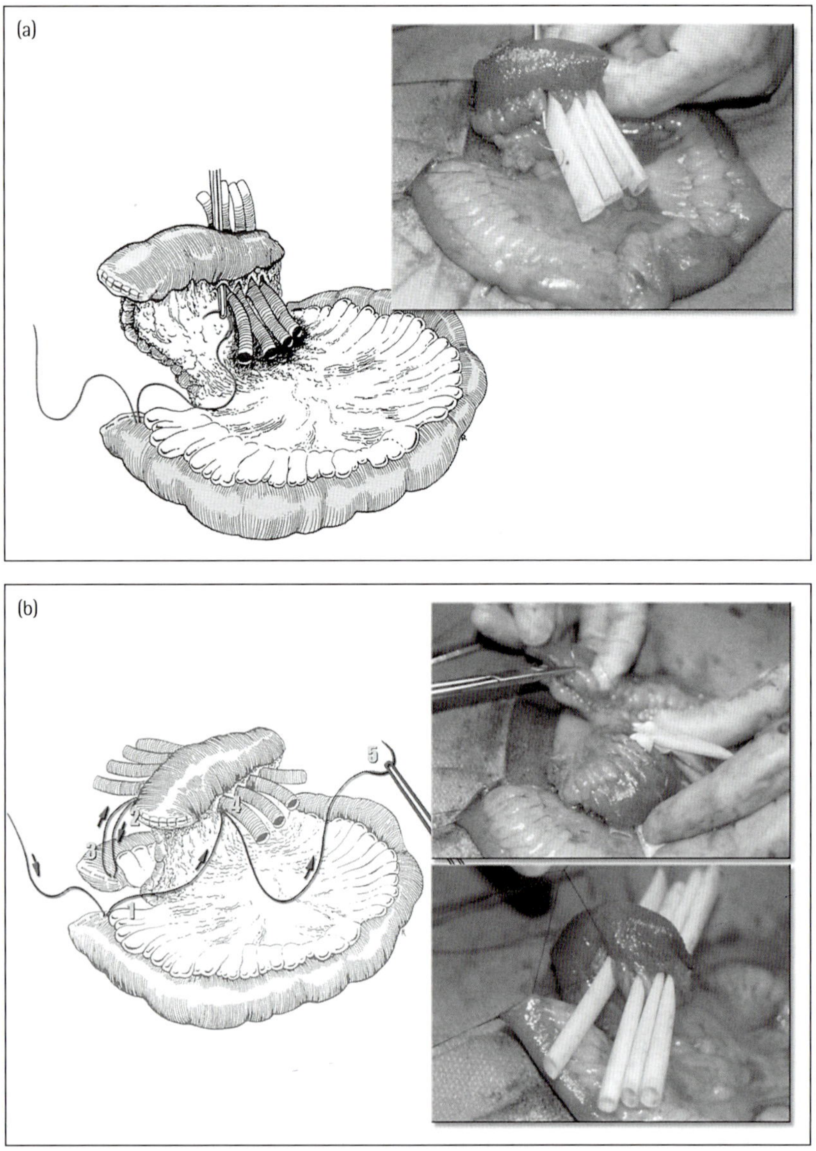

Figure 23.16 (a) A series of interrupted silk sutures are use to approximate the serosa of the base of the two adjacent 22 cm ileal segments. Note these sutures are brought through the windows of Deaver facilitated by the use of the Penrose drains (¼ inch). (b) After passing the silk suture through the window of Deaver, it is placed at a corresponding site on the adjacent 22 cm ileal segment. This suture is brought back through the same window of Deaver and tied down.

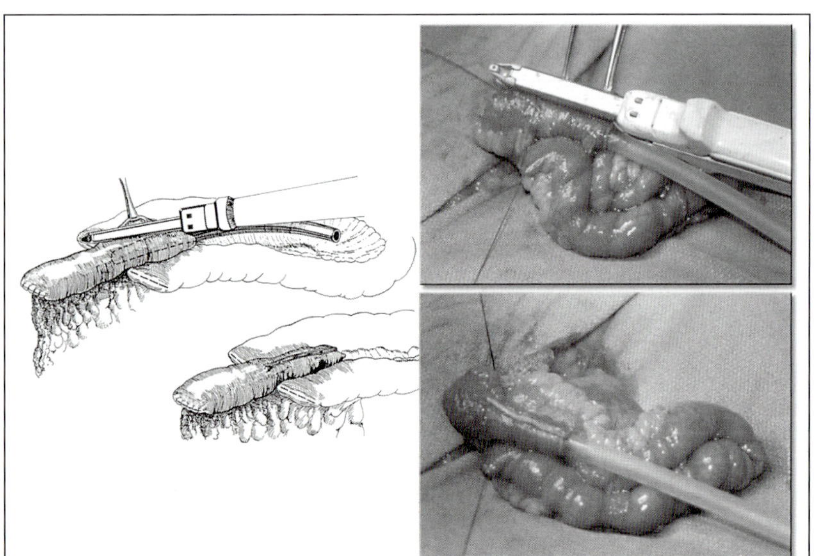

Figure 23.17 The previously anchored distal 4 cm afferent ileal segment is tapered over a 30-Fr catheter on the antimesenteric boarder. Note that the author prefers to use a GIA55 stapler to taper this distal 3–4 cm afferent segment.

the tunnel length to lumen diameter ratio; providing a more effective flap valve mechanism.

After the distal 4 cm of the afferent ileal segment has been tapered, the remaining portion of the adjacent 22-cm ileal segments are approximated together with a side-to-side 3-0 PGA suture. This suture line is placed adjacent to the mesentery (Figure 23.18) and can be placed in a running or interrupted fashion.

Starting at the apex of the 'U', the bowel is then opened immediately adjacent to the serosal suture line using electrocautery. This incision is carried upward toward the base where the afferent limb is anchored (Figure 23.19). Once this incision reaches the level of the afferent ostium, it is extended directly lateral to the antimesenteric border of the ileum, and carried upward (cephalad) to the base of the ileal segment. An incision is then made in a similar manner on the adjacent 22-cm ileal segment. This incision provides wide flaps of ileum that will ultimately be brought over the tapered afferent ileal segment to create the antireflux mechanism in a flap valve technique (Figure 23.20).

The previously incised ileal mucosa is then oversewn with two layers of a running 3-0 PGA suture starting at the apex and running upward to the afferent limb (Figure 23.21). Once the ostium of the afferent limb is reached, the running suture is tied. An interrupted mucosa-to-mucosa anastomosis is then performed between the ostium of the afferent ileal limb and the incised intestinal ileal flaps with 3-0 PGA sutures (Figure 22a, b). The mucosal edges of the ileal flaps are then approximated over the tapered portion of the afferent ileal limb (4 cm) with a running suture in two layers (Figure 23.23). This suture line completes the posterior wall of the reservoir and creates the antireflux mechanism.

The reservoir is then completed by folding the ileum in half, in an opposite direction to which it was opened (Figure 23.24). This effectively creates a low-pressure, high-capacity urinary reservoir. The anterior wall is closed with a running, two layer 3-0 PGA suture that is water tight (Figure 23.25). This anterior suture line is stopped just prior to the end of the right side to allow insertion of an index finger. This is the most mobile and dependent portion of the reservoir and will later be anastomosed to the urethra (Figure 23.26).

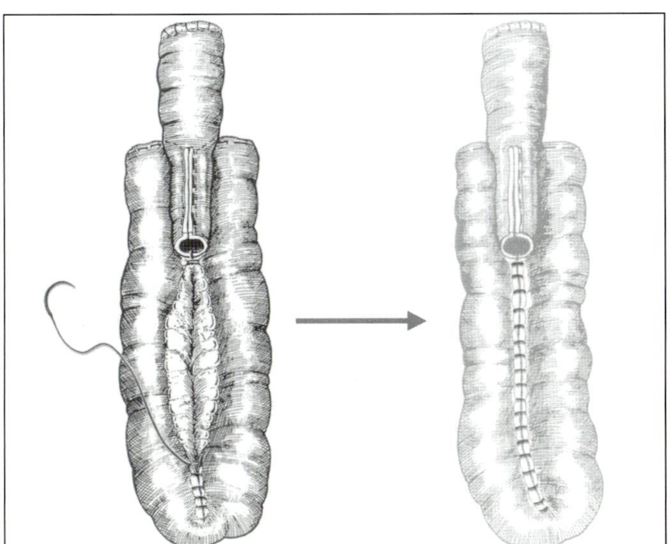

Figure 23.18 The adjacent 22-cm ileal segments are joined by a running suture. This suture is placed adjacent to the mesentery and runs from the apex to the ostium of the afferent ileal segment.

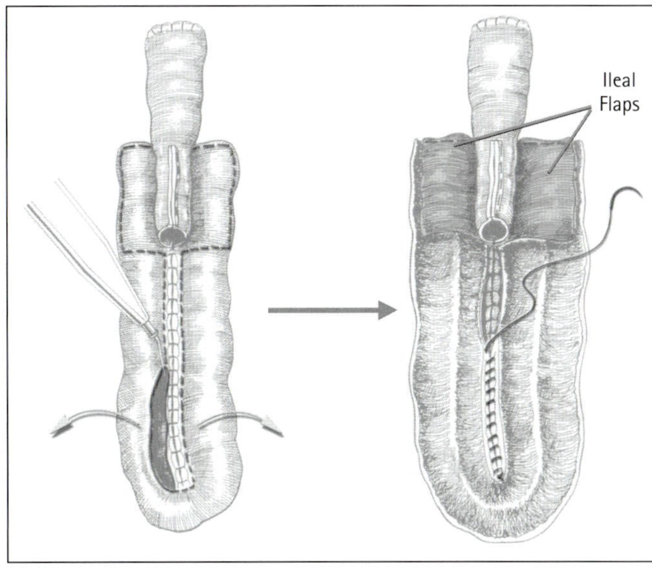

Figure 23.19 The adjacent 22-cm ileal segments are opened immediately next to the serosal suture line beginning at the apex and carried upward to the ostium of the afferent segment. Note, once the incision reaches the ostium it is then directed lateral (to the antimesenteric boarder) and cephalad to the base. The dotted line depicts the incision line.

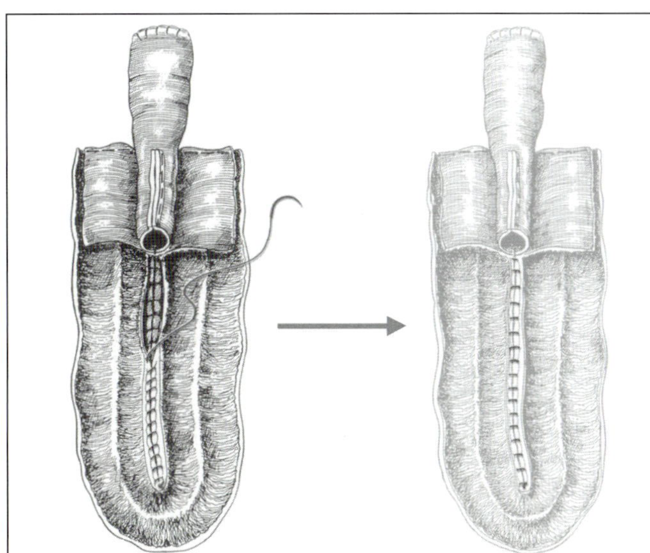

Figure 23.20 Completing the incision of the bowel. Note the incision provides wide flaps of ileum that can easily be brought over and cover the tapered distal afferent ileal segment to form the antireflux mechanism in a flap valve technique.

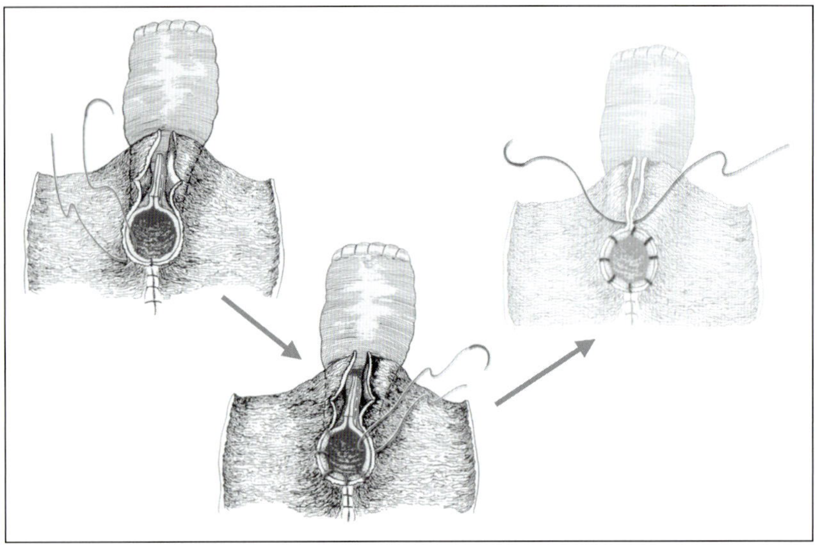

Figure 23.21 The incised ileal mucosa is oversewn in two layers beginning at the apex and continuing toward (cephalad) the ostium of the afferent ileal segment.

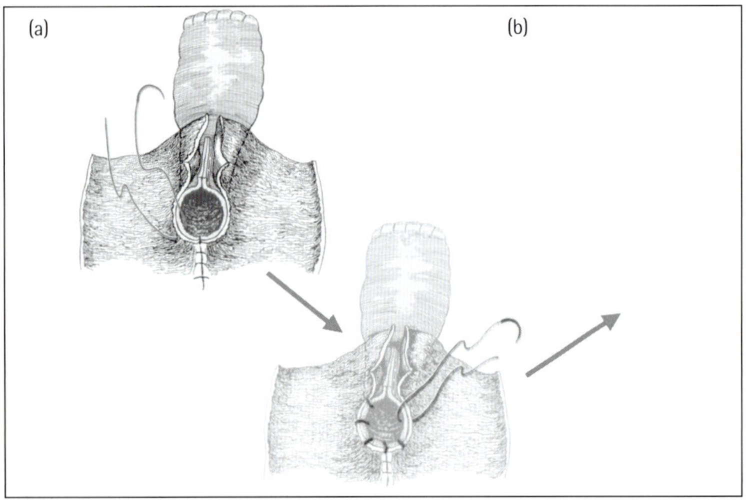

Figure 23.22 (a) A mucosa-to-mucosa, ileal-to-ileal anastomosis is performed between the ostium of the afferent segment and the edges of the ileal flaps. Note this is performed with interrupted 3-0 PGA suture. (b) Completion of the ileal-to-ileal anastomosis.

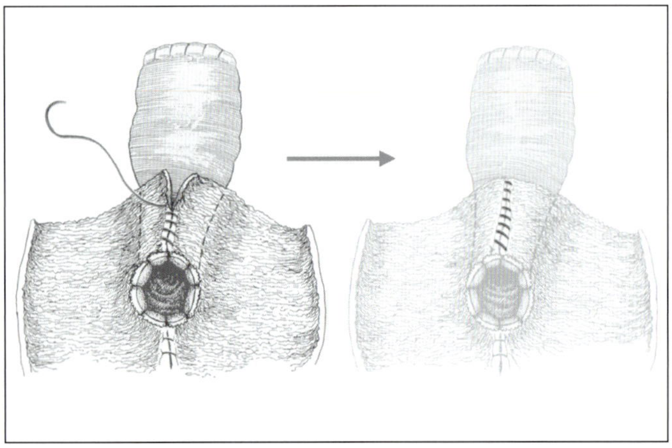

Figure 23.23 The mucosal edges of the ileal flaps are brought over the tapered distal portion of the afferent ileal segment. Note this will exclude the staple line from the reservoir.

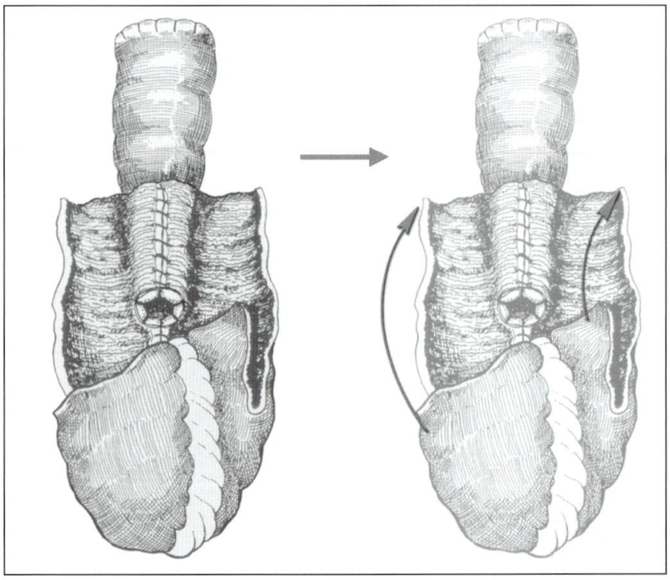

Figure 23.24 The reservoir is folded and closed in an opposite direction to which it was opened.

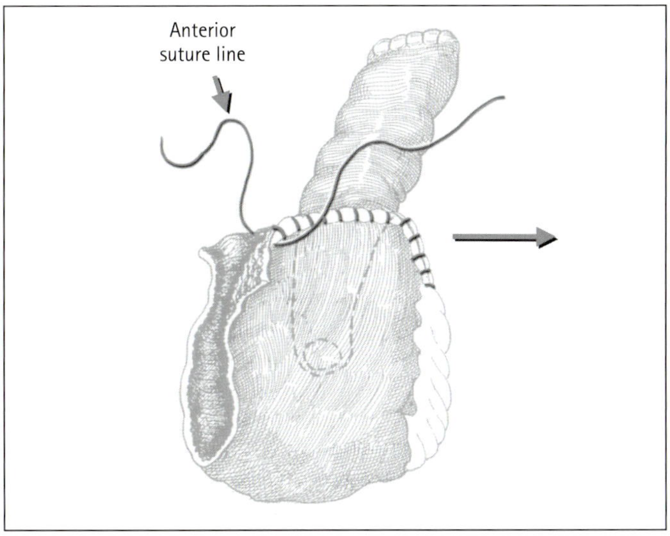

Figure 23.25 The anterior suture line is completed in a two-layer closure with a continuous 3-0 PGA suture. The anterior suture line is stopped just short of the right side to allow insertion of an index finger which will become the neourethra. Note the most mobile and dependent portion of the reservoir (neobladder neck) will be anastomosed to the urethra following the ureteroileal anastomosis.

After the reservoir has been closed, each ureter is spatulated and a standard bilateral end-to-side ureteroileal anastomosis is performed using interrupted 4-0 PGA. These anastomoses are stented with no. 8 infant feeding tubes which are directed from the ipsilateral renal pelvis (kidney), across the ureteroileal anastomosis through the afferent limb into the reservoir and out of the neourethra. A 24-Fr hematuria catheter is placed per urethra to provide adequate drainage of the reservoir. The ureteral stents are secured to the end of the urethral catheter with a 3-0 nylon suture. This facilities removal of the stents at 3 weeks along with the urethral catheter. A tension free mucosa-to-mucosa urethroileal anastomosis is performed.

Double-T-pouch continent cutaneous ileal reservoir

The double-T-pouch continent cutaneous ileal reservoir is based on similar techniques and principles as the T-pouch orthotopic neobladder. The flap valve T-mechanism is constructed to form both the antireflux and the continent, catheterizable efferent limb in the double-T-pouch.

The double-T-pouch ileal reservoir is constructed from approximately 66 cm of the terminal portion of ileum (Figure 23.27). The distal mesenteric division is again made along the avascular plane of Treves between the ileocolic artery and the terminal branches of the superior mesenteric artery. This division extends deep into the avascular plane of the mesentery, which is essential for adequate mobility to the reservoir. The proximal mesenteric division is short, providing a broad vascular blood supply to the reservoir. A small window of mesentery and 3–5 cm of small bowel proximal to the overall ileal segment is discarded.

The double-T-pouch is created from a 44-cm segment of ileum placed in a 'W' configuration (Figure 23.28). Each limb of the 'W' measures 11 cm. Two additional segments of ileum (proximal and distal) flank the 44-cm ileal segment: a proximal (oral) 10–12-cm ileal segment used to construct the afferent antireflux limb; and a distal (aboral) 10–13-cm ileal segment is used to create the efferent continence limb. If ureteral length is short or compromised, a longer proximal afferent ileal segment may be selected.

The ileum is divided between the flanking afferent and efferent ileal segments, and the middle (reservoir) 44-cm portion of ileum. The mesentery between the afferent ileal (oral) segment and the 44-cm segment is incised 2 cm, while the mesentery between the efferent ileal (aboral) segment and the 44-cm segment is incised 4 cm. Care is taken to preserve the major vascular arches with these incisions. These mesenteric incisions

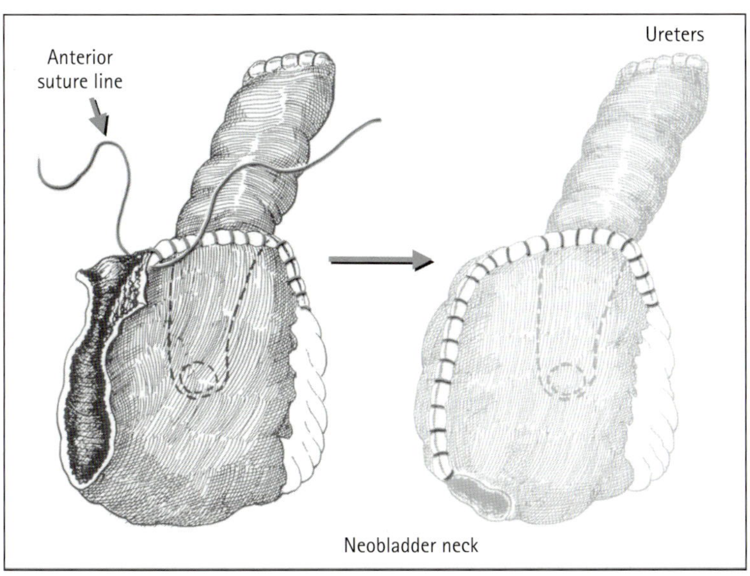

Figure 23.26 Completion of the orthotopic T-pouch ileal neobladder.

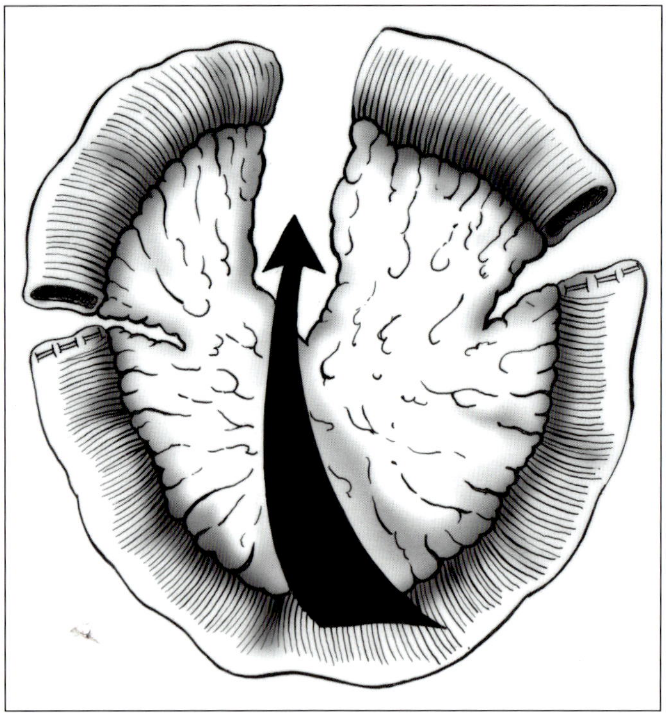

Figure 23.27 The double-T-Pouch cutaneous ileal reservoir is constructed from approximately 66 cm of terminal ileum: a 44-cm segment of ileum placed in a 'W' configuration. Note the proximal (oral) 10–12-cm ileal segment used to construct the afferent antireflux limb and the distal (aboral) 10–13-cm ileal segment used to create the efferent continence limb.

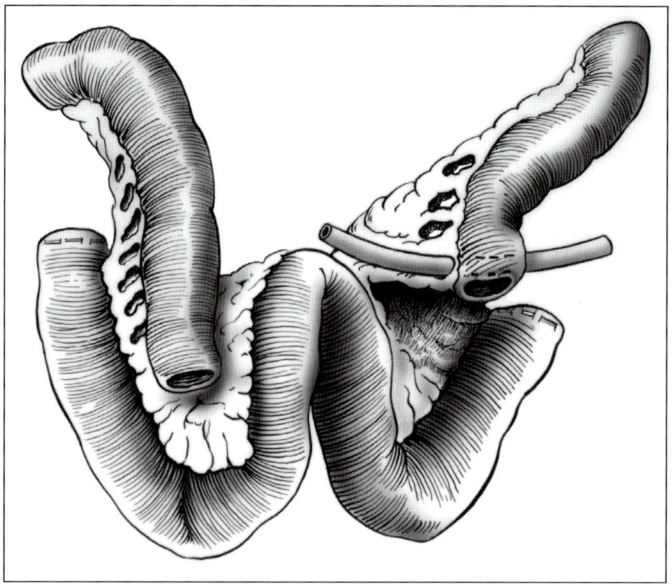

Figure 23.28 The isolated 44-cm ileal segment is placed in a 'W' configuration. Each ileal limb of the 'W' is approximately 11 cm in length. The proximal serous-lined ileal trough will form the antireflux mechanism. The distal serous-lined ileal trough will form the continence mechanism. The afferent antireflux mechanism is constructed by opening the mesenteric windows of Deaver between the vascular arcades for 4 cm along the distal most portion of the isolated afferent ileal segment. The efferent continence mechanism is made by opening the mesenteric windows of Deaver between the vascular arcades for 8–9 cm of the proximal portion of the isolated efferent ileal segment. Preserving these arches maintains the vascularized ileal segments and allows permanent fixation of the limbs into their respective serosal-lined ileal troughs. Penrose drains (¼ inch) placed through each window of Deaver facilitate identification and easy passage of the silk suture back and forth through the mesentery.

provide the necessary mobility to the afferent and efferent ileal segments, which will be advanced and permanently anchored in the proximal and distal serous-lined ileal troughs, respectively. These serous-lined ileal troughs are formed by the base (cephalad portion) of the 'W' configuration.

The proximal end of the afferent ileal segment is closed with a running Parker-Kerr suture of 3-0 chromic, and a third layer of interrupted 3-0 silk sutures. The bowel anastomosis is performed and the mesenteric trap is closed. The isolated 44-cm ileal segment is then placed in the 'W' configuration. The proximal serous-lined ileal trough will form the afferent antireflux mechanism, and the distal serous-lined ileal trough will form the efferent continence mechanism. Specifically, the afferent antireflux mechanism is created by anchoring the distal 4 cm of the afferent ileal segment into the base of the proximal serous-lined ileal trough formed by the first two adjacent 11-cm ileal segments. The efferent continence mechanism is created by anchoring the proximal 8–9 cm of the efferent ileal segment into the base of the distal serous-lined ileal trough formed by the adjacent third and fourth 11-cm ileal segments.

The afferent antireflux mechanism is constructed by first opening mesenteric windows of Deaver between the vascular arcades (adjacent to the serosa of the bowel) for 4 cm along the distal most portion of the isolated afferent ileal segment. In similar fashion, the efferent continence mechanism is made by opening windows of Deaver between the vascular arcades (adjacent to the serosa of the bowel) for 8–9 cm of the proximal portion of the isolated efferent ileal segment. Preserving these arches maintains a well-vascularized ileal segment, allowing for the permanent fixation of both limbs into their respective serous-lined ileal troughs. Again, Penrose drains (¼ inch) are placed through each window of Deaver to facilitate identification and easy passage of the silk sutures through the mesentery.

A series of 3-0 silk sutures are then used to approximate the serosa of each ileal trough. The sutures are passed through the previously opened windows of Deaver and anchor the 4 cm of the afferent limb, and 8–9 cm of efferent limb. Specifically, a silk suture is placed in the seromuscular portion of the ileum (adjacent to the mesentery), brought through the window of Deaver and placed at a corresponding site on the adjacent ileal segment. The suture is then brought back through the same window of Deaver and tied down (Figure 23.29). This process is repeated for each window of Deaver until the distal 4 cm of the afferent, and 8–9 cm of the efferent ileal segments are anchored in the serosal-lined ileal troughs. The Penrose drains are systematically removed as the respective limb is fixed within the serosal-lined trough. It is important that several (2–4) silk sutures are used for each window of Deaver. This will help permanently anchor the limbs in the serous-lined trough and

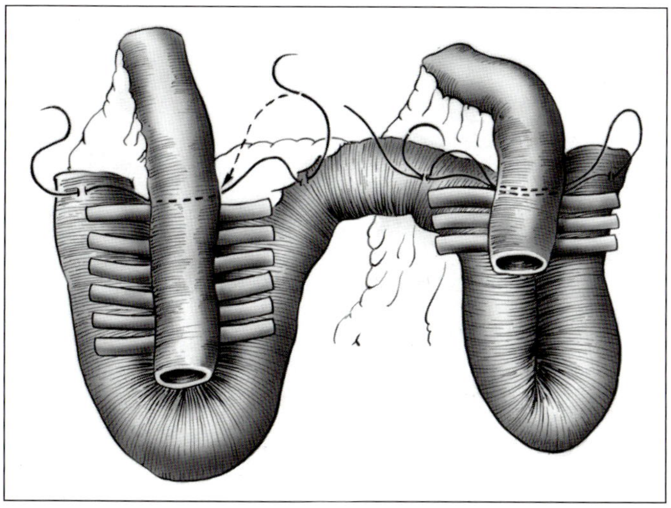

Figure 23.29 A series of 3-0 silk sutures are used to approximate the serosa of each ileal trough; the sutures are passed through the previously opened windows of Deaver and anchor the afferent and efferent limbs. Note, a silk suture is placed in the seromuscular portion of the ileum adjacent to the mesentery, brought through the window of Deaver and placed at a corresponding site on the adjacent ileal segment. The suture is then brought back through the same window of Deaver and tied. This process is repeated two to four times for each window of Deaver until the distal 4 cm of the afferent, and 8–9 cm of the efferent ileal segments are anchored in their respective serous-lined ileal troughs.

maintain the posterior wall (backboard) of the reservoir. The posterior wall forms the so-called backboard of the flap valve technique. If the posterior wall (serous trough) separates the compressive effect of the flap valve technique is lost and reflux or incontinence may occur.

The anchored portions of the afferent (4 cm) and efferent (8–9 cm) segments are then tapered on the antimesenteric border over a 30-Fr and 14-Fr catheter, respectively (Figure 23.30). Tapering these portions of the anchored ileal segments reduces the bulk and luminal diameter of the limb and facilitates later coverage with the ileal flaps. After the ileal tapering, the remaining portion of each serous-lined trough is reapproximated with a side-to-side running or interrupted 3-0 PGA suture. The serosa of the ileum in the midline (between the two serous-lined ileal troughs) is then reapproximated.

The bowel is opened with electrocautery beginning at the apex (caudal) of each 11-cm ileal segment immediately adjacent to the serosal suture line. The incision is carried upward to the anchored afferent and efferent limbs. Once the incision reaches the ostium of these anchored limbs, the incision is directed lateral to the antimesenteric border and then carried upward to the base (cephalad) of each 11-cm ileal segment. These incisions provide wide, viable flaps of ileum that will be brought over the tapered afferent and efferent ileal segments to create the flap valve antireflux and continence mechanism, respectively (Figure 23.31).

The incised ileal mucosa is then oversewn in two layers of running 3-0 PGA suture starting at the apex and running

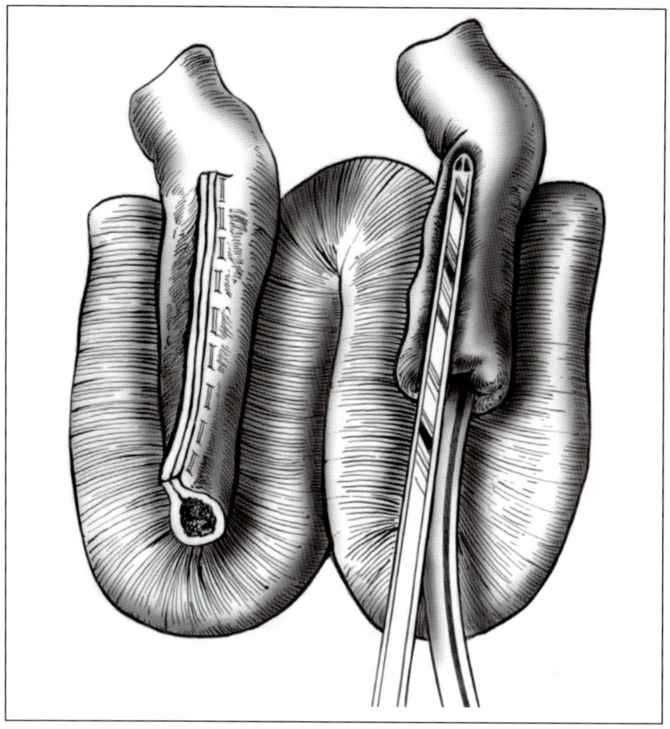

Figure 23.30 The anchored portions of the afferent (4 cm) and efferent (7–8 cm) ileal segments are tapered on the antimesenteric border over a 30-Fr and 14-Fr catheter, respectively. Note, tapering these portions of the ileal segments reduces the bulk and luminal diameter of the anchored limb and facilitates later coverage with the ileal flaps.

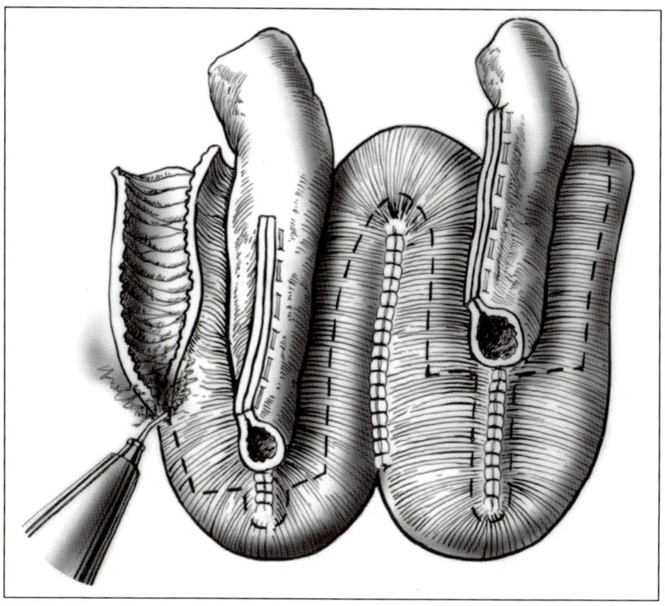

Figure 23.31 The bowel is incised beginning at the apex (caudal) of each 11-cm ileal segment immediately adjacent to the serosal suture line, and is carried upward to the anchored afferent and efferent limbs. Once the incision reaches the ostium of these anchored limbs, the incision is directed lateral to the antimesenteric border and carried upward to the base (cephalad) of each 11-cm ileal segment. Note these incisions provide wide, viable flaps of ileum that will be brought over the tapered afferent and efferent segments to create the antireflux and continence mechanism, respectively.

upward to the ostium of the afferent and efferent limbs. Once the ostium of these limbs is reached, the running suture is tied. An interrupted mucosa-to-mucosa anastomosis is then performed between each ostium and the incised intestinal ileal flaps with 3-0 PGA suture (Figure 23.32). The mucosal edges of the ileal flaps are then reapproximated over the tapered portion of the afferent and efferent ileal segment in two layers. The incised mucosa in the midline (between the two ileal troughs) is then reapproximated which completes the posterior wall of the reservoir (Figure 23.33).

The reservoir is then folded in a side-to-side manner creating a low-pressure urinary reservoir. The pouch is closed with a two-layer, water-tight 3-0 PGA suture (Figure 23.34). Once the pouch is closed, each ureter is spatulated and a standard bilateral (stented) end-to-side ureteroileal anastomosis is performed to the proximal portion of the afferent ileal segment.

A cutaneous stoma site is then identified and a small plug of skin removed. The subcutaneous fat and anterior rectus fascia are incised, and the rectus muscle split large enough to accommodate two fingers. Two horizontal mattress sutures (no. 1 PGA) are passed through the anterior rectus fascia on either side of the stoma, and placed at the junction of the efferent limb and reservoir. The efferent limb is brought through the abdominal wall foramen and the sutures securely fashioned. No redundant efferent limb is left intra-abdominally; the reservoir should be immediately adjacent/beneath the abdominal wall. The redundant ileum at the skin level is excised, and a flush

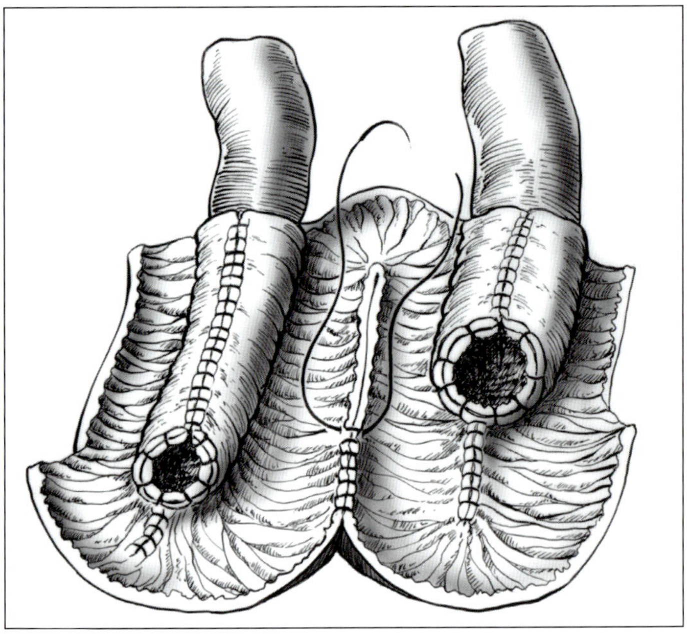

Figure 23.33 The mucosal edges of the ileal flaps are then reapproximated over the tapered portion of the afferent and efferent ileal segment. The incised mucosa in the midline (between the two ileal troughs) is reapproximated, completing the posterior wall of the reservoir.

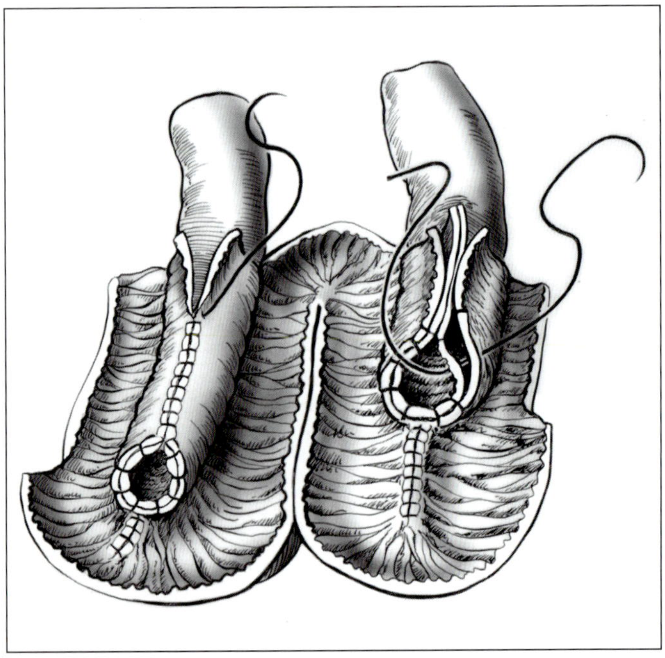

Figure 23.32 The incised ileal mucosa is oversewn with two layers of running 3-0 PGA suture starting at the apex and running upward to the ostium of the afferent and efferent limbs. Once the ostium of these limbs is reached, the running suture is tied. An interrupted mucosa-to-mucosa anastomosis is then performed between each ostium (afferent and efferent) and the incised intestinal ileal flaps with 3-0 PGA suture.

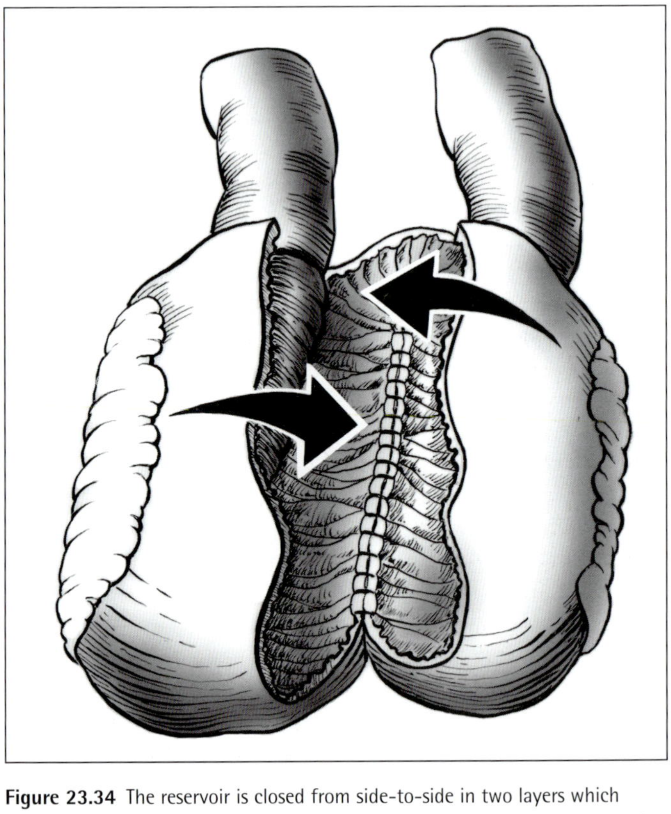

Figure 23.34 The reservoir is closed from side-to-side in two layers which completes the creation of the reservoir. Once closed, each ureter is spatulated and a standard bilateral, stented end-to-side ureteroileal anastomosis is performed to the proximal portion of the afferent ileal segment.

stoma is matured to the skin with 3-0 PGA suture. An 18-Fr catheter is placed through the stoma and efferent limb into the reservoir. A 24-Fr hematuria catheter is placed into the reservoir through a separate site below the cutaneous stoma to provide adequate irrigation and drainage of the reservoir.

Alternatively, the umbilicus may be used as the cutaneous stoma site. The proximal umbilical skin is anastomosed to the end of the efferent segment of ileum. Again, the reservoir adjacent to the efferent limb is secured to the posterior rectus fascia. Construction of the stoma site is facilitated by elevating the subcutaneous tissue off the anterior rectus fascia. This allows the reservoir and the efferent limb to pass directly through the umbilical defect under direct vision. The incised proximal umbilical skin can then be easily anastomosed to the ileum with 3-0 PGA suture. The advantage of the umbilical stoma is that it is well concealed. Furthermore, it is particularly helpful in obese patients with a thick abdominal wall pannus. A small suction subcutaneous drain (Blake) is placed over the fascia under the subcutaneous flap for several days.

Discussion

Critical components to the success of lower urinary tract reconstruction include the ability to create a large-capacity, low-pressure reservoir, with an effective antireflux mechanism to protect the upper urinary tracts, and an adequate continence mechanism to store urine. In general, continence and antireflux mechanisms in urinary diversions are dependent on the relationship between the outlet resistance and internal reservoir pressure. This mechanism should not only exceed intrareservoir pressures at rest, but also during change of position, posture, or under Valsalva pressure.

Kock's landmark report in 1982[3] renewed enthusiasm toward a continent form of urinary diversion and stimulated the development and improvement of a wide variety of continent cutaneous outlet mechanisms. Kock's initial report was based on his previous clinical experience with the intussuscepted nipple valve in patients with a continent ileostomy[27] and experimental work with the intussuscepted nipple in urinary diversion.[28] The evolution of urinary diversion logically proceeded with the continent cutaneous urinary reservoir logically evolving to an orthotopic form of reconstruction. Orthotopic diversion eliminated the cutaneous urostomy, stoma and the need for catheterization in most patients and arguably improved the quality of life of patients.[6]

Beginning in 1982, the intussuscepted nipple valve was employed as an antireflux mechanism in all forms of continent urinary diversion at our institution.[5–8,29] The basic surgical premise for the Kock ileal reservoir is sensible: a low-pressure, large-capacity reservoir, employing the intussuscepted antirefluxing and continent nipple valves. The Achilles' heel of the Kock ileal reservoir, however, remains the intussuscepted nipple valve. Despite several surgical modifications to improve upon the construction of the intussuscepted nipple valve, there remains complications and a certain reoperation rate.[16,17] It became apparent that improvements were required to develop an effective mechanism that could prevent urinary reflux, and provide a continent catheterizable mechanism in continent forms of urinary diversion without the significant morbidity related to the intussuscepted nipple.

Based on clinical[19,20] and experimental[18] studies, Abol-Enein and Ghoneim described an antireflux technique incorporating an extramural serous-line ureteral tunnel. We modified this technique and developed a novel extramural serous-lined ileal flap valve technique coined the T-mechanism. This technique was developed to eliminate the inherent problems with the intussuscepted nipple valve and may represent a small advance in the evolution of urinary diversion. This T-mechanism was initially applied as an antireflux technique in the T-pouch ileal neobladder.[21] Subsequently it was applied to a continent cutaneous ileal reservoir – creating an afferent antireflux, and continent efferent catheterizable mechanism called the double-T-pouch.[32] The evolution from the intussuscepted nipple valve to the T-mechanism is obvious. Future developments in lower urinary reconstruction will require an understanding of the history and technical aspects of each method.

In general, all flap valve techniques for continence or antireflux rely on the dynamic principle that the channeled segment (appendix, ureter, or intestine) is fixed and tunneled along the inner wall of the reservoir. As reservoir filling occurs, the channel is compressed against the wall (backboard) of the pouch, and continence or reflux prevention is thus achieved. This concept is based on similar principles for reimplantation of the ureter into the bladder. Keys to success of the flap valve technique include an appropriate tunnel-length to lumen-diameter ratio. Furthermore, the wall of the reservoir must be sufficiently capable to allow compression of the tunneled channel as the pouch fills.

The unique aspect of the T-mechanism (antireflux and continence) is the ability to create a reliable and effective flap valve system. Maintenance of the vascular arcades (opening the windows of Deaver) provides complete preservation of the mesentery and blood supply to the limb which should eliminate problems with ischemia or stenosis of the ostium or the bowel segment. Permanent fixation of the limb into the serous-lined ileal trough should also eliminate problems associated with prolapse or extussusception of the limb. Importantly, no exposed metallic staples exist within the reservoir which should reduce the incidence of stone formation typically associated with exposure of metallic foreign bodies to urine. Furthermore, if necessary the afferent limb can be easily lengthened when there are shortened or compromised ureters. A longer proximal afferent segment may be harvested to bridge any ureteral defect and/or maintain a tension-free ureteroileal anastomosis.

Several technical points regarding the specifics of the construction of the flap valve T-mechanism (antireflux, continence) deserve mention. An effective afferent antireflux valve can be created from a 4-cm segment of anchored ileum, while the efferent continence mechanism should include an 8–9-cm segment of ileum anchored within the serous-lined ileal trough. Permanently anchoring these portions of ileum in their respective trough is critical to fix the limb and prevent any valve slippage or prolapse. In addition, the silk sutures used to anchor the valve (passed through the windows of Deaver) should be placed adjacent to the mesentery, and incorporate a generous portion of the seromuscular ileum to prevent potential separation of the serous-lined ileal troughs. These ileal troughs form the so-called 'backboard' (posterior wall of the reservoir) of the flap valve technique and are critical to the continence and antireflux mechanism as the reservoir fills. Placement of two to four sutures within in each window of Deaver will help prevent separation of these ileal troughs.

The antimesenteric tapering of the valves is also an important component to the flap valve T-mechanism. Tapering of the afferent limb over a 30-Fr catheter has been effective in preventing reflux of urinary constituents and protection of the upper tracts in patients undergoing an orthotopic T-pouch ileal neobladder, and in the limited series of continent cutaneous urinary diversions. Tapering of the longer efferent limb should be done over a 14-Fr catheter. This effectively increases the tunnel-length to lumen-diameter ratio and has provided an excellent efferent continence mechanism.

The flap valve T-mechanism provides an effective and reliable antireflux and continence mechanism and should eliminate the observed complications associated with the intussuscepted nipple valve. The long-term results of the T-pouch and double-T-pouch are yet to be determined, but the initial and intermediate results have been good. Furthermore, this technique can be learned with a little experience. The T-mechanism is a versatile flap valve technique that has evolved from the intussuscepted nipple valve. It would be beneficial for all surgeons interested in reconstructive urology to have a basic understanding of the history and technical aspects of both surgical techniques, and ultimately incorporate these in their surgical armamentarium.

References

1. Bricker EM. Bladder substitution after pelvic evisceration. Surg Clin North Am 1950; 30: 1511–21.
2. Gilchrist RK, Merricks JW, Hamlin HH, Rieger IT. Construction of a substitute bladder and urethra. Surg Gynecol Obstet 1950; 9: 752.
3. Kock NG, Nilson AE, Nilsson LO, Philipson BM. Urinary diversion via a continent ileal reservoir: clinical results in 12 patients. J Urol 1982; 128: 469–75.
4. Rowland RG, Mitchell ME, Bihrle R et al. Indiana continent urinary reservoir. J Urol 1987; 137: 1136–9.
5. Skinner DG, Boyd SD, Lieskovsky G. Clinical experience with the Kock continent ileal reservoir for urinary diversion. J Urol 1984; 132: 1101–7.
6. Skinner DG, Boyd SD, Lieskovsky G et al. Lower urinary tract reconstruction following cystectomy: experience and results in 126 patients using the Kock ileal reservoir with bilateral ureteroileal urethrostomy. J Urol 1991; 146: 756–60.
7. Stein JP, Stenzl A, Esrig D et al. Lower urinary tract reconstruction following cystectomy in women using the Kock ileal reservoir with bilateral ureteroileal urethrostomy: initial clinical experience. J Urol 1994; 152: 1404–8.
8. Elmajian DA, Stein JP, Esrig D et al. The Kock ileal neobladder: updated experience in 295 male patients. J Urol 1996; 156: 920–5.
9. Studer UE, Ackermann D, Casanova GA et al. A newer form of bladder substitute based on historical perspectives. Semin Urol 1988; 6: 57–65.
10. Hautmann RE, Egghart G, Frohneberg D et al. The ileal neobladder. J Urol 1988; 139: 39–42.
11. Stein JP, Skinner DG. Orthotopic urinary diversion. In: Walsh PC, Retick AB, Vaughan ED, Wein AJ (eds). Campbell's Urology, 8th Edn. Vol. 4. Philadelphia: WB Saunders, 2002: 3835–67.
12. Skinner DG. Intussuscepted ileal nipple valve – development and present status. Scand J Urol Nephrol 1992; 142 (Suppl): 63–5.
13. Lieskovsky G, Boyd SD, Skinner DG. Management of late complications of the Kock pouch form of urinary diversion. J Urol 1987; 137: 1146–50.
14. Lieskovsky G, Skinner DG, Boyd SD. Complications of the Kock pouch. Urol Clin North Am 1988; 15: 195–205.
15. Ginsberg D, Huffman JL, Lieskovsky G et al. Urinary tract stones: a complication of the Kock pouch continent urinary diversion. J Urol 1991; 145: 956–9.
16. Stein JP, Huffman JL, Freeman JA et al. Stenosis of the afferent antireflux valve in the Kock pouch continent urinary diversion: diagnosis and management. J Urol 1994; 151: 338–40.
17. Stein JP, Freeman JA, Esrig D et al. Complications of the afferent antireflux valve mechanism in the Kock ileal reservoir. J Urol 1996; 155: 1579–84.
18. Abol-Enein H, Ghoneim MA. Optimization of uretero-intestinal anastomosis in urinary diversion; an experimental study in dogs. III. A new anti-reflux technique for uretero-ileal anastomosis; a serous-lined extramural tunnel. Urol Res 1993; 21: 135.
19. Abol-Enein H, Ghoneim MA. A novel uretero-ileal reimplantation technique: the serous lined extramural tunnel. A preliminary report. J Urol 1994; 151: 1193–7.
20. Abol-Enein H, Ghoneim MA. Further clinical experience with the ileal W-neobladder and a serous-lined extramural tunnel for orthotopic substitution. Br J Urol 1995; 76: 558–64.
21. Stein JP, Lieskovsky G, Ginsberg DA et al. The T pouch: an orthotopic ileal neobladder incorporating a serosal lined ileal antireflux technique. J Urol 1998; 159: 1836–42.
22. Perl JJ. Intussuscepted conical valve formation in jejunostomies. Surgery 1949; 25: 297.
23. Basso DE. The efficacy and applicability of an intussuscepted conical valve in preventing regurgitation and leakage of intestinal contents. Ann Surg 1951; 133: 447.
24. Mathisen W. A new method for ureterointestinal anastomosis. Surg Gynecol Obstet 1953; 86: 255.
25. Grey DN, Flynn P, Goodwin WE. Experimental methods of ureterocystostomy: experience with the ureteral intussusception to produce a nipple or valve. J Urol 1957; 77: 154.

26. Smith GI, Hinman F Jr. The intussuscepted ileal cystostomy. J Urol 1955; 73: 261.
27. Kock NG. Continent ileostomy. Progr Surg 1973; 12: 180.
28. Kock NG, Nilson AE, Norlen L, Sundin T, Trasti H. Changes in renal parenchyma and the upper urinary tracts following urinary diversion via a continent ileum reservoir: an experimental study in dogs. Scand J Urol Nephrol (Suppl) 1978; 49: 11–22.
29. Skinner DG, Lieskovsky G, Boyd SD. Technique of creation of a continent internal ileal reservoir (Kock pouch) for urinary diversion. Urol Clin North Am 1984; 11: 741–9.
30. Stein JP, Grossfeld GD, Freeman JA et al. Orthotopic lower urinary tract reconstruction in women using the Kock ileal neobladder: updated experience in 34 patients. J Urol 1997; 158: 400–5.
31. Stein JP, Daneshmand S, Dunn M et al. A continent right colon reservoir utilizing a cutaneous appendicostomy Urology 2004; 63: 577–80.
32. Stein JP, Skinner DG. T-mechanism applied to urinary diversion: the orthotopic T-pouch ileal neobladder and cutaneous double-T-pouch ileal reservoir. Tech Urol 2001; 7: 209–22.
33. Nichols RL, Broido P, Condon RE, Gorbach SL, Nyhus LM. Effect of preoperative neomycin-erythromycin intestinal preparation on the incidence of infectious complications following colon surgery. Ann Surg 1973; 178: 453–62.

24 Continent urostomy with hydraulic valve

Abdellatif Benchekroun

Introduction

During the past two decades there has been a surge of interest in continent urinary diversion, most reports being of the Kock, Indiana and Mainz pouch-type procedures. There has been a particular interest in continent diversion in Morocco where incontinent diversions have been poorly accepted, primarily because of the cost of complex appliances and the difficulties of social reintegration for the patients. Hence, in 1975, a hydraulic ileal valve system was developed which is adaptable for use with various types of urinary reservoir. This chapter discusses the construction of this system and results of its use with 28 years of follow-up.

The ideal urinary diversion comprises a capacious internal reservoir and a predictably continent skin stoma, and the success of these depends on a variety of factors. The continence mechanism should be easy to construct and reliable in function. The reservoir should have good capacity and compliance without high-pressure characteristics during fill and the upper urinary tract should be protected against reflux and metabolic problems. Additionally, there should be no nutritional or dietary changes required in relation to the intestinal exclusion for this use.

In 1988, we noticed that the same result could be obtained by using the hydraulic valve when adapted to the ileal pouch, what we describe as valve in continuity. This technique is easy to follow and a description of two aspects of ileal hydraulic valve is given in this chapter: the independent valve and the valve in continuity.

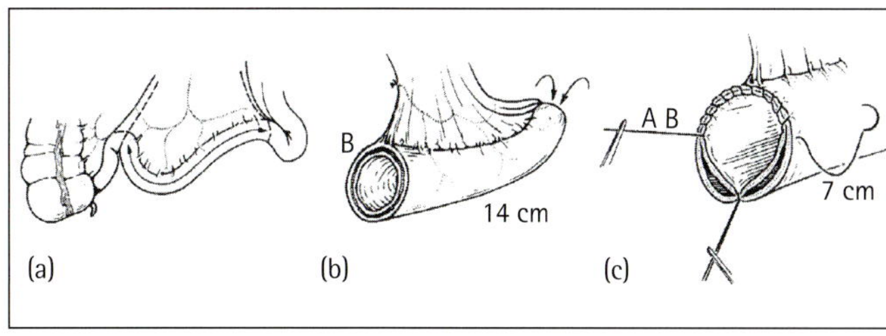

Figure 24.1 (a) Ileal loop for the hydraulic valve. (b) Ileal invaginated loop. (c) Spaces on either side of the posterior median point.

Surgical technique

Construction of the independent hydraulic valve

The hydraulic valve is constructed from a 14-cm length of terminal ileum taken 8 cm from the ileocecal valve (Figure 24.1).[1–7] This isolated segment of ileum is then folded inward upon itself along its entire length, forming an intussusception with the serosal surface rather than the mucosal surface forming the outer and inner layers of the tube. The two open ends of the bowel segment come to lie one inside the other, and these are now approximated in a watertight fashion using continuous 3-0 polyglycolic acid (PGA) suture around the anterior half of the opening. The sutures encompass all layers of the two bowel walls. An additional single mattress suture through the entire thickness of both bowel walls is placed in the posterior midline. As a result of this closure, two distinct openings are left between the layers of the inverted ileum. The internal surface of the inverted ileal segment is lined with mucosa and these openings are meant to allow the mucus secreted by the inverted mucosa to flow into the reservoir. Additionally, these openings allow urine from the reservoir to pass into the invaginated ileal segment when the reservoir is full. This provides compression along the full length of the hydraulic valve, increasing resistance to leakage over and above that offered by the intussusception alone.

Construction and technique of the hydraulic valve in continuity

In the last 200 cases we have used the detubularized ileal pouch and the valve in continuity. It is very easy to do with the use of a double J stent and the fixation of the valve directly to the pouch. Without doing a transverse ileotomy we

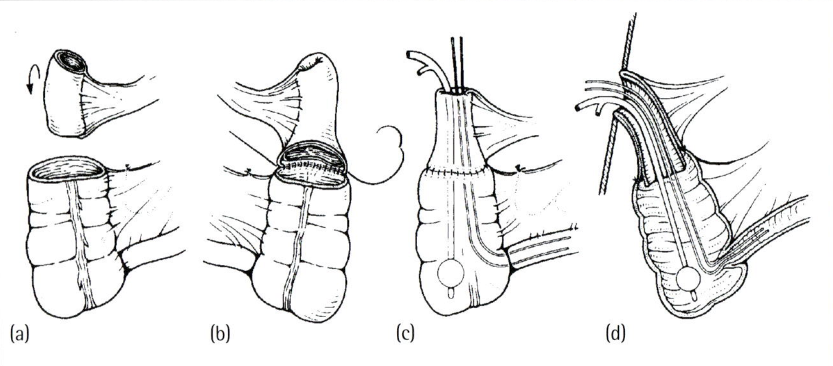

Figure 24.2 (a–d) Hydraulic valve and ileocecal reservoir.

avoid unnecessary operative time and the valve is fixed more tightly directly to the pouch.

An ileal segment 50–55 cm long is isolated, 40 cm is detubularized for the construction of Hautmann pouch. The afferent loop from the reservoir should measure 10–12 cm. From within the reservoir lumen the loop is folded inward upon itself to create the internal invagination along its entire length. The urostomy half-circle anastomosis and placement of the opposing suture is then done through the pouch, instead of what we did earlier, when we fixed the invagination through a transverse ileostomy. With this new approach, we reduce the operative time and the valve, fixed directly to the pouch, is more secure.

The urinary reservoir

The ileal valve can be adapted to all types of reservoirs, its open/sutured end being anastomosed to the reservoir in such a fashion that urine will fill the invaginated ileal segment in the manner described above. The other end of the ileal segment is matured to the skin as the continent catheterizable stoma. We have used this valvular system with a variety of reservoirs, most commonly with a non-detubularized ileocecal reservoir (Figure 24.2).

In this procedure the terminal ileum is transected 22 cm above the ileocecal valve, and the right colon segment measures 15 cm from the base of the cecum. Ileotransverse colostomy is accomplished in the standard fashion to re-establish bowel continuity and the 14-cm ileal segment is detached from the terminal ileum for construction of the hydraulic valve. The ureters are anastomosed to the remaining ileal tail, reflux being prevented by the ileocecal valve. In 12 cases, a detubularized ileocecal reservoir was used in an attempt to reduce reservoir pressure (Figure 24.3). We have modified this technique further to allow the hydraulic valve to be formed in continuity with the reservoir, rather than as a detached system (Figure 24.4). In this latter event, the ureters are anastomosed to the reservoir wall by tunneled non-refluxing reimplants for the ileocecal valve lost in the process of detubularization.

The hydraulic valve can be used with a sigmoid reservoir as shown in Figure 24.5, the stoma being exteriorized in the left ileal fossa. In two cases this procedure was used to convert a wet colostomy into a continent sigmoidostomy. Ideally the sigmoid is detubularized as shown in Figure 24.6, and in this event 30 cm of bowel is selected for reservoir construction. After detubularization and remodeling, a 5-cm opening should remain for attachment of the hydraulic valve, and the ureters are reimplanted using a tunnelled antireflux technique. Figure 24.7 illustates the technique by which the hydraulic valve had been used to convert a rectal bladder into a continent abdominal-wall stoma system. The rectal bladder was sectioned close to the anus, and the site of the section closed to create the reservoir. This procedure was performed for the management of urinary leakage following rectal bladder construction. The hydraulic ileal valve can be used in the construction of an ileal reservoir, either being constructed in continuity with the

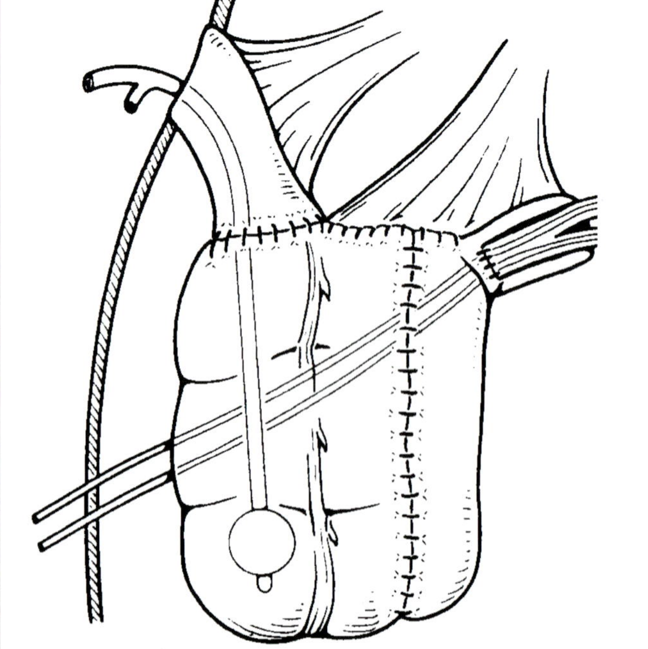

Figure 24.3 Detubularized ileocecum with independent hydraulic valve and antireflux valve.

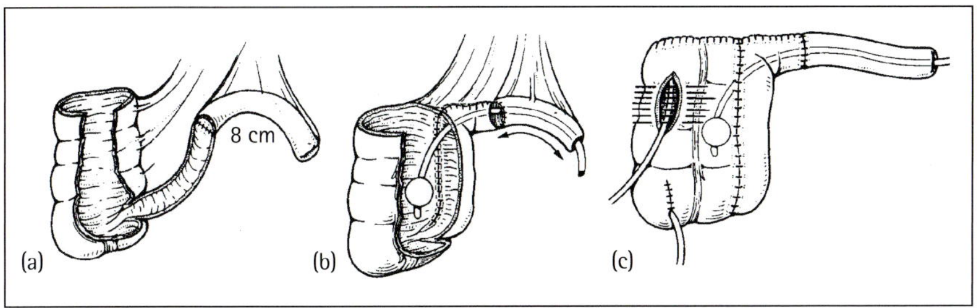

Figure 24.4 (a–c) Detubularized ileocecum with hydraulic valve in continuity.

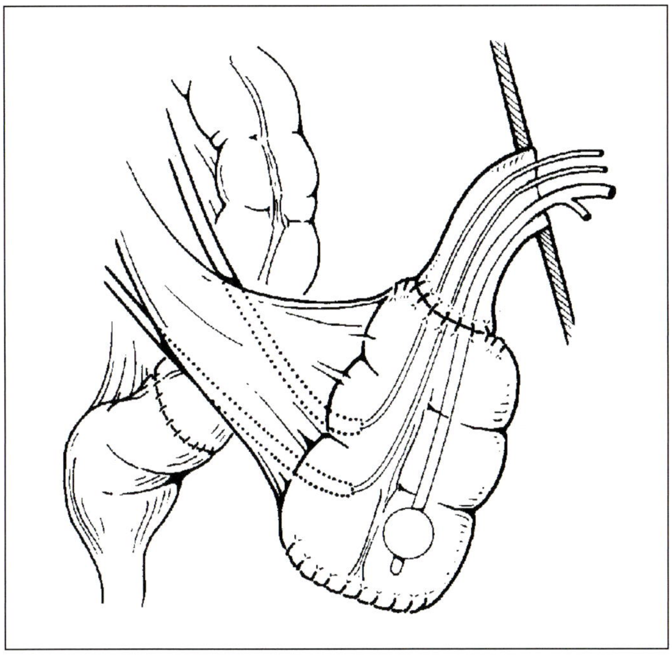

Figure 24.5 Hydraulic valve and sigmoid reservoir (continent sigmoidostomy).

reservoir (Figure 24.8) or as a detached continence mechanism (Figure 24.9).

Any of the various ileal reservoir systems can be adapted to this construction including the Kock and Hautmann pouches.[6,8,9] When used with the Kock system, the ureters may be implanted into the afferent ileal limb to the reservoir using the Camey–LeDuc method, providing the ureters are not wide. Wide ureters may be anastomosed using the new technique. When constructing the hydraulic ileal valve in continuity with the reservoir the efferent ileal loop from the reservoir should measure 16 cm. A transverse ileotomy is made 14 cm from the distal end of this loop, and from within the bowel lumen the loop is folded inward upon itself to create the internal invagination along its entire length. The customary half-circle anstomosis and placement of the opposing suture is then done through the transverse ileotomy, which is then closed to render the system watertight.

The hydraulic valve has been used to create a continent cystostomy in patient in whom the bladder neck was closed and

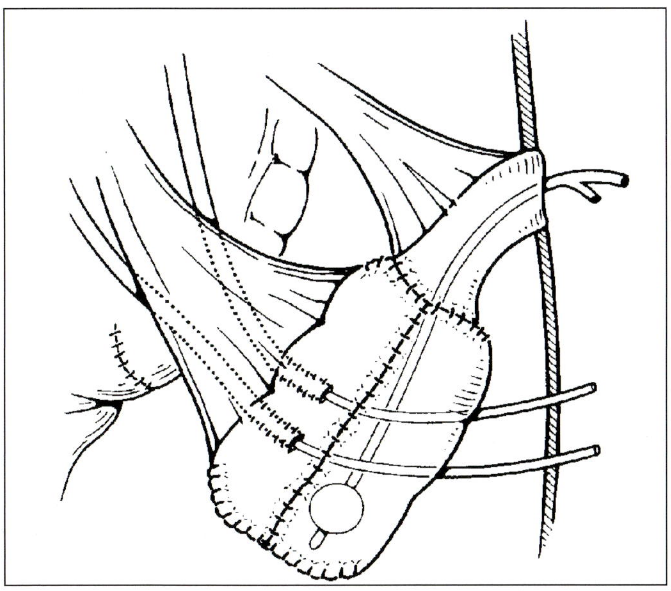

Figure 24.6 Hydraulic valve and detubularized sigmoid reservoir.

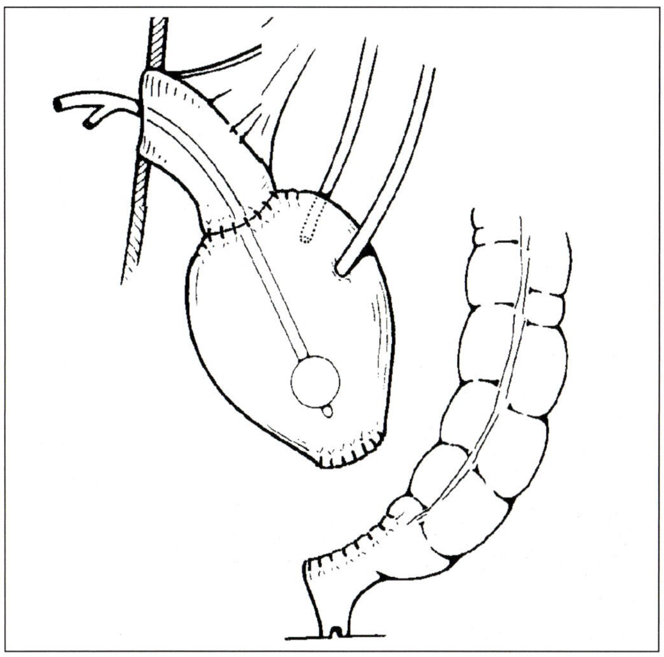

Figure 24.7 Hydraulic valve and rectum reservoir (continent rectostomy).

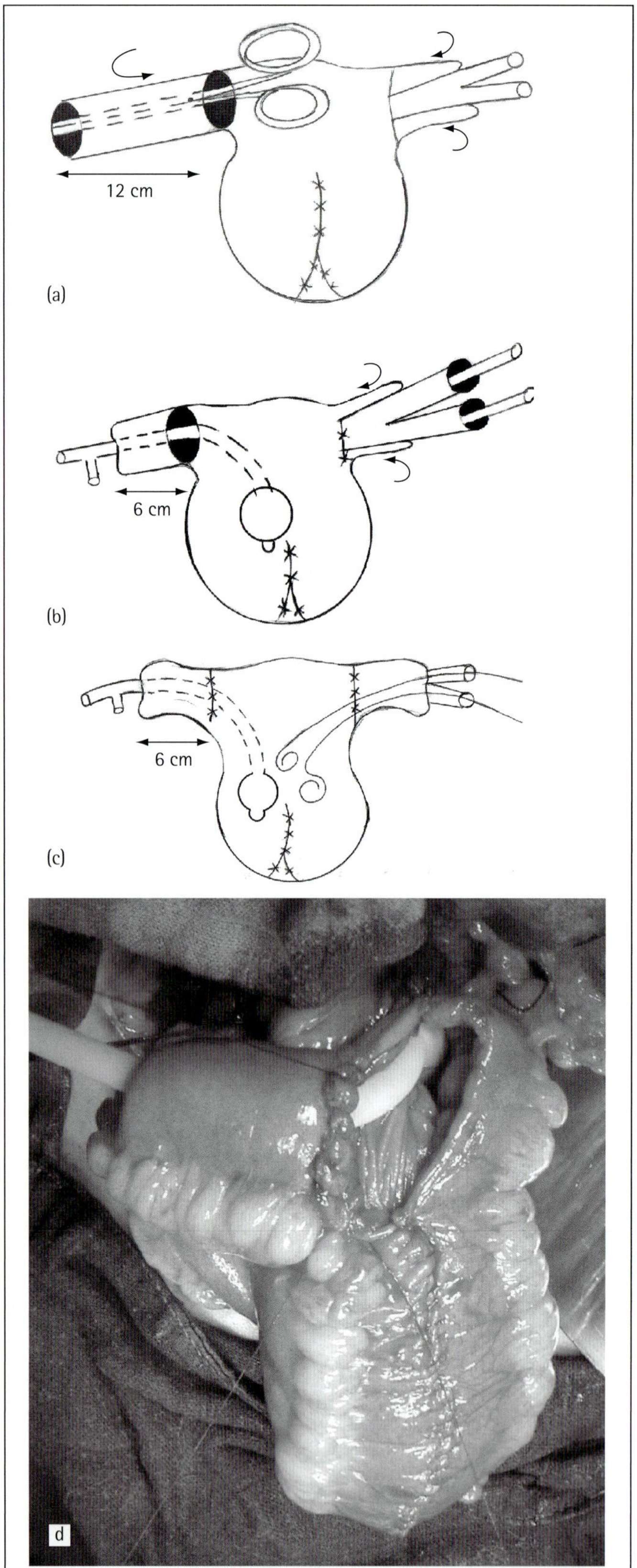

Figure 24.8 (a–c) Hydraulic valve and ileal reservoir (Kock or Hautmann). Continent ileal pouch with antireflux valve. (d) Ileal pouch with the valve in continuity.

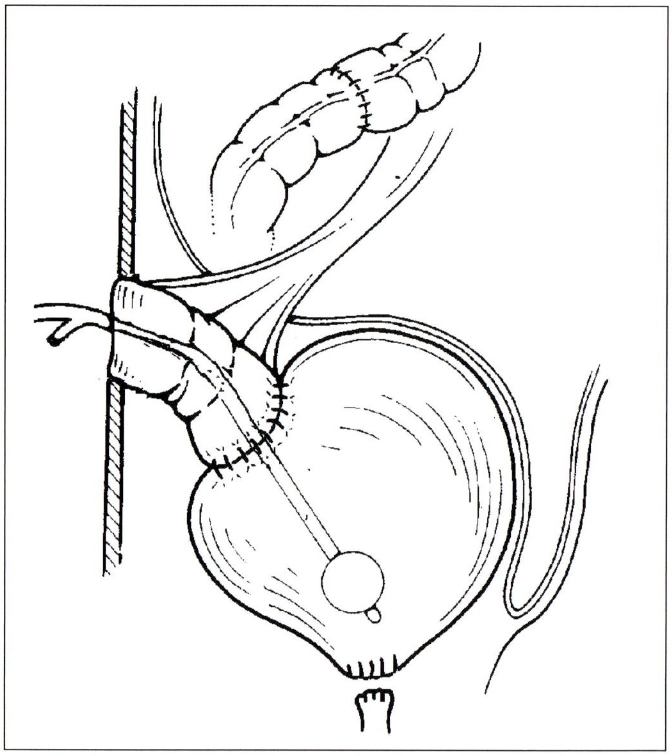

Figure 24.9 Hydraulic valve and bladder (continent cystostomy).

the valve was placed to the bladder dome and a cutaneous stoma formed.

Ureteral reimplantation

As mentioned earlier, when constructing an ileocecal continent reservoir, the ureters are anastomosed to the short segment of terminal ileum, protected by the ileocecal valve. There are four variations of this technique

- Ureteral ileal anastomosis with eversion of 1 cm of ureter.
- Uretero-ileal reimplantation using the Camey–LeDuc method.
- Ureterocecal implantation using the tunneled Leadbetter antireflux technique.
- Uretero-ileal reimplantation using an antireflux valve (Figure 24.10).

With regard to the technique of ureteral reimplantation, our policy now is to implant directly the ureters with a sleeve technique, unless they are wide – in these cases we prefer the hydraulic antireflux valve. For this purpose, we use about 10 cm of afferent limb of the ileum. This latter technique is depicted in Figure 24.10 and it creates a characteristic radiographic appearance as shown in Figure 24.11. The distal ends of the two ureters are spatulated for 2–3 cm and anastomosed side to side to create a wide caliber common opening. This common opening is anastomosed to the open end of the afferent ileal limb,

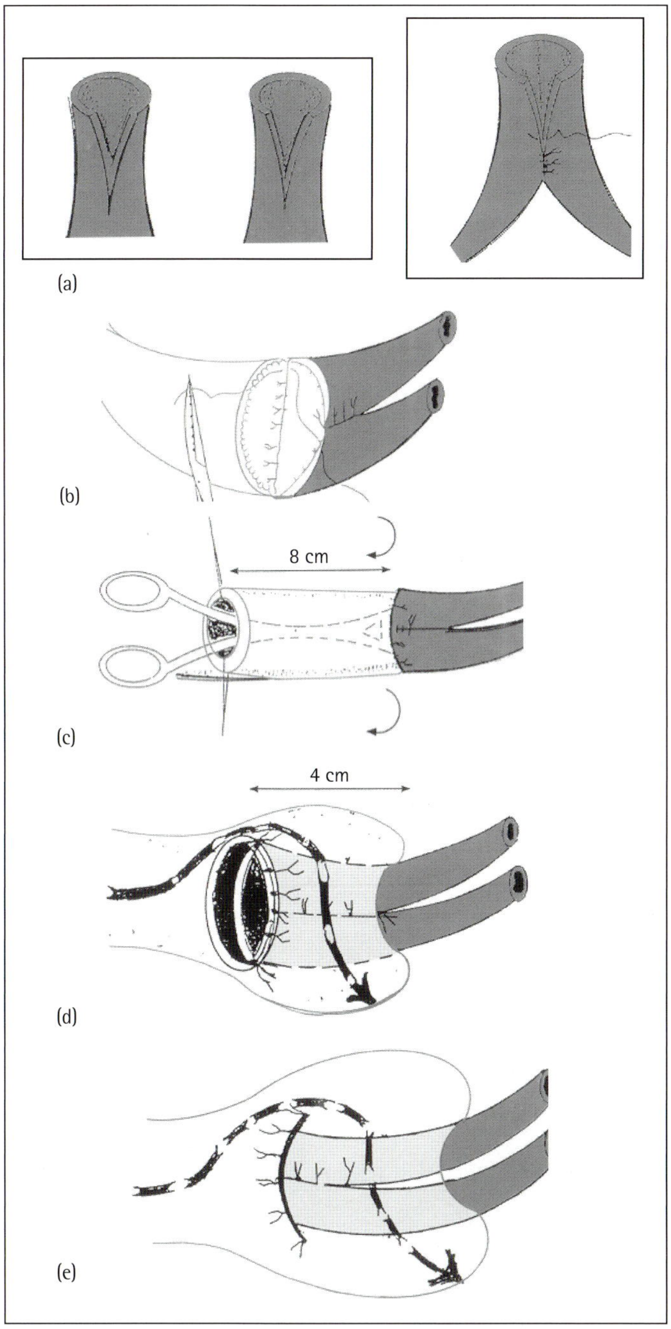

Figure 24.10 Hydraulic antireflux valve in continent urinary diversion. (a) Ureteroureteral anastomosis. (b) Ureteroileal anastomosis. (c) Ureteroileal intussusception through the ileotomy. (d) Fixation of the intussesception (running suture). (e) Closure of the ileotomy.

and then a transverse ileostomy is made 8 cm from the ureteroileal anastomosis. A 4-cm long ileal invagination is then created by pushing the ureteroileal anastomosis intraluminally, its progress monitored through the ileotomy. The invaginated ureteroileal segment is then attached to the proximal labium of the transverse ileotomy by a three-quarter circumferential 3-0 PGA continuous suture. Finally, the ileotomy is closed with the distal labium of the ileotomy on one side and the proximal

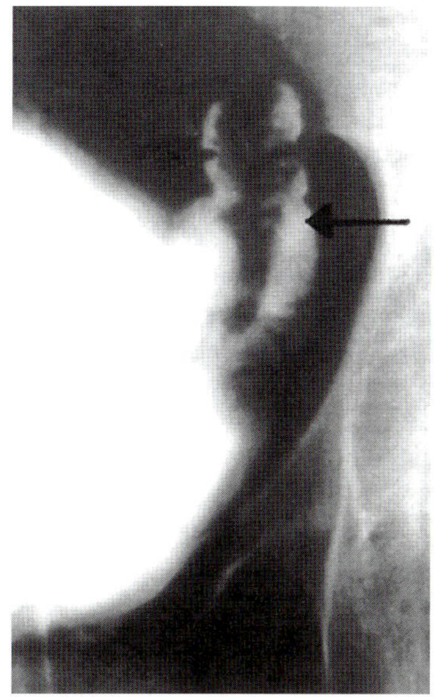

Figure 24.11 Pouchogram showing the ureteral trajectory in a filled hydraulic antireflux valve.

labial complex of the ileotomy and ureteroileal anastomosis on the other side. Since 1987, we have used this technique in 30 patients.

Patients and results of use of the hydraulic valve continence system

Between 1975 and 2002, this ileal valve continence system was used in 500 cases (399 male and 101 female), 5–76 years old (average age 49 years). Initially, it was envisioned that this procedure would be used only in patients with benign disorders such as irreparable vaginal fistulas. However, given the dependability of the continence system, the indications for its use were gradually extended, ultimately to diversions in patients with carcinoma of the bladder. Our current patient group includes 64% with bladder carcinoma, 17% with complex vesicovaginal fistulas, 9.2% with neurogenic bladder, 6.2% with vesical exstrophy and 3.6% with miscellaneous disorders including prostate carcinoma, extensive urethral stricture, 'malignant' lithiasis of the bladder and vesico-urethrorectal fistulas (Table 24.1). Of the 500 patients, 45 (9%) had an existing poorly tolerated diversion, including 20 internal diversions (17 ureteroneosigmoidostomies and 3 rectal bladders) and 25 external diversions (8 Bricker procedures, 5 cystostomies, 9 cutaneous ureterostomies, 2 nephrostomies and 1 wet colostomy).

Preoperatively, renal function was acceptable in all patients. Blood urea nitrogen (normal 0.30 g/1) and serum creatinine (normal 10 mg/1) were a maximum of 0.8 g/l and 20 mg/1, respectively (mean 0.46 g/1 and 12.4 mg/l, respectively).

Routine excretory urography was performed preoperatively, 952 renal units being examined in the 500 patients. Only 571

Table 24.1 Indication for cystectomy and type of reservoir constructed in patients receiving a hydraulic valve

Reservoirs	Ileocecum	Ileum	Bladder	Sigmoid	Rectum	Colon	Total %
Bladder cancer	99	202	0	15	1	3	320 (64)
Vesicovaginal fistulas	58	15	10	1	1	0	85 (17)
Neurogenic bladder	18	16	11	1	0	0	46 (9.2)
Bladder exstrophy	13	10	5	3	0	0	31 (6.2)
Miscellaneous	9	5	3	1	0	0	18 (3.6)
Total	197	248	29	21	2	3	500 (100)

renal units (60%) appeared to be normal. There were 152 (15.96%) cases of ureteral atonia (a state between normal and dilated), 171 (17.97%) cases of hydronephrosis, 29 (3.05%) cases of pyelonephritic kidneys and there were 18 destroyed kidneys and 11 kidneys with stone disease.

Of our 500 patients, 82 (16.5%) had urinary diversions that were tolerated poorly, including internal diversion in 16 (14 ureteroneosigmoidostomies and 2 rectal bladders) and external diversions in 17 (7 Bricker procedures, 3 cutaneous ureterostomies, 3 cystostomies, 3 nephrostomies and 1 wet colostomy).

Complications

A total of 400 patients (80%) had no postoperative complications and established effective urinary continence (defined as no loss of urine between emptying of the reservoir by self-catheterization); 100 patients developed a complication. Serious postoperative complications occurred in 17 patients (3.4%). These included irreversible septic shock in six, fatal uro-intestinal fistulas in three, intestinal fistulas in five (one fatal), an ileal pouch fistula which resolved spontaneously in one and two fatal pulmonary emboli. There were a total of 12 deaths. Valve failure occurred in 75 patients (15%) and required surgical reintervention for its correction. Three patients had valve necrosis, 30 developed external devagination and valve fistulas occurred in 42 patients. Following the second repair, 465 patients (93%) were continent. This is a global appreciation for all cases since 1975.

If we consider only the last 200 detubularized ileal pouch patients, there were no postoperative complications in 180 patients (90%).

Major electrolyte problems did not occur, blood urea nitrogen ranging from 0.2 g/l to 1 g/l (mean 0.4 g/l) and serum creatinine ranging from 5 mg/l to 20 mg/1 (mean 10 mg/1). Serum chloride was generally normal; however, in two cases, hyperchloremia was observed, one in a patient with an ileal pouch and one in a patient with an ileocecal reservoir. Alkaline reserve showed a slight tendency towards acidosis in some patients (in four with an ileal reservoir and two with an ileocecal reservoir) and was corrected by administration of 5 g of sodium bicarbonate daily.

In 465 patients, upper tracts were studied postoperatively, allowing for the evaluation of 850 kidneys: 419 units (49.2%) were normal; 330 (38.8%) showed atonia and 85 (10%) showed hydronephrosis. There were 16 pyelonephritic kidneys (1.9%). When compared with preoperative studies, it is notable that all normal kidneys remained normal; however, there was definite improvement in hydronephrosis, these moving into the category of atonia (Figure 24.12). The excretory urography study was complemented by a loopogram/pouchogram in many cases. In 425 cases studied, reservoir capacity was more than 300 ml and in some undisciplined patients, the capacity reached almost 1 liter! Reflux was observed in only 12 patients (a total of 19 kidneys). Ureters in these patients were markedly dilated preoperatively and the ureteroileal reimplant performed was a

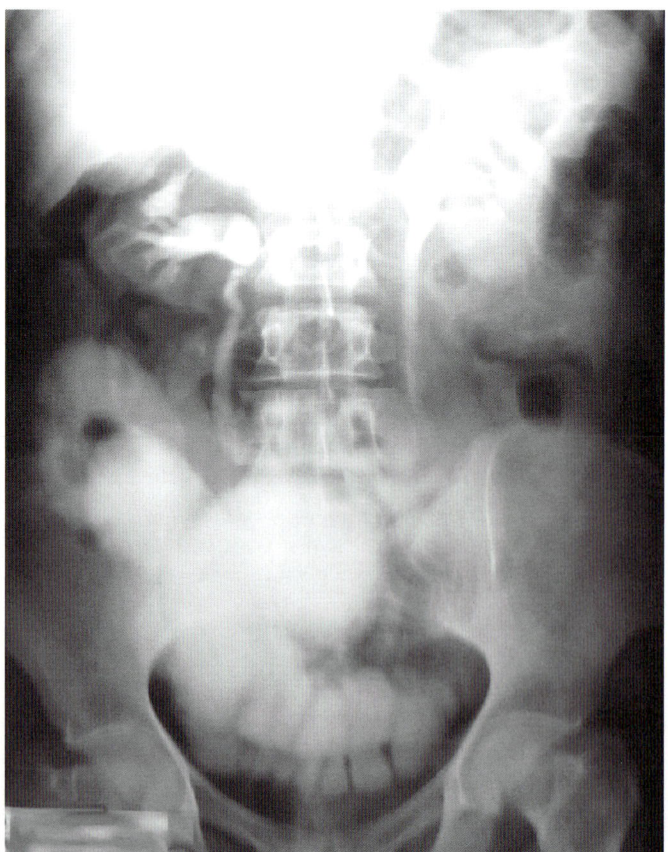

Figure 24.12 Intravenous pyelogram 27 years postoperatively.

ureteral flap/eversion technique in six, the two others having been implanted by the previously described Benchekroun antireflux valve.

Urodynamic studies were performed in some patients, and it is to be noted that the pressure profile of the valve is determined by fullness of the reservoir (Figure 24.13). When the reservoir is full, the maximum closing pressure in some cases approximated 80 cmH_2O, this being due to the urine accumulating between the two mucosally lined ileal walls within the invaginated valve, compressing the inner ileal segment. Ileocecal reservoirs made up the majority of this series and pressure peaks of 30 cmH_2O were noted during early postoperative months, but this hyperactivity tended to disappear with time.

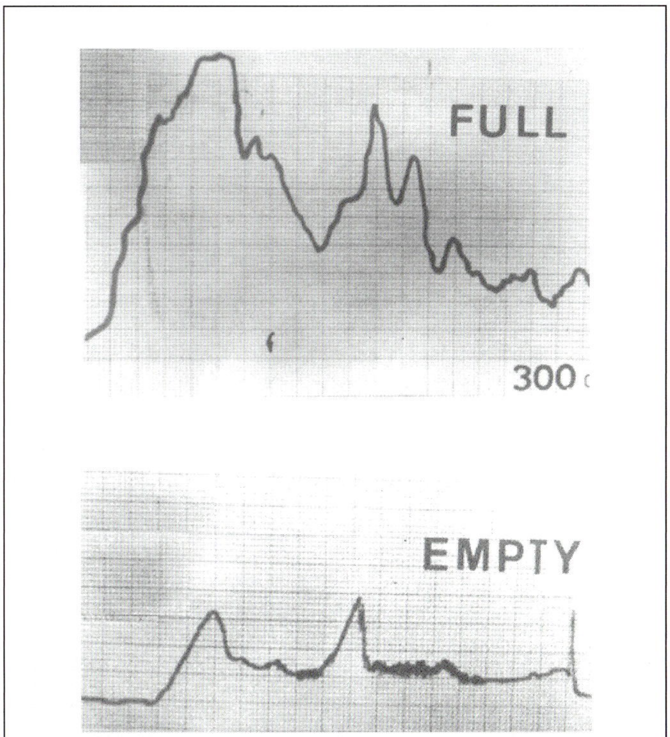

Figure 24.13 Valve profile with empty reservoir (below) and with full reservoir (above).

Re-operations

During the 28 years follow-up; we have had to deal with many kinds of complications, mainly with fistulas of the valve and disinvagination. These occurred during the first decade of using the hydraulic valve system. Fistulas occurred when we passed the ureteral catheters through the stomy because of problems with infection. When we passed the ureteral catheter through the pouch or since recently when we have been using the double J stent, the number of fistulas has reduced dramatically.

The internal disinvagination is easy to treat, we reinvaginate the same loop, and we fixed it through the pouch.

For the major complication, stoma stenosis, we recommend all our patients to use a 40-Fr catheter. When the stenosis is critical we make a small peristomal incision and dilate it with a dilatator and we recommend letting the catheter drain continuously for a few days. Re-operations for valve failure early (40 patients) or late (14 patients), and valve fistulas (20 patients) occur within 2 weeks postoperatively. Valve fistulas may be suture-repaired, and disinvaginated valves may be reinvaginated, but in some, a new ileal segment must be used for new valve creation (Figure 24.14). Stomal stenosis occurred in 52 patients and was treated by dilatation, as for urethral strictures, and maintained on catheter drainage for several days. Stones were removed endoscopically unless large. A total of 20 open surgical removals were necessary for large calculi which had formed in patients who had failed to attend for follow-up.

Discussion

As is evident from our presentation, the hydraulic valve has proved to be versatile, simple to construct and reliable. A number of other workers have experience with this technique, including Leonard and Quinlan,[9] Quinlan et al.[10] and Ronzoni et al.[11] Ronzoni has reported his experience with a selected population of paraplegics using the hydraulic valve and an ileal pouch. In his series of 10 cases, there were no complications and the mean follow-up was 18 months.[11] Leonard and Quinlan reported the ileal valve with a detubularized ileocecal segment in eight males and seven females ranging in age from 7 to 63 years (mean 25.2 years).[9] All patients achieved both daytime

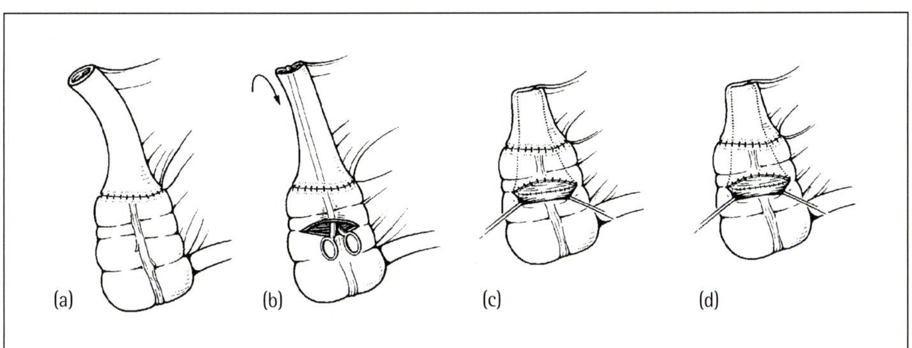

Figure 24.14 Reinvagination of the same ileal loop. (a) Hydraulic valve disinvagination. (b) Reinvagination through transverse cecotomy. (c) Fixation of the invaginated anterior ileal layer to the proximal cecotomy section. (d) Final aspect.

and night-time continence; however, they have reported some complications including stomal stenosis in six and an internal disinvagination requiring surgical correction. Jeffs has used the hydraulic valve in nine patients and reports daytime and night-time continence and acceptable pouch volumes with a follow-up of 11 to 20 months.[10] He describes the technique as his preferred continence mechanism because of its simplicity and versatility and there being no need for staples. The large lumen afforded is also cited as an advantage.

Conclusion

After a follow-up of 28 years, our first patients are still alive. The continent urostomy with Benchekroun's hydraulic valve is indicated for benign pathologies like vesicovaginal fistulas, bladder extrophy and neurogenic bladder. With time the pouch capacity increases, and the continence is always secure.

Acknowledgement

The author thanks his urologic staff for their contribution, in particular, Professor A Iken and Dr H El Sayegh.

References

1. Benchekroun A. The ileo-cecal continent bladder. In: King LR, Stone AR, Webster GB (eds). Bladder Reconstruction and Continent Urinary Diversion. Chicago: Year Book Medical Publishers, 1987.
2. Benchekroun A. Continent caecal bladder. Br J Urol 1982; 54: 505–6.
3. Benchekroun A. Urostomie continente utilisant le caecum. J Urol 1985; 10: 704–5.
4. Benchekroun A, Marzouk M, Hachimi M et al. Cystostomie continente. Acta Urol Belg 1988; 51: 74–80.
5. Benchekroun A, Faik M, Essakalli HN et al. Urostomie continente: poche iléale et valve de Benchekroun. Acta Urol Belg 1988; 51: 55–63.
6. Benchekroun A, Essakalli HN, Faik M et al. Urostomie continente: douze annees d'ex. perience avec la vessie ileo-caecale continente. Ann Urol 1989; 23: 188–96.
7. Hautman R, Egghart G, Frohnenberg DIH, Miller K. The ileal neo-bladder. Communication Societé Francaise D'Urologie, Paris, 1986.
8. Kock NG, Myrvold HE, Nilsson LO. Construction of a stable nipple valve for the continent ileostomy. Ann Chir Gynecol 1980; 69: 132.
9. Leonard MP, Quinlan DM. The Benchekroun ileal valve. Partial and total bladder reconstruction. Urol Clin North Am 1991; 18: 717–24
10. Quinlan DM, Leonard MP, Brendler CB, Gearhart JP, Jeffs RD. Use of the Benchekroun hydraulic valve as a catheterizable continence mechanism. J Urol 1991; 145: 1151–5.
11. Ronzoni G, De Vechis M, Rizzotto A, Raschi R, Cuneo L. Dérivation-urinaire continente utilisant un greffon iléal prepéritonéal et la valve hydraulique de Benchekroun. Ann. Urol 1989; 23(5), 426–9.

25 Right colon reservoir using a tapered ileal outlet

Randall G Rowland and Andrew C McGregor

Introduction

The first continent urinary diversion was a ureterosigmoidostomy performed by Simon in 1851.[1] Although several other types of continent urinary diversion have been described in the literature, it was not until the late 1970s and early 1980s that significant success was achieved. This success has, in turn, stimulated interest in adopting and adapting continent urinary diversions.

The Indiana continent urinary diversion described in this chapter grew out of the Gilchrist procedure which was first reported in 1950.[2] The ileocecal valve and efferent limb were modified by plication in an effort to improve continence.[3] In the initial 10 patients the right colonic segment was not detubularized. Half of the patients required revision to correct incontinence due to high pressure within the reservoir.[4] After that initial experience, all subsequent reservoirs have been detubularized by addition of an ileal segment or reconfiguration of the right colon. The reliability of the efferent limb and continence mechanism has been improved by using a stapling technique to taper the efferent limb prior to suture plicating the ileocecal valve. Since 1993, the reservoir has been reconfigured (detubularized) using the GIA stapler with absorbable staples if it is available. Since 1998, the ureterocolonic anastomoses have been done end-to-side.

This chapter reports a series of 50 consecutive patients with a right colonic reservoir who had a stapled-plicated efferent limb, hand-sewn detubularization, and tunneled tenial ureterocolonic anastomoses and a series of 29 patients with a right colonic reservoir who had a stapled-plicated efferent limb, a reservoir detubularized and closed with absorbable staples, and end-to-side ureterocolonic anastomoses. All patients had a serum creatinine <2 mg/dl or a creatinine clearance >50 ml/min, normal or nearly normal bowel function, the willing-

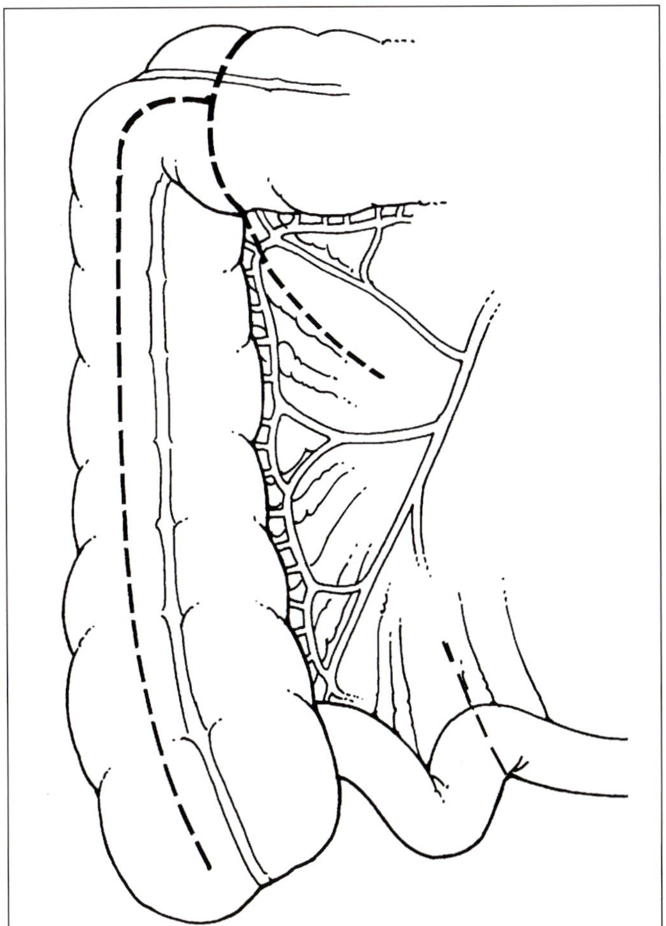

Figure 25.1 A 25–30-cm segment of cecum and ascending colon and a 6–10-cm segment of terminal ileum are isolated. The dashed lines indicate incision sites including the antimesenteric portion of the cecum and ascending colon to detubularize this segment by cauterization or by absorbable staple technique. This segment will be used to form the reservoir.

ness and ability to perform self-catheterization to be a candidate for an Indiana continent urinary reservoir.

Surgical technique

Prior to surgery, the patient has mechanical and antibiotic bowel preparation over a 48-hour period. Patients who are debilitated or become dehydrated from the bowel preparation are admitted the night before the surgery for intravenous hydration. Those with neurologic disorders will often require admission to the hospital for 1 day before the surgery to assure that the bowel preparation has been complete.

After the cystectomy or other primary procedure has been completed, an ileocecal segment is isolated as shown in Figure 25.1. Between 25 cm and 30 cm of cecum and ascending colon and 6–10 cm of terminal ileum are isolated and supported by the ileocolic and right colic arteries. An ileocolostomy is performed either using hand-sewn or an end-to-side stapled anastomotic technique. When a stapled technique is used for the anastomoses, a 25-mm EEA stapler is usually the correct size. The open end of the colon is usually closed with a TA55 or TA60 4.8-mm stapler. The mesenteric defect is closed with 3-0 silk sutures to prevent potential internal herniation. Any remaining fecal material is irrigated out of the isolated bowel segment. If an appendix is present, it is removed in the standard fashion. The entire colonic segment will be detubularized either by using absorbable staple cartridges (GIA and TA55) if available or cautery to incise the antimesenteric border of the segment, folding the segment over, and using 3-0 braided, absorbable suture to close the segment transversely.

Prior to performing the reconfiguration of the colonic segment, the efferent limb and continence mechanism are created as shown in Figure 25.2. GIA55 or GIA60 staple cartridges with 3.5-mm metal staples are applied sequentially to narrow the efferent limb over a 12-Fr catheter which has been placed adjacent to the mesentery of the bowel segment. Excess antimesenteric ileum is removed by the GIA stapler. The last application

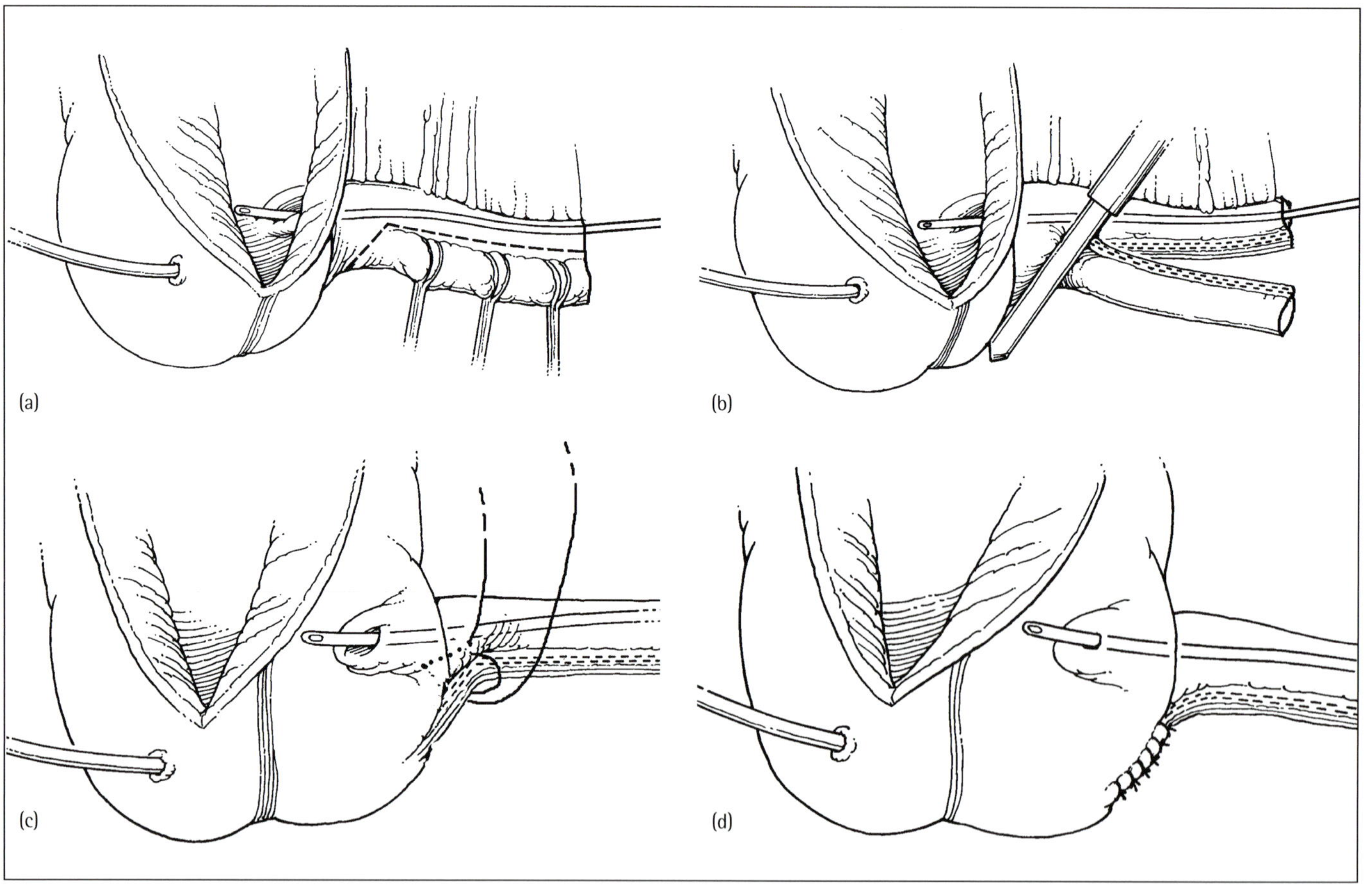

Figure 25.2 (a) A 12-Fr catheter is passed through the efferent limb adjacent to the mesentery. Babcock clamps are used to grasp the antimesenteric edge of the ileum. A GIA55 or GIA60 stapler is used to trim away the excess antimesenteric bowel wall as indicated by the dashed line. Depending on the length of the efferent limb segment, a second application of the stapler parallel to the mesentery may be needed. (b) The last application of the GIA stapler is made at an angle to avoid entering the cecal wall. (c) Silk Lembert sutures are placed to plicate the ileocecal valve. Each successive suture has a wider base to invert more tissue as the sutures progress toward the cecal wall (see row of dots). A total of five to seven sutures are used. (d) When the plication sutures are tied, the funneled area at the ileocecal junction is converted into a right angle. The valve is narrowed and resistance should be felt when an 18-Fr catheter is passed through this area.

of the GIA stapler is placed at an angle to prevent stapling into the wall of the cecum (see Figure 25.2b). A total of two or three applications of the stapler will be needed depending on the length of the efferent which is determined by the body wall thickness.

After narrowing the efferent limb, the ileocecal valve area is plicated with five to seven Lembert stitches of 3-0 silk suture (see Figure 25.2c,d). Care is taken to avoid having the sutures enter the lumen of the bowel. Each Lembert stitch is progressively wider beginning at the junction of the angled staple line and the straight staple line on the efferent limb and working toward the cecal wall. This increases the amount of tissue that is plicated the closer one gets to the cecal wall. In general the stitches are placed about 5 mm apart.

The tightness of the plication sutures is tested by passing an 18-Fr catheter through the efferent limb. If the catheter does not pass through the valve, the first stitch at the junction of the angled and straight stapled lines should be removed. If no resistance is felt as the catheter passes through the valve, additional stitches should be placed proximal to the first stitches placed to further narrow the ileocecal junction area. The feeling of resistance or a slight 'pop' as the catheter passes through the valve correlated with a good continence result.

Once the efferent limb and continence mechanism have been completed, the reservoir is reconfigured. If a hand-sewn technique is chosen, the entire antimesenteric line of the colonic segment is incised using the coagulation current of the electrocautery unit. The line of incision is shown by the dashed line between the two lateral teniae on the colon in Figure 25.1. The folding of the detubularized segment is shown in Figure 25.3. The colonic segment is then closed in a transverse manner as shown in Figure 25.4 using 3-0 braided, absorbable suture material. Every other or every third stitch is locked to prevent shortening of the suture line. Prior to the final closure of the reservoir, a 22-Fr Malecot catheter is placed in the cap of the cecum to act as a drain for the reservoir in the postoperative period. The flanges of the Malecot catheter must be away from the wall of the bowel by 1–2 cm to avoid blockage of the catheter by bowel mucosa. This can be accomplished by the use of a purse-string suture of 3-0 chromic catgut.

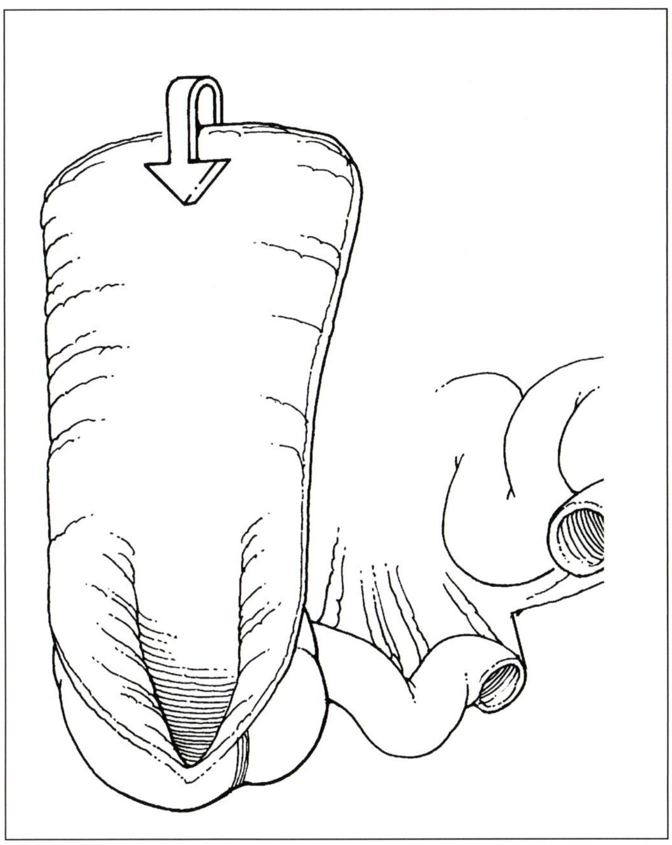

Figure 25.3 The arrow indicates that the cephalad end of the detubularized right colonic segment which will be folded caudally to the apex of the antimesenteric incision when a hand-sewn closure is planned.

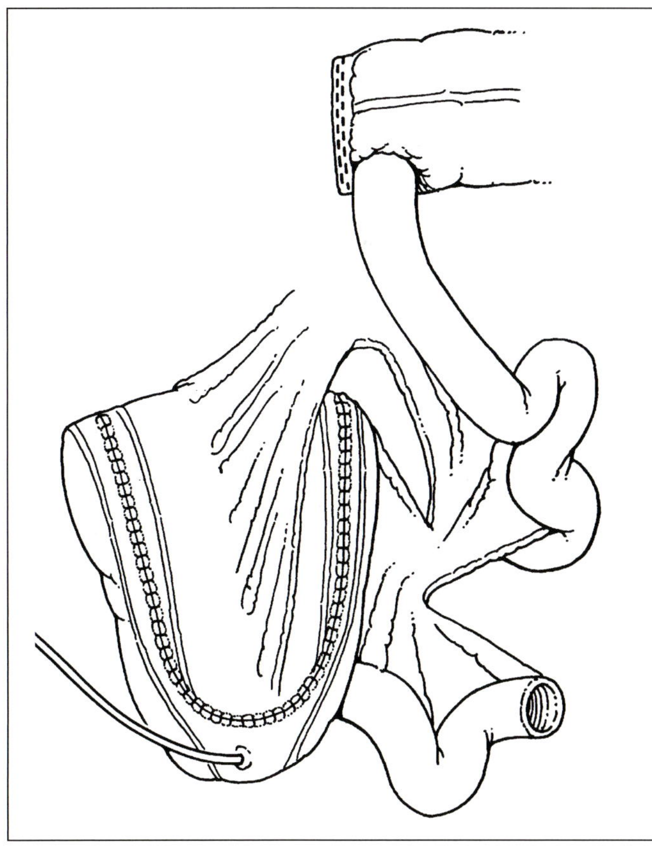

Figure 25.4 An end-to-side ileocolostomy is performed using 25-mm EEA and TA55 4.8-mm staple devices. As an alternative, an end-to-side hand-sewn anastomosis can be performed after spatulating the terminal ileum to compensate for the size discrepancy between the two bowel segments. A 22-Fr Malecot catheter is placed in the dependent portion of the cecum prior to closing the reservoir.

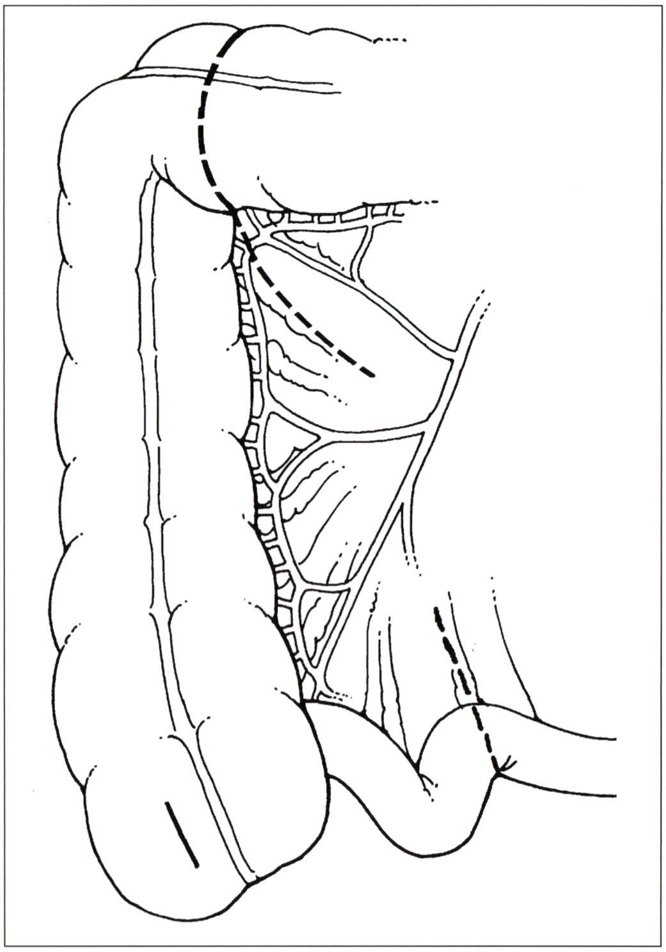

Figure 25.5 When absorbable staples on a GIA stapler are going to be used to detubularize the reservoir, the ileocecal segment is isolated by making incisions along the dashed lines. A 2-cm antimesenteric cecotomy is made as illustrated by the solid line near the cap of the cecum.

The use of absorbable staples on a GIA stapler for the detubularization and reconfiguration of the colonic segment, as in our second series of patients, is illustrated in Figures 25.5 and 25.6. Initially the colonic segment is configured into an inverted 'U' with 3-0 braided, absorbable sutures. The antimesenteric surface at the open distal end of the colonic segment is aligned with the cecotomy made to construct the efferent limb and continence mechanism. A 75-mm stapler with absorbable staples is inserted into the open end of the colon and the cecotomy incision (see Figure 25.6b). Care is exercised to avoid rotation of the bowel segment to the extent that the teniae would be incorporated into the staple line. The stapler which staples to 75 mm and cuts to 70 mm is fired. Usually one or two more applications of the stapler will be needed to complete the detubularization. In contrast with metal staples, absorbable staple lines cannot overlap. Overlapping of absorbable staple lines causes breakage of the staples. To avoid overlapping, it is necessary to incise the remaining uncut 5 mm of tissue between the previously applied staples and extend this full-thickness incision for another 5–6 mm to get the ends of the previous staples at least 1 cm apart to allow application of the next stapler without crushing any staples. Prior to applying the second and/or third staplers, a 3-0 braided, absorbable suture is placed under the end of each distal staple row. The needles should be retained on the sutures to allow the holding stitches to be used as figure-of-eight stitches to close the small gap that will be present between the absorbable staple rows (see Figure 25.6c).

After completion of the detubularization of the reservoir and placement of a cecostomy tube as described earlier, the reservoir is closed by either hand-sewing the remainder with 3-0 braided-absorbable suture or closing all but the areas where the detubularization staples intersect the opening of the pouch with an absorbable TA55 cartridge using 0.060 inch staples (Figure 25.6e). The remaining areas need to be closed with sutures.

Once the reservoir has been detubularized and closed, it is tested for leaks by instilling 200–300 ml of fluid through the cecostomy tube. Any leaks that are present are closed with interrupted or figure-of-eight sutures.

At this point the location of the reservoir must be selected. The location of the stoma (right or left lower quadrant or in the umbilicus), length of the ureters and the length of the mesentery are all factors that determine the final location of the reservoir. Both ureters should be mobilized to the level of the lower pole of the kidneys while care is taken to preserve their blood supply. The left ureter should be led through the retroperitoneum to the right side of the abdomen by passing it through the descending colonic mesentery cephalad to the inferior mesenteric artery. This allows for extra length without kinking as the ureter passes through the mesentery. The left ureter may also be passed through the mesentery of the reservoir if needed to make a smooth course for the ureter to the wall of the reservoir. The right ureter is led to the reservoir with a gentle sweep to avoid kinking.

Both ureters are implanted into the reservoir using an end-to-side technique. Each ureter is cut obliquely or spatulated to increase the size of the anastomosis which helps avoid stenosis (Figure 25.7). The anastomosis is begun at the apex of the spatulation or the short side of the obliquely cut ureter, and 5-0 monofilament, absorbable interrupted stitches are placed with the knots on the outside of the anastomosis. A full thickness bite should be taken on the colonic side to assure that there is good approximation of the mucosa of the ureter and the mucosa of the colon. An 8-Fr pediatric feeding tube is introduced into the reservoir about 1–2 cm in front of the anastomosis and is passed up the ureter to the level of the renal pelvis. A 'Z' stitch of 3-0 chromic catgut is used to secure the stent to the wall of the reservoir. The remainder of the anastomosis is completed with the 5-0 sutures. Usually six to eight stitches are used.

The stoma site is created by making a 1.5-cm hole through all layers of the abdominal wall. The anterior rectus sheath is incised in a cruciate manner and 3-0 braided, absorbable holding stitches are placed from the outside in on the tip of each tab of sheath formed by the cruciate incision. The efferent limb is led as directly as possible through the abdominal wall defect.

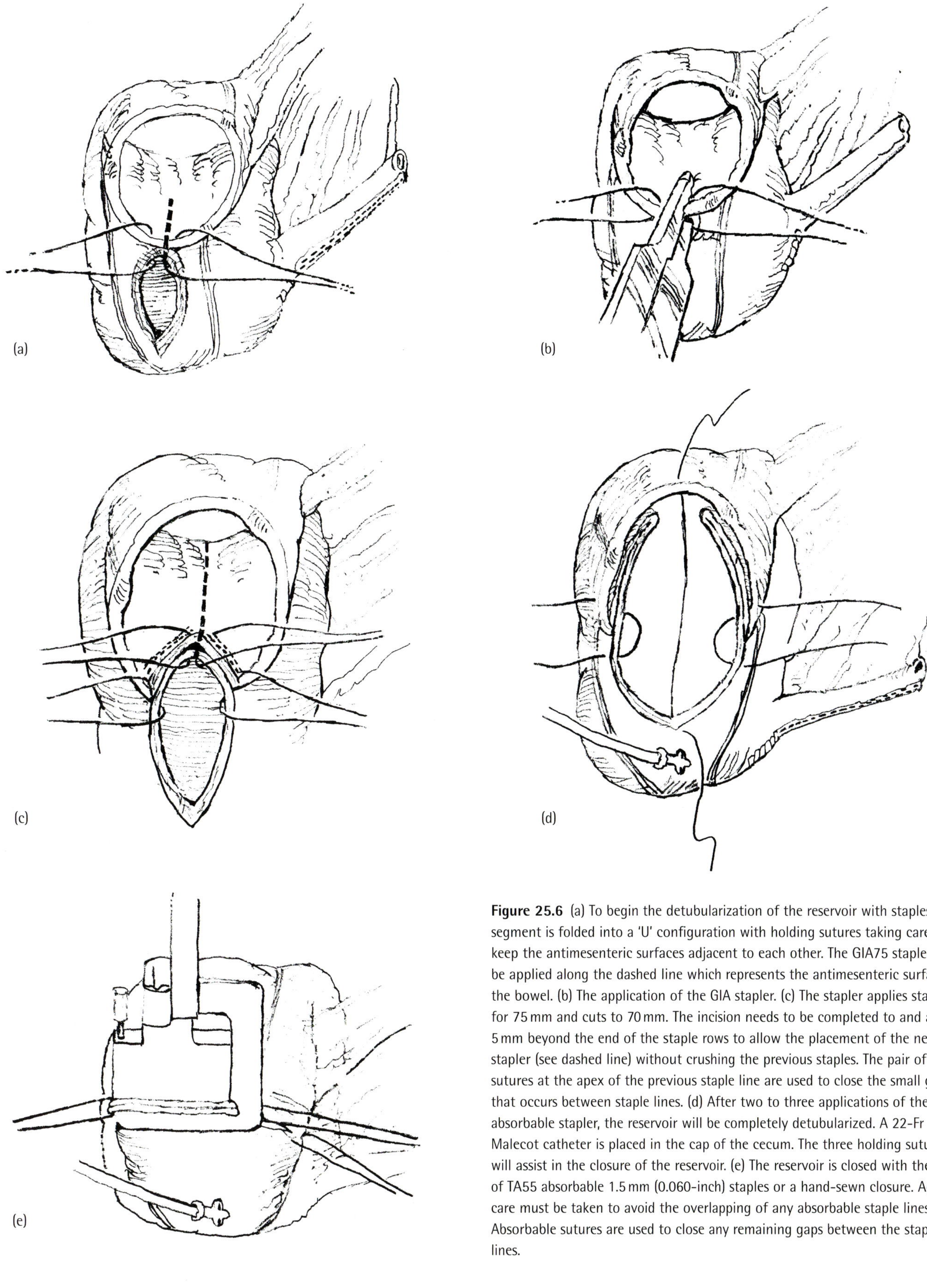

Figure 25.6 (a) To begin the detubularization of the reservoir with staples, the segment is folded into a 'U' configuration with holding sutures taking care to keep the antimesenteric surfaces adjacent to each other. The GIA75 stapler will be applied along the dashed line which represents the antimesenteric surface of the bowel. (b) The application of the GIA stapler. (c) The stapler applies staples for 75 mm and cuts to 70 mm. The incision needs to be completed to and about 5 mm beyond the end of the staple rows to allow the placement of the next stapler (see dashed line) without crushing the previous staples. The pair of sutures at the apex of the previous staple line are used to close the small gap that occurs between staple lines. (d) After two to three applications of the absorbable stapler, the reservoir will be completely detubularized. A 22-Fr Malecot catheter is placed in the cap of the cecum. The three holding sutures will assist in the closure of the reservoir. (e) The reservoir is closed with the use of TA55 absorbable 1.5 mm (0.060-inch) staples or a hand-sewn closure. Again, care must be taken to avoid the overlapping of any absorbable staple lines. Absorbable sutures are used to close any remaining gaps between the staple lines.

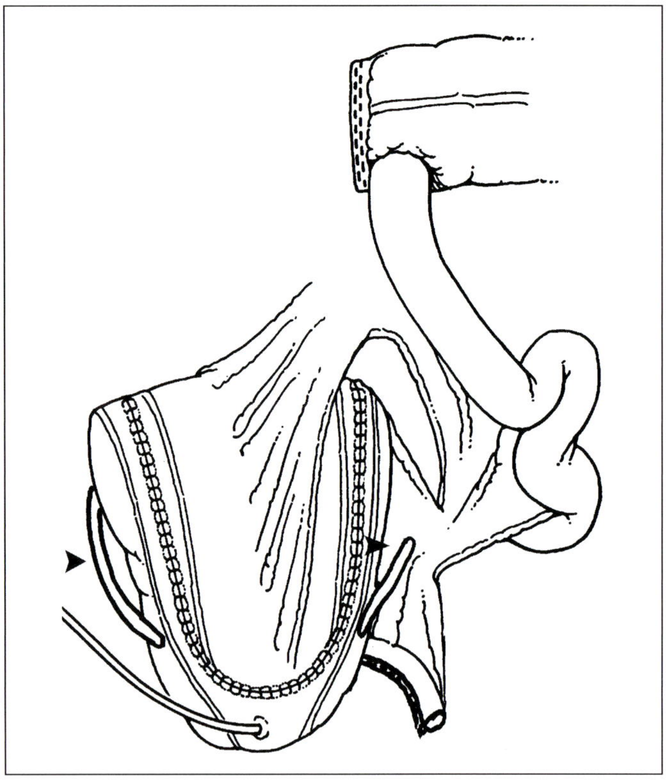

Figure 25.7 The completed reservoir. The ureters, indicated by the arrowheads, have been led to the reservoir in a manner to avoid kinking. The left ureter is led through the sigmoid mesentery cephalad to the inferior mesenteric artery to gain additional length. It may also be passed through the mesentery to the reservoir if needed to achieve a direct path to the anastomosis. Ureteral stents, which are not shown, are led out through the wall of the reservoir approximately 1–2 cm in front of each anastomosis.

The holding stitches are used to secure the anterior rectus sheath to the efferent limb. Any excess length of efferent limb is resected to yield a flush stoma. Usually eight stitches of 3-0 braided, absorbable suture are used to approximate the stoma to the skin.

The cecostomy tube and the stents are led through the abdominal wall using separate stab wounds caudal to the efferent limb. A closed suction drain is usually led through a contralateral stab wound. All tubes are sutured in place with 2-0 silk sutures. Usually catheters or stents are not left through the efferent limb. A petroleum jelly gauze is placed over the stoma in the immediate postoperative period to prevent the mucosa from drying out.

Post-operative care

Beginning immediately after surgery, the cecostomy tube is irrigated with 60–120 ml of saline four times daily to prevent obstruction with mucus. The ureteral stents are placed to straight drainage and are irrigated only as needed to ensure free drainage.

At 1 week postoperatively, radiographs of the stents are taken by injecting contrast under fluoroscopic control. If free drainage of contrast around the stents into the reservoir is noted, the stents are removed. The cecostomy tube is left in place. If pelvic drainage is <100 ml/day, the drain is removed prior to discharging the patient.

At 3 weeks postoperatively, the patient is evaluated with a pouchogram which is performed by filling the reservoir with contrast material through the cecostomy tube by gravity flow. The reservoir is assessed for leakage and the presence or absence of ureteral reflux is noted. An intravenous pyelogram (IVP) is taken to evaluate the upper tracts for any signs of obstruction. Assuming that the radiologic studies are satisfactory, the cecostomy tube is plugged and the patient is taught how to perform self intermittent catheterization. After the patient has done this successfully on several occasions, the cecostomy tube is removed. Leakage from the cecostomy tube site is rarely a problem.

The patient begins a catheterization schedule every 2 hours during the day and every 3 hours during the night. Over a 4–6-week period, the patient is usually able to increase the catheterization intervals to 4–6 hours. Irrigation of the pouch is continued on a less frequent basis as mucus production decreases. Daily irrigation is recommended permanently.

Renal function, electrolytes, and complete blood counts are monitored at 3, 6 and 12 months and then annually if the patient is stable. An IVP is obtained at 3–6 months if no upper tract changes were present on the 3-week postoperative films. The IVP is done again at 1 and 2 years and every 2–3 years thereafter if upper tract changes are absent.

The risk of developing a secondary malignancy in the pouch, which is isolated from the fecal stream seems to be quite low;[5] however, isolated cases have been reported.[6,7] Pouchoscopy and/or cytology may be prudent in the long-term follow-up.

Results of right colon reservoir surgery in the two series of patients

The mean age of first series of 50 patients (27 male and 23 female) was 45.8 years (range 13–76). The indications for surgery are shown in Table 25.1. Note that the most common indication for surgery was a pelvic malignancy. Patients with a previous diversion in this group are listed in Table 25.2. Serum blood urea nitrogen (BUN), creatinine and electrolytes obtained preoperatively, 3 weeks postoperatively, and at least 2.5 years postoperatively are shown in Table 25.3. There were no significant changes in any of these parameters.

Functional results are presented in Table 25.4. The mean and maximum volume of catheterization increased with time. Continence was defined as the ability to remain dry for 4 hours at a time in the day or night without having to catheterize. It should be noted that by 2 years, about three-quarters of the

Table 25.1 Indications for surgery in the first series of 50 patients who underwent right colon reservoir surgery

Bladder cancer	58%
Cervical cancer	4%
Congenital anomalies	16%[a]
Neurogenic bladder	14%[a]
Interstitial cystitis	12%

[a] Two patients had both congenital anomalies and neurogenic bladder.

Table 25.2 Previous urinary diversion in the first series of 50 patients who underwent right colon reservoir surgery

Ileal conduit	12%
Colon conduit	2%
Vesicostomy	6%
Other	10%
Total	30%

Table 25.3 Metabolic studies in the 50 patients who underwent right colon reservoir surgery

Study	Preoperative	First postoperative visit	Last postoperative visit
BUN (mg/dl)	13.9 ± 6.0	14.0 ± 6.5	16.0 ± 8.3
Creatinine (mg/dl)	1.0 ± 0.3	1.0 ± 0.4	1.2 ± 0.3
Na^+ (mEq/l)	139.7 ± 2.7	140.6 ± 2.9	139.4 ± 1.8
K^+ (mEq/l)	4.3 ± 0.4	4.4 ± 0.4	4.3 ± 0.2
Cl^- (mEq/l)	103.0 ± 3.6	104.3 ± 3.3	104.0 ± 1.6
CO_2 (mEq/l)	26.2 ± 4.0	25.1 ± 2.7	27.0 ± 1.8

BUN, blood urea nitrogen.

patients were able to sleep their normal interval without having to catheterize or be wet.

Early complications are those that occur within the first 30 days postoperatively. The incidence and reoperation rates for pouch-related and non-pouch-related complications are presented in Table 25.5. The overall early reoperation rate was 4%. The late (>30 days) post-operative complications are presented in Table 25.6. The overall reoperation rate for late complications was 14%.

In the second series of 29 patients with end-to-side ureterocolonic anastomoses, there were 20 males and 9 females with a mean age of 50.9 years (range 33–68). There was a total of 57 renal units. The obstruction rate was 3/29 patients (10.3%) and 3/57 renal units (5.3%). Two patients had open repairs (one had ureteral reimplantation and one had ileal ureter). One patient had an endoscopic balloon dilatation. All obstructions in this group of patients occurred on the left side. Renal function was not significantly altered postoperatively in any patient. The three patients with unilateral ureteral obstruction had a mean rise of serum creatinine of 0.23 mg/dl. By 1 year, 98% of the patients were dry for at least 4 hours at a time day and night and 85% were sleeping their normal sleep interval without having to catheterize or having leakage.

Discussion

The right colon reservoir using a tapered, plicated ileal efferent limb (Indiana continent urinary reservoir or pouch) described in this chapter meets the requirements for a satisfactory continent cutaneous urinary reservoir. This method creates a high capacity, compliant reservoir with a reliable continence mechanism. The tunneled tenial group had no reflux and had a 6% incidence of pyelonephritis. This group had a 4% incidence of ureteral obstruction with half of these patients (2%) requiring operative intervention for the ureteral obstruction. The group with the end-to-side anastomoses had an obstruction rate of 10.3% with all patients requiring either open or endoscopic intervention. None of the latter group has had pyelonephritis or

Table 25.4 Functional results in the first series of 50 patients who underwent right colon reservoir surgery

	Intraoperative	3-6 months	9–12 months	>24 months
Pouch volume (ml)	484 ± 145			
Mean catheter volume	–	433 ± 143	472 ± 80	500 ± 100
Maximum catheter volume (ml)	–	687 ± 156	731 ± 255	733 ± 378
Day catheter interval (hours)	–	4.2 ± 1.1	4.9 ± 1.3	4.8 ± 1.2
Night catheter interval (hours)	–	4.7 ± 1.5	5.4 ± 1.7	5.3 ± 1.7
Day dry >4 hours	–	73%	94%	94%
Night dry >4 hours	–	75%	94%	94%
Night sleep interval without catheter	–	41%	58%	71%

Table 25.5 Early postoperative complications in the first series of 50 patients who underwent right colon reservoir surgery

Complication	Incidence (%)	Reoperation (%)
Pouch-related		
Pouch leak	4	0
Incontinence	0	0
Inability to catheterize	2	2
Stomal stenosis	0	0
Peristomal hernia	0	0
Ureteral obstruction		
Mild	4	0
Moderate/severe	0	0
Reflux, all grades	0	0
Not pouch-related		
Bowel obstruction	6	0
Wound related	4	2
Total		4

Table 25.6 Late postoperative complications in the first series of 50 patients who underwent right colon reservoir surgery

Complication	Incidence (%)	Reoperation (%)
Pouch-related		
Pouch leak	2	2
Incontinence	4	2
Inability to catheterize	2	0
Stomal stenosis	2	2
Peristomal hernia	0	0
Obstruction		
Mild	0	0
Moderate/severe	4	2
Reflux, all grades	0	0
Not pouch-related		
Bowel obstruction	8	2
Wound related	4	2
Pyelonephritis	6	2
Total		14

loss of a kidney. The higher rate of obstruction in the end-to-side group is hard to explain other than the series had fewer patients than the first series. One possible explanation is that the ureter may receive some additional new blood supply from the submucosal tenial tunnel.

The continence rates were very good in both groups. The first group has a 94% continence rate and the second, a 100% rate. Of the three patients in the first group who were unable to go at least 4 hours between catheterizations two went at least 3.5 hours between catheterizations and chose not to have any intervention. The only patient in the first group who had significant and frequent incontinence had a high pressure reservoir despite complete detubularization and required an ileal cup patch augmentation to the reservoir to achieve continence.

The tapered ileal segment provides a very satisfactory efferent limb. Other than the first patient who had the stapled efferent limb in whom the efferent was made too long (15 cm), no other patient has required revision of the efferent limb with the exception of stomal revision for stenosis in about 5% of the patients. A report from the University of Kansas observed a 15.2% stomal stenosis rate and a 14.4% reoperation rate for this cause.[8] Other reports in the literature have observed complication rates and reoperation rates similar to those reported in this series.[9,10]

A report from the Robert Wood Johnson Medical School looked specifically at comparing non-refluxing ureteroenteric anastomoses versus end-to-side anastomoses.[11] These authors reported a 13% obstruction rate in the non-refluxing group and 1.7% in the end-to-side group. This was statistically significant at the $P<0.05$ level. There was no statistically significant difference in the rate of hydronephrosis, pyelonephritis, upper tract stones, or renal insufficiency. The present authors plan to continue with the end-to-side technique unless a statistically significant difference is shown between the two techniques.

As the types of urinary diversion and reconstruction evolve, the continent cutaneous urinary reservoir will probably always have a place in some patients. In patients without a good continence mechanism or an unsatisfactory or non-existent urethra, the continent cutaneous technique offers the patients an opportunity to avoid wearing an appliance.

The right colonic continent cutaneous urinary reservoir has a short learning curve for surgeons who are accustomed to doing any bowel work. The use of staples for the efferent limb tapering has significantly reduced the operating time and improved the reliability of the efferent limb. Absorbable staples when used to detubularize and close the reservoir decrease the operating time by approximately 1 hour and eliminate the most tedious portion of the procedure.

References

1. Simon J. Ectopia vesicae (absence of the anterior walls of the bladder and public abdominal parietes): operation for directing the orifices of the ureters into the rectum; temporary success; subsequent death; autopsy. Lancet 1852; ii: 568.
2. Gilchrist RH, Merricks JW, Hamlin JW, Reiger IT. Construction of a substitute bladder and urethra. Surg Gynecol Obstet 1950; 90: 752–60.
3. Rowland RG, Mitchell ME, Bihrle R et al. The cecoileal continent urinary reservoir. World J Urol 1985; 3: 185–90.
4. Rowland RG, Mitchell ME, Bihrle R et al. The Indiana continent urinary reservoir. J Urol 1987; 137: 1136–9.
5. Rowland RG, Regan JS. The risk of secondary malignancies in urinary reservoirs. Internationale d'Urologie Reports: Continent Urinary Diversion 1992; 2: 299.

6. Lisle D, Cataldo P, Bibawi SE, Wood M. Colonic adenocarcinoma occurring in an Indiana pouch: report of a case and review of the literature. Dis Colon Rectum 2000; 43: 864–7.
7. L'Esperance JO, Lakshmanan Y, Trainer AF et al. Adenocarcinoma in an Indiana pouch after cystectomy for transitional cell carcinoma. J Urol 2001; 165: 901–2.
8. Holmes DG, Trasher JB, Park GY, Kueker DC, Weigel JW. Long-term complications related to the modified Indiana pouch. Urology 2002; 60: 603.
9. Ahlering TE, Weinbert AC, Razor B. Modified Indiana pouch. J Urol 1991; 145: 1156–8.
10. Dolezal J, Pacik D. Our early experience with the Indiana pouch – cecoileal continent urinary reservoir. Central European Symposium on Coloproctology. 1993; Abstract 9a: 6.
11. Pantuck AJ, Han KR, Perrotti M, Weiss RE, Cummings KB. Ureteroenteric anastomosis in continent urinary diversion: long-term results and complications of direct versus non-refluxing techniques. J Urol 2000; 163: 450–5.

26 The Mitrofanoff principle in continent urinary diversion

Christopher S Cooper and Howard M Snyder, III

Introduction

Mitrofanoff reported the use of appendix implanted into the bladder as a continent catheter conduit in 1980.[1] In this series the bladder neck was routinely closed to achieve continence. The appendix was first used as a continent catheterizable channel in children in the USA at the Children's Hospital of Philadelphia in 1982 and was subsequently named by Drs John W Duckett and Howard M Snyder, III as the 'Mitrofanoff principle'.[2] Since then, many institutions have reported application of the appendicovesicostomy using the Mitrofanoff principle in the pediatric population,[2–9] and it has become the most widely used alternative continence mechanism in the world.[3–6,10,11] It has been used in exstrophy and epispadias patients who are reluctant to perform intermittent catheterization due to a sensitive urethra. It is also useful in spina bifida patients who may find it difficult to access their urethra due to obesity or wheelchair dependence. Mitrofanoff originally reported the use of either the appendix or ureter as the catheterizable channel and others have reported their use of ileum, fallopian tube, cecum and stomach.[7,8,12] Furthermore, this technique has also been applied to reconstructive surgery in adults, and for achieving a continent stoma for antegrade enemas.[13]

The principle

The Mitrofanoff principle describes the creation of a flap valve using a small diameter, supple conduit, such as the appendix or ureter, tunneled into a reservoir. The small diameter of such a continence channel facilitates catheterization. The continence channel runs along the inner wall of the reservoir and is fixed in place. As filling of the reservoir occurs, the continence channel is compressed, leading, by hydraulic principles, to a higher resistance to flow than the pressure produced in the reservoir (Figure 26.1). This is the same mechanism employed in ureteral reimplantation to prevent reflux. A supple conduit may be more effectively compressed against a firm reservoir wall, such as the bladder, compared with the same length of conduit implanted into the intestine.[8]

A high percentage of Mitrofanoff's original patients developed bilateral upper tract deterioration or incontinent stomas.[14] These patients underwent their operations before recognition of the need for a low-pressure reservoir became established. With time and experience, the importance of a low-pressure reservoir became apparent. Storage of urine in the reservoir at

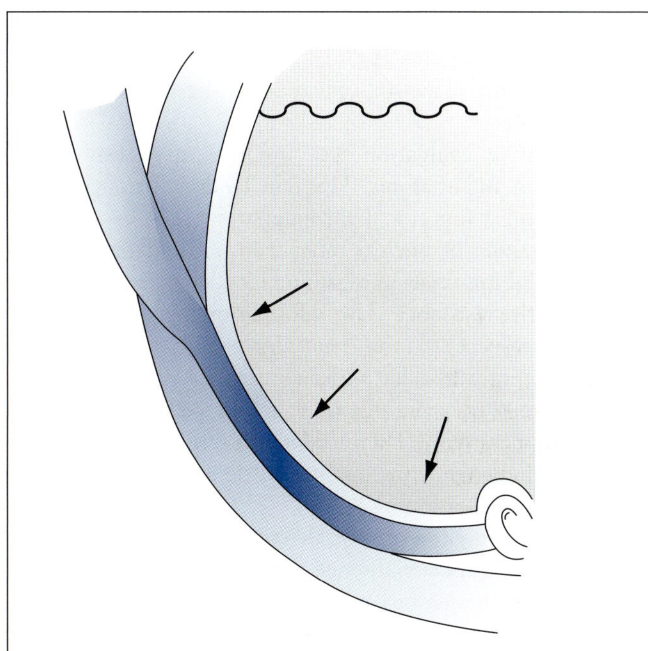

Figure 26.1 Flap valves create continence by having a segment compressed by reservoir filling, as for a reimplanted ureter.

pressures of less than 35–40 cmH_2O is critical to avoid damage to the upper tracts.[15,16] In Mitrofanoff's original series, bladder neck closure effectively eliminated a 'pop-off' mechanism for elevated reservoir pressures. The capacity of the reservoir also relates to the storage pressure since over-distension of any bladder results in elevated pressures. Catheterization more than every 4 hours is difficult to achieve so the reservoir size must be adequate to permit low-pressure storage of urine volume corresponding to a patient's emptying frequency of four to six times a day. This is frequently accomplished by augmentation cystoplasty at the time of creating an appendicovesicostomy.

Preoperative evaluation

Prior to performing a continence procedure along with the Mitrofanoff principle, the patient's compliance with intermittent catheterization must be ensured. Lapides et al introduced the concept that low-pressure emptying is more important than sterility in maintaining urinary tract health.[17] One of the consequences of intermittent catheterization is bacterial colonization of the lower urinary tract. As long as storage pressures are maintained at a low level and emptying is complete, symptomatic episodes of infection appear to be rare in children and adults.[18,19] Non-compliance with catheterization increases the chance for infection and upper tract deterioration from elevated storage pressures. Furthermore, the flap valve mechanism is so continent that bladder or reservoir rupture may occur before stomal incontinence if compliance with catheterization is lacking. Postoperative rates of infection, stomal stenosis and revision are statistically higher in non-compliant patients compared with compliant patients, highlighting the importance of preoperative patient selection and education regarding catheterization.[20] In this regard, the surgeon must remember that a technically successful operation in the wrong patient is destined to fail.

Preoperative evaluation also involves an assessment of renal function and anatomy. This may be done through serum creatinine and a functional imaging study, such as an intravenous pyelogram or nuclear renal scan. A urodynamic study provides useful information regarding bladder capacity, compliance and outlet resistance. This information may guide the surgeon with respect to the need for simultaneous bladder augmentation or a bladder outlet continence procedure, however, it serves as no guarantee that such procedures will not be needed postoperatively. The bladder and sphincter muscles are dynamic and change with time, requiring a lifetime of routine postoperative evaluation.

If available, fluoroscopic urodynamics provide information regarding the presence or absence of reflux. Alternatively, a cystogram may be obtained to evaluate reflux. Although the cessation rate of reflux after bladder augmentation is high, we routinely perform a ureteral reimplant at the time of augmentation in patients with a history of reflux to avoid the unpleasant predicament of persistent reflux in a patient with chronic bacteriuria.

Surgical technique

We routinely perform a mechanical and antibiotic bowel preparation in patients undergoing anticipated appendicovesicostomy in case the appendix is not suitable for use and an alternative segment of bowel is required. Precautions regarding latex serve to minimize exposure to latex allergens. The appendicovesicostomy is performed through either a midline incision or Pfannenstiel's incision. The midline incision curves widely around the umbilicus, leaving enough fascia lateral to the umbilicus to permit closure away from the appendicovesicostomy stoma, which may be placed in the depths of the umbilicus. The cecum is widely mobilized so that the base of the intact appendix reaches the umbilicus or anterior abdominal wall beneath the location of the planned stoma. This mobilization prevents stretching of the vascular pedicle to the appendix. By mobilizing the cecum the appendix can be easily placed to the umbilicus or elsewhere on the abdominal wall without tension. Placement of the appendix has also been described in an orthotopic urethral location in female patients.[21] Since the blood supply of the appendix is at the end of the superior mesenteric artery it has great mobility. By moving the appendix with the cecum there is no need to widely separate the appendix from the cecum and this, in turn, protects the appendix blood supply.

Following removal of the peritoneum from the bladder dome, the ability of the bladder to reach the umbilicus is tested by traction on the dome of the bladder. If the bladder reaches the umbilicus, it is opened along the anterior surface, usually to the left of the midline, which permits the right side of the bladder to be more easily stretched to the umbilicus. This incision also facilitates access to the opened bladder for sigmoid cystoplasty. If needed, a ureteral reimplant or bladder neck continence procedure is performed at this time.

The bladder can virtually always be stretched to reach the umbilicus, especially if the bladder is opened on the left side, permitting a flap to be stretched on the right side to reach the umbilicus. Additional mobility may be gained by incising the left side of the bladder wall transversely. Leaving a portion of the cephalad anterior bladder wall intact as a cap permits manual elevation from inside of the bladder toward the umbilicus (Figure 26.2). The umbilicus represents an advantageous site for the stoma not only from a cosmetic standpoint, but its depth often makes it the easiest place to reach as it traverses the subcutaneous tissue in an obese abdomen.

The site of the bladder hiatus is identified and made large enough to easily admit a finger. The path of the intended appendiceal tunnel is identified and injected submucosally with a mixture of lidocaine and epinephrine (1:100 000). The path of the appendix should be off the midline to prevent future catheterization of the urethra via the appendicovesicostomy. If

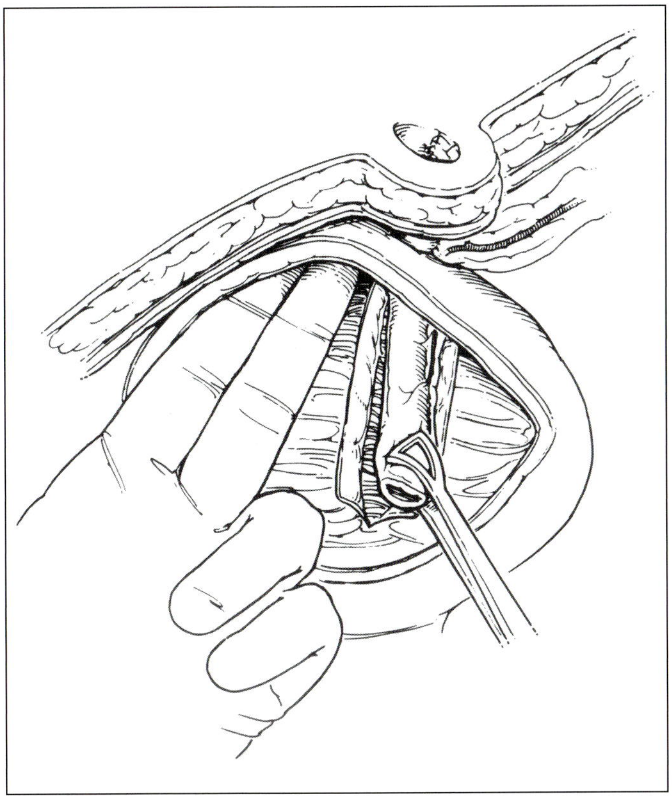

Figure 26.2 Leaving an anterior cap of bladder facilitates manual positioning of the bladder against the anterior abdominal fascia.

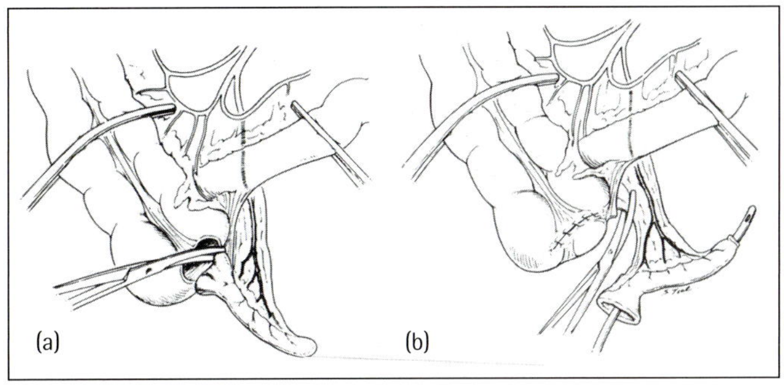

Figure 26.3 (a) The appendix is isolated with small cuff of cecum. (b) Care is taken to preserve the vasculature.

the trigone is sensate it is wise to direct the path of the appendix such that catheterization does not irritate the trigone. Mucosal flaps are elevated broadly around the hiatus and along the intended path of the appendix prior to fixation of the bladder to the abdominal wall.

The umbilical stoma is created with a U-shaped skin flap incision in the depths of the umbilicus from the 3 o'clock to the 9 o'clock positions. The flap is sharply elevated from the fascia to which it is adherent. The fascia is opened vertically and wide enough for a finger to be inserted from below to ensure no compression of the appendix mesentery. A similar laterally based skin flap can also be used at other sites along the abdominal wall and interdigitated with a spatulated appendix.

A minimal separation of the appendix mesentery at the cecal junction is carried out to expose the cecal wall. The appendix is harvested by taking a small cuff of cecum (Figure 26.3). In the rare situation where the appendix is short (less than 5 cm long) a few centimeters of a strip of the cecum may be tubularized to lengthen the appendix.[22]

The cecal end of the appendix is brought through the fascial and umbilical opening and spatulated (to interdigitate with the skin flap of the bottom of the umbilicus) taking care to avoid the mesentery. The appendix is approximated to the edges of the skin of the umbilicus or an alternative skin flap with multiple interrupted absorbable sutures (5-0 vicryl) placed at 2–3 mm intervals, taking solid bites of the full thickness of the appendix. This skin-to-appendix anastomosis is facilitated by doing it before attaching the appendix to the bladder so that the anastomosis can be carried out above the skin level (Figure 26.4). A well-lubricated catheter should be repeatedly passed at this time, and following each of the subsequent steps, checking for any evidence of obstruction.

Following creation of the appendicovesicostomy stoma, the appendix is passed through the bladder hiatus and pulled down, causing the disappearance of the stoma into the depths of the umbilicus (Figure 26.5). The bladder is manually elevated to the umbilicus or the alternative fascial hiatus in the abdominal wall. By fixing the bladder reservoir as close as possible to the conduit stoma, the length of the conduit and chance for subsequent catheterization difficulties are minimized. The bladder or reservoir is pexed to the fascia on the lateral side of the umbilicus so that the hiatus in the bladder and fascia are aligned (Figure 26.6). Our preference has been to do this with permanent 2-0 prolene sutures, however, others do this with absorbable sutures.[8] With several more sutures the medial and anterior aspects of the hiatus are attached to the abdominal wall. A gap in the pexing sutures is left along the posterior side to avoid compression of the appendiceal mesentery. During the attachment of the bladder to the abdominal wall, a lubricated feeding tube is repeatedly passed into the appendix to ensure that no obstructing edge of fascia or bladder wall has been created that can later interfere with catheterization. If the catheter does not pass easily at the time of the operation, it is unlikely to improve postoperatively and the cause of the obstruction should be identified and remedied.

The appendix is stretched to the distal end of the mucosal trough helping to ensure a straight appendix for catheterization. A tunnel length of at least 2.5 cm has been suggested for continence.[23] The fixation of the appendix at the umbilicus and distally to the detrusor keeps it straight and helps to avoid kinks in the course of the appendix. Kinks of the appendix as it traverses the abdominal fascia or bladder wall can lead to deflection of the catheter with resultant distortion and sacculation of the appendix, that may result in difficulty with catheterization.

The distal appendix is amputated and the bladder end spatulated over 3–4 mm to prevent a stenosis occurring through

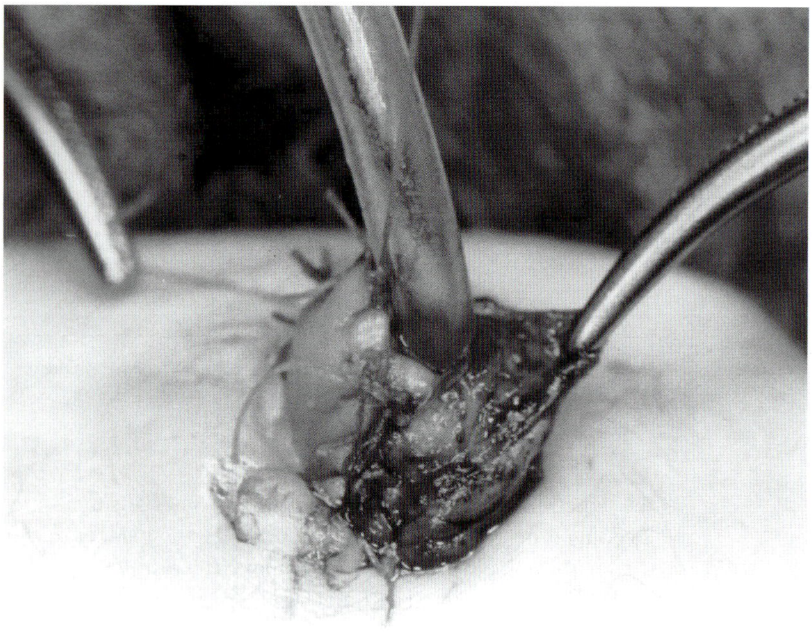

Figure 26.4 The appendix is sutured to the everted umbilical skin flap. The feeding tube is demonstrated entering the appendix. (Reprinted from Harris CF et al. J Urol 2000; 163: 1922–6[9] with permission from Lippincott Williams & Wilkins.)

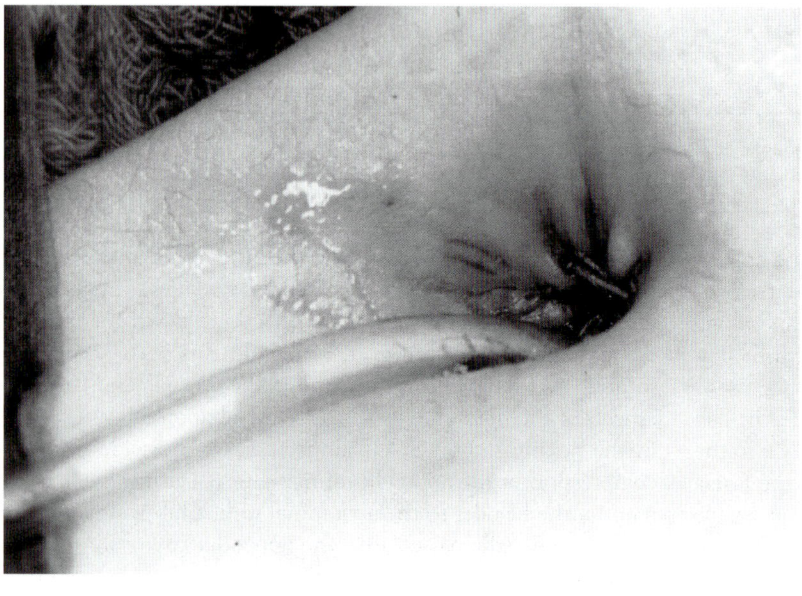

Figure 26.5 After completion of the stoma, traction on the distal aspect of the appendix results in the disappearance of the appendicovesicostomy in the depths of the umbilicus. (Reprinted from Harris CF et al. J Urol 2000; 163: 1922–6[9] with permission from Lippincott Williams & Wilkins.)

wound contracture at the distal anastomosis of the appendix to the bladder. The distal appendix is attached with two or three interrupted polyglycolic or polyglycan sutures, catching a solid bite of the detrusor muscle at the edge of the apical incision in the mucosa. The back wall of appendix may be sutured in several places to the detrusor to relieve tension and help maintain the position of the appendix in the trough. Care must be taken not to rotate the appendix with these sutures, which could create a mucosal fold in the appendix capable of interfering with catheterization. The mucosal flaps are approximated over the appendix. Having completed the appendicovesicostomy, catheterization is repeated to ensure a smooth course has been created. If augmentation of the bladder is to be performed it is carried out last.

A suprapubic tube is routinely used as well as a drain in the perivesical space. Filling of the bladder through the suprapubic tube permits the surgeon to check the continence of the appendicovesicostomy. A 10-Fr polyethylene catheter is left in the appendix as a stent for 2–3 weeks. Three weeks after surgery a cystogram is performed and then catheterization of the appendicovesicostomy is started with a 12-Fr polyethylene catheter. Long-term catheterization is carried out with a 12- or 14-Fr catheter, which has a blunter tip than the 10-Fr catheter. A 14-Fr catheter improves emptying of intestinal mucus if an entero-

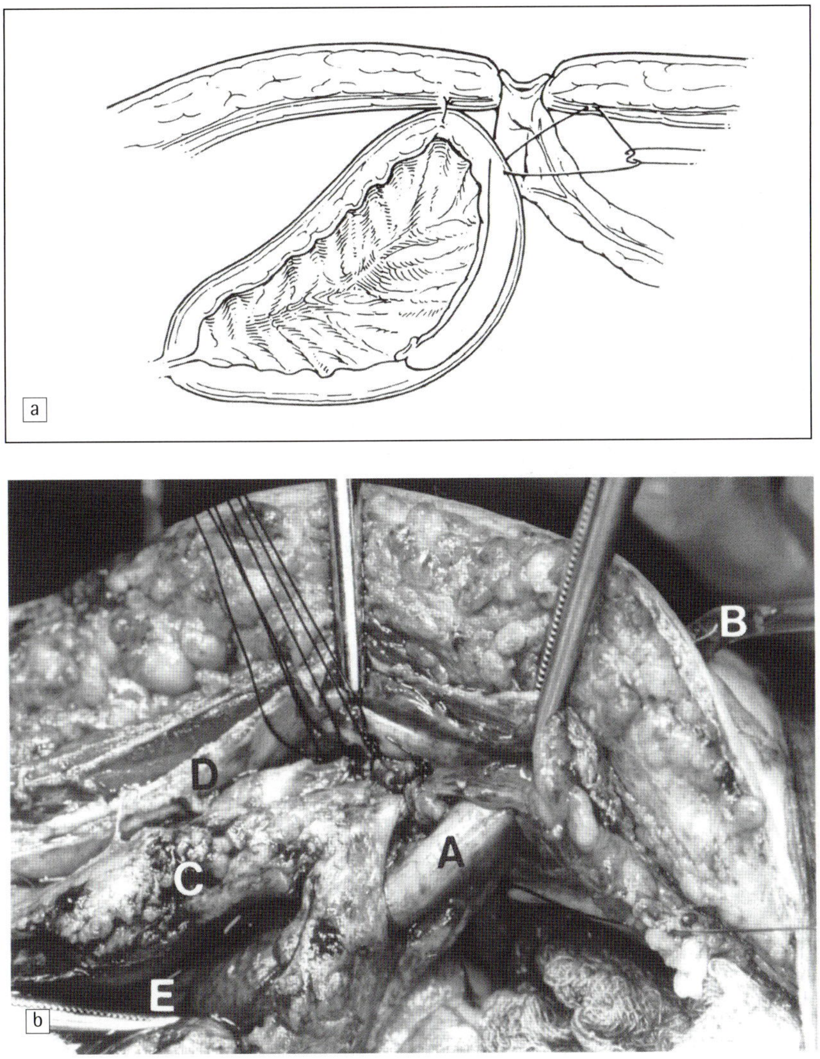

Figure 26.6 (a) The appendix with feeding tube inserted via the umbilical stoma traversing fascial and bladder openings. (b) The appendix (A) with feeding tube (B) inserted via the umbilical stoma is demonstrated traversing the fascial and bladder openings. The sutures are fixing the bladder wall (D) to the anterior abdominal fascia (C) along the lateral side of the hiatus. The bladder lumen is demonstrated (E). (Reprinted from Harris CF et al. J Urol 2000; 163: 1922–6[9] with permission from Lippincott Williams & Wilkins.)

cystoplasty has been done. The suprapubic tube is removed when catheterization is reliably established. Office bladder ultrasound permits assessment of the efficacy of catheterization by measurement of post-catheterization residual urine.

Instead of the appendix, several other tissues may be used with the Mitrofanoff principle. Some of the reported options are ileum, fallopian tube, cecum and stomach.[7,8,12] As originally described, the ureter was also used, although results with this technique appear less satisfactory than with the appendix.[24] If the ureter is employed and reflux needs to be corrected, an extravesical reimplantation offers the potential advantage of preserving the distal blood supply.

Recently, the use of a short, transversely retubularized segment of bowel to create a conduit similar to the appendix has been used and is discussed in further detail in Chapter 28.[25,26] Success rates with this technique appear to be similar to those with the appendix, which some have suggested reserving for use with an antegrade enema stoma.[27] Others describe dividing the appendix for use with bladder and bowel.[28]

Outcome and complications

Success of the appendicovesicostomy has led to its widespread use with good early follow-up.[3,4,7,12] Minimal complications have been reported. The most common complication has been stomal stenosis and, rarely, appendiceal necrosis or stricture. The technique of interdigitating a U-shaped flap of skin into a spatulated appendix minimizes the incidence of stomal stenosis.[9] Mobilization of the cecum and the root of the mesentery and avoidance of dissection separating the appendix from the cecum should reduce injury to the vascular supply of the appendix and also decrease stenosis as well as ischemic stricture occurrence.

Published series report appendicovesicostomy stomal stenosis rates between 7 and 45% with mean follow-up ranging from 13 to 240 months (Table 26.1). Stomal stenosis is generally considered an early complication of appendicovesicostomy, but has occurred as late as 71 months following the operation.[7] Unless the stenosis is mild, dilation of stomal stenosis usually

Table 26.1 Published reports and series of the Mitrofanoff procedure in children and adults: stomal stenosis and other complications

Investigators	Patients with appendix used	Age in years mean (range)	Follow-up in months mean (range)	Stomal stenosis	Mean time to stomal stenosis occurrence	Appendiceal stoma continence	Stones	Necrosis	Stricture	Revisions (no. of patients)
Dykes et al[3]	19	10.1 (1–19)	13 (median) (2–45)	4/19 (21%)	NA	100%	NA	1/19	0/19	5/19 (26%)
Keating et al[4]	14	9 (4–15)	17 (6–29)	0		NA	NA	0	0	0
Duckett and Lofti[10]	25	13 (median) (5–25)	38.4 (6–96)	3/41 (7%)	NA	NA	13/41 (32%)	1/26	3/41 (7%)	3/41 (7%)
Sumfest JM et al[5]	26	11 (3–31)	28.8 (2–72)	4/26 (15%)	NA	25/26 (96%)	0	0	1/26	2/26
Woodhouse and MacNeily et al[12]	54	29.3 (median) (13.6–82.3)	30 (median) (2–98)	24/100 (24%)	7 months (median)	49/54 (91%)	NA	0	0	13/54 (24%)
Jayanthi et al[29]	25	8.7 (18 months–18.6)	29 (6–63)	4/25 (16%)	NA	25/25 (100%)	5/28 (18%)	0	0	4/25
Van Savage et al[6]	48	8.8 (3 days–20)	36	6/48 (13%)	NA	48/48 (100%)	5/66 (8%)			7/66 (11%)
Suzer O et al[7]	36	10 (3–21)	36 (0.5–78)	3/36 (8%)	15.4 months	NA	2/43 (5%)	0	6/36	6/36 (17%)
Kaefer and Retik[8]	17	13.7 (3–38)	62.4 (1–122)	5/50 (10%)	NA	NA	6/50 (12%)	NA	1/50	NA
Cain et al[11]	57	11 (2–23)	30.5			56/57 (98%)				12/57 (21%)
Harris et al[9]	50	13.1 (4–25)	52 (3–196)	5/50 (10%)	13 months	49/50 (98%)	7/50 (14%)	1	2/50 (4%)	8/50 (16%)
Liard et al[14]	20	8 (3–16)	240 (180–276)	9/20 (45%)	NA	15/20 (75%)	5/20(25%)	1/20	0	10/20 (50%)

fails and repair requires surgical revision with advancement of a cutaneous flap into a spatulated conduit.[23] If the stenosis is at the junction of the conduit and reservoir it may be revised by endoscopic incision.

Besides stomal stenosis, difficulty with catheterization can result from angulations in the course of the catheterizable channel. Hitching the bladder to the abdominal wall and use of an umbilical stoma decreases the requirement for a long appendix. This technique also decreases the length of the extravesical appendix and reduces the likelihood of kinking the appendix. Frequent catheterization of the appendix throughout the operative procedure helps ensure an easily catheterizable appendix postoperatively.

The flap-valve mechanism at the appendicovesical junction provides excellent continence at the stoma. Stomal continence rates range from 75[15] to 100%[29] in the literature. Because of the successful continence mechanism generated with the Mitrofanoff principle, rupture of the bladder or reservoir may occur without catheterization. Even in patients compliant with daily catheterization, the dynamic nature of the bladder may lead to hypertrophy and altered storage characteristics. Elevated storage pressures may subsequently lead to hydronephrosis and renal damage, so routine lifetime follow-up requires periodic renal imaging most often accomplished with renal sonography.

Significant leakage of urine through the stoma should prompt a complete urodynamic study. If there is low-pressure leakage, treatment options include injection of submucosal bulking agents, artificial sphincter placement around the conduit, or revision of the conduit with creation of a longer submucosal tunnel.[23]

Bladder stones are a complication most likely related to incomplete bladder emptying. Bacterial colonization and pooling of mucus in a dependent region of the bladder predispose to stone formation in the patient with an appendicovesicostomy. This is most likely to occur in the patient with an augmented bladder emptied only through the appendicovesicostomy. Periodic bladder irrigation should help reduce the risk of bladder stones, however, occurrence of stones has been reported 20 years following the operation.[14] The potential for stones requires lifetime follow-up with bladder sonography at the time of routine renal sonography. Treatment alternatives include extracorporeal shock wave lithotripsy, endoscopic lithotripsy or cystolithotomy.

References

1. Mitrofanoff P. Cystostomie continent trans-appendiuclaire dans le traitement des vessies neurologiques. Chir Pediatr 1980; 21: 297–305.
2. Duckett JW, Snyder HM III. Continent urinary diversion: variations on the Mitrofanoff principle. J Urol 1986; 136: 58–62.
3. Dykes EH, Duffy PG, Ransley PG. The use of the Mitrofanoff principle in achieving clean intermittent catheterisation and urinary continence in children. J Pediatr Surg 1991; 26: 535–8.
4. Keating MA, Rink RC, Adams MC. Appendicovesicostomy: a useful adjunct to continent reconstruction of the bladder. J Urol 1993; 149: 1091–4.
5. Sumfest JM, Burns MW, Mitchell ME. The Mitrofanoff principle in urinary reconstruction. J Urol 1993; 150: 1875–7.
6. Van Savage JG, Khoury AE, McLorie GA, Churchill BM. Outcome analysis of Mitrofanoff principle applications using appendix and ureter to umbilical and lower quadrant stomal sites. J Urol 1996; 156: 1794–7.
7. Suzer O, Vates TS, Freedman AL, Smith CA, Gonzalez R. Results of the Mitrofanoff procedure in urinary tract reconstruction in children. Br J Urol 1997; 79: 279–82.
8. Kaefer M, Retik AB. The Mitrofanoff principle in continent urinary reconstruction. Urol Clin North Am 1997; 24: 795–811.
9. Harris CF, Cooper CS, Hutcheson JC, Snyder HM III. Appendicovesicostomy: the Mitrofanoff procedure – a 15-year perspective. J Urol 2000; 163: 1922–6.
10. Duckett JW, Lotfi AH. Appendicovesicostomy (and variations) in bladder reconstruction. J Urol 1993; 149: 567–9.
11. Cain MP, Casale AJ, King SJ, Rink RC. Appendicovesicostomy and newer alternatives for the Mitrofanoff procedure: results in the last 100 patients at Riley Children's Hospital. J Urol 1999; 162: 1749–52.
12. Woodhouse CR, MacNeily AE. The Mitrofanoff principle: expanding upon a versatile technique. Br J Urol 1994; 74: 447–53.
13. Malone PS, Ransley PG, Kiely EM. Preliminary report: the antegrade continence enema. Lancet 1990; 336: 1217–18.
14. Liard A, Séguir-Lipszyc, Mathiot A, Mitrofanoff P. The Mitrofanoff procedure: 20 years later. J Urol 2001; 165: 2394–8.
15. McGuire EJ, Woodside JR, Borden TA, Weiss RM. Prognostic value of urodynamic testing in myelodysplastic patients. J Urol 1981; 126: 205–9.
16. Churchill BM, Gilmour RF, Williot P. Urodynamics. Pediatr Clin North Am 1987; 34: 1133–57.
17. Lapides J, Diokno AC, Silber SM, Lowe BS. Clean intermittent self-catheterization in the treatment of urinary tract disease. J Urol 1972; 107: 458–61.
18. Kass EJ, Koff SA. Bladder augmentation in the pediatric neuropathic bladder. J Urol 1983; 129: 552–5.
19. Månsson W. Continuing experience with the right colon as a continent reservoir for urine. In: King LR, Stone AR, Webster GD (eds). Bladder Reconstruction and Continent Urinary Diversion. 2nd edn. Chicago: Mosby, 1991: 283–98.
20. Clark T, Pope JC IV, Adams MC, Wells N, Brock JW III. Factors that influence outcomes of the Mitrofanoff and Malone antegrade continence enema in reconstructive procedures in children. J Urol 2002; 168: 1537–40.
21. Barroso U Jr, Duel B, Barthold JS, Gonzalez R. Orthotopic urethral substitution in female patients using the Mitrofanoff principle. J Urol 1999; 161: 251–3.
22. Bruce RG, McRoberts JW. Cecoappendicovesicostomy: conduit-lengthening technique for use in continent urinary reconstruction. Urology 1998; 52: 702–4.
23. Mitrofanoff P, Liard A. Continent diversions. In: Gearhart JP, Rink RC, Mouriquand PDE (eds). Pediatric Urology. Philadelphia: WB Saunders, 2001; 947–55.

24. Mor Y, Kajbafzadeh AM, German K et al. The role of ureter in the creation of Mitrofanoff channels in children. J Urol 1997; 157: 635–7.
25. Yang WH. Yang needle tunneling technique in creating antireflux and continent mechanisms. J Urol 1993; 150: 830–4.
26. Monti PR, Lara RC, Dutra MA, de Carvalho JR. New techniques for construction of efferent conduits based on the Mitrofanoff principle. Urology 1997; 49: 112–15.
27. Cain MP, Casale AJ, King SJ, Rink RC. Appendicovesicostomy and newer alternatives for the Mitrofanoff procedure: results in the last 100 patients at Riley Children's Hospital. J Urol 1999; 162: 1749–52.
28. Kajbafzadeh AM, Chubak N. Simultaneous Malone antegrade continent enema and Mitrofanoff principle using the divided appendix: report of a new technique for prevention of stoma complications. J Urol 2001; 165: 2404–9.
29. Jayanthi VR, Churchill BM, McLorie GA, Khoury AE. Concomitant bladder neck closure and Mitrofanoff diversion for the management of intractable urinary incontinence. J Urol 1995; 154: 886–8.

27 In situ modification of the Mitrofanoff principle in adult patients

Elmar W Gerharz and Hubertus Riedmiller

Introduction

Ever since Bardenheuer of Cologne performed the first cystectomy for a tumor of the bladder in 1887,[1] the surgical challenge has not been to remove the diseased organ but to replace its function appropriately: the first patient died 14 days after his ureters were left to drain the urine into the pelvis. More than a hundred years later, the optimal form of urinary diversion after cystectomy for muscle invasive bladder cancer remains a highly controversial issue. Some authors suggest that orthotopic bladder substitution allows a quality of life similar to that of individuals with a native lower urinary tract.[2] In fact, a recent study comparing recurrence-free Danish patients after orthotopic reconstruction with a frequency matched control population in the same geographical region using a non-established questionnaire found similar wellbeing and subjective quality of life in both groups.[3] In a Cochrane review,[4] however, an evidence-based approach to determine the best way of improving or replacing the function of the lower urinary tract using intestinal segments did not find any evidence that continent diversion was better than conduit diversion, or vice versa. The authors were also critical about the absence of good quality data in the literature despite the fact that such surgery has been commonplace for so many years.

Among the different techniques, the versatile Mitrofanoff principle[5] has attained significant popularity predictably providing continence and allowing easy catheterization in more than 90% of cases. Although the French urologist with the exotic Russian name was neither the first nor the last to use the appendix as a channel for evacuation of a urinary reservoir his paper undisputedly has become a modern classic in reconstructive urology. While Paul Mitrofanoff himself basically described a surgical technique Duckett and Snyder[6] and Woodhouse and MacNeily[7] elaborated on the subject and actually defined what is referred to as the 'principle' nowadays. In 1990 Riedmiller et al[8] introduced the Mitrofanoff theme to the ileocecal reservoir significantly reducing the length of the Mainz pouch procedure.

Diagnosis

The most common indication for continent cutaneous diversion is bladder replacement after anterior pelvic exenteration for malignant disease, followed by functional or morphological bladder loss for other reasons. Diagnostic modalities therefore should be directed at the underlying pathology and definitive treatment.

In every case of urinary diversion or conversion preoperative anatomic evaluation must provide maximum information. Excretory urography, voiding cysturethrography, loopogram, urethrography, endoscopy and retrograde injection of ureteral stumps may be useful investigations especially in patients with urogenital abnormalities, in patients with multiple prior surgeries and before complex conversion procedures. In upper urinary tract dilatation functional assessment may include diuresis isotope renography.

Indications for surgery

This chapter is written in a time that is witnessing an 'indication shift' away from continent cutaneous diversion towards orthotopic substitution challenging some of the long-held oncologic beliefs in the surgical management of transitional cell carcinoma (TCC) of the bladder. For very obvious reasons the advent of neobladder construction has stimulated an increased interest in the 'fate of the urethra'[9] after definitive treatment of invasive TCC. While the fear of urethral tumor recurrence was the rationale for prophylactic en bloc urethrectomy at the time of cystectomy there is now a strong tendency to preserve the urethra wherever possible. The exclusion criteria for orthotopic reconstruction in men, however, remain contentious. While previous or synchronous urethral TCC is an absolute contraindication to urethral preservation the role of multifocality, associated carcinoma in situ, bladder neck and prostatic involvement in urethral recurrence are less well defined. In these cases, continent cutaneous diversion still is a safe alternative in the appropriate patient. In women with TCC orthotopic reconstruction is possible, but can hardly be considered a standard procedure yet as experience with this approach is largely confined to a few highly specialized centers.

Although bladder cancer undoubtedly accounts for the majority of cases in urinary diversion there is still a broad spectrum of clinical situations in which continent cutaneous diversion remains the method of choice. Whenever the native sphincter mechanism is lacking, destroyed or dysfunctional, or urethral catheterization is painful or technically impossible cutaneous diversion is the only alternative to modified ureterosigmoidostomy and ileal loop. As a salvage procedure in failed exstrophy reconstruction, other complicated congenital abnormalities of the urinary tract, neurogenic bladder dysfunction (wheelchair-bound myelomeningocele patients), otherwise intractable urinary incontinence, severe pelvic trauma and complicated fistulae, the continent cutaneous reservoir provides excellent results even in extremely complex cases. Until recently, a small but significant group of patients was widely excluded from the benefits of continent urinary diversion: if an abnormality of the native lower urinary tract has resulted in endstage renal disease and the same fate was likely to affect the transplant kidney either an ileal conduit or a cutaneous ureterostomy was established in the majority of cases. Recently, several authors reported encouraging experiences with kidney transplantation into continent urinary intestinal reservoirs as a planned two-stage procedure in patients with functional or morphological bladder loss (see Results later).[10]

Contraindications include impaired renal function with serum creatinine >2 mg/l, inflammatory bowel disease, large bowel malignancy, or previous history of multiple bowel ablative procedures, with or without history of diarrhea.

Surgical technique

Selection of the technique in the individual patient is based on objective (age, prognosis of underlying disease, comorbidity, urinary and anal sphincter competence, manual dexterity, renal function and upper urinary tract configuration on the intravenous urogram) and subjective (motivation, compliance, expectation of social support, emotional capability of dealing with clean intermittent catheterization) criteria. Patient priorities are considered whenever medically justifiable and technically feasible.

While there is a broad consensus among reconstructive urologists regarding detubularization and spherical reconfiguration of bowel as basic principles in the creation of a low-pressure high-capacity reservoir the issues of reflux prevention (afferent limb) and continence (efferent limb) are more controversial. The still growing number of techniques described for achieving continence in urinary reconstruction indicates that a universally applicable procedure with a low complication rate has not yet evolved. The principal methods for construction of a continence mechanism depend either on the formation of a nipple valve, utilization of the ileocecal valve or construction of a flap valve.

Although a general enthusiasm for the healthy appendix as the first choice for a Mitrofanoff conduit has even stimulated some pediatric urologists to state a strong case against incidental appendicectomy, its attachment to the reservoir (reversed, in situ; imbricated, embedded, unaltered), the location of the stoma (umbilicus, lower abdomen) and appropriate alternatives are rather controversial issues. It is known that the success of the Mitrofanoff principle is not dependent upon the underlying pathologic condition, the type of tube and its possible peristalsis, the type and configuration of the reservoir or the patient's age but the maintenance of a pressure gradient between the channel lumen and the reservoir. It is therefore the availability of the required material and the simplicity of a technique that determine its popularity. Recent variations of the Mitrofanoff theme have aimed at its simplification and reduction of long-term complications.

Ileocecal pouch (Mainz pouch I)

After mobilization of cecum, ascending colon and the right colonic flexure the mesentery is divided between the right colic and the ileocolic arteries.[11] A 15-cm segment of cecum and ascending colon is isolated along with two equal-sized limbs of distal ileum (Figure 27.1). The excluded bowel segment is split antimesenterically. These three opened bowel loops are folded in the form of an incomplete W, and their posterior aspects are sutured to one another to form a broad posterior plate. Both ureters are implanted into the large bowel segment of the pouch plate, forming submucosal tunnels for reflux prevention. The bowel is then folded on itself in a side-to-side fashion thus creating a low-pressure high-capacity reservoir. Ureteral stents (6 Fr or 8 Fr) and a 10-Fr pouchostomy are led through the abdominal wall at separate sites.

Intussuscepted ileal nipple

If the vermiform appendix is absent as in cloacal exstrophy, completely obliterated, immobile, insufficient in diameter and length or had been removed beforehand we usually isolate an

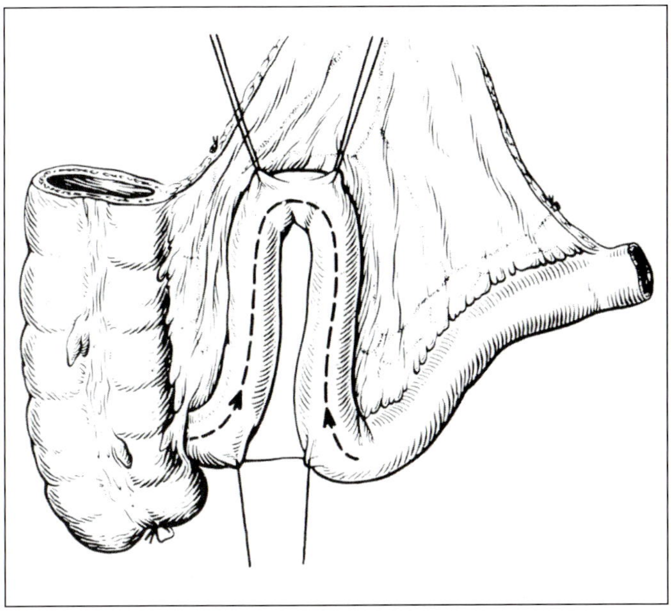

Figure 27.1 Ileocecal pouch (Mainz pouch I) with intussuscepted ileal nipple valve. Isolation of cecum/ascending colon (10–15 cm) and two equal-sized ileal loops (10–15 cm each) for reservoir formation and an additional ileal segment (8–10 cm) for nipple formation. (Reproduced with permission from Hohenfeller R (ed). Ausgewählte urologische OP-Techniken. Stuttgart: Thieme, 1994.)

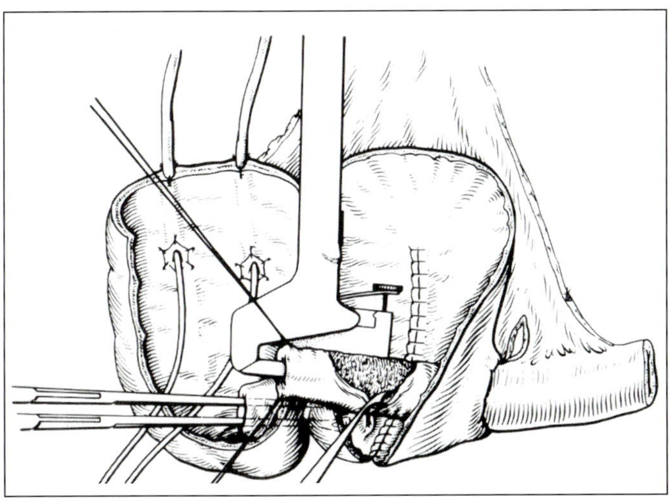

Figure 27.2 Ileocecal pouch (Mainz pouch I) with intussuscepted ileal nipple valve. After anti-mesenteric splitting of the bowel, side-to-side anastomosis of the terminal and next proximal ileal loop with subsequent detubularization of the ascending colon the mesentery of the mid-portion of the oral ileal segment (4–5 cm) is removed in preparation for intussusception. Intussusception of the ileal segment and stabilization by applying one row of staples. (Reproduced with permission from Hohenfeller R (ed). Ausgewählte urologische OP-Techniken. Stuttgart: Thieme, 1994.)

additional portion of ileum measuring 8–10 cm which is left tubularized. The mid-portion of the intact ileal segment is freed of its mesentery for a distance of 4–5 cm to allow its intussusception. In contrast to the original description, we apply only one row of staples to stabilize the intussusception itself (Figure 27.2). Thereafter the intussuscepted nipple is pulled through

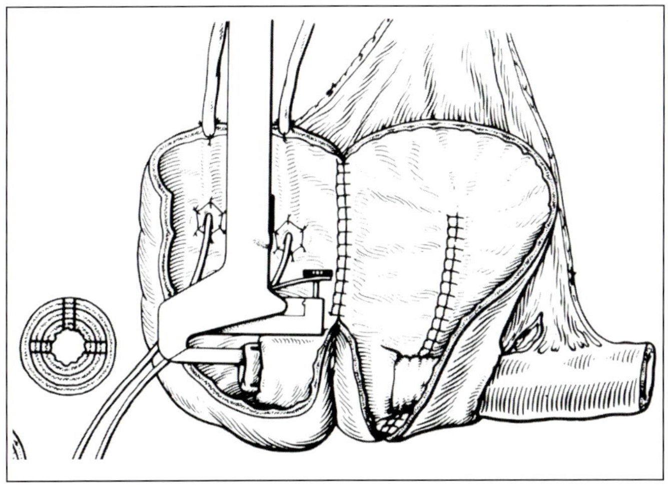

Figure 27.3 Ileocecal pouch (Mainz pouch I) with intussuscepted ileal nipple valve. The intussuscepted ileal nipple is pulled through the ileocecal valve and two additional rows of staples are used to attach the nipple to the valve. (Reproduced with permission from Hohenfeller R (ed). Ausgewählte urologische OP-Techniken. Stuttgart: Thieme, 1994.)

the intact ileocecal valve and two rows of staples are applied to attach the nipple to the ileocecal valve (Figure 27.3). After the mucosa of the intussucepted nipple and the colonic aspect of the ileocecal valve have been removed the circumferences are joined.

Appendix stoma

If present, the appendix is carefully inspected and dilated to accommodate a 16–18-Fr catheter to ensure sufficient postoperative drainage of mucus. In this case, the lower 5 cm of the cecum (cecal pole) is left tubularized and intact.[8] The seromuscular layer of the intact cecal pole is divided along the tenia down to the mucosa analogous to the Lich–Gregoir procedure for vesicoureteral reflux (Figure 27.4). By careful dissection of the seromuscular tissue, a broad submucosal bed (5 cm) is created for the appendix. The appendicular mesentery is freed of its excessive fatty tissue. Windows in the mesoappendix are excised between the branches of the appendicular artery without compromising the blood supply (Figure 27.5). Anatomical variations of the appendicular artery have to be respected and an additional branch of the anterior or posterior cecal artery supplying the base of the appendix should be preserved. After the appendix is correctly positioned the seromuscular layer is closed over the embedded in situ appendix with interrupted 4-0 polydioxanone sutures. A short mobile portion of the distal appendix remains for creation of the appendico-umbilical stoma (Figure 27.6). The entire pouch is rotated so as to bring the distal appendix to the region of the umbilicus. A small button of skin is removed from the depth of the umbilical funnel. The pouch is carefully attached to the posterior fascia with interrupted non-absorbable sutures to prevent the pouch from rotating and kinking. The appendix is then connected to the umbilical funnel with interrupted absorbable sutures. If no umbilicus is present (as in the case of exstrophy), it is created

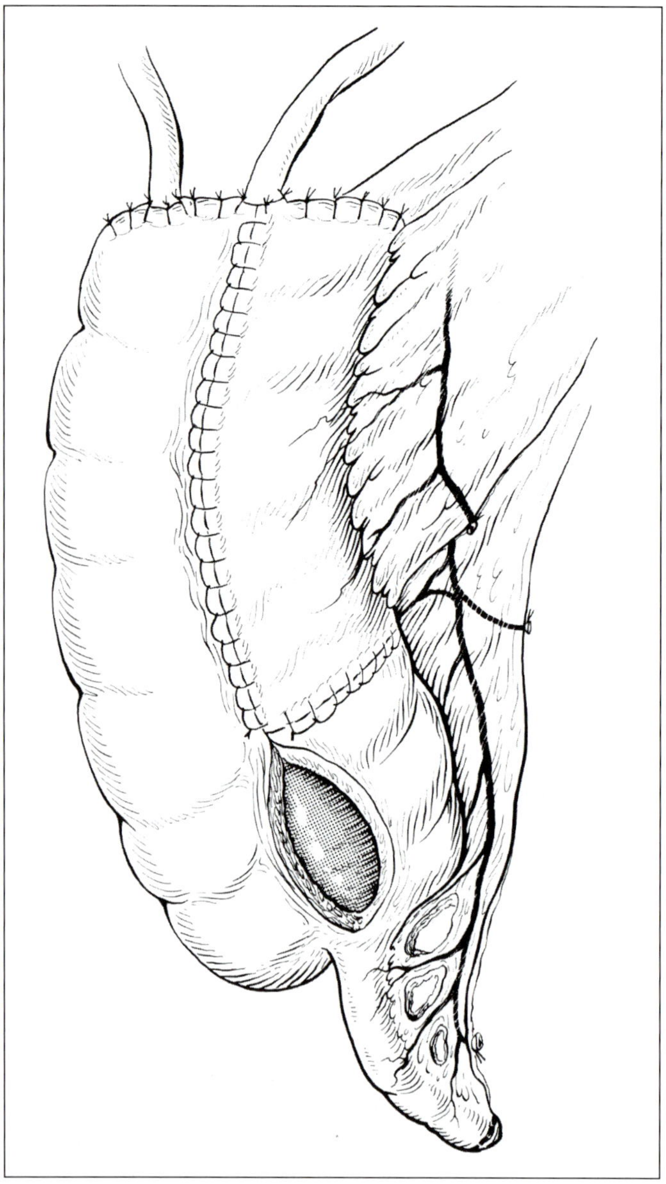

Figure 27.4 Ileocecal pouch (Mainz pouch I) with appendix stoma. Seromuscular layer of the intact cecal pole is split along the tenia down to the mucosa, a broad submucosal bed for the appendix is created. (Reproduced with permission from Hohenfeller R (ed). Ausgewählte urologische OP-Techniken. Stuttgart: Thieme, 1994.)

by tubularizing a V-shaped cutaneous flap and connecting it to the appendicular stump. A vigorous wash-out regimen is started early in the postoperative course. Ureter stents are removed after 10–14 days. Clean intermittent catheterization is usually started at the end of the third postoperative week after leakage and reflux has been ruled out by pouchogram.

Alternative techniques for construction of continence mechanism

More recent techniques use a small-caliber conduit fashioned from the cecal wall. One technique uses a full-thickness tube lined by mucosa (Figure 27.7) and the other a seromuscular

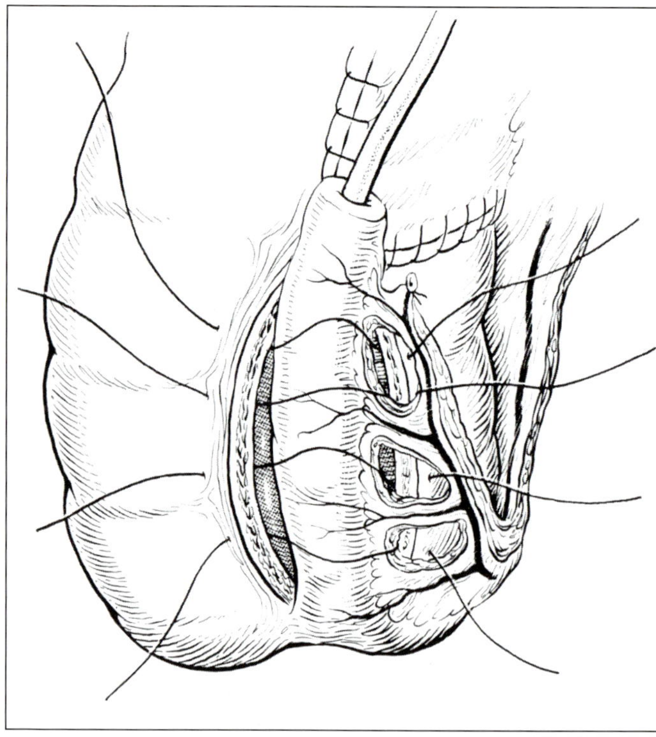

Figure 27.5 Ileocecal pouch (Mainz pouch I) with appendix stoma. Windows in the meso-appendix are excised between the branches of the appendicular artery without compromising the blood supply. (Reproduced with permission from Hohenfeller R (ed). Ausgewählte urologische OP-Techniken. Stuttgart: Thieme, 1994.)

tube lined by serosa (Figure 27.8).[12] Other authors have described transversely retubularized ileum to create a tunneled access into the right colon.[13]

Outcomes of modified Mitranoff procedures

Surgical complications

While continence using the appendix, once established, is durable with late onset failure of 1–2% at about 4 years the notorious drawback of that technique is impaired catheterization due to a gradually stenosing stoma with a true incidence between 8–28% depending on the length of follow-up. It has been assumed that Mitrofanoff channels only remain patent because of regular catheterization. Although stenosis represents a minor technical problem the subsequent inability to insert the catheter is a distressing complication with potentially serious consequences in patients in whom the Mitrofanoff channel is the only route of evacuation. In these cases the reservoir must be immediately emptied percutaneously, which is facilitated by fixation of the pouch to the abdominal wall.

Skin stenosis may be dilated, incised or repaired by open surgery, carefully removing the fibrotic tissue. All reports so far

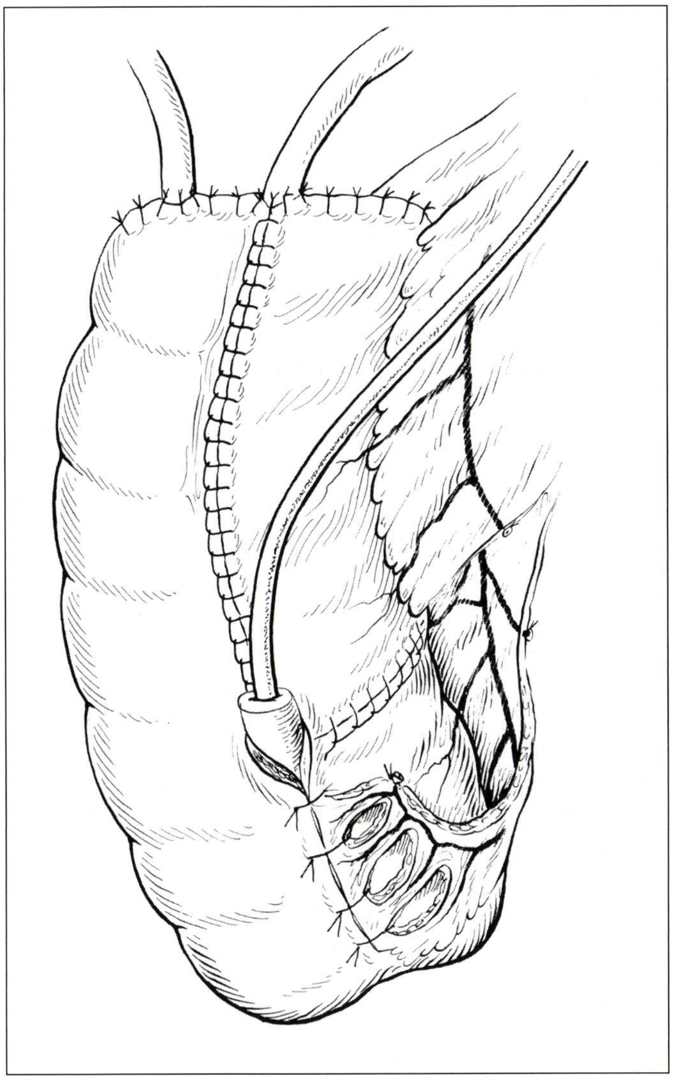

Figure 27.6 Ileocecal pouch (Mainz pouch I) with appendix stoma. After the appendix is correctly positioned the seromuscular layer is closed over the embedded in situ appendix. (Reproduced with permission from Hohenfeller R (ed). Ausgewählte urologische OP-Techniken. Stuttgart: Thieme, 1994.)

state that a proportion of such stenoses can be treated conservatively. According to our experience dilatation alone seldom produces a lasting improvement. We therefore tend to early intervention. Although revisions are usually successful prevention of stenosis is desirable. According to our latest experience with a technique described by Woodhouse and MacNeily[7] stomal stenosis can be avoided by incorporation of a V-shaped flap of umbilical funnel into the spatulated appendix.

To prevent recurrence we have developed a cone-shaped metal dilator.[14] Its effective length was designed to cover only the known critical segment of the channel. Directly before inserting the catheter for evacuation of the reservoir, the stoma is gently dilated for a few minutes once or twice daily. A similar effect might be produced by occasionally leaving the catheter in the pouch at night.

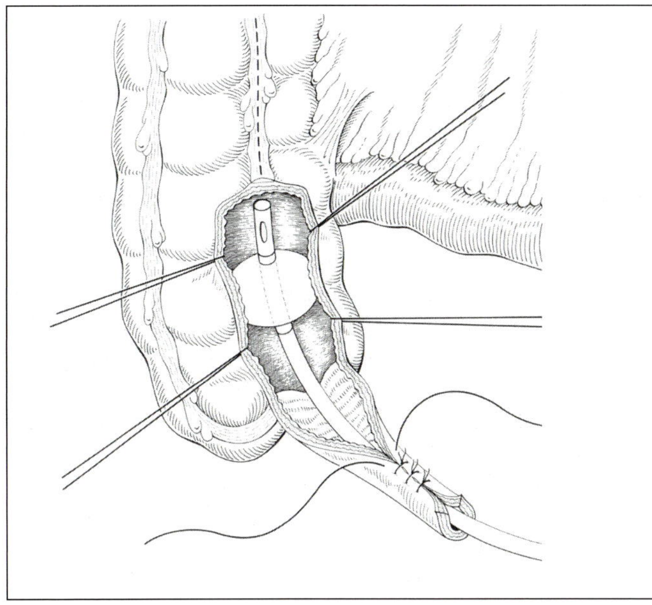

Figure 27.7 Full thickness bowel flap tube. U-shaped incision (3 x 6 cm) of all layers of bowel wall resulting in pedicled bowel flap at lower pole of cecum. Tubularization of pedicled flap over 18 F Foley catheter and incision of seromuscularis of tenia omentalis (5 cm) for submucosal embedding starting at pedicle of bowel flap tube. (Reproduced with permission from Operative Techniken, Aktuelle Urologie 1998; 29: V.)

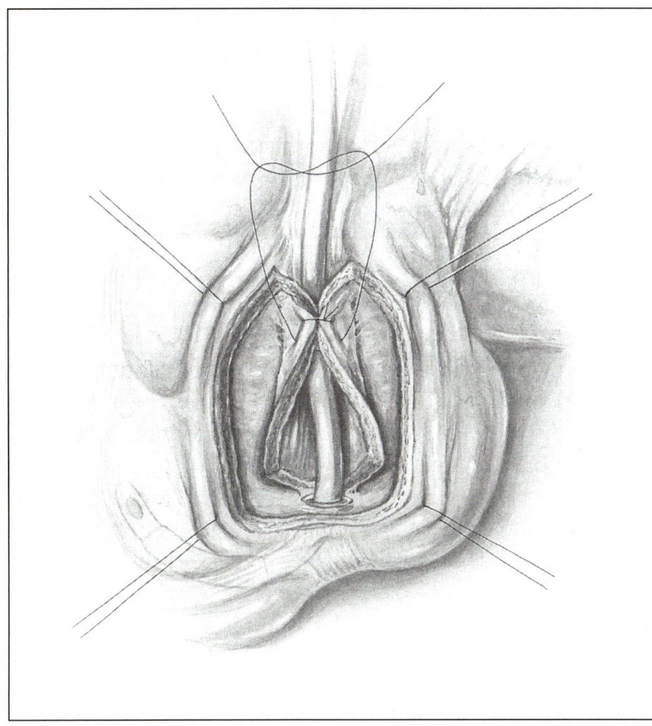

Figure 27.8 Seromuscular bowel flap tube. U-shaped incision (3 x 5 cm) of seromuscular layer at lower pole of cecum and transverse incision of mucosa (0.5 cm) at oral end of flap for insertion of 18 F Foley catheter into lumen of reservoir. Tubularization of seromuscular bowel flap over 18 F Foley catheter. Suturing of anterior circumference of seromuscular tube to margin of mucosa. (Reproduced with permission from Hohenfeller R (ed). Ausgewählte urologische OP-Techniken. Stuttgart: Thieme, 1994.)

Results of the authors' experience with continent reservoirs

Between 1990 and 2002, 765 patients underwent urinary diversion at our department with creation of continent reservoirs in more than 65%. The most common indication for urinary diversion was bladder replacement after anterior exenteration for pelvic malignancies (84.5%). Continent urinary diversion was performed as a primary surgical approach, in conversion procedures and salvage maneuvers after failure of previous reconstruction. The spectrum of applied techniques included orthotopic bladder substitution (n = 103), sigma rectum pouch (n = 41), and ileal and colonic conduit (n = 263); in 358 patients, an ileocecal pouch with umbilical stoma was created in a standardized fashion that has been described in detail above (mean follow-up 63.6 months, range 1–122 months). As a continence mechanism the submucosally embedded in situ appendix could be utilized in 159 cases. In 196 cases an ileal intussuception valve was established. The Yang–Monti technique (transversely retubularized ileum) and a Lampel–Thüroff tube (full-thickness bowel flap) have been used in three salvage procedures with major loss of bowel in earlier operations. For antirefluxing ureterointestinal anastomosis the Goodwin technique (submucosal tunnel) was used in most instances (85%), a serous-lined extramural tunnel (Abol-Enein) was created in grossly dilated ureters and after irradiation. In 25 cases the ureter had to be replaced totally or in part by ileum.

Perioperative morbidity was 0.8% in the patients with continent diversion. Five major stoma-related complications were observed in patients with in situ appendix (3.1%). Due to ischemic necrosis with total incontinence upon removal of the peroperatively inserted catheter the appendix had to be replaced by either an intussuscepted ileal nipple (n = 4) or a Yang–Monti tube. Minor complications (outlet stenosis at skin level) were recorded in 20 out of 159 patients with appendix stoma (12.6%) (including two exstrophy patients with a neo-umbilicus) after a mean follow-up of 20.4 months (range 1.9–50.6 months). In these patients 26 reinterventions, either surgical removal of scar tissue or star-shaped incision, were required. All but 10 procedures could be performed under local anesthesia on an outpatient basis. An indwelling catheter was left in place for 1–3 days. All patients with clinically relevant appendico-umbilical stenosis have been instructed to use a modified Dittel device at least once a day before catheterization. The incidence of stoma-related complications has declined over time with only three minor revisions within the past 24 months. In 34 patients with intussuscepted ileal nipple (17.3%) a second operation became necessary; among the 13 patients with partial/complete necrosis of the efferent limb with subsequent incontinence a secondary ileal nipple was created in 11 patients and a Yang–Monti tube in two. In 13 patients with dislocation of the nipple from the ileocecal valve and/or detachment from the fascia the original nipple could be restored in the original position. Fibrotic stomal stenosis was incised in eight patients. At the time of our investigation all patients with umbilical stoma were completely continent day and night with easy catheterization.

Ureterointestinal stenosis was encountered in 30 out of 358 patients (all patients with continent cutaneous reservoir) (8.4%). Diagnosis was usually based on a urogram and confirmed by diuresis scintigraphy. After disappointing experiences with dilatation and stenting, early reimplantation was performed in most cases and nephrectomy in five patients due to a significant loss of renal function. Rupture of the continent reservoir occurred in three patients out of 358 (all patients with continent cutaneous reservoir) (0.8%), in all cases related to catheter trauma during intermittent self-catheterization.

Urodynamic evaluation in a random subset of patients with ileocecal reservoir and appendiceal continence mechanism (n = 14; ≥6 months postoperatively) resulted in a maximum median capacity of 654 ml (range 420–790 ml) with a mean reservoir pressure of 24 cmH_2O (range 18–29 cmH_2O) at 50% capacity and a mean of 33 cmH_2O (range 23–47 cmH_2O) at 100% capacity. Maximum median closure pressure of the appendix was 121 cmH_2O (range 79–169 cmH_2O).

Whereas no calculi were observed in the appendix group, stones had to be removed from seven patients (2%) with ileal nipple. Although the serum concentration of vitamin B_{12} did not drop below normal in any patient, there was a tendency for it to decrease over time. Mild hyperchloremic metabolic acidosis occurred in 23% requiring alkalizing medication. In 4.3% of all patients with continent cutaneous reservoirs (358) a slight transient diarrhea was observed in the early postoperative period and in only two patients medical treatment with cholestyramine was necessary for up to 9 months. Mucus production varied enormously intra- and interindividually but never led to clinically significant problems.

In 12 patients with absent or dysfunctional lower urinary tract, a continent urinary reservoir has been created in preparation for renal transplantation. Within a mean follow-up of 26.1 months after kidney transplant renal function was stable with serum creatinine values ranging from 0.9 mg/dl to 1.8 mg/dl. Performed as a staged procedure with urinary diversion as the first step, this strategy successfully combines the advantages of two clinically well-established therapeutic principles obviating external urine collecting devices and chronic hemodialysis.

Both in situ appendix and intussuscepted ileum valve are very satisfactory techniques for providing continence in an ileocecal urinary reservoir. Besides the advantages of the appendix in the primary reconstructive approach – a straightforward and relatively quick procedure, minimized risk of stone formation and reduced functional loss of bowel – the treatment of subsequent complications is usually simple. Thus, whenever an appropriate appendix is encountered it should be the intestinal segment of choice in forming a continence mechanism in cutaneous diversion.

Quality of life

When continent cutaneous diversion and orthotopic bladder substitution became realistic alternatives in clinical urology it was a priori assumed that these measures should considerably improve the patient's adjustment after radical cystectomy for bladder carcinoma compared with conduit diversion. Over the past 10 years numerous reports have been published on the quality of life after cystectomy using different methods for reconstructing the urinary tract; it comes with some surprise and disappointment that there is no clear evidence that the new methods give a better quality of life. The available data regarding directly stoma-related issues (urine leakage, urine odor, practicality of stoma care), however, clearly support the concept of continent diversion when compared with the traditional ileal conduit.[15] A high acceptance rate for patients receiving a continent catheterizable stoma was demonstrated by Horowitz et al.[16] All patients who had the potential to catheterize either the Mitrofanoff tube or their native urethra preferred to use the artificial channel. No differences were found in a recent comparison of quality of life in men after radical cystectomy who had either a continent cutaneous diversion or orthotopic bladder substitution.[17]

References

1. Murphy LJT. The History of Urology. Springfield, USA: Charles C Thomas 1972: 354–5.
2. Hautmann RE. Urinary diversion: ileal conduit to neobladder. J Urol 2003; 169: 834–42.
3. Henningsohn L, Steven K, Brohm Kallestrup E, Steineck G. Distressful symptoms and well-being after radical cystectomy and orthotopic bladder substitution compared with a matched control population. J Urol 2002; 168: 168–75.
4. Yong SM, Dublin N, Pickard R et al. Urinary diversion and bladder reconstruction/replacement using intestinal segments for intractable incontinence or following cystectomy. Cochrane Database Syst Rev 2003; 1: CD-003306.
5. Mitrofanoff P. Cystostomie continente transappendiculaire dans le traitement des vessies neurologiques. Chir Pediatr (Paris) 1980; 21: 297–305.
6. Duckett JW, Snyder HM III. Continent urinary diversion: variations on the Mitrofanoff principle. J Urol 1986; 136: 58–62.
7. Woodhouse CRJ, MacNeily AE. The Mitrofanoff principle: expanding upon a versatile technique. Br J Urol 1994; 74: 447–53.
8. Riedmiller H, Bürger R, Müller S et al. Continent appendix stoma: a modification of the Mainz pouch technique. J Urol 1990; 143: 1115–16.
9. Bell CR, Gujral S, Collins CM, Sibley GN, Persad RA. The fate of the urethra after definitive treatment of invasive transitional cell carcinoma of the urinary bladder. BJU Int 1999; 83: 607–12.
10. Riedmiller H, Gerharz EW, Kohl U et al. Continent urinary diversion in preparation for renal transplantation: a staged approach. Transplantation 2000; 70: 1713–17.
11. Thüroff JW, Alken P, Riedmiller H et al. The Mainz pouch (mixed augmentation ileum and cecum) for bladder augmentation and continent diversion. J Urol 1986; 136: 17–26.
12. Lampel A, Hohenfellner M, Schultz-Lampel D et al. In situ tunneled bowel flap tubes: 2 new techniques of a continent outlet for Mainz pouch cutaneous diversion. J Urol 1995; 153: 308–15.
13. Monti PR, Lara RC, Dutra MA, de Carvalho JR. New techniques for construction of efferent conduits based on Mitrofanoff principle. Urol 1997; 49: 112–15.
14. Köhl U, Gerharz EW, Weingärtner K, Riedmiller H. A simple device in the prevention of recurrent appendico-umbilical stenosis. Br J Urol 1996; 77: 603–4
15. Gerharz EW, Weingärtner K, Köhl U, et al. Quality of life following cystectomy and urinary diversion – an interdisciplinary retrospective study. J Urol 1997; 158: 778–85.
16. Horowitz M, Kuhr CS, Mitchell ME. The Mitrofanoff catheterizable channel: patient acceptance. J Urol 1995; 153: 771–2.
17. Mansson A, Davidsson T, Hunt S et al. The quality of life in men after radical cystectomy with a continent cutaneous diversion or orthotopic bladder substitution: is there a difference? BJU Int 2002; 90: 386–90.

28 The Monti principle in continent urinary diversion

Padraig SJ Malone, Ramesh Babu and Martin A Koyle

Introduction

The Mitrofanoff principle has been extensively discussed in Chapter 26. The appendix remains the first choice for the Mitrofanoff tube, because of its supple nature, adequate lumen and reliable blood supply.[1] However the appendix is not always available because of scarring, short length, poor blood supply, or previous surgical removal.[2,3] Furthermore many patients with neuropathic bladder also have bowel problems in the form of constipation and or incontinence. With the popularization of the Malone Antegrade Continence Enema (MACE) procedure to treat the above, the appendix may be less available and therefore other alternatives are required for the Mitrofanoff procedure.[4,5]

Since Mitrofanoff described his procedure in 1980,[3] using the appendix, several other options and modifications of continent catheterizable conduits have been described.[6–9] The different structures used for these techniques include: ureter, longitudinally tapered ileum, large bowel, bladder, stomach, fallopian tube, vas deferens and prepucial skin. Adequate vascularity, mobility and lumen size have been difficult to achieve with the above and many are surgical curiosities without clinical relevance.[10,11] Yang was the first to describe the technique of transverse retubularization of the ileum to create a continent catheterizable conduit, using the needle tunneling technique.[6] In 1997, Monti et al developed this technique further to create a neo-appendix in a canine model.[7] Two alternative techniques were described, where a single or two small ileal segments were opened longitudinally and retubularized transversely to create a small caliber conduit. In the canine model the tube was continent, easily catheterizable and the main complication was stomal stenosis attributed to infrequent catheterization. Since then this procedure has been studied in the clinical setting, and successful outcomes have been reported.[1,2,9–13] In addition, further modifications of the initial Yang–Monti technique have been introduced and evaluated.[14,15]

The Yang–Monti principle

The Yang–Monti principle creates a 'neo-appendix' using a segment of ileum. The principle involves the following:

- isolation of a short segment of ileum (2–4 cm), which is usually freely available, and has good mobility and blood supply (Figure 28.1a). The circumference of the bowel used will determine the tube length
- detubularization along the longitudinal axis with transverse retubularization, after which the mucosal folds are rearranged longitudinally facilitating easy catheterization (Figure 28.1b)
- no mesentery is left at the ends of the tube aiding creation of a continence mechanism and transit through the abdominal wall (Figure 28.1c)
- the continence mechanism is created by implantation of the tube into the bladder using a submucosal tunnel or by imbricating the tube in a bowel wrap
- the length of the bowel segment isolated (2–4 cm) will determine the diameter of the refashioned tube (1 cm or 14 Fr). Longer segments will result in a wider channel for catheterization, but will also require a longer tunnel in the bladder because of its bulk
- if the length of the single Monti tube is not adequate, two Monti tubes can be joined together 'The Full Monti' (Figure 28.2)
- when a concomitant ileocystoplasty is created, the adjacent bowel segment is used for the Monti tube, obviating the need for additional bowel anastomoses.

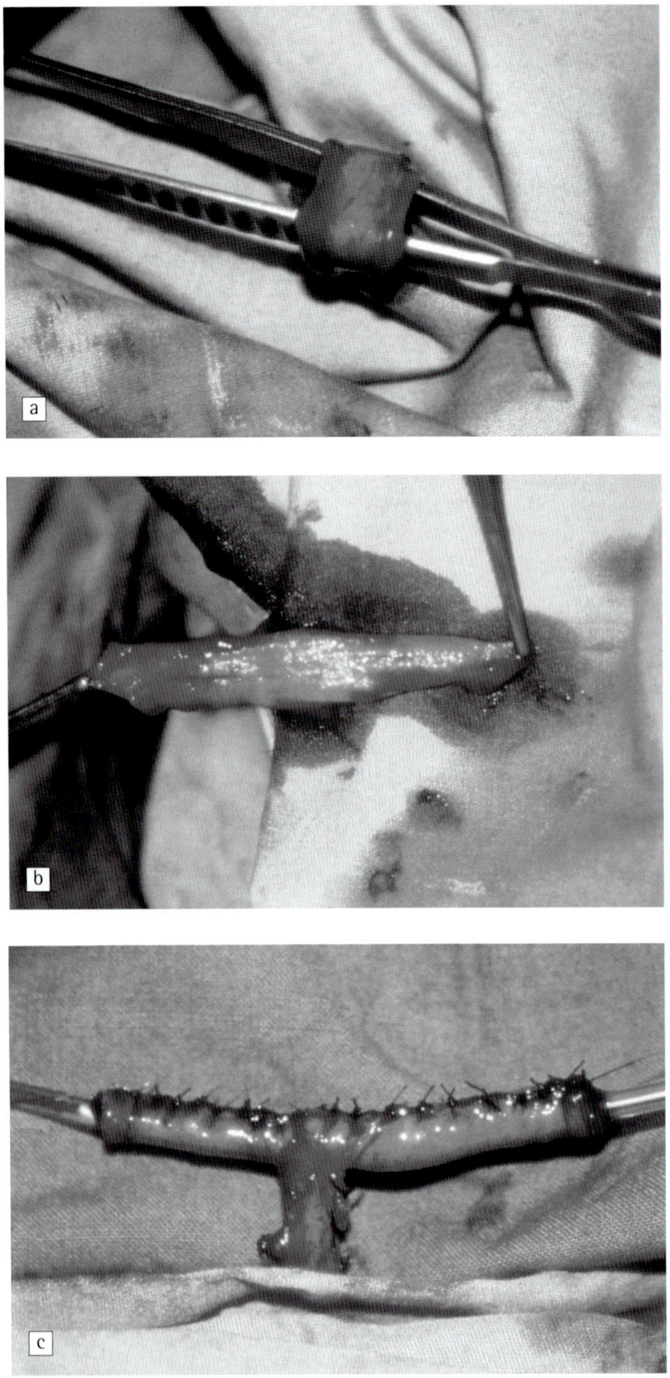

Figure 28.1 The Monti technique. (a) A single 2 cm ileal segment is isolated on its pedicle. (b) The detubularized ileal segment 7 cm long; note the longitudinal axis of the valvulae conniventes. (c) The 7-cm tubularized conduit; note the free ends, with the pedicle in the middle. (Reproduced from Sugarman ID et al. Br J Urol 1998; 81: 253–6[16] with permission from Lippincott Williams & Wilkins.)

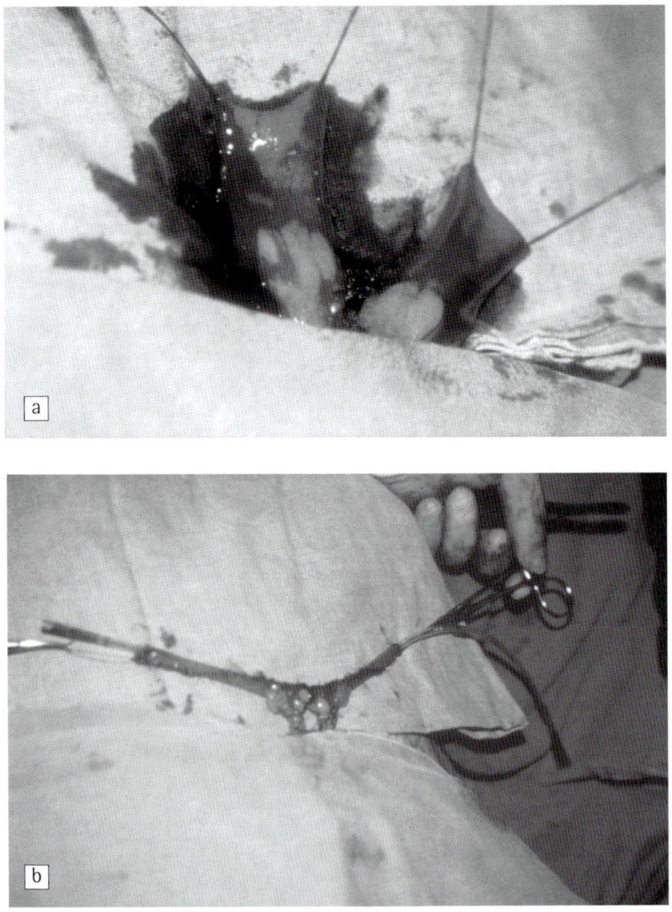

Figure 28.2 The Double Monti or 'Full Monti'. (a) Two 2-cm ileal segments are isolated. (b) A double segment 14-cm conduit. (Reproduced from Sugarman ID et al. Br J Urol 1998; 81: 253–6[16] with permission from Lippincott Williams & Wilkins.)

Patient selection and preparation

The indications for a Monti procedure are the same as those for a Mitrofanoff. The situations where the Yang–Monti procedure is required include where the appendix:

- has been removed
- has been used for other procedures (MACE)
- is unsuitable.

Preoperative evaluation should include urinary tract ultrasonography, cystography and isotope and urodynamic studies as indicated. To determine patient suitability for catheterization, psychological assessment and counseling should be carried out by the nurse-specialist. Failure to counsel and prepare patients adequately can result in failure to catheterize. When dealing with children, it is equally important to educate and counsel parents and all other support workers such as those who help the child at school for a successful outcome. Bowel preparation is required when an associated augmentation is performed. Perioperative antibiotic prophylaxis is used and continued while catheters are in situ.

The Yang–Monti operative technique

The abdominal incision is based on the concomitant procedures that will be performed and on previous scars. Classically, a 2–4 cm ileal segment is isolated (at least 10 cm from the ileocecal valve) with its pedicle being carefully preserved. An end-to-end ileal anastomosis restores bowel continuity. In the original Yang–Monti technique the excluded bowel segment was opened longitudinally about 1 cm from the mesentery creating a long limb, which was used for the continence mechanism. More recently, the ileum has been opened along the antimesenteric border in the middle.[9,12,17,18] This creates equal afferent and efferent limbs, keeps the mesentery in the middle and ensures good blood supply for both the limbs. The resulting pedicled rectangular segment is retubularized over a 14-Fr catheter in the transverse direction (see Figure 28.1). Fine absorbable sutures are used to approximate the mucosa, followed by a second serosal layer or a single-layer extramucosal interrupted suture can also be used according to the surgeon's preference. The closure is facilitated by maintaining tension on the stay sutures at both ends of the ileal patch. A sigmoid colonic segment has also been used for the Monti tube with successful results.[15]

For creation of the antireflux flap valve the tube is implanted into a submucosal tunnel in the native bladder. Alternatively, it can be implanted in the intestinal segment of an augmented bladder by imbricating the tube in a bowel wrap. It is important to achieve an adequate tunnel length:tube width ratio (5:1) to ensure continence. In addition it is vital to avoid tension, torsion or angulation on the pedicle and the tube to avoid complications such as stenosis or necrosis. It is important to ensure easy catheterization at the end of each step of the procedure because it is easy to kink the Monti tube as it enters the submucosal tunnel. Stoma formation is similar to the Mitrofanoff procedure and has been discussed in Chapter 26.

Modifications

Double or 'Full Monti'

In patients in whom there is a long distance between the reservoir and the abdominal wall two adjacent ileal segments of 2–4 cm can be isolated and retubularized (see Figure 28.2).[7,8,12] The segments are opened on the opposite sides of the antemesenteric border and the shorter limbs are joined together. This creates a long Monti tube with the mesentery in the middle. Both the afferent and efferent limbs are long and therefore can be used for creation of the stoma and the antireflux mechanism. When a simultaneous ileocystoplasty is performed, the Monti segments can be harvested from both ends of the ileal segment used for cystoplasty, thereby facilitating a single ileal anastomosis. It is essential to align the two tubes correctly and ensure smooth catheterization at the end, as angulation can result in pouch formation and creation of a false passage.

Casale's procedure

This is an alternative to the full Monti. A long continent ileovesicostomy can be created using a single piece of bowel.[8,14] The isolated ileal segment is divided half way, approximately 80% of the circumference, leaving the bowel intact over the mesentery. The two segments are opened on opposite sides, leaving a strip intact over the mesentery (Figure 28.3). The unfolded bowel is straightened, reconfigured and retubularized. Like the double Monti, this procedure also leaves long afferent and efferent limbs and is suitable in obese patients.

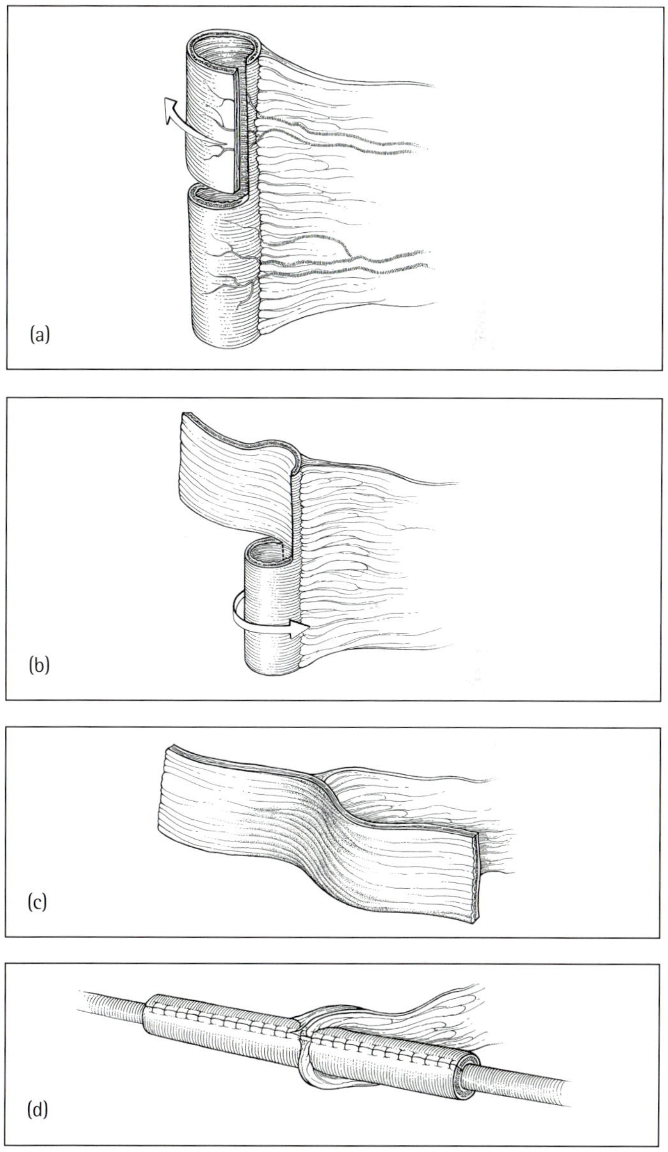

Figure 28.3 (a–d) Casale's long continent ileovesicostomy. The two bowel segments are not totally divided in the area of mesentery. The segments are detubularized 180° from each other and retubularized over a catheter. (Reproduced with permission of the artist Rong-zeng Li, MD from Furness PD et al. Contemp Urol 2003; 15: 30–45.[8])

Composite Monti (Monti tube + appendix)

A Monti tube can be anastomosed to the appendix to create a composite Monti in the following situations:

- as a primary procedure during a Mitrofanoff, when after reimplanting the appendix the length is found to be inadequate
- when it is difficult to catheterize the initial Mitrofanoff tube because of complications such as stomal stenosis, stricture or false passage, but the continence mechanism is still intact. A Monti tube is added to the Mitrofanoff and a new stoma created, avoiding the need for a difficult re-creation of the continence mechanism.

The Monti tube can be simply anastomosed to the appendix using full thickness interrupted absorbable sutures.

Monti MACE

The Monti technique has been applied successfully for the MACE procedure when the appendix has been used earlier for the Mitrofanoff procedure.[4,16] The Monti tube, created as described above, is implanted into a 4–5-cm submucosal tunnel along a tenia. The tube can also be implanted in the left colon and brought out as a stoma in the left lower quadrant, the left Monti–MACE procedure.[19,20] Tackett et al[21] compared appendiceal and Monti–MACE procedures and reported no significant difference in continence or complication rates. In patients who require simultaneous Mitrofanoff and MACE procedures, a split appendix technique has been described if the appendix is of adequate length.[22,23] Otherwise, it is best to use the appendix for an in situ MACE[24] and the Monti tube for the Mitrofanoff. Double continence rates of up to 76% are reported using this approach.[23]

Postoperative care

A 10–14-Fr silastic catheter is left indwelling for about 4–5 weeks. It is essential to secure this well, as early attempts to reintroduce catheters into the newly formed Monti channel before its complete healing can result in postoperative complications. Antibiotic prophylaxis is continued during this period. At the end of the 5 weeks, intermittent catheterization is started with a latex-free catheter.

Results from different series

Since the introduction of the Monti procedure, there have been a number of series reporting successful outcomes.[1,2,9,11,12,18,21] Only one study comparing the Monti procedure with the Mitrofanoff using the appendix reported a higher complication rate with the Monti.[1] McAndrew and Malone reported that there were no significant differences in complication rates between the Monti and the Mitrofanoff.[2] Tackett et al, who compared the Monti technique with the native appendix for the MACE procedure, also reported no significant differences in complication rates or continence.[21] Table 28.1 summarizes and compares the results from different series of the Monti Procedure.

Stomal complications

Stomal complications are the most common problems encountered after a continent urinary diversion. McAndrew and Malone reported a 31% overall stenosis rate with 33% for the appendix and 24% for the Monti tube.[2] There was a lower incidence of stenosis for an umbilical stoma (21%) compared with an abdominal stoma (38%), however, there was no significant difference relating to the conduit used, the reservoir or the stoma type.[2] Narayanaswamy et al reported a stenosis rate of 15% for the appendix stoma and 16% for the Monti tube.[1] Van Savage et al suggested that the stomal location could play a role in the development of stenosis with an incidence of 13% at the umbilicus and 4% at a lower quadrant location.[25] The incidence of stomal ischemia, retraction, prolapse, and parastomal hernia can be reduced by avoiding angulation of the efferent limb, fixing the reservoir to the anterior abdominal wall, and incorporating a vascularized skin flap at the stoma.[8]

Table 28.1 Outcome following the Monti procedure in various series

Authors	Year	N	Follow-up in months (mean)	Stomal stenosis	Conduit stenosis/loss	Stomal leak	Dry
McAndrew and Malone[2]	2002	21	1–120 (34)	5	–	0	21
Tackett et al[22]	2002	17	4–65 (26)	2	1	–	–
Narayanaswamy et al[1]	2001	25	6–66 (25)	4	5	3	17
Van Savage et al[18]	2000	8	18–60 (36)	0	0	0	6
Castellan et al[12]	1999	29	3–26 (13)	0	3	2	–
Cain et al[9]	1999	21	(8)	–	1	1	–
Gerharz et al[11]	1998	16	1–9 (4)	–	–	2	13

Conduit complications

In addition to stomal stenosis, conduit stenosis or kinking at the substomal, mid conduit or bladder level can result in problems with catheterization.[1] These complications can be prevented by paying particular attention to preserving the vascularity and avoiding any tension or kinking on the vascular pedicle or the tube. Mid-stomal stenosis is a unique complication associated with the double Monti technique, which can be prevented by paying attention to the anastomosis of the two Monti tubes. Preserving the vascularity and making the Monti tube less bulky can prevent bladder level stenosis.

Pouch formation has been reported as another complication associated with the Monti technique.[1] Rearrangement of the muscularis propria, unequal wall tension, angulation at mid-channel and weakness at the suture line have all been described as the factors responsible for pouch formation. Early postoperative difficulties in catheterization and a false passage can aggravate the tendency towards pouch formation. Achieving uniform wall tension, avoiding redundancy in length or angulation and ensuring an easy straight path for catheterization at the end of the operation are essential for preventing these complications.

Spontaneous lengthening of the Monti tube can occur with time producing angulation or kinking. In one author's (PSM) experience, one patient had this complication after a double Monti procedure. One complete length of the Monti tube was excised and the stoma refashioned to solve the problem.

Incontinence

Stomal incontinence presenting as a leak may be the result of any one of the following problems:

- inadequate flap valve mechanism
- breakdown of the implanted Monti tube resulting in an internal fistula
- inadequate reservoir.

Harvesting too wide an ileal segment could result in a bulky Monti tube and create difficulties in achieving 5:1 tunnel:channel width ratio. Failure to pay attention to the vascularity can result in complete Monti tube breakdown. The long suture line of the Monti tube itself makes it prone to internal fistula if the mucosa of the reservoir is damaged during creation of the submucosal tunnel. A cystoscopy or cystogram can identify these problems, which can be addressed by either reimplantation at a different site or creation of a new Monti tube. Urodynamic evaluation is essential to detect an inadequate reservoir and repeat augmentation may be required to correct this.

Advantages and disadvantages of the Monti technique

The advantages of the Yang–Monti technique include constant availability, need for only a short segment of small bowel, adequate mobility of the conduit and its mesentery, reliable vascularity, adequate channel length with a wide diameter, and the ability to undertake repeat procedures. It does not require an additional bowel anastomosis when combined with an ileocystoplasty. The rearranged tube has longitudinal folds making it easier to catheterize. The main disadvantage is the long suture line, which makes it more prone to breakdown or fistula formation. Angulation, lack of uniform lumen size and mid-channel stenosis can make the Monti tube more prone to difficulties with catheterization, false passage and pouch formation. The bulkiness of the implanted Monti tube can be the cause of an inefficient flap valve mechanism that can cause incontinence. However most of the latter disadvantages can be overcome by a careful operative technique. Table 28.2 summarizes the advantages and disadvantages of the Monti technique.

Conclusion

Although the appendix is still agreed by most urologists to be the conduit of choice for a Mitrofanoff conduit, in its absence, the Monti tube has become a very successful second-line

Table 28.2 The advantages and disadvantages of the Yang-Monti technique

Advantages	Disadvantages
Constant availability	Long suture line
Reliable vascularity	Lack of uniform diameter
Adequate mobility	Angulation (catheterization difficulties)
Wide diameter	Bulk (needs long tunnel)
Ability to repeat	
Longitudinal folds (easier to catheterize)	
Adequate channel length (with double Monti)	
Only a short segment of ileum required	
No need for additional bowel anastomosis (when combined with ileocystoplasty)	

option. The advantages of a Monti tube far outweigh the disadvantages and reports suggest a good success rate. The Yang–Monti technique is a useful addition to the reconstructive urologist's armamentarium and is likely to gain wider acceptance with longer follow-up.

References

1. Narayanaswamy B, Wilcox DT, Cuckow PM, Duffy PG, Ransley PG. The Yang-Monti ileovesicostomy: a problematic channel? BJU Int 2001; 87: 861–5.
2. McAndrew HF, Malone PS. Continent catheterizable conduits: which stoma, which conduit and which reservoir? BJU Int 2002; 89: 86–9.
3. Mitrofanoff P. Cystostomie continente trans-appendiculaire dans le traitement des vessies neurologiques. Chir Pediatr 1980; 21: 297–305.
4. Malone PS, Curry JI, Osborne A. The antegrade continence enema procedure why, when and how? World J Urol 1998; 16: 274–8.
5. Curry JI, Osborne A, Malone PS. The MACE procedure: experience in the United Kingdom. J Pediatr Surg 1999; 34: 338–40.
6. Yang WH. Yang needle tunneling technique in creating antireflux and continent mechanisms. J Urol 1993; 150: 830–4.
7. Monti PR, Lara RC, Dutra MA, de Carvalho JR. New techniques for construction of efferent conduits based on the Mitrofanoff principle. Urology 1997; 49: 112–15.
8. Furness PD, Malone PSJ, Barqawi A, Koyle MA. The Mitrofanoff principle. Innovative applications in continent urinary diversion. Contemp Urol 2003; 15: 30–45.
9. Cain MP, Casale AJ, King SJ, Rink RC. Appendicovesicostomy and newer alternatives for the Mitrofanoff procedure: results in the last 100 patients at Riley Children's Hospital. J Urol 1999; 162: 1749–52.
10. Gerharz EW, Woodhouse CR. The transverse ileal tube as second-line modification of the Mitrofanoff principle. World J Urol 1998; 16: 231–4.
11. Gerharz EW, Tassadaq T, Pickard RS et al. Transverse retubularized ileum: early clinical experience with a new second line Mitrofanoff tube. J Urol 1998; 159: 525–8.
12. Castellan MA, Gosalbez R Jr, Labbie A, Monti PR. Clinical applications of the Monti procedure as a continent catheterizable stoma. Urology 1999; 54: 152–6.
13. Gerharz EW, Roth S. Transversely tubularized ileal segments for the Mitrofanoff or Malone antegrade colonic enema procedures: the Monti principle. Br J Urol 1998; 82: 460–1.
14. Casale AJ. A long continent ileovesicostomy using a single piece of bowel. J Urol 1999; 162: 1743–5.
15. Van Savage JG, Yepuri JN. Transverse retubularized sigmoidovesicostomy continent urinary diversion to the umbilicus. J Urol 2001; 166: 644–7.
16. Sugarman ID, Malone PS, Terry TR, Koyle MA. Transversely tubularized ileal segments for the Mitrofanoff or Malone antegrade colonic enema procedures: the Monti principle. Br J Urol 1998; 81: 253–6.
17. Cain MP, Casale AJ, Rink RC. Initial experience using a catheterizable ileovesicostomy (Monti procedure) in children. Urology 1998; 52: 870–3.
18. Van Savage JG, Chancellor MB, Slaughenhoupt B. Transverse retubularized ileovesicostomy continent urinary diversion to the umbilicus. Tech Urol 2000; 6: 29–33.
19. Mouriquand P, Mure PY, Feyaerts A. The Left Monti-Malone. BJU Int 2000; 85 (Suppl 4): 65.
20. Liloku RB, Mure PY, Braga L, Basset T, Mouriquand PD. The left Monti-Malone procedure: preliminary results in seven cases. J Pediatr Surg 2002; 37: 228–31.
21. Tackett LD, Minevich E, Benedict JF, Wacksman J, Sheldon CA. Appendiceal versus ileal segment for antegrade continence enema. J Urol 2002; 167: 683–6.
22. Kajbafzadeh AM, Chubak N. Simultaneous Malone antegrade continent enema and Mitrofanoff principle using the divided appendix: report of a new technique for prevention of stoma complications. J Urol 2001; 165: 2404–9.
23. Wedderburn A, Lee RS, Denny A, Steinbrecher HA, Koyle MA, Malone PS. Synchronous bladder reconstruction and antegrade continence enema. J Urol 2001; 165: 2392–3.
24. Gerharz EW, Vik V, Webb G, Woodhouse CR. The in situ appendix in the Malone antegrade continence enema procedure for faecal incontinence. Br J Urol 1997; 79: 985–6.
25. Van Savage JG, Khoury AE, McLorie GA, Churchill BM. Outcome analysis of Mitrofanoff principle applications using appendix and ureter to umbilical and lower quadrant stomal sites. J Urol 1996; 156: 1794–7.

29 Ureterosigmoidostomy and Mainz pouch II

Margit Fisch, Joachim W Thüroff and Rudolf Hohenfellner

Introduction

The first urinary diversion using the anus for continence was published over 140 years ago by Simon.[1] Since that first description, more than 60 modifications of ureterosigmoidostomy have been published.[2] It was the method of choice for urinary diversion until the late 1950s, when electrolyte imbalances and secondary malignancies arising at the ureteral implantation site were observed.[3,4] However, secondary malignancies were later also reported in other forms of urinary diversion.[5] The development of new absorbable suture material, modern ureteric stents, antibiotics and alkalinizing drugs served in solving many of the traditional shortcomings of ureterosigmoidostomy and have rekindled the interest in this technique. Critics of ureterosigmoidostomy tend to quote publications dealing with complications in patients operated on before the 1950s.[6]

Another major drawback of ureterosigmoidostomy was frequency and urgency especially at night.[4,7,8] Urodynamic investigations showed that bowel contractions with rise in pressure in the bowel/reservoir are responsible for the incontinence.[8,9] By interrupting the circular contractions (antimesenteric opening of the bowel and 'reconfiguration') a low-pressure reservoir can be created thus improving continence rates and protecting the upper urinary tract. The era of low pressure anal reservoirs began.

Kock was the first who applied these principles to ureterosigmoidostomy.[9] Reports on similar techniques either augmenting the sigma with ileal[10] or ileocecal[11] segments followed. The sigma-rectum pouch[12,13] (Mainz pouch II) represents an equally effective but more simple operative procedure for creation of a low-pressure rectal reservoir. The idea was not new, the first description dates back to Kocher in 1907.[14] As standard technique for ureteral implantation the submucosal tunnel is used – the same technique as for classical ureterosigmoidostomy. However, in dilated or ureters with thickened walls it is associated with an increased complication rate. For these the technique published by Abol-Enein and Ghoneim for ureteral implantation into an ileal neobladder represents an alternative[15,16] It is also applicable for the sigma-rectum pouch.[17] During the past years modifications of the original technique have been described.[18,19] These represent an increasing interest in the procedure. Today, the techniques of low-pressure anal reservoirs have completely replaced classical ureterosigmoidostomy.[20–22]

Indications and contraindications

The sigma-rectum pouch is suitable for primary urinary diversion, revision of ureterosigmoidostomy and conversion of incontinent diversion. The procedure is indicated in patients with functional or actual loss of the urinary bladder. The main indications at the University of Mainz are urinary diversion in patients with bladder exstrophy or after radical cystectomy for bladder cancer. A competent anal sphincter is prerequisite for the sigma-rectum pouch as it is for ureterosigmoidostomy. There should be no renal insufficiency.

Contraindications are an incompetent anal sphincter, irradiation of the pelvis, diverticulosis of the sigmoid colon, polyposis and a serum creatinine >1.5 mg/dl.

Preoperative investigations and preparation

The anal sphincter function should be checked by a water tap enema (per anal instillation of 200–300 ml saline, which the patient should retain for at least 3 hours) and a rectodynamic investigation (no incontinence during measurement, anal sphincter profile: resting closure pressure >60 cmH_2O, closure pressure under stress >100 cmH_2O). Bowel disease like polyposis or diverticulosis have to be excluded.

For bowel preparation oral administration of 4–7 l of Fordtran's solution can be used on the day before the operation (alternatively 8–10 l of Ringer`s lactate solution via a gastric tube). Metronidazole in combination with a cephalosporine, alternatively piperacillin-sodium and an aminoglycoside is given at the beginning of surgery. A gastric tube or gastrostomy and a rectal tube are placed. For parenteral nutrition a central venous catheter has to be inserted.

Surgical technique

Instruments and suture material

- Basic abdominal set, suction, basin containing prepared iodine solution (disinfection).
- Two ureteral stents (6 Fr), 1 rectal tube.
- suture material: see Box 29.1.

> **BOX 29.1 SUTURE MATERIALS FOR URETEROSIGMOIDOSTOMY/SIGMA-RECTUM POUCH**
>
> **Bowel/pouch wall**
> absorbable synthetic suture material, e.g. polyglyconic acid
> 5-0 (mucosa)
> 4-0 (seromuscular layer)
>
> **Ureteral implantation**
> absorbable synthetic suture material, e.g. polyglycolic acid or polyglactin
> 5-0 and 6-0 (submucous tunnel)
> non-absorbable suture material, e.g. polypropylene 4-0 and absorbable material, e.g. polyglyconic acid 5-0 and 4-0 (serous lined extramural tunnel)
>
> **Stent fixation**
> polyglactin 4-0 with short reabsorption time

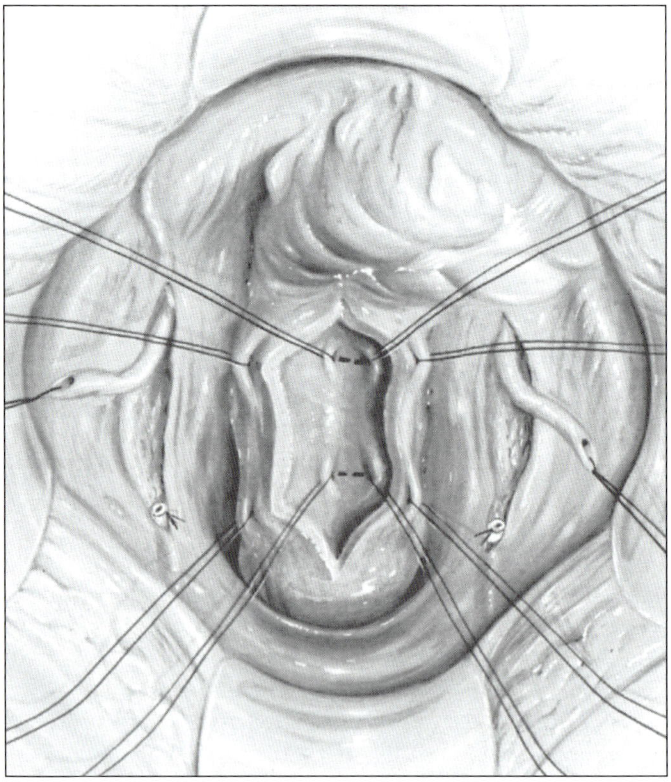

Figure 29.1 Open transcolonic ureterosigmoidostomy: both ureters have been cut at their entrance into the bladder and mobilized. The sites of the planned ureteral implantations in the posterior sigmoid wall are outlined by stay sutures.

Classical ureterosigmoidostomy

After median laparotomy the peritoneum is incised lateral to the descending colon and the left ureter is identified. A peritoneal incision is made on the contralateral site lateral to the ascending colon with identification of the right ureter. Both ureters are dissected respecting the longitudinal vessels running inside the Waldeyer's sheet. The dissection is extended caudally to the ureterovesical junction. The ureters are cut as distal as possible and stay sutures are placed at the 6 o'clock position. The ureteral stumps are ligated. The colon is slightly elevated at the rectosigmoid junction by four stay sutures. After opening of the sigmoid colon over a length of 4 cm by an incision of the anterior tenia, four mucosal stay sutures are placed in the mucosa of the posterior aspect of the sigmoid (Figure 29.1). The bowel mucosa is incised between the proximal stay sutures and a buttonhole type of excision of posterior bowel wall is performed. A straight or slightly curved clamp is

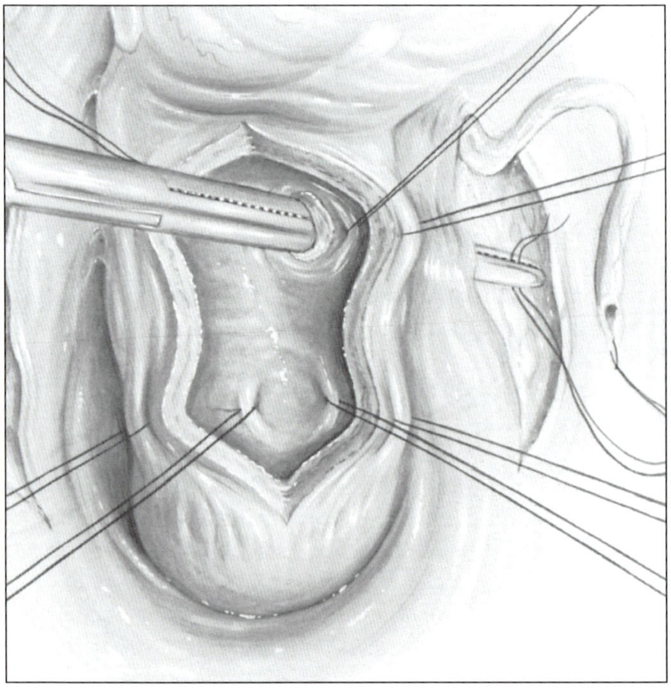

Figure 29.2 After incision of the mucosa and button-hole type of excision of the posterior bowel wall site, the ureter is to be brought through the intestinal wall, a subperitoneal tunnel is modeled bluntly from this point to the left incision in the peritoneum. The curved clamp is advanced precisely below the peritoneum.

advanced through the opening and a tunnel is created by blunt dissection below the visceral peritoneum of the mesosigmoid (Figure 29.2). The ureter is pulled into the lumen of the intestine. After creation of a submucosal tunnel of about 3 cm in length the ureter is threaded through this tunnel, carefully avoiding torsion (Figure 29.3). The anterior wall of the ureter is spatulated for a length of 1 cm. For uretero-intestinal anastomosis an anchor suture is placed at the 6 o'clock position grasping intestinal mucosa and musculature (absorbable synthetic suture material 5-0) and the anastomosis is completed by several uretero-mucosal single stitches (absorbable synthetic suture material 6-0). A 6-Fr silastic stent is inserted into the ureter and fixed to the mucosa by a polyglactin 4-0 suture with short reabsorption time (Figure 29.4 a, b). The contralateral ureter is implanted about 3 cm lateral and proximal or distal to the first anastomosis using the same technique (Figure 29.5). The ureteral stents are inserted into the rectal tube and pulled out through the anus. Thereafter the rectal tube is reinserted. The anterior sigmoid colon is closed in one layer using interrupted stitches of absorbable synthetic suture material 4-0 or in two layers using running sutures (absorbable synthetic material 5-0 for the mucosa and 4-0 for the seromuscularis). The peritoneal incisions are closed. At the end of surgery, separate fixations of the rectal tube and ureteral stents to the skin of the anus are performed.

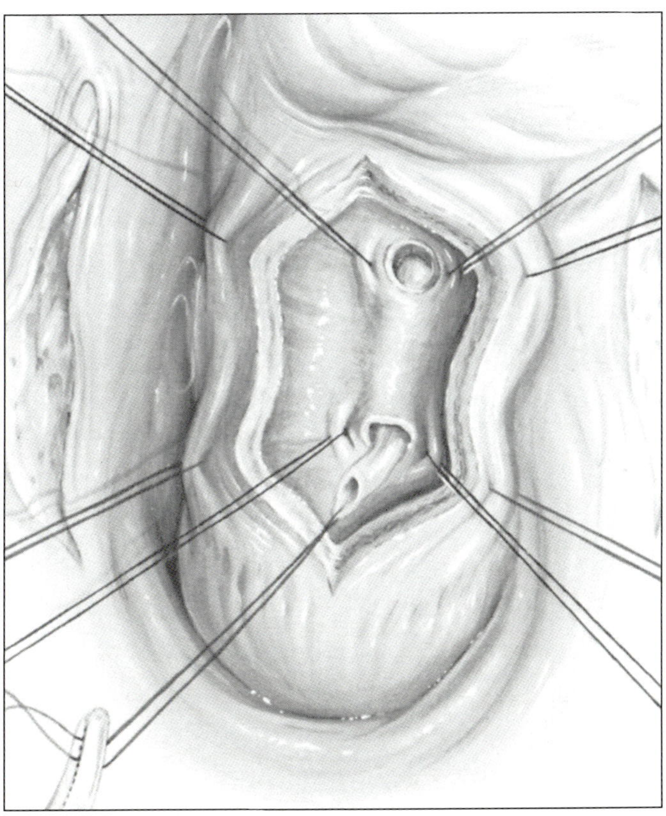

Figure 29.3 The ureter has been pulled into the bowel and through a submucous tunnel reaching from the proximal to the distal stay sutures.

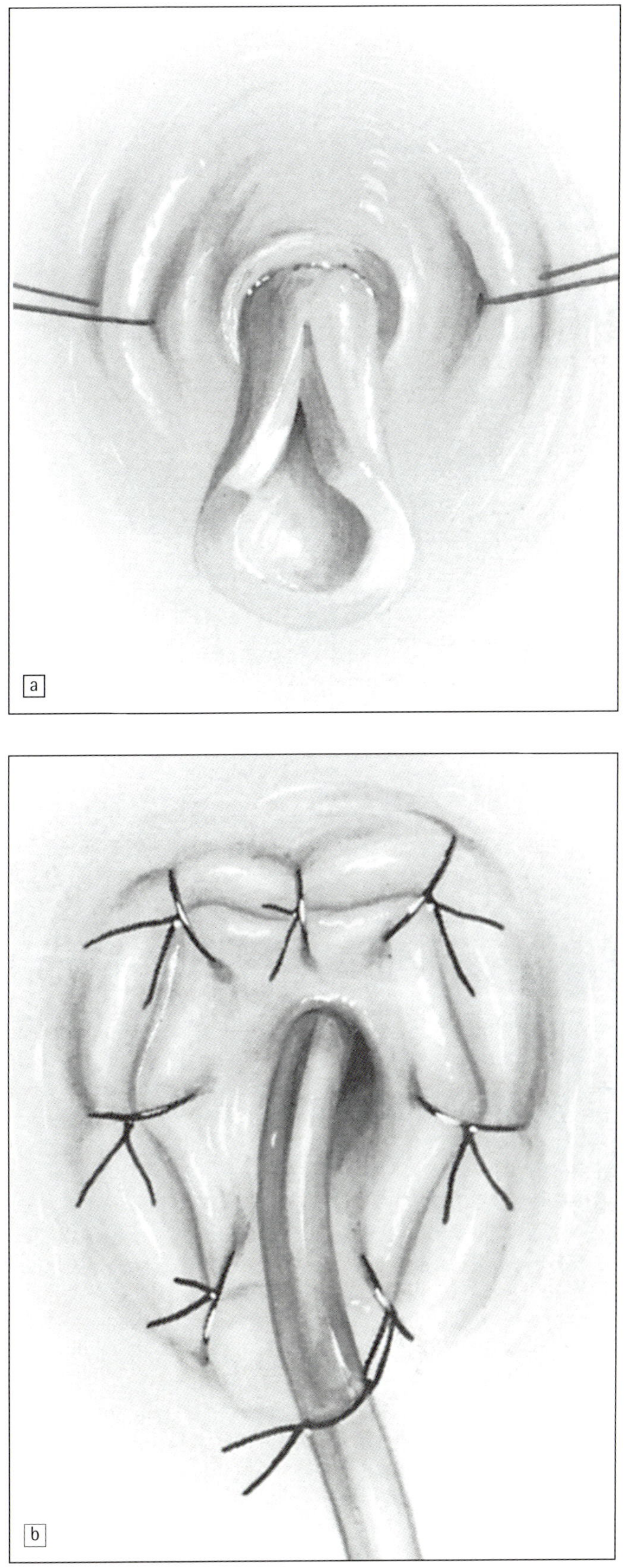

Figure 29.4 Spatulation of the anterior wall of the ureter (a) and uretero-mucosal anastomosis between ureter and intestinal wall. (b) The ureter is stented.

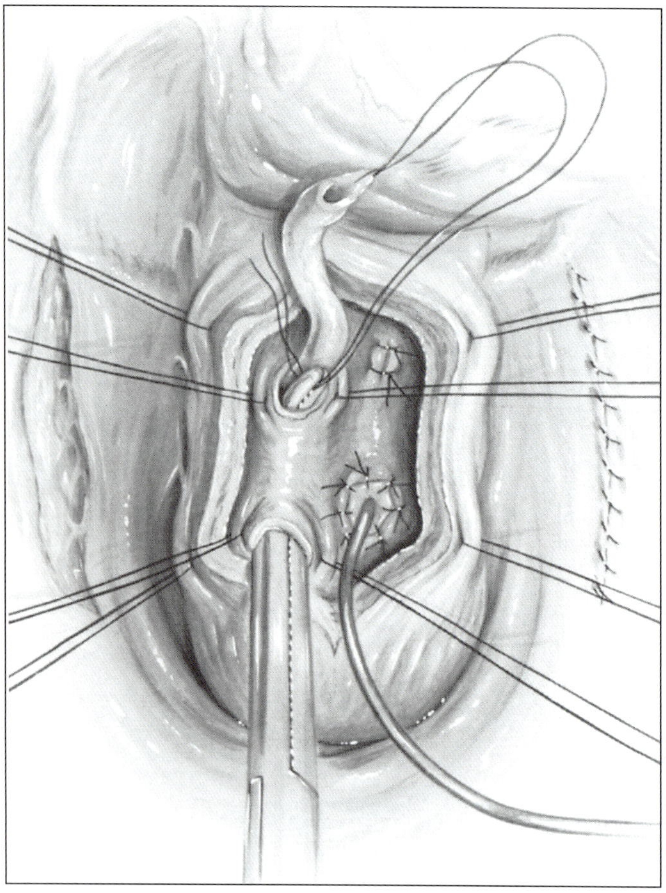

Figure 29.5 Identical implantation of the right ureter 3 cm lateral and proximal or distal of the first anastomosis.

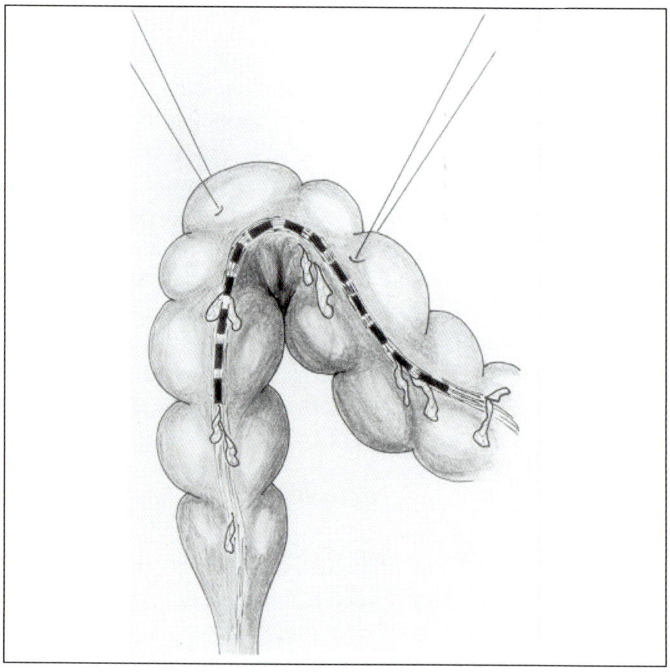

Figure 29.6 Identification of the rectosigmoid junction.

Sigma-rectum pouch (Mainz pouch II)

Access is gained by a median laparotomy as for ureterosigmoidostomy. The rectosigmoid junction is identified and two stay sutures are placed. The peritoneum is incised lateral to the descending colon and the left ureter is identified. Another peritoneal incision is made lateral to the ascending colon and the right ureter is identified. Both ureters are dissected down to the uretero-vesical junction respecting the longitudinal vessels running inside the Waldeyer's sheet. The ureters are cut as distal as possible, stay sutures are placed at the 6 o'clock position and the ureteral stumps are ligated.

For creation of the pouch, the intestine is opened at the anterior tenia starting from the rectosigmoid junction over a total length of 20–24 cm distal and proximal of this point (Figure 29.6). By placing two stay sutures in the middle of the incision at the right side of the opened rectosigmoid the intestine is positioned in a shape of an upside-down U. The posterior wall of the pouch is closed by side-to-side anastomosis of the medial margins of the U using two-layers of running sutures of absorbable synthetic suture material 4-0 for the seromuscular layer and 5-0 for the mucosa (Figure 29.7). Subsequently, the left ureter is pulled through retromesenterically

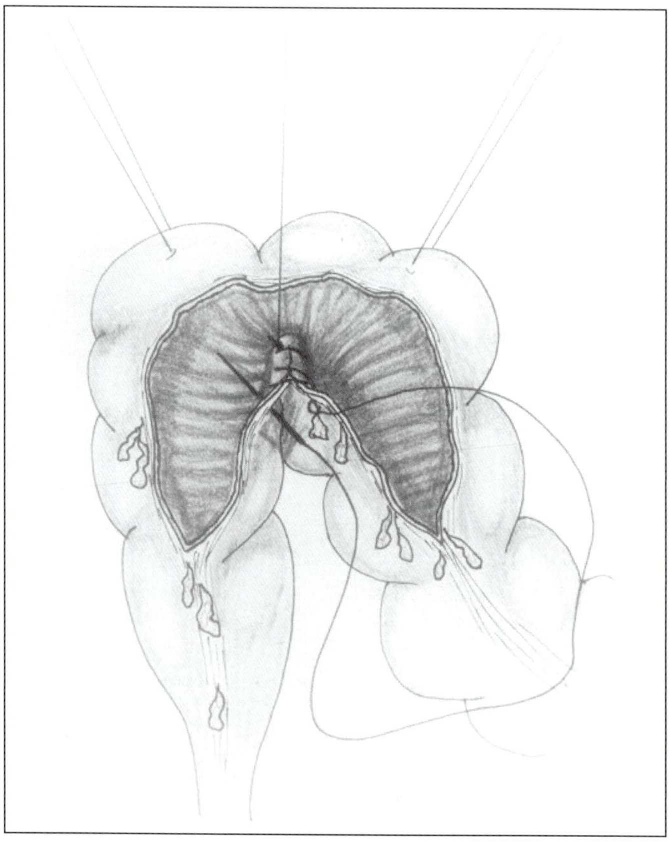

Figure 29.7 Opening of the rectosigmoid at the anterior tenia starting from the rectosigmoid junction over a total length of 20–24 cm distal and proximal of this point. Side-to-side anastomosis of the medial margins of the cut bowel edges by two-layer closure using running sutures of absorbable synthetic suture material 4-0 for the seromuscular layer and 5-0 for the mucosa.

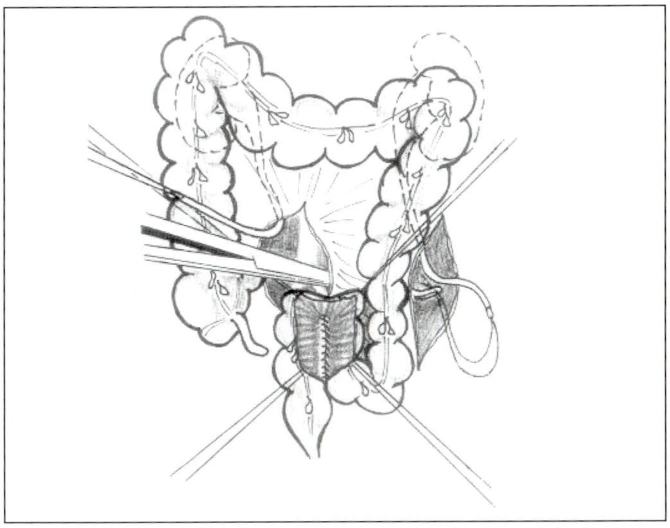

Figure 29.8 The left ureter is pulled through retromesenterically to the right side.

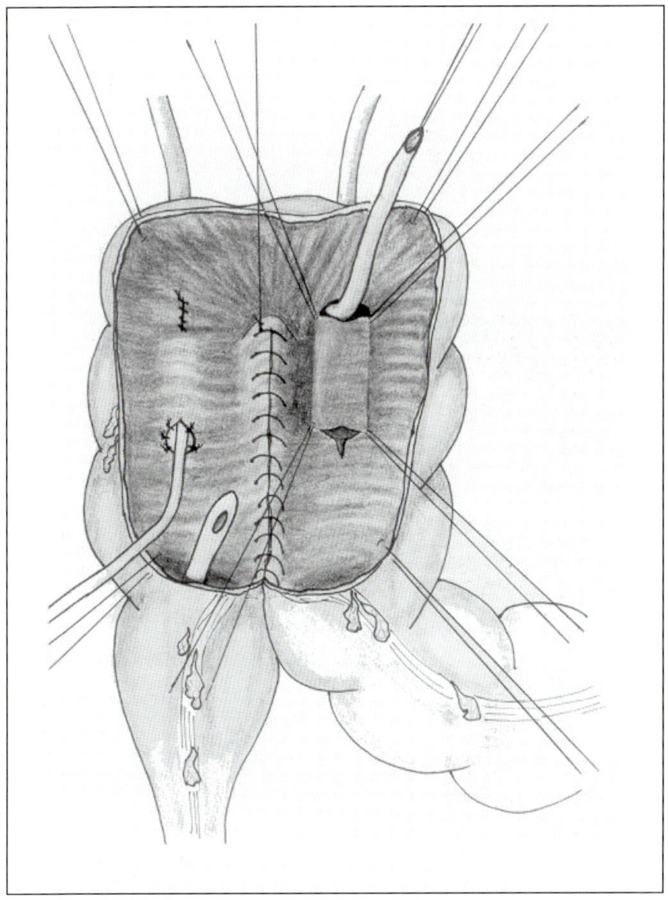

Figure 29.9 Creation of a wide entrance of the ureter into the pouch and preparation of a submucosal tunnel (2–2.5 cm in length). Incision of the mucosa at its end and pull through of the ureter. Ureteral implantation by an anchor suture at the 6 o'clock position and single stitch uretero-mucosal sutures. Closure of the cranial mucosal incision by a running suture with absorbable synthetic suture material 6-0.

above the inferior mesenteric artery from the left to the right side (Figure 29.8).

For ureteral implantation four mucosal stay sutures are placed parallel right and left to the medial running suture. The mucosa is incised and the seromuscular layer is excised between the two cranial stay sutures to create a wide buttonhole type of opening as an entrance of the ureter into the pouch. The dissection of the submucous tunnel starts from this incision downwards over a length of 2–2.5 cm. The mucosa is incised at the distal end of the tunnel and the ureter is pulled into the tunnel. After having resected the ureter to an adequate length, implantation is completed by placing an anchor suture at the 6 o'clock position (absorbable synthetic suture material 5-0) and several interrupted uretero-mucosal sutures (absorbable synthetic suture material 6-0).

Sufficient spatulation of the ureters is of utmost importance to avoid a nipple-like protrusion of the ureters. To drain an incidental hematoma of the submucosal tunnel, the mucosa covering the tunnel can be selectively incised at different points. After having finished the ureteral implantation, the cranial mucosal incision is closed by a running suture with polyglactin 4-0 (short reabsorption time). The contralateral ureter is implanted in the same manner (Figure 29.9). Six French ureteral stents are inserted into the ureters and are pulled out through the anus with the rectal tube, which is afterwards reinserted.

The pouch is fixed to the anterior longitudinal ligament of the spine at the promontory in the region of the proximal end of the posterior medial running sutures by two Bassini sutures with non-absorbable suture material 3-0 (Figure 29.10). To facilitate fixation of the pouch to the promontory, one sutured end of the dorsal running suture can be pulled through dorsally outside of the pouch and knotted with the fixation suture placed in the anterior band at the promontory.

The anterior pouch wall is closed by two-layers of sutures (5-0 absorbable synthetic suture material for the seromuscular and 4-0 absorbable synthetic suture material for the mucosal layer). Alternatively, single-layer closure using interrupted stitches can be done (Figure 29.11). When the anastomosis reaches deep down to the rectum, it is easier to suture the pouch starting caudally, as the deepest point of the anastomosis is the most critical part and is easier to reach at the beginning of the anastomosis. The peritoneal incisions are closed and the anastomotic site of the pouch is covered by omentum. The rectal tube and the ureteral stents are separately fixed to the skin of the anus (non-absorbable material).

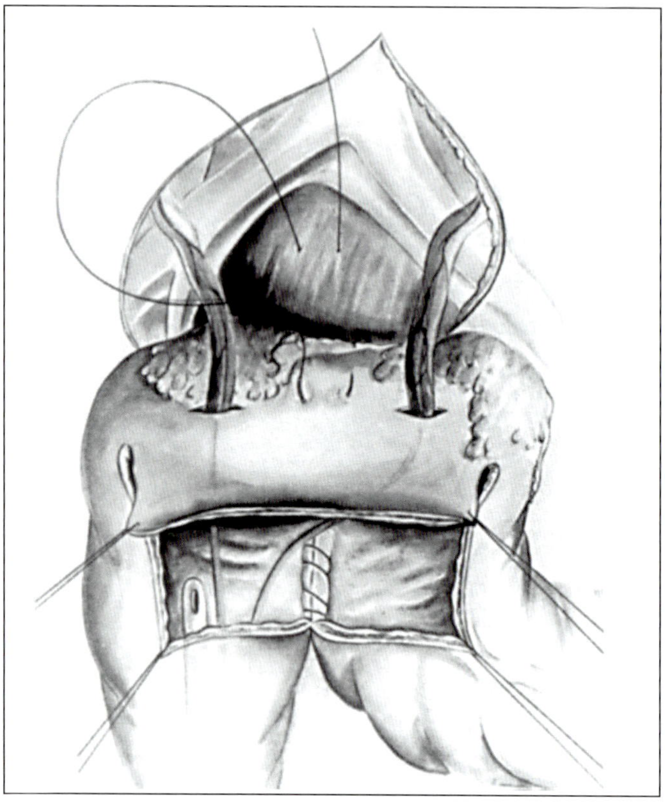

Figure 29.10 After having inserted a 6-Fr stent in each ureter, which are pulled out through the anus with the rectal tube, the pouch is fixed to the anterior longitudinal ligament of the spine in the region of the proximal end of the posterior medial running suture to be fixed to the anterior longitudinal ligament of the promontory by two Bassini sutures.

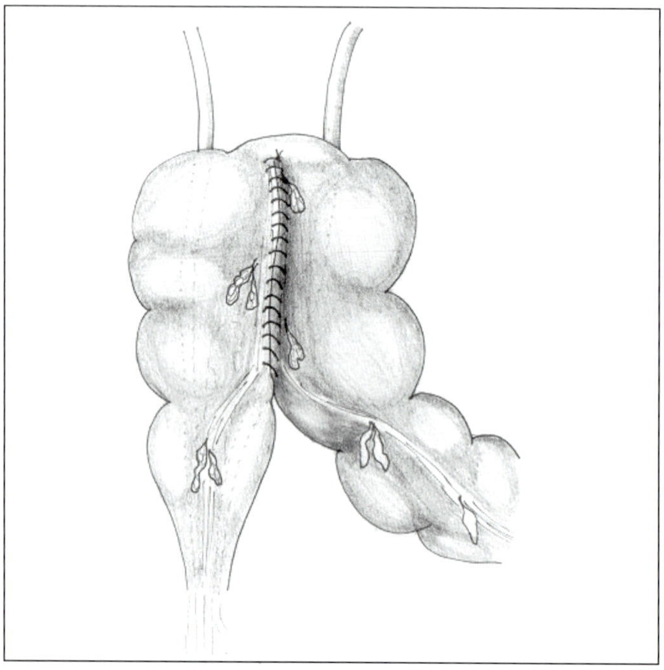

Figure 29.11 Closure of the anterior pouch wall by seromuscular single stitches with absorbable synthetic suture material 4-0. Closure of the peritoneal incisions.

Ureteral implantation through a serosal-lined extramural tunnel

Mobilization of the bowel includes the left colonic flexure (in cases of a short sigmoid). Dissection of the ureters is identical to the standard technique (Figure 29.12). An S-shaped sigmoid segment is outlined by stay sutures, each limb of 10–12 cm length resulting in a total length of 30–36 cm (Figure 29.13).

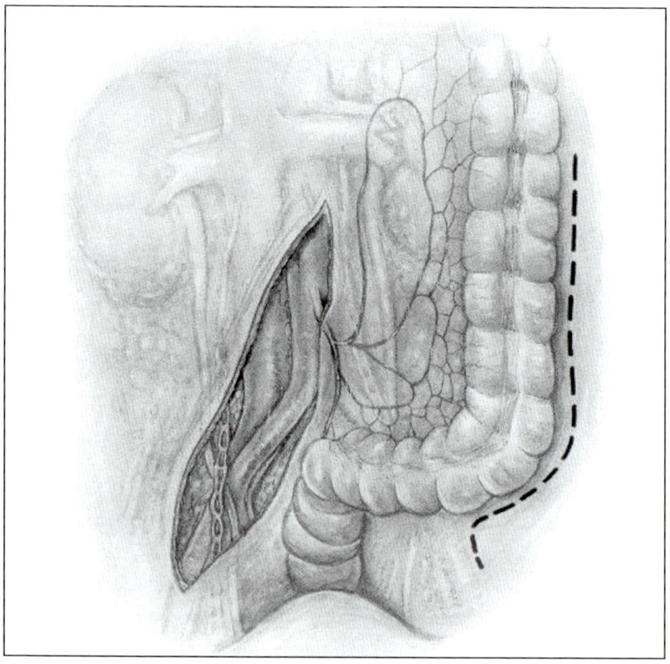

Figure 29.12 Right and left paracolonic incisions, identification and dissection of the ureters.

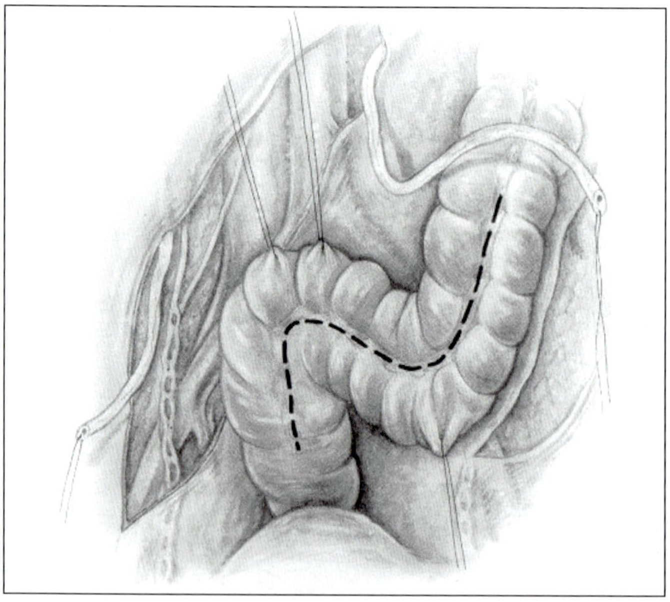

Figure 29.13 S-shaped sigmoid segment is outlined by stay sutures, the length of each segment is 10–12 cm, starting at the rectosigmoid junction (same as standard technique) adding another segment of 10–12 cm of ascending colon.

After antimesenteric opening of the S-shaped sigmoid colon (Figure 29.14) in the area of the anterior tenia a side-to-side adaptation of the seromuscularis of both limbs is obtained by single stitch sutures close to the mesentery (non-absorbable suture material). Thereby two-serosal lined channels are created. On the right side an entrance for the right ureter is left at the cranial aspect of the sutures. The mesentery cranial to the left sutures is incised and the left ureter pulled through. The ureters are placed in their respective channels (Figure 29.15) and the cut edges of the bowel are sutured above the ureter by all-layer running suture thus converting the channel into a tunnel. The length of the tunnel should be four times the diameter of the ureter. For implantation of the ureter, it is cut to its required length and spatulated. Four anchor sutures are placed at the 11 and 1 o'clock and the 5 and 7 o'clock positions through all layers of the ureter as well as all layers of the bowel wall (absorbable synthetic suture material 4-0). Uretero-mucosal stitches are placed inbetween the anchor sutures to complete the anastomosis (absorbable synthetic suture material 5-0, Figure 29.16). Two ureteral stents are inserted and pulled out through the anus with the rectal tube after having been fixed to the bowel mucosa (polyglactin 4-0 with short reabsorption time). The anterior pouch wall is closed by interrupted seromuscular sutures (absorbable synthetic suture material 4-0, Figure 29.17).

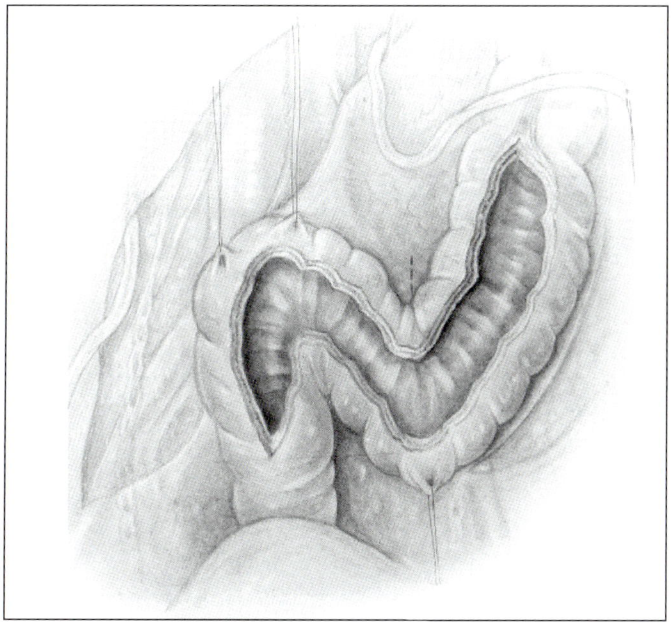

Figure 29.14 The marked segments are opened in the area of the anterior tenia. Incision of a mesenteric window for pull through of the left ureter.

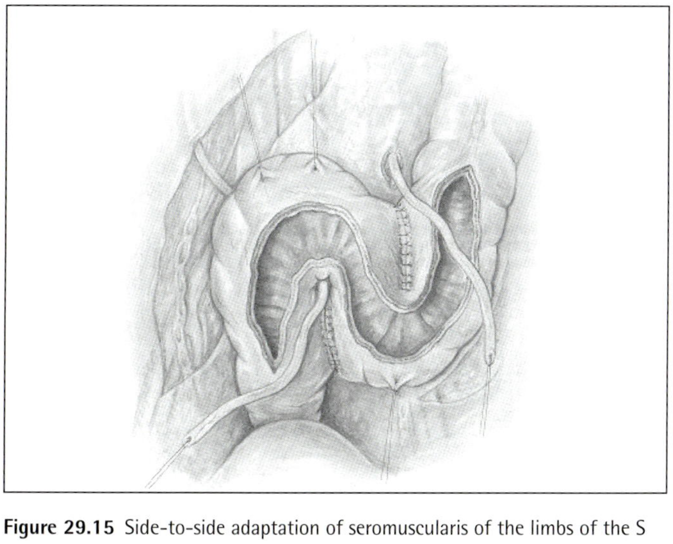

Figure 29.15 Side-to-side adaptation of seromuscularis of the limbs of the S by two interrupted suture lines close to the mesentery (non-absorbable suture 4-0) thereby creating two serosal-lined channels. On the right side, an entrance for the right ureter is left at the cranial aspect of the sutures and the ureter is pulled through. One ureter is placed in each channel created between the segments of the S.

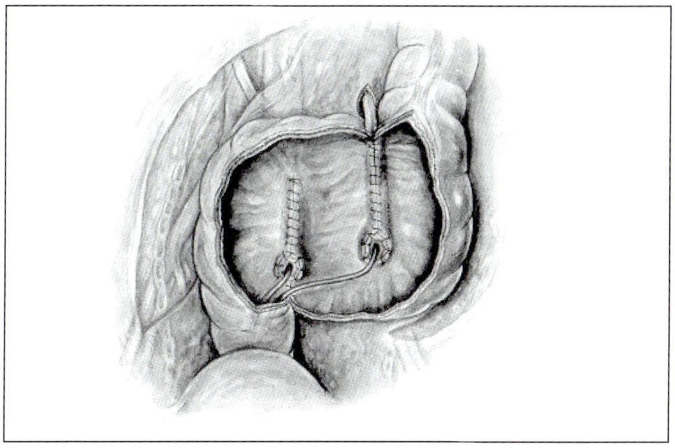

Figure 29.16 Ureteral implantation in the area of the continuous suture line. Insertion of ureteral stents.

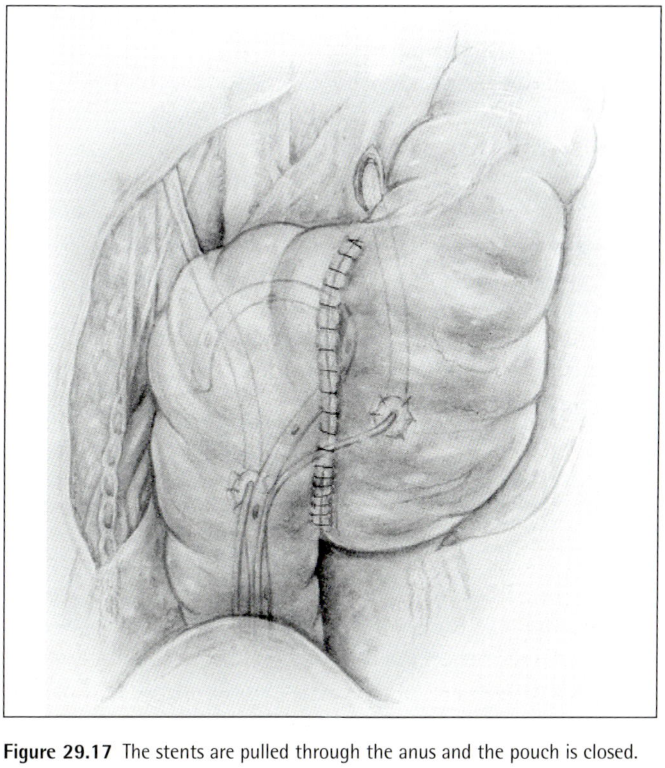

Figure 29.17 The stents are pulled through the anus and the pouch is closed.

Clinical experience

Of utmost importance for the outcome is patient selection. A functioning anal sphincter is prerequisite. Also important are technical details such as ureteral implantation, side-to-side anastomosis by two layers as well as the fixation to the promontory.

Between 1990 and 1999 a sigma-rectum pouch was performed in 123 patients at the Mainz University hospital. There were 94 adults and 29 children. The mean age was 44 years (10 months–73 years). Indications were malignancy (n = 92), bladder exstrophy and incontinent epispadias (n = 26), trauma (n = 4) and sinus urogenitalis (n = 1). Of the 123 patients 102 were followed with a mean follow-up of 46 months (1–9 years). Eight patients died during follow-up due to their primary malignant tumor, another two died unrelated to the underlying disease, eleven were lost to follow-up. Four early pouch-related complications were encountered: two dislodged ureteral stents requiring temporary nephrostomy and one ileus treated by operative intervention. One patient developed severe complications as a result of anastomotic leakage from a pouch fistula requiring revision and colostomy. Stenosis at the ureteral implantation site was the most common complication (7% = 14 renal units). Eleven renal units required surgical reimplantation. During follow-up, pyelonephritis was observed in 3% of patients. Of the 102 patients who were followed-up 99 were completely continent postoperatively, nighttime continence was 97%. The majority of the patients (70/102, 69%) use alkalinizing drugs to prevent metabolic acidosis.

Other reports of the sigma-rectum pouch mirror our own experience. A significant rise in capacity with decrease in rectal pressures was confirmed by Gumus et al[23] and Gilja.[24] Capacity improved from a mean of 150 ml preoperatively to 520 ml postoperatively.[23] Voiding frequency was described to be lower as after classical ureterosigmoidostomy and in the series of Obek et al[25] was 5.1 ± 1.1 per day and 1.9 ± 0.7 per night. In all series day and nighttime continence was high, ranging from 97 to 100%.[25–28] Early complications were low, 3.3% in a series of 60 patients.[25] Also late complications were comparable with other methods of continent urinary diversion.[25,29,30] In the series of Gerharz of 34 patients only one conversion to another form of urinary diversion became necessary.[26] Besides bladder cancer, bladder exstrophy represents an indication for the procedure.[31] The first 11 patients are reported in whom laparoscopic radical cystectomy and intracorporal creation of the sigma-rectum pouch was performed.[32]

Conclusion

Low-pressure rectal reservoirs have replaced classical ureterosigmoidostomy. The main indication is infiltrating bladder cancer. The technique is excellent for continent diversion in women and is very much accepted in countries in which catheter material or stoma bags are difficult to obtain or do not find patient acceptance.[8,18–20,22] Another indication is bladder exstrophy, especially in those patients in whom bladder reconstruction has failed.[22,31,33] However, secondary malignancies have to be considered and lifelong surveillance with rectoscopy starting from the fifth postoperative year is mandatory. A quite new indication is laparoscopic cystectomy with removal of the specimen through the rectum during laparoscopic creation of a sigma-rectum pouch.[32]

References

1. Simon J. Ectropia vesica (absence of the anterior walls of the bladder and pubic abdominal parieties); operation for directing the orifices of the ureters into the rectum; temporary success; subsequent death; autopsy. Lancet 1852; ii: 568.
2. Hinman F, Weyrauch HM Jr. A critical study of the different principles of surgery which have been used in uretero-intestinal implantation. Trans Amer Assoc Genitourin Surg 1936; 29: 15.
3. Wear JB, Barquin OP. Ureterosigmoidostomy: long-term results. Urology 1973; 1: 192–200.
4. McConnell JB, Steward WK. The long-term management and social consequences of ureterosigmoid anastomosis. Br J Urol 1975; 47: 607.
5. Kälble T, Tricker AR, Friedl P et al. Ureterosigmoidostomy: long-term results, risk of carcinoma and etiological factors for carcinogenesis. J Urol 1990; 144: 1110–14.
6. Connor JP, Hensle TW, Lattimer JK, Burbige KA. Long-term followup of 207 patients with bladder exstrophy: an evolution in treatment. J Urol 1989; 142: 793–6.
7. Boyce WH. A new concept concerning treatment of exstrophy of the bladder: 20 years later. J Urol 1972; 107: 476–89.
8. Ghoneim MA, Shebab-El-Din AB, Ashamallah AK, Gaballah MA. Evolution of the rectal bladder as a method for urinary diversion. J Urol 1981; 126: 737–40.
9. Kock NG, Ghoneim MA, Lycke KG, Mahrab MR. Urinary diversion to the augmented and valved rectum: preliminary results with a novel surgical procedure. J Urol 1988; 140: 1375–9.
10. Miller K, Matsui U, Hautmann R. Functional, augmented rectal bladder: early clinical experience. Eur Urol 1991; 19: 269–73.
11. Kato T, Sato K, Miyazaki H et al. The uretero-ileoceco-proctostomy (ileocecal rectal bladder): early experiences in 18 patients. J Urol 1993; 150: 326–31.
12. Fisch M, Hohenfellner R. Der Sigma-Rektum Pouch: Eine Modifikation der Harnleiterdarmimplantation. Akt Urol 1991; 22: I-IX.
13. Fisch M, Wammack R, Müller SC, Hohenfellner R. The Mainz Pouch II (Sigma Rectum Pouch). J Urol 1993; 149: 258–63.
14. Kocher. Chirurgische Operationslehre. Jena, Germany: Verlag Gustav Fischer, 1907.
15. Abol-Enein H, Ghoneim MA. Optimization of uretero-intestinal anastomosis in urinary diversion: an experimental study in dogs. III A new antireflux technique for uretero-ileal anstomosis: a serous-lined extramural tunnel. Urol Res 1993; 21(2): 135–9.
16. Abol-Enein H, Ghoneim MA. A novel uretero-ileal reimplantation technique: the serous lined extramural tunnel. A preliminary report. J Urol 1994; 151: 1193–7.

17. Fisch M, Abol-Enein H, Hohenfellner R. Ureterimplantation mittels serösem extramuralem Tunnel in Mainz-Pouch I und Sigma-Rektum Pouch (Mainz Pouch II). Akt Urol 1995; 26: I–X.
18. Sundin T, Mansi MK. The valved s-shaped rectosigmoid pouch for continent urinary diversion. J Urol 1993; 150: 838–42.
19. Dzamic Z, Hadzi-Djokic J, Tulic C et al. Quality of life in patients with modified Mainz pouch II urinary diversion. Acta Chir Iugoslavica 1999; 46: 11–13.
20. Obek C, Kural AR, Ataus S et al. Complications of the Mainz pouch II. Eur Urol 2002; 39: 204–11.
21. Fisch M, Macedo A, Klinkowski U, Fichtner J, Hohenfellner R. The Sigma rectum pouch (Mainz Pouch II): Clinical experience of 4.5 years. Abstract Book Continent Urinary Reconstruction, Second International Meeting, Mainz, Germany. 1998: 114.
22. Hafez AT, Elsherbiny MT, Dawaba MS, Abol-Enein H, Ghoneim M. Long-term outcome analysis of low pressure rectal reservoirs in 33 children with bladder exstrophy. J Urol 2001; 165(6 Pt 2): 2414–17.
23. Gumus E, Miroglu C, Saporta L et al. Rectodynamic and radiological assessment in modified Mainz Pouch II cases. Eur Urol 2000; 38: 316–22.
24. Gilja I, Kovacic M, Radej M, Kosuta D, Bakula B, Goles L. The sigmoidorectal pouch (Mainz pouch II). Eur Urol 1996; 29: 210–15.
25. Obek C, Kural AR, Ataus S et al. Complications of the Mainz pouch II. Eur Urol 2001; 39: 204–11.
26. Gerharz EW, Kohl UN, Weingärtner K et al. Experience with the Mainz modification of ureterosigmoidostomy. J Urol 1999; 162: 846–8.
27. Venn SN, Mundy AR. Continent urinary diversion using the Mainz-type ureterosigmoidostomy – a valuable salvage procedure. Eur Urol 1999; 36: 247–51.
28. Woodhouse CRJ, Christofides M. Modified ureterosigmoidostomy (Mainz II) – technique and early results. Br J Urol 1998; 81: 247–52.
29. Pajor L, Kelemen Z. Our experience with the Mainz Pouch II: 40 patients; follow-up and complications. Ann Urol 1995; 29: 246–9.
30. Golbano Ablanque JM, Serrano Pascual A, Otero Tejero I et al. [Detubularized ureterosigmoidostomy Mainz II: a diversion with a future?] [Article in Spanish]. Arch Esp Urol 2001; 54: 123–8.
31. Mingin GC, Stock JA, Hanna MK. The Mainz II pouch: experience in 5 patients with bladder exstrophy. J Urol 1999; 162: 846–8.
32. Türk I, Davis JW, Deger S et al. [Laparoscopic radical cystectomy with intracorporeal creation of a continent urinary diversion. Future or present?] [Article in German]. Urologe A 2002; 41: 107–12.
33. Stein R, Fisch M, Stöckle M, Hohenfellner R. Urinary diversion in bladder exstrophy and incontinent epispadias: 25 years of experience. J Urol 1995; 154: 1177–81.

30 Urinary diversion to the modified rectal bladder: an anal sphincter-controlled bladder substitute

Hassan Abol-Enein and Mohamed A Ghoneim

Introduction

Attempts to create a bladder substitute controlled by the anal sphincter go back over 100 years when ureterosigmoidostomy was first introduced by Simon.[1] Thereafter, the procedure has undergone many technical modifications, more than 60 methods being cited by Hinman and Weyrauch.[2] These operative approaches include the following categories:

- without fecal exclusion
- with total fecal exclusion
- with partial fecal exclusion.

Anal sphincter controlled bladder substitutes without fecal exclusion

Ureterosigmoidostomy

In the early 1950s, the results of ureterosigmoidostomy were the subject of two main reports. On behalf of the British Urological Association, Jacobs and Stirling[3] reviewed the results of 1763 cases. The US experience was reported by Clarke and Leadbetter[4] who reviewed the results of 2897 patients. The discouraging results reported in these two reviews, as well as the introduction of Bricker's ileal loop, led to a sharp decline in the use of this procedure. However, during the late 1960s and 1970s, ureterosigmoidostomy underwent a revival.[5–8] In all of these contributions, the postoperative mortality and morbidity were remarkably reduced as a result of improved surgical technique, and the availability of a wide range of antimicrobial agents. Nevertheless, the incidence of delayed complications still remained significant. Pyelonephritis was encountered in 26–50% of cases, stenotic problems in 33–50% and hyperchloremic acidosis in 30–50% (Table 30.1).

While the pathogenesis of hyperchloremic acidosis was the subject of many investigations, two observations are relevant to this contribution. Stamey[9] provided objective evidence that profound hyperchloremic acidosis could develop from urine enemas in patients with normal renal function. It was also observed that urine placed in the rectum freely refluxes to fill the entire colon and does not completely empty with defecation. Irvine et al,[10] working with dogs, demonstrated that the severity of this disorder is directly related to the surface area of colonic mucosa exposed to urine as well as the time of contact with the colonic mucosa.

Adenocarcinoma of bowel arising in juxtaposition of the site of the ureterocolic implantation was repeatedly reported in the literature. Although it is difficult to determine accurately the incidence of this complication, Leadbetter et al,[11] reported that about 5% of patients with a ureterosigmoidostomy were likely to develop a tumor. Husman and Spence[12] collected 94 such cases from among patients who had ureterosigmoidostomy

Table 30.1 Mortality and morbidity after ureterosigmoidostomy

Series	No. of cases	Pyelonephritis (%)	Abnormal pyelogram (%)	Hyperchloremic acidosis (%)
Mathisen[5a]	45	50	50	38.8
Williams et al[6b]	51	45	35	31.3
Wear and Barquin[7c]	24	57	33	50
Zincke and Segura[8d]	173	26	36	30

[a]Whole series had bladder cancer, 20.6% had palliative diversion.
[b]Most cases had bladder carcinoma. An open transcolonic approach was utilized.
[c]Results of cases with bladder cancer and ureterosigmoidostomy – Leadbetter technique.
[d]88% had carcinoma of the bladder. Leadbetter technique was utilized.

for bladder exstrophy. Almost without exception the growth originated at, or in proximity with, the anastomotic sites of the ureters to the colon. The pathogenesis of this complication is not clearly defined. Using a rat model, Crissey et al,[13] proved experimentally that the development of bowel tumors after urinary diversion was due to the effect of urine and fecal matter on the colonic mucosa. It is very interesting to note that these investigators have also observed that an initial proximal colostomy for 1–3 months offered some protection against later development of tumors. Stewart et al,[14] suggested that urinary nitrates are converted by fecal bacterial into nitrosamines which act as active carcinogens. This contention has been challenged, however, by Stribling et al,[15] and Shands et al,[16] who reported a significant decrease in the production of nitrosamines in urine by ascorbic acid. Nevertheless, urocolonic tumors continued to appear in treated animals.

In summary, although the mortality and initial morbidity following ureterosigmoidostomy have been significantly reduced, some inherent chronic complications remain problematic.

Anal sphincter controlled bladder substitutes with total fecal exclusion

Rectal bladder with terminal colostomy

In 1895, Mauclaire[17] first described isolated rectum as a bladder substitute in dogs. He diverted the fecal stream by a proximal colostomy (Figure 30.1). The first clinical experience was reported in in 1906 by Remedi.[18] The method of Mauclaire was reintroduced into clinical practice by Creevy and Reiser[19] and later advocated by others.[20–22] The use of an isolated rectal pouch as a urinary reservoir following cystectomy was favored in view of some theoretic considerations: it is a continent method of diversion; there is no need for a sophisticated external appliance; the colostomy soon acquires a regular habit for emptying and a simple colostomy belt is all that is needed; the operation is technically simple and can be staged;[23] and the isolated rectum presents a limited absorbent surface area, reducing the chances of biochemical disturbances.[10] Furthermore, since the fecal and urinary streams are separated, the incidence of ascending infection is minimized. The result is a minimum incidence of pyelonephritis and hydronephrosis, with subsequent low incidence of renal failure and acidosis.

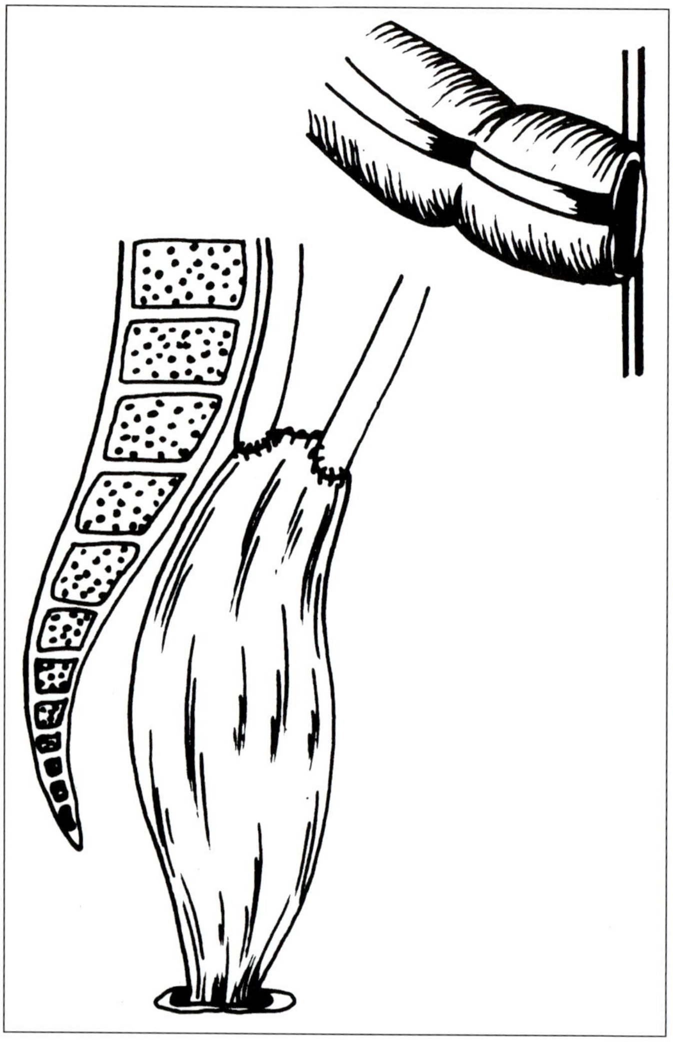

Figure 30.1 An isolated rectal bladder with terminal colostomy (Mauclaire).

In view of these possible advantages, the rectal bladder was utilized as the principal method for urinary diversions in the Department of Urology, University of Mansoura, Egypt, throughout the 1960s and early 1970s.[24] In 1974, Ghoneim and Ashamallah[25] reported that this method of urinary diversion had two main problems, namely loss of renal units due to pyelonephritis in ~30% of their cases, and nocturnal urinary leakage in 40%. These two problems were addressed in a subsequent report.[26] A submucosal tunnel ureteral reimplantation was utilized for reflux prevention whenever the ureters were of normal caliber and imipramine hydrochloride was given for the treatment of enuresis.

In summary, although the isolated rectal bladder offers some advantages, it is a non-compliant reservoir with a significant incidence of enuresis. Furthermore, any advantages over ureterosigmoidostomy are at the expense of the presence of a terminal colostomy.

Rectal bladder with perineal colostomy

Gersuny, in 1898,[27] devised a surgical procedure intended to maintain fecal and urinary continence. The trigone was implanted into an isolated rectal pouch.

The proximal sigmoid was mobilized and pulled down through the perineum in front of the anus so that the anal sphincter would control the newly formed rectal bladder as well as the sigmoid now functioning as an artificial anus (Figure 30.2a). In 1912, Heitz-Boyer and Hovelacque[28] modified Gersuny's original operation. They brought the sigmoid colon down posterior to the rectum and passed it directly underneath the anal mucosa to obtain full control of both the internal and external anal sphincters (Figure 30.2b).These concepts were revived by Lowsely and coworkers in 1953.[29] They claimed that when this procedure was employed, urinary and fecal continence could be achieved. This was followed later by sporadic reports of good results.[30,31] It is intriguing to note that none of these reports was followed up by a larger series with a satisfactory outcome.

In 1974, Ghoneim and Shoukry,[32] used the Gersuny–Lowsley procedure in eight patients. Cystectomy for carcinoma of the bladder was the indication for diversion in six cases and vesical exstrophy in two. All patients achieved good urinary continence indicating that manipulation of the external anal sphincter did not interfere with its integrity. In addition, successful creation of a properly sited well-vascularized artificial anus was achieved in seven out of eight cases. In spite of the presence of a functioning sphincter, flatus and/or feces could pass suddenly without prior warning.

Distension of the sigmoid colon in normal subjects produces a purely abdominal sensation of flatulent discomfort, whereas rectal distension causes a feeling of fullness interpreted by the patient as a need to pass gas or stool. Thus the sigmoid does not function as an ideal reservoir since it is unable to mediate afferent sensations that can be interpreted easily by the patients as a need for defecation.

In summary, although the operation is technically feasible, the patients have what is, in effect, an often incontinent perineal colostomy.

Anal sphincter controlled bladder substitutes with partial fecal exclusion

Rectal bladder with sigmoidoproctostomy

In 1903 Borelius[33] was the first to consider the possibility of partial exclusion of the sigmoid colon. The objective was to separate the urinary and fecal contents after ureterosigmoidostomy. He devised a method whereby a short-circuited loop of the sigmoid was partially excluded by a side-to-side anastomosis at its base (Figure 30.3a). The ureters were anastomosed to the dome of the loop. In 1909, Descomps[34] working with a cadaver, sectioned the upper rectum and carried out a terminolateral

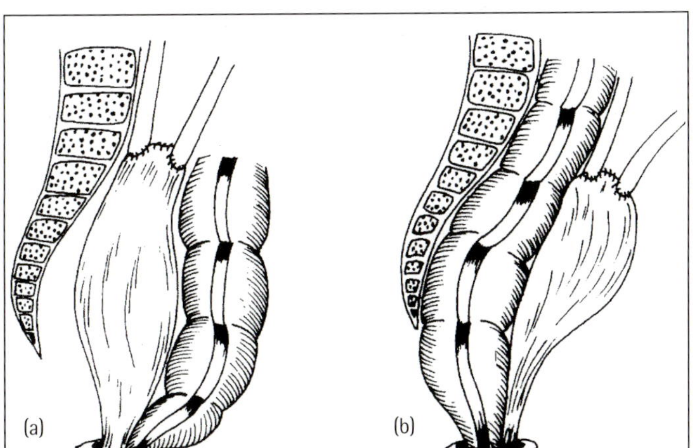

Figure 30.2 An isolated rectal bladder with perineal colostomy. (a) The Gersuny operation. (b) Heitz-Boyer and Hovelacque procedure.

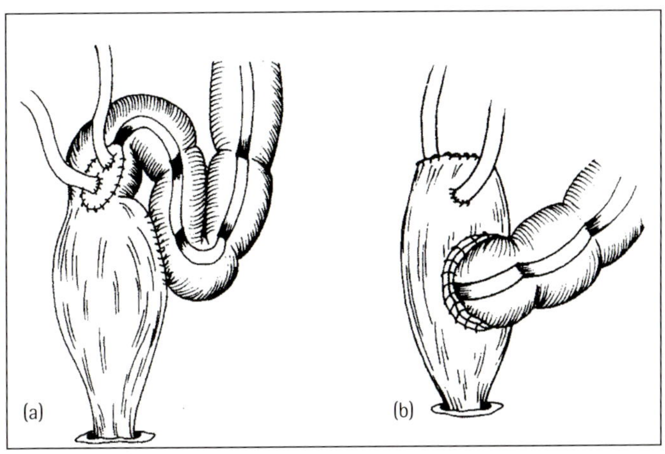

Figure 30.3 A rectal bladder with sigmoidoproctostomy: (a) The Borelius operation. (b) The Descomps procedure.

implantation of the sigmoid to the anterior surface of the rectum lower down. The ureters were implanted in the superior portion of the excluded rectum (Figure 30.3b). In 1962, Modelski[35] utilized the same principle. While operating on a 6-year-old boy, he was unable to obtain an adequate length of the sigmoid to form a perineal colostomy. The sigmoid stump was anastomosed end to side to the distal segment of the rectum above the anal sphincter. The same procedure was later reported by Leiter and Brendler in 1964[36] and Chargi et al in 1965.[37]

Functionally, the procedure does not provide a clear advantage over conventional methods of ureterosigmoidostomy since the accumulating urine can readily regurgitate to the proximal colon. Consequently, biochemical imbalances resulting from absorption of urine through a large surface area cannot be eliminated.[38]

The problem

An isolated rectal bladder with a terminal colostomy is superior to other methods aimed at construction of a bladder substitute controlled by the anal sphincter. Nevertheless, all its advantages must be weighed against the necessity of having a terminal colostomy. Furthermore, in view of the limited capacity of the rectum and the viscoelastic properties of its wall, a significant proportion of patients have nocturnal urinary incontinence.

The proposal

A surgical procedure incorporating the following three concepts was considered:

1 The rectum is functionally isolated by an isoperistaltic intussuscepted nipple valve at the colorectal junction: an idea initially proposed in 1975 by Knox and Jago[39] in animal experiments using piglets.
2 The ureters are implanted into this isolated rectal bladder by an antireflux mechanism.
3 The urodynamic qualities of the neo-reservoirs are improved by patching with an open sheet of ileum.

Experimental verification

These concepts were tested in a series of elaborate experiments (on dogs) in the animal laboratories of the Department of Surgery, University of Göteborg.[40] The investigation provided the following evidence:

- The intussusception valve constructed at the colorectal junction effectively prevented regurgitation of fluid from the rectum to the proximal colon without obstruction of the fecal stream in an aboral direction.
- The rectal augmentation with a patch of ileum increased the capacity of the reservoir 4–5 fold within 6 months postoperatively and the intraluminal pressures did not exceed 18 cmH_2O with maximal filling. As an indication of the good compliance of the rectal reservoir, no leakage through the anus was ever seen and no masceration around the anus was observed.
- Incorporation of the ureters within the intussusception valve provided an efficient antireflux mechanism.

These observations were later reproduced and supported by the animal experiments carried out by Miller and coworkers.[41–43]

Clinical trial

Patients

Encouraged by the favorable experimental findings, we started a clinical trial at the Urology-Nephrology Center, Mansoura, Egypt. Our initial clinical experience was the subject of a preliminary report.[44] Up to December 1992, 115 of such procedures had been performed in 77 adult females, 28 adult male, and 10 children. The indications are outlined in Table 30.2.

Operation

The anterior wall of the rectum is incised longitudinally from the rectosigmoid junction to a level 3–5 cm distal to the level of the peritoneal reflection. The incision is approximately 15 cm in length. The mesentry of the distal 10 cm of the sigmoid is mobilized, defatted, and the appendices epiploicae removed. Through the opened lumen of the rectum, the sigmoid is grasped by a pair of Babcock's clamps and pulled down to form a 5 cm intussusception valve. The intussuscepted position is maintained by three or four rows of metallic staples applied at the base of the valve with an automatic stapling device (Figure 30.4a). One row of staples is placed on each side of the mesentery and the other two in the opposite quadrants. An additional row is further applied to anchor the valve to the wall of the rectum, providing additional stability and support.

The ureters are anastomosed to the isolated rectal pouch using an antirefluxing system. A buttonhole is cut at the summit of the nipple valve. A straight clamp is introduced between the two layers of the intussusception and parallel to the staple rows. The ureters are then pulled down through these tunnels (Figure 30.4b). A stented mucosa-to-mucosa anastomosis is carried out between the ureter and the sigmoid mucosa using interrupted sutures of absorbable 4-0 material (Figure 30.4c). While

Table 30.2 Indications for diversion using a modified rectal bladder

Indication	Cases (n = 115)
Bladder extrophy	5
Irrepairable urinary fistulas	12
Contracted bladder	2
Sarcoma of the bladder	2
Carcinoma of the bladder	94

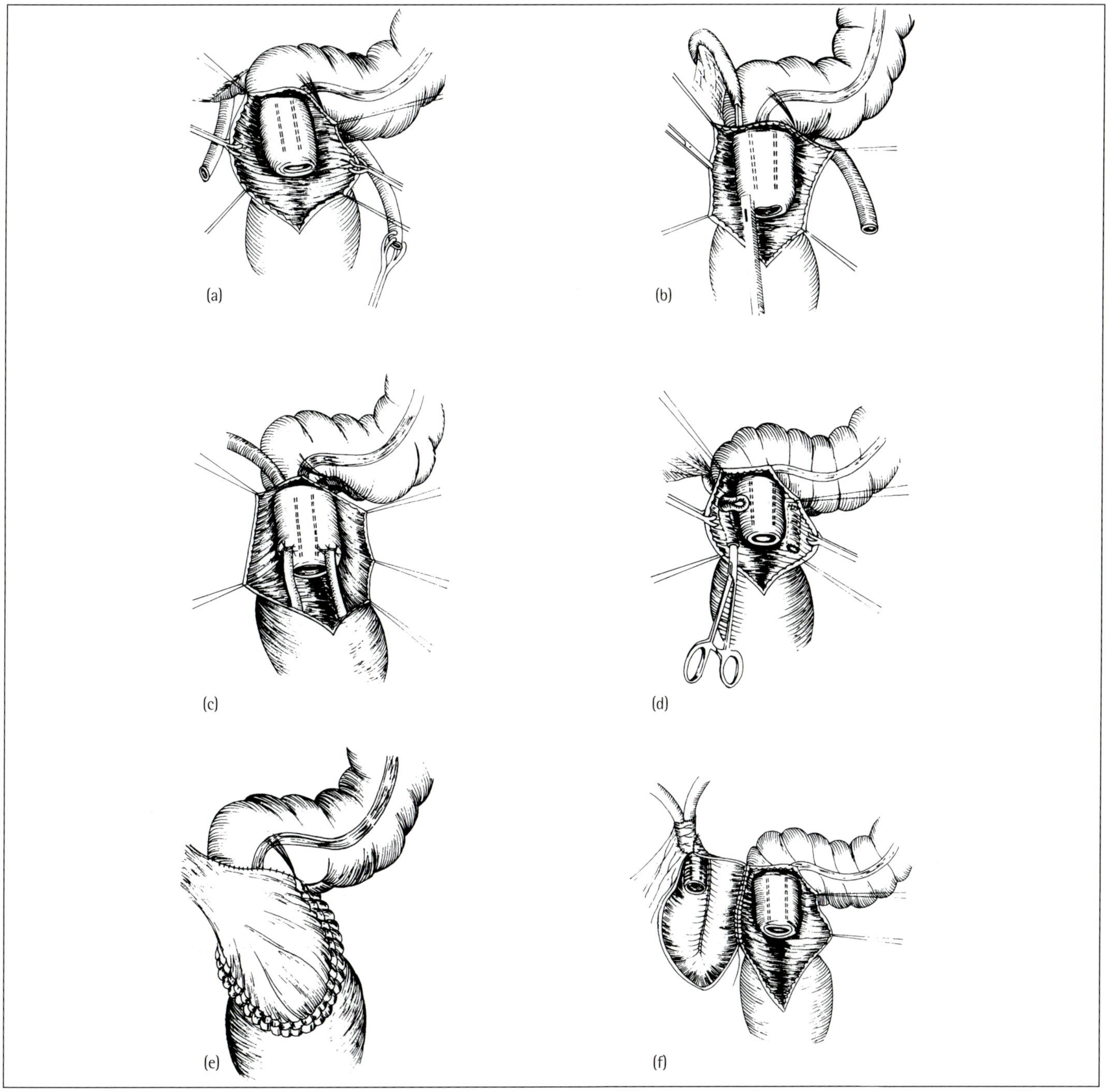

Figure 30.4 (a) The anterior wall of the rectosigmoid is opened and a colorectal intussusception valve is created. (b) The ureter is passed between the two layers of the intussusception. (c) A stented mucosa-to-mucosa anastomosis is completed on both sides. (d) An alternative (currently the method of choice), is to reimplant the ureters through a submucous tunnel following Goodwin's technique. (e) The opened rectum is closed with an ileal patch. (f) With dilated ureters a second intussusception valve from ileum is used for reflux prevention.

this method was used initially,[44] an alternative technique is readily available. A standard submucous tunnel following the procedure originally described by Goodwin et al,[45] can also be adopted (Figure 30.4d). For rectal augmentation, a 20 cm segment of distal ileum is isolated. Its antimesentric border is opened, folded into a U, and the two adjacent borders are sutured together. This intestinal plate is then patched on the anterior wall of the open rectum (Figure 30.4e).

If the ureters are grossly dilated, the two methods mentioned above are unsuitable for reimplantation. Under such circumstances, a second antireflux valve is created from the ileum in connection with the patch used for augmentation (Figure 30.4f). The ureters are then anastomosed to the afferent limb of this valve. For this procedure, the isolated segment of ileum should be 30–35 cm in length to provide adequate material for construction of the patch as well as the nipple valve.

Finally, a temporary transverse colostomy is made; this is closed after 6–8 weeks. More recently a tube cecostomy is performed for proximal colonic decompression. The cecostomy tube is removed two weeks postoperatively. The rectal pouch is drained by a tube for 3 weeks. Ureteric stents are removed after 10 days.

Results

Early complications

There was no postoperative mortality. The early complications are listed in Table 30.3. Sixteen complications were seen in 11 patients; all but three were treated conservatively.

Follow-up and evaluation

The patients were followed-up for periods ranging from 11 to more than 16 years (median 13 years). During the observation period 30 patients died from cancer, two were awaiting closure of their colostomy and one was not followed. Eighty-four patients are currently fully evaluable. The evaluation of patients included symptom analysis for daytime continence, nocturnal enuresis and frequency of voiding. Urographic studies and ascending proctograms were carried out to assess the renal function and configuration and the efficiency of the nipple valve in reflux prevention. A slow-fill (10 ml/min) water proctometry was obtained to measure the volume–pressure relationship in the neobladder.

During the observation period, all patients were continent during the day with an emptying frequency of two to five times. Similarly, all patients but eight were dry at night with a voiding frequency of nought to two times. It must be noted that of the eight enuretics, two were children and all responded favorably to treatment with imipramine hydrochloride given orally before bedtime.

None of the patients complained of constipation or abdominal distension following closure of their colostomies. In the initial phase of the work, an antegrade barium study through the temporary colostomy was carried out to ensure unobstructed flow of material through the anorectal valve. Thereafter, it was judged that this investigation was unnecessary and it was abandoned (Figure 30.5).

Table 30.3 Early complications of an anal sphincter controlled bladder substitute

Complication	No. of cases
Mortality	0
Prolonged ileus	4
Sepsis	5
Deep vein thrombosis	2
Intestinal obstruction	1[a]
Internal hemorrhage	1[a]
Rectovaginal fistula	3[b]

[a]Required surgical intervention.
[b]One required surgical intervention; the others were treated by prolonged drainage with a rectal tube.

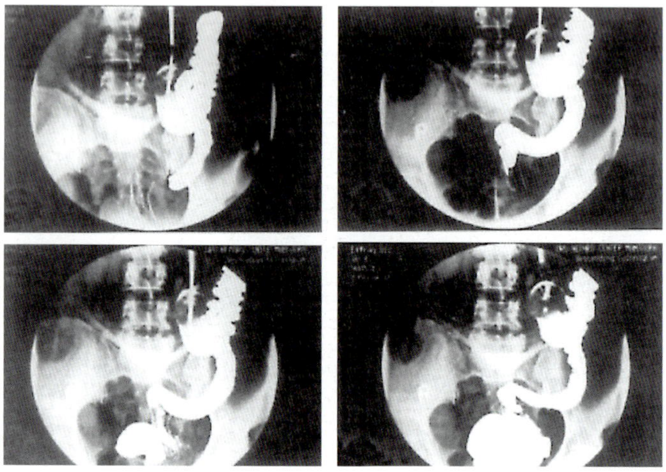

Figure 30.5 Antegrade barium study showing free flow of barium through the colorectal valve.

Table 30.4 Urographic evaluation

	Renal units		
Finding	Right	Left	Total (%)
Decompression	11	14	25 (15%)
Stability	62	63	125 (75%)
Deterioration	10	7	17 (10%)
Total	84	84	167

Urographic studies demonstrated an improvement or stabilization of upper urinary tract function in the majority of cases (Table 30.4). An example case with a longitudinal follow-up of 4 years is demonstrated in Figure 30.6. A case incorporating a second ileal intussusception valve, to provided an antireflux mechanism for dilated ureters otherwise unsuitable for submucosal reimplantation, is shown in Figure 30.7.

The causes of deterioration of renal functions relative to the method of ureteral reimplantation are given in Table 30.5. It may be noted that implantation of the ureters through a second intussusception ileal nipple valve was followed by the least incidence of complications. It is now routinely employed as our method of choice.

Ascending proctography provided evidence that the colorectal intussusception valve was efficient in reflux prevention to the proximal colon in all but five patients. In four of these, antireflux was also observed to the upper tract, due to the incorporation of the ureters in the colorectal valve; surgical correction of these was carried out prior to the closure of the transverse colostomy. Revision was successful in three cases while, in the

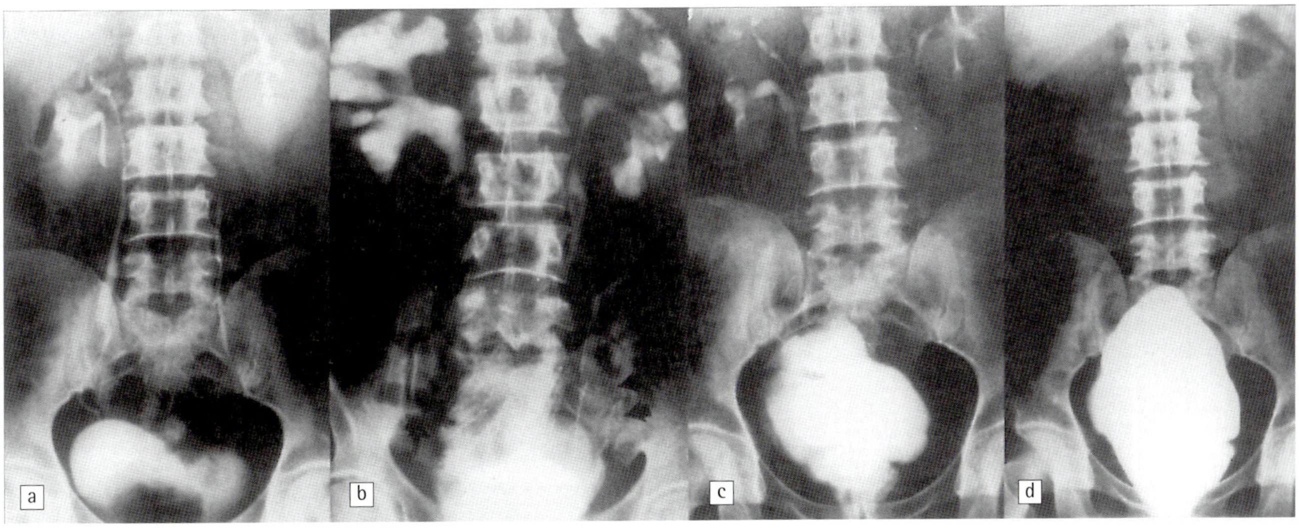

Figure 30.6 (a) Preoperative intravenous pyelogram (IVU). (b) IVU 3 months after surgery. Ureters were implanted by Goodwin's technique. (c) IVU 48 months after surgery. (d) Ascending study: no regurgitation to the colon or reflux to the ureters.

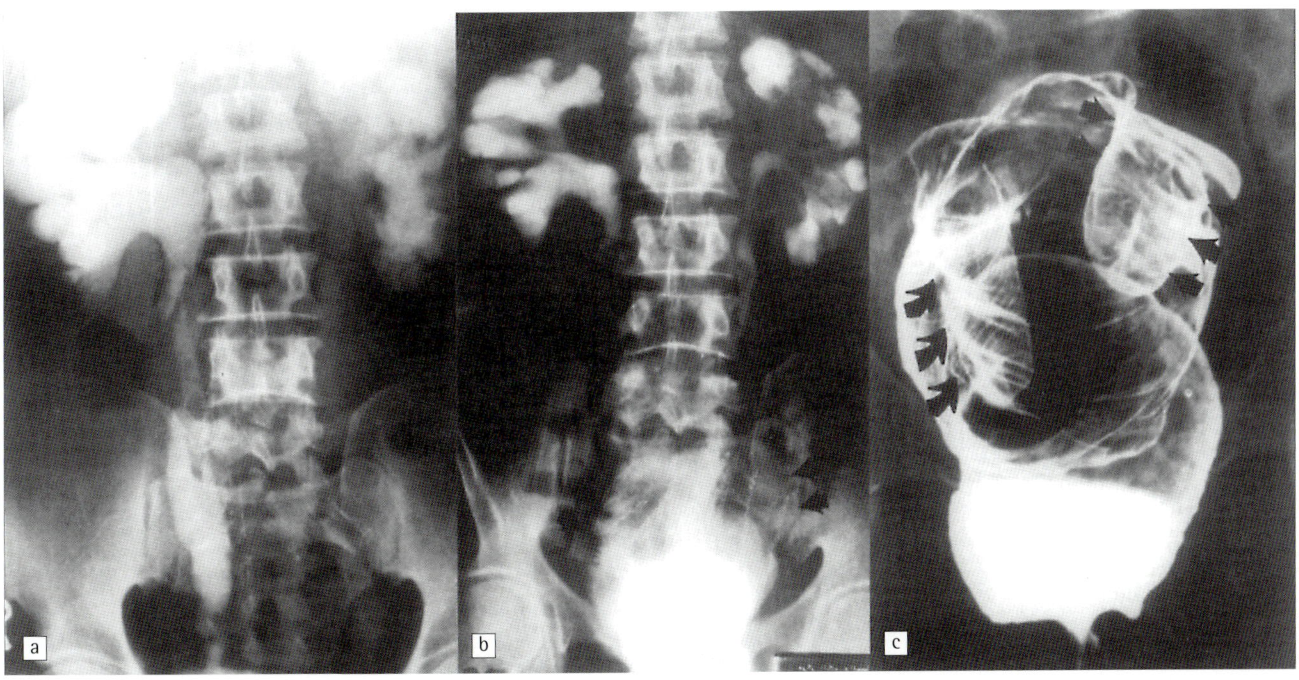

Figure 30.7 (a) Preoperative intravenous pyelogram (IVU) showing dilated ureters. (b) Postoperative IVU, showing decompression on both sides. (c) Ascending study (air and contrast). Two valves are seen: the colorectal valve on the left side and the ileal intussusception valve on the right.

fourth, the attempt was abandoned in view of detection of extensive local tumor recurrence on surgical exploration.

Filling proctometry revealed an adequate reservoir capacity ranging between 480 ml and 800 ml, 6 months postoperatively. Filling was achieved at low pressure without any segmental contractions (Figure 30.8). The pressure at maximum capacity did not exceed 30 cmH_2O. Figure 30.9 illustrates a simultaneous tracing of the subtracted intrarectal pressure during voiding as well as urine flowmetry. This study demonstrates that the driving force of voiding in this system is the function of a voluntary increase in the intra-abdominal pressure, rather than due to intrinsic contractions of the rectal musculature. Furthermore, it shows that peak flow of <20 ml/s may be achieved.

Additional studies

A study was performed in which 3 μCi of technetium-99 diluted in 300 ml saline was instilled into the rectum of a patient with ureterosigmoidostomy or with a modified rectal bladder. The solution was kept for 1 hour and then the patients were asked to evacuate their rectal contents. Scintigraphs were taken

Table 30.5 Causes of deterioration of renal function relative to method of ureteral reimplantation

	Renal units			
	Stricture	Reflux	Total	Deterioration (%)
Sigmoid valve	5	3	8/58	14
Submucous tunnel	6	2	8/87	9
Ileal valve	2	0	2/36	5
Total	13	5	18/181	

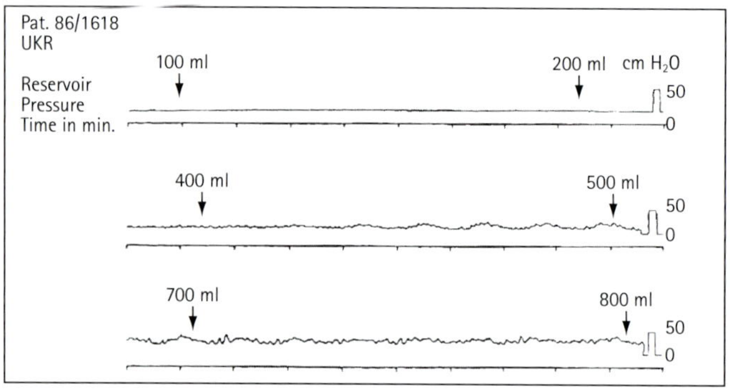

Figure 30.8 A slow fill proctometry shows a reservoir of large capacity, low pressure without segmental contractions.

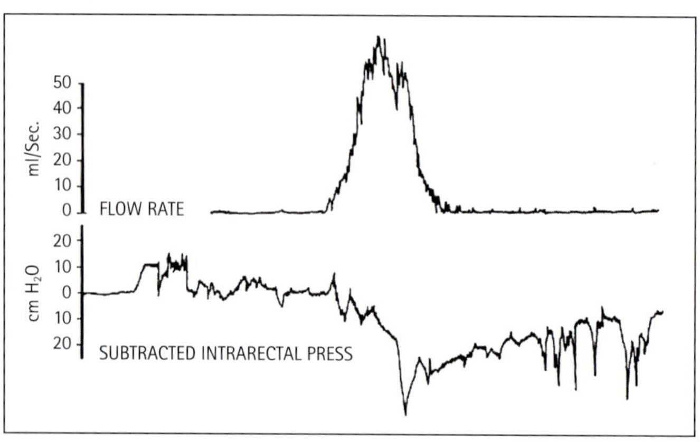

Figure 30.9 Combined uroflometry and recording of the subtracted intrarectal pressure. Flow is achieved by increasing the intra-abdominal pressure.

before and after evacuation using a γ-camera (Figure 30.10) . In patients with a modified rectal bladder, the reservoir could be emptied completely. On the other hand, in cases with a ureterosigmoidostomy, rectal contents were partly voided and partly refluxed back to fill the entire colon. Thus in such cases a large surface area of colonic mucosa is not only exposed to urine but also a longer time is allowed for contact. These two factors acting together would explain the significantly higher levels of absorption following ureterosigmoidostomy and underline the central importance of the anorectal valve.[46]

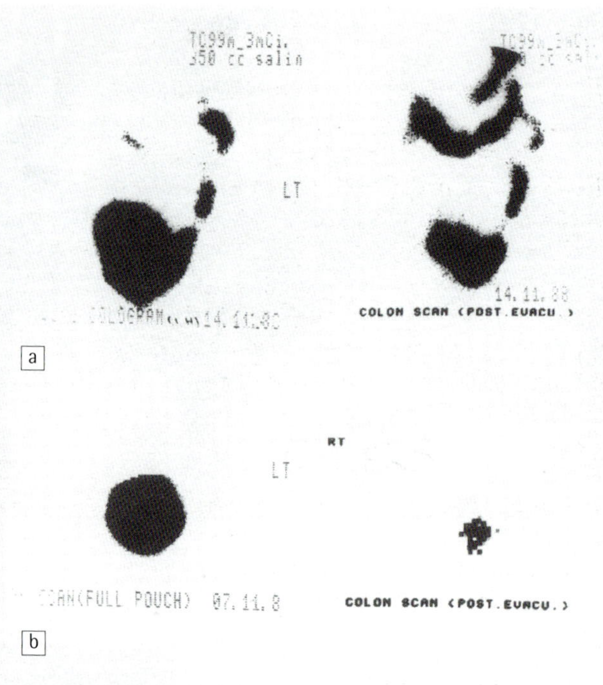

Figure 30.10 (a) Ascending scintigraphy and postvoiding pictures of a case of ureterosigmoidostomy. (b) Ascending scintigraphy and postvoiding pictures of a case of modified rectal bladder.

Summary

The modified rectal bladder seems to provide several significant improvements over the simple rectal bladder on the one hand and ureterosigmoidostomy on the other. There is no need for a terminal colostomy. Regurgitation of the rectal contents into the proximal colon is prevented by an efficient colorectal intussusception valve. Furthermore, the urodynamic qualities of the rectal bladder are improved by patching with ileum. Its volume capacity and compliance are increased. Filling is achieved at a low pressure without segmental contractions, which explains continence during the day and night, observations and potential merits also reported by Skinner et al in 1989[47] and Miller et al in 1990.[48]

Two questions remain unanswered: (i) What will be the incidence of pyelonephritis?, and (ii) How much will renal function be affected in the long run? We know that the reported incidence of pyelonephritis after ureterosigmoidostomy in which an antireflux procedure has been employed is of the order of 30%.[5–8] However, it could be postulated that the projected incidence of pyelonephritis following the modified rectal bladder could be significantly reduced as we are dealing with a very low pressure system.

What will be the incidence of tumors in this system where the stools and urine are mixed? It may also be argued that in view of the experimental observations of Grissey et al.[13] some protection is offered by the temporary transverse colostomy. The suture line is allowed to heal without exposure to the fecal stream.

Variations on the theme

Modification and refinement aimed at simplifying of this procedure have been proposed by several investigators. Sundin and coworkers[49] introduced the valved S-shaped rectosigmoid pouch. Instead of patching the rectal bladder with ileum they folded the rectosigmoid region, incised its antimesenteric border and joined the adjacent flaps. This would increase the volume capacity without a need for using an additional segment of ileum. The creation of an intussusception valve at the rectosigmoid junction was eliminated by Baron et al[50] due to its complexity. They suggestd that any metabolic consequence can be easily avoided by oral bicarbonate.

Fisch et al in 1993 created a low-pressure rectal reservoir by single folding of the rectosigmoid colon. The ureters were reimplanted using Goodwin submucosal tunnel for reflux prevention.[51] El-Mekresh et al double folded the rectosigmoid colon to improve its urodynamic characteristics. The ureters were reimplanted using the serous-lined extramural tunnel principle as an antireflux technique (Figure 30.11).[52] They reported their results in 64 patients. All patients were continent by day and night with reasonable frequency of emptying, but four children had noctunral enuresis. The upper urinary tract was maintained or improved in 95% of the patients. Within the observation period no clinical evidence of acidosis was observed, since all patients were kept on prophylactic oral alkalinization.

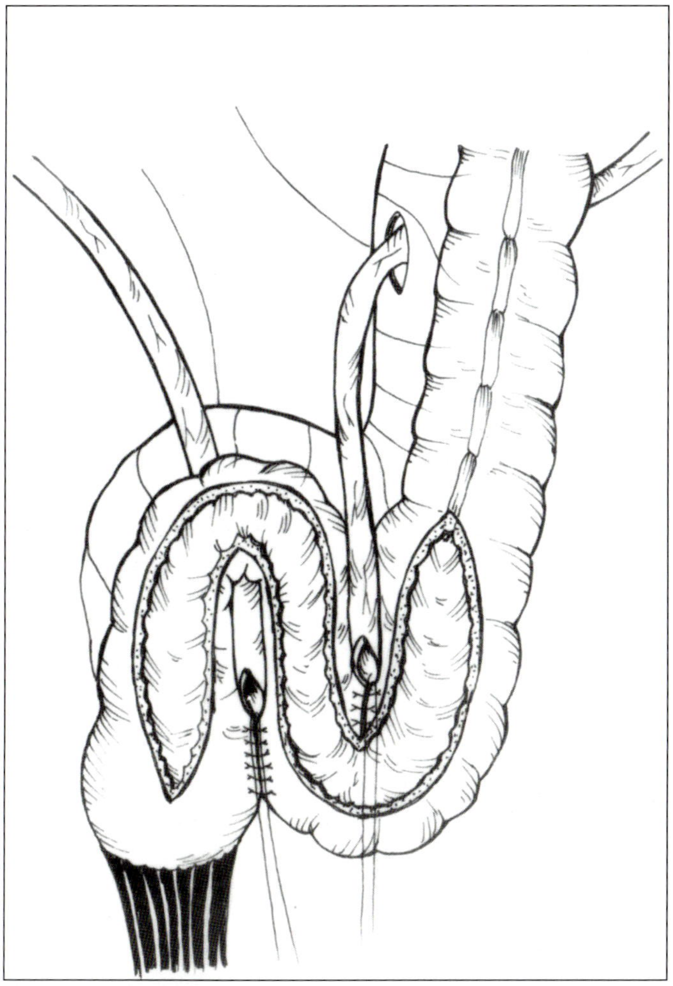

Figure 30.11 The rectosigmoid is folded into an S-shaped configuration and incised at its antimesentric border. The ureters are implanted in serous-lined tunnels created between the adjacent colonic flaps.

The functional significance of creating a colorectal valve was studied by Shoma et al.[53] Eighty-seven patients were included in a retrospective study that compared 42 patients with a modified rectal bladder with 45 with a double-folded rectosigmoid pouch without an intussucepted valve. They reported that 69% of patients with a sigmoid valve had an acid–base profile within normal compared with only 12.6% of those without a valve.

Long-term follow-up of the outcome of rectal reservoirs was studied by Hafez et al in 33 children.[54] The mean follow-up was 66 months (range 24–148). All patients were continent by day and night. The upper tract improved or stabilized in 64 of 66 renal units. No patients had reflux to the upper urinary tract. Hyperchloremia was noted in 57% of patients. Arterial blood gases showed subclinical metabolic acidosis in 55%. Supine height measurements at last follow-up revealed that 19 of the 33 patients (57%) had decreased linear growth. All patients had significant reduction in bone density. The mean bone density corrected for age was 70%.[54]

The augmented valved rectum and double s-folded rectosigmoid bladder provide preservation of the upper urinary tract with excellent continence rates. Nevertheless, the rectal reservoir is becoming less popular. This trend is due to the increasing use of orthotopic reservoirs in men and women, successful construction of continent cutaneous urinary reservoirs and emphasis on primary reconstructive surgery and/or undiversion in children.

Acknowledgement

This work has been realized in collaboration with Professor Nils G Kock from Göteborg, Sweden. His efforts were always stimulating and his thoughts inspiring.

References

1. Simon J. Ectopia vesicae; Operation for directing the orifices of the ureters in the rectum, success, subsequent death, autopsy. Lancet, 1852; ii: 568–70.
2. Hinman F, Weyrauch HM. A critical study of the different principles of surgery which have been used in uretero-intestinal implantation. Trans Am Assoc Genitourin Sur 1936; 29: 15–156.
3. Jacobs A, Stirling WB. The late results of ureterocolic anastomosis. Br J Urol 1952; 24: 259–90.
4. Clarke BG and Leadbetter WF. Ureterosigmoidostomy: Collective review of results in 2897 reported cases. J Urol 1955; 73: 999–1008.

5. Mathisen W. Clinical and experimental studies on ureterocolic anastomosis. Universitetsforlaget Tryk, Ningssentral, Oslo, 1969.
6. Williams DF, Burkhoider GV, Goodwin WE. Uretero-sigmoidostomy, a 15 years experience. J Urol 1969; 101: 168–70.
7. Wear JB, Barquin OP. Ureterosigmoidostomy, Long term results. Urology 1973; 1: 192–200.
8. Zincke H, Segura JW. Ureterosigmoidostomy: Critical review of 173 cases. J Urol 1975; 113: 324–7.
9. Stamey TA. The pathogenesis and implications of the electrolyte imbalance in ureterosigmoidostomy. Surg Gynecol Obstet 1956; 103: 736–58.
10. Irvine WT, Allan C, Webster DR. Prevention of late complications of ureterosigmoidostomy by methods of foecal exclusion. Br J Surg 1956; 43: 650–8.
11. Leadbetter GW Jr, Zickerman P, Pierce E. Uretero-sigmoidostomy and carcinoma of the colon. J Urol 1964; 92: 37–41.
12. Husman DA and Spence HM. Current status of tumour of the bowel following ureterosigmoidostomy: a review. J Urol 1990; 144: 607–10.
13. Crissey MM, Steele GD and Gittes RF. Rat model for carcinogenesis in ureterosigmoidostomy. Science 1980; 207: 1079–80.
14. Stewart M, Hill MJ, Pugh RCB, Williams P. The role of N-nitrosamine in carcinogenesis at the ureterocolic anastomosis. Br J Urol 1981; 53: 115–18.
15. Stribling MD, Cohen MS, Fagan JD et al. The effect of ascorbic acid on urinary nitrosamines and tumour developement in a rat animal model for ureterosigmoidostomy. J Urol 1989; 141: 304 A.
16. Shands C III, McDougal WS, Wright EP. Prevention of cancer at the urothelial enteric anastomotic site. J Urol 1989; 141: 178–81.
17. Mauclaire P. De quelques essais de Chirurgie experimental applicables au traitment de L'extrophie de la vessie et des anus contre nature. Complexes. Ann Mol Org 1895; 13: 1080–1.
18. Remedi V. Un caso diestrofia della vescica. La clinica Chirmgica. 1906; 14: 608–40.
19. Creevy CD, Reiser MP. Observations upon the absorption of urinary constituents after ureterosigmoidostomy. The importance of renal damage. Surg Gynecol Obstet 1952; 95: 589–96.
20. Boyce WH, Vest SA. A new concept concerning treatment of extrophy of the bladder. J Urol 1952; 67: 503–17.
21. Paul DP, Hodges CV. The rectosigmoid colon as a bladder substitute. J Urol 1955; 74: 360–7.
22. Hanely HG. The rectal bladder. Br J Urol 1967; 39: 693–8.
23. Pyrah LN. The recto-sigmoid bladder as a method of urinary diversion. J Urol 1963; 90: 189–92.
24. Ghoneim MA. The rectosigmoid bladder for urinary diversion. Br J Urol 1970; 42: 429–33.
25. Ghoneim MA, Ashamallah A. Further experience with the rectosigmoid bladder. Br J Urol 1974; 46: 511–19.
26. Ghoneim MA, Shehab El-Din AB, Ashamallah A, Gaballah MA. Evolution of the rectal bladder as a method for urinary diversion. J Urol 1981; 126: 737–40.
27. Gersuny R. Cited by Foges. Officielles Protokll der KK Gesellschaft der aerzte in Wien. Wien Klin Wochenschr 1898; 11: 990.
28. Heitz-Boyer M, Hovelacque A. Creation d'une nouvelle vessie et d'une nouvel uretre. J d'Urol 1912; 1: 237–58.
29. Lowsely OS, Johnson TH, Rueda AE. A new operation for diversion of the urine with voluntary control of feces and urine. J Int Coll Surg 1953; 20: 457–64.
30. Stonington OG, Eiseman B. Perineal sigmoidostomy in cases of total cystectomy. J Urol 1956; 76: 74–82.
31. Hinman F Jr. The technique of the gersuny operation (uretero-sigmoidostomy with perineal colostomy) in vesical extrophy. J Urol 1959; 81: 126–9.
32. Ghoneim MA, Shoukry I. The rectal bladder with perineal colostomy for urinary diversion. Urology 1974; 4: 511–19.
33. Borelius J. Eine neue modifikation der Maydl'schen operations methode bei angeborener blasenektopie, Zentralbl F Chir 1903; 30: 780–2.
34. Descomps P. Abouchement ureteral dans le rectum exclu. Ureterorectostomie haute terminale apres sigmoido-rectostomie basse termino-laterale. Arch Gen de Chir 1909; 4: 892–909.
35. Modelski W. The transplantation of ureters into the partially excluded rectum. J Urol 1962; 87: 122–4.
36. Leiter E, Brendler H. A method of urinary diversion which preserves continence. J Urol 1964; 92: 37–41.
37. Chargi A, Charbonneau J, Cholette JP, Gauthier GE. A method of urinary diversion by anastomosis of the ureters into a sigmoid pouch. J Urol 1965; 94: 376–9.
38. Kamidono S, Oda Y, Hamami G, Hikosaka K, Katoaka V, Ishigami J. Urinary diversion: anastomosis of the ureters into a sigmoid pouch and end to side sigmoido-rectostomy. J Urol 1985; 133: 391–4.
39. Knox AJS, Jago RH. The value of intestinal valves in urinary diversion: an experimental study. Br J Urol 1975; 47: 391–7.
40. Kock NG, Berglund B, Ghoneim MA et al. Urinary diversion to the augmented and valved rectum. An experimental study in dogs. Scand J Urol Nephrol 1988; 22: 227–33.
41. Miller K, Hautmann R. The functional rectal-bladder. An experimental study in dogs on continent urinary diversion. J Urol 1988; 139: 312 A.
42. Miller K, Hautmann R. Urodynamic evaluation of the functional rectal-bladder. An experimental study. J Urol 1989; 141: 351 A.
43. Miller K, Matsui U, Hautmann R. The functional rectal bladder-prevention of hyperchloremic acidosis following vesico-sigmoidostomy in dogs. J Urol 1990; 144: 375–80.
44. Kock NG, Ghoneim MA, Lycke KG, Mahran MR. Urinary diversion to the augmented and valved rectum. Preliminary results with a novelle surgical procedure. J Urol 1988; 140: 1375–9.
45. Goodwin WE, Harris AP, Kauffman JJ, Beal JM. Open transcolonic uretero-intestinal anastomosis, a new approach. Surg Gynecol Obstet 1953; 97: 295–300.
46. El-Mekresh MM, Shehab El-Din AB, Fayed SM et al. Bladder substitute controlled by the anal sphincter: a comparison of the different absorption potentials. J Urol 1991; 146: 970–2.
47. Skinner DG, Lieskovsky G, Boyd S. Continent urinary diversion. J Urol 1989; 141: 1323–7.
48. Miller K, Matsui M, Hautmann R. The augmented functional rectal bladder. First clinical experience. J Urol 1990; 143: 398 A.
49. Sundin T, Rafiq S, Norlen BJ, Ahlgren G. Current procedures for bladder substitution and urinary diversion at King Faisal Special-

ist Hospital and Research Centre. Ann Saudi Med 1991; 11: 276–83.
50. Baron JC, Arhan P, Boccon-Gibod L, Boccon-Gibod L. Ureterorectal diversion with rectal augmentation. Morphological and manometric study in the dog. Urol Res 1992; 20: 247–51.
51. Fisch M, Wammack R, Muller SC, Hohenfellner R. The Mainz pouch 11 (Sima Rectum Pouch). J Urol 1993; 149: 258–63.
52. El-Mekresh MM, Hafez AT, Abol-Enein H, Ghoneim MA. Double folded rectosigmoid bladder with a new ureterocolic antireflux technique. J Urol 1997; 157: 2082–9.
53. Shoma AM, Ashamallah A, Ghoneim MA. Rectosigmoid urinary diversion: the functional significance of creating an intussuscepted colorectal valve. J Urol 1999; 161: 415–17.
54. Hafez AT, El-Shirbiny MT, Dawaba MS, Abol-Enein H, Ghoneim MA. Long term outcome analysis of low pressure rectal reservoirs in 33 children with bladder exstrophy. J Urol 2001; 156: 2414–17.

31 Is reflux prevention important in urinary diversion?

Michael L Guralnick

Introduction

Since the very first urinary diversion performed by Simon in 1852,[1] an issue that has been a matter of significant debate is the need for reflux prevention. In this chapter, we shall discuss the arguments for and against reflux prevention in urinary diversion by reviewing the evidence regarding the possible adverse effects of reflux as well as the results of experimental and clinical studies that have looked at the issue of the need for reflux prevention in urinary diversion. We shall briefly review the different types of ureterointestinal anastomoses with respect to reflux prevention and the complications thereof, and the clinical results of different urinary diversions that have and have not incorporated reflux prevention.

Historical aspects

The first form of urinary diversion was a ureterosigmoidostomy to divert the urine into an intact sigmoid colon.[1] No attempt was made to prevent reflux and it was soon realized that this form of diversion was associated with significant complications including recurrent pyelonephritis and sepsis, ureteral obstruction, secondary malignancy, electrolyte imbalances, renal deterioration and death.[2–4] This led to modifications in ureterointestinal anastomoses to incorporate an antireflux mechanism, which did result in a reduction of these complications.[2,5] In the 1950s Bricker[6] introduced the ileal conduit with refluxing ureterointestinal anastomoses and this revolutionized urinary diversion with its simplicity such that it became the diversion of choice. The complications seen with ureterosigmoidostomies did seem to be lessened with ileal conduits but on long-term follow-up, still occurred, possibly related to the adverse effects of reflux of infected urine.[7] This led to the use of colon as a conduit with the incorporation of antirefluxing ureterointestinal anastomoses, but as will be discussed, the long-term results of these are not much different from those of ileal conduits. In the past 20 years, continent urinary diversion has become popular either in the form of a catheterizable reservoir or an orthotopic neobladder, and it initially incorporated antirefluxing ureterointestinal anastomoses. However, more recently the need for reflux prevention with these types of diversion has come into question thus continuing the debate.

Effects of reflux

Ureteral reflux, or the retrograde flow of urine through the ureters, is not a normal finding in the urinary tract. It is more common in children and often associated with urinary tract infections (UTIs). It is also associated with renal parenchymal scarring such that the extent of renal scarring correlates with the severity of reflux.[8,9] Reflux nephropathy is the term used to describe the pathologic changes seen in kidneys with chronic pyelonephritis secondary to reflux. On intravenous urograms these changes typically include thinning of the renal cortex associated with dilated calyces, particularly at the polar regions. In animal models it appears to be related to the presence of intrarenal reflux which seems to occur predominantly in the polar regions of the kidneys secondary to the morphology of the renal papillae.[10] There is evidence that scar formation in these kidneys occurs after the first significant infection and this usually occurs in infancy.[11] The development of new scars is generally a rare event, possibly because the surviving renal parenchyma has non-refluxing papillae and thus is not exposed to intrarenal reflux. This fits the clinical observation in humans that most patients with reflux nephropathy have their scars when first seen and rarely develop new scars irrespective of the frequency or pattern of urinary tract infections.[9,12] It is noteworthy that vesicoureteral reflux in adults is generally well tolerated and surgical correction of reflux in the adult appears to have no beneficial effect on renal size, scarring, proteinuria or the preservation of renal function.[13–15] Furthermore, in his review of the literature, Stamey noted that in the absence of obstruction, it is very rare for infection to cause significant renal damage in adults.[16] It appears therefore, that the infant kidney is more susceptible to damage from reflux and infection than the adult kidney.

An issue that has yet to be resolved is whether sterile reflux can cause renal damage. In the animal model, it has been shown by some that infection must be present with reflux before renal damage occurs,[17] although others have found that sterile reflux can cause renal damage in the face of bladder outlet obstruction and elevated intravesical pressures.[18,19] However, generally the renal damage is seen only in infant kidneys that are still developing. When adult kidneys were exposed to sterile reflux associated with elevated intravesical pressures caused by outlet obstruction, no evidence of renal damage was identified.[20] It is also noteworthy that when adult dog kidneys were directly exposed to unobstructed bladder pressures by a sterile refluxing pyelovesicostomy, no renal damage was identified, again confirming that at least in the animal model, sterile reflux is not harmful to the adult kidney.[21] This is consistent with the clinical results of medical management of vesicoureteral reflux in children: by and large, renal function is preserved while on antibiotic prophylaxis and the development of new renal scarring is not significantly different from that which occurs following ureteroneocystostomy.[22]

The presence of reflux may actually be beneficial in certain patients. With the majority of urinary diversions being performed following surgery to remove the bladder for malignancy, one concern in the follow-up of these patients is the development of recurrent cancer in the upper urinary tract. The presence of refluxing ureterointestinal anastomoses allows for the relatively easy performance of retrograde contrast studies of the upper tracts that avoids the need for intravenous contrast administration and potentially simplifies surveillance.

Animal models

The most compelling evidence favoring the use of antireflux ureterointestinal anastomoses comes from animal experiments. Richie and Skinner created both an ileal conduit and a colon conduit in dogs and then anastomosed one ureter to the ileal conduit in a refluxing fashion and the contralateral ureter to the colon conduit in a tunneled, antireflux fashion.[23] After 3 months, they noted histologic evidence of pyelonephritis in 83% of kidneys connected to ileal conduits but only 7% of kidneys connected to colon conduits. There was no significant difference in the bacterial growth between the ileal and colon conduits nor was there any difference in the resting pressures or emptying properties of either conduit. However, the ileal conduits were noted to have more peristalsis with higher pressures, particularly when they were acutely occluded. It was concluded that the prevention of infected reflux by colon conduits resulted in less pyelonephritis, thereby making colon conduits more advantageous. In a similar vein, Kristjansson and Mansson studied whether or not reflux prevention was important in low pressure enterocystoplasties in dogs.[24] They noted significantly more bacteriuria and pyelonephritis as well as renal scarring in upper tracts that had direct, refluxing anastomoses versus those that had antireflux anastomoses. However, there was no difference in the glomerular filtration rate (GFR) of these kidneys as measured by DTPA renal scans. Based on these studies, it is reasonable to conclude that reflux prevention should be a primary consideration in urinary diversion. However, clinical studies in humans are less conclusive.

Clinical studies

Issues of assessment

To compare the results of different types of ureterointestinal anastomotic techniques, one must consider the methods of assessment. The endpoints generally reported are the preservation of renal function, radiographic appearance of the upper tracts (i.e. presence of hydronephrosis, renal scarring), presence or absence of ureteral reflux, development of UTI/pyelonephritis and ureteral obstruction. Unfortunately, most studies on urinary diversion are retrospective, often lacking adequate means to compare pre- and postoperative results and furthermore, often only relying on blood chemistries (e.g. serum creatinine) and urographic imaging to make all of these assessments. The sensitivity of serum creatinine for detecting early renal impairment is low owing to ongoing renal tubular secretion.[25] As well, while urography provides a gross anatomic picture of the upper tracts and a crude estimate of renal function based on the excretion of contrast, the presence of ureteral dilatation on urographic imaging is neither sensitive nor specific for ureteral obstruction.[25] On the other hand, nuclear renography is very useful in determining information on total and separate GFR, effective renal plasma flow, upper tract dilation with or without obstruction and the presence of renal scarring, but most studies on urinary diversion do not incorporate nuclear renal scans.[25] The determination of ureteral reflux may also be fraught with inaccuracies that may be related to technical factors including the volume and pressure within the diversion as well as the presence of a diuresis.[25,26] It is noteworthy that several studies using direct, refluxing ureterointestinal anastomoses had low incidences of demonstrable reflux postoperatively,[27–29] a finding that has also been noted in experiments using a canine model.[24,30] Furthermore, the significance of reflux demonstrated on loopography has been questioned because the technique of loopography results in non-physiologic conditions. When a more physiologic method of reflux assessment was performed using a radioisotope technique, Woodside et al found that only approximately half of ureterointestinal anastomoses in ileal conduits that had reflux on standard loopgraphy actually refluxed.[31] With respect to ureterointestinal anastomotic complications, the definition of a stricture is variable, and often only so-called obstructions that either required surgery or resulted in renal loss are included.[25] Furthermore, it has been repeatedly reported that the timing of investigation of ureterointestinal anastomotic obstructions is important: upper tract dilation (often thought to result from obstruction secondary to edema) is not uncommon in the first year following a urinary diversion but may be associated with a significant spontaneous resolution rate.[32–34] In addition, the left ureter, which is usually tunneled under the bowel mesentery to the right side for anastomosis, is at risk for obstruction, often related to excessive mobilization and adventitial thinning and/or kinking under the inferior mesenteric artery.[7,35] Most reports on the complications of ureterointestinal anastomoses fail to distinguish between the side of the obstruction and the exact location in the ureter, which may result in erroneously attributing a negative outcome to the type of anastomosis performed. Furthermore, in many studies reporting complications of urinary diversion, there is no differentiation between upper tract deterioration secondary to obstruction versus that secondary to reflux (they are grouped together) and therefore it is difficult to ascertain which of the two is actually responsible for the renal deterioration.[36] Lastly, when trying to compare outcomes between different studies, one must be cognizant of differences between patient populations with respect to age, underlying pathologies, use of radiation and duration of follow-up.[37]

Ureterointestinal anastomoses

A variety of techniques for ureterointestinal anastomosis exist and that no single type of anastomosis is universally used emphasizes the fact that we have yet to identify the ideal type of anastomosis. The ideal ureterointestinal anastomosis is one that is easy to construct, has a low rate of anastomotic leakage and stenosis, and prevents reflux. Anastomotic leakage may be minimized by the use of soft, silicone stents and stenosis can be minimized by careful handling of the ureters, avoiding excessive thinning of the ureteral adventitia, with enough mobilization to minimize tension on the anastomosis.[7] The different types of anastomoses are discussed elsewhere in this book and will be reviewed briefly herein.

Refluxing ureterointestinal anastomoses are performed by directly anastomosing the ureters to the intestine either singly as described by Nesbit[38] and Bricker[6] or conjoined as described by Wallace.[39] They are the simplest anastomoses to perform with no attempt being made to prevent reflux. The direct Nesbit/Bricker anastomosis has a reported stricture rate of 4–22% with an average of 7%, while the Wallace conjoined technique appears to have the lowest rate of anastomotic obstruction of approximately 3%.[7] However, the Wallace anastomosis may theoretically put both kidneys at risk when a complication such as recurrent tumor or stone affects one ureter.

The purpose of antireflux anastomoses is the prevention of reflux of urine and its potential adverse effects on the kidneys as discussed earlier. In general, they usually accomplish the goal of preventing reflux with most studies reporting rates of reflux using an antirefluxing ureterointestinal anastomosis of less than 5–10%. However, the benefits of reflux prevention may be outweighed by complications associated with the technique of antireflux anastomosis, especially stenosis. Antireflux ureterointestinal anastomoses generally involve either modifications in the way the ureter is anastomosed to the intestinal reservoir or incorporate a modification of the intestine itself. The oldest form of antireflux anastomosis is based on the flap valve principle elucidated by Coffey in 1911.[40] By exposing the distal ureter to the internal pressures of the urinary reservoir, a flap valve is created such that as the pressure within the urinary diversion increases (such as by filling with urine), there is compression and occlusion of the distal ureter thus preventing reflux. This can be accomplished by tunneling the ureter submucosally,[2,5] a task that is much easier to perform when using colon as opposed to ileum, or, as described by Le Duc et al, by placing the distal ureter in a mucosal trough in the intestinal wall, leaving its anterior surface exposed, to be ultimately covered by intestinal mucosa with time.[41] The literature on submucosal tunneling suggests it is an effective method for reflux prevention but is associated with anastomotic stenosis in up to 15% of patients.[28,42–44] One of the concerns about the Le Duc mucosal trough technique is the fact that one surface of the distal ureteral adventitia is exposed to urine until the intestinal mucosa ultimately covers it. It is thought that this may result in scarring of the ureter with resultant stenosis, a fact that might explain the up to 31% incidence of stricturing with this type of anastomosis.[45–47] However, others have reported excellent results with this technique and stricture rates of less than 5%.[32,35,41] While one would like to blame surgical technique and experience for the poor outcomes that have been associated with the Le Duc technique, Roth et al found that the higher risk of stenosis associated with a Le Duc anastomosis (20% vs. 3.6% with a direct, refluxing anastomosis) was independent of surgeon experience.[46]

Another way to accomplish the effect of distal ureteral compression by intrareservoir pressures is by creating a ureteral nipple valve. The distal ureter is everted (split-cuff nipple) and then implanted into the intestine such that the everted ureteral end is exposed to intrareservoir pressures.[48] This technique does appear to be effective for reflux prevention and has a low stenosis rate, at least in the short term.[48,49]

Reflux may also be prevented by making modifications to the intestine itself. In these anastomoses, the ureters are implanted into the intestine in a direct, refluxing fashion, and then the intestine is manipulated to prevent reflux. One method is the intussuscepted intestinal nipple valve in which a segment of ileum (to which the ureters are directly anastomosed) is intussuscepted into the urinary reservoir (held in place by metallic staples) thus forming a nipple valve.[50] This is the mechanism of reflux prevention in catheterizable Kock pouches and orthotopic hemi-Kock neobladders. Alternatively, one can take advantage of the peristaltic properties of the ileum for reflux prevention. The use of an isoperistaltic limb of ileum as a dynamic valve is based in part on experiments by Hinman and Oppenheimer who demonstrated that a long length of ileum (≥18 cm) was able to prevent reflux of urine when interposed between bladder and skin as an ileocystostomy in dogs.[51] However, shorter segments of ileum were not able to do so and thus there appears to be a minimum length of ileum required for effective reflux prevention. This has been confirmed in animal experiments as well as clinical studies of ileal ureteral replacements.[52,53] As such, the Studer neobladder incorporates a 20-cm isoperistaltic limb of non-detubularized ileum into which the ureters are directly implanted in a refluxing fashion.[54]

Criticism of intussuscepted intestinal nipple valves includes their complexity and complications, including afferent nipple stones related to exposed metallic staples (5%), nipple stenosis (4%), and nipple prolapse (1%) requiring reoperation in about 10% of patients.[55] On the other hand, the advantages of an isoperistaltic afferent limb include its simplicity and low stenosis rate (3%), since direct, refluxing ureterointestinal anastomoses are performed. Studer et al compared antireflux nipples (either split-cuff ureteral nipples or intussuscepted ileal nipple valves) to an afferent isoperstaltic ileal limb in patients with an ileal neobladder and found a 13% versus 3% anastomotic stricture rate, respectively.[56] They also performed reservoir videourodynamics combined with simultaneous renal pelvic pressure monitoring and noted that with standard filling, reflux was not identified in either group during abdominal straining, coughing or voiding (a finding noted by others[57]) and similar pressure spikes were recorded simultaneously in the neobladder, rectum and renal pelvis. However, in both groups, when the neobladder was overfilled, elevated pressures were noted (with pressures spikes up to 80 cmH_2O) that were transmitted to the renal pelvis. With the afferent isoperistaltic limb, this occurred with visible reflux but in patients with a nipple valve, the pressure transmission was noted in the absence of visible reflux. In these patients the elevated intrareservoir pressure resulted in compression (as would be expected) of the nipple valve and resultant obstruction to upper tract drainage, and this combined with ongoing diuresis resulted in elevated renal pelvic pressures. It was argued, however, that because these elevated pressures were seen only experimentally in an unphysiologic fashion, their significance on a day-to-day basis is minimal.

Yet another technique for reflux prevention involving a modification to the intestine is the serous-lined extramural tunnel.[58] This is a flap valve mechanism in which an intestinal reservoir is fashioned such that serous-lined tunnels are created into which the ureters are placed and direct ureter–intestine anastomoses are performed. Midterm results with this technique show a low rate of reflux (3%) and stenosis (3.8%) with upper tract preservation in 96%.[59]

Results in conduit diversions

In the 1950s, Bricker introduced the ileal conduit with refluxing ureterointestinal anastomoses[6] and soon after this became the diversion of choice as it was easy to perform and the severe complications seen after ureterosigmoidostomy were reduced. However, with long-term follow-up, a significant number of patients have been shown to have renal damage. Pitts and Muecke followed patients for up to 20 years after ileal conduit diversion and noted that 11% of all kidneys showed some damage postoperatively including 14% of adult kidneys and 9% of pediatric kidneys.[60] They noted two important facts with respect to renal damage: (i) previously damaged kidneys were at greater risk for further damage postoperatively and (ii) with increasing follow-up intervals there was a greater proportion of kidneys damaged such that at 16–20-year follow-up, 35% of all preoperatively normal kidneys showed evidence of damage. Noteworthy is the fact that 45% of the kidneys that sustained renal damage had evidence of ureteral obstruction. Only 24% of kidneys had deterioration without obstruction and all were noted to have damage preoperatively or had a history of calculi. Madersbacher et al recently reported their long-term follow-up of 131 patients with ileal conduit diversion.[61] They noted renal deterioration in 27% of patients overall and similarly noted that after prolonged follow-up (greater than 10–15 years) there was a greater risk for renal deterioration (50% of patients surviving greater than 15 years). Ureterointestinal anastomotic obstruction was reported in 10% and stomal complications in 24% of patients but unfortunately no information is given on how many patients with renal deterioration had anastomotic or stomal complications. This long-term deterioration in the function and radiographic appearance of the upper tracts following ileal conduit diversion has been reported by others.[62,63] However, it is unclear whether this is actually due to the presence of reflux per se or other factors. What is clear is that the presence of ureteral obstruction (either at the ureterointestinal anastomosis or more proximal) can definitely harm the kidneys.

Some studies have suggested that obstruction or dysfunction in the conduit itself (e.g. stomal stenosis) may play an important role in upper tract dilatation and deterioration.[64,65] It has been shown that the non-obstructed ileal conduit with refluxing ureterointestinal anastomoses but without dilated upper tracts, has low resting and emptying pressures whereas conduits with dilated upper tracts and clinical evidence of conduit outlet obstruction have higher resting pressures and empty with large peristaltic contractions.[66,67] Furthermore, when presumed obstructed conduits were revised, 53% of patients had a reduction in their conduit pressures and improvement in the radiologic appearance of their upper tracts.[67] This suggests that it is the obstruction to conduit outflow with resultant elevated intraconduit pressure and urinary stasis that causes upper tract deterioration, rather then ureteral reflux per se.[66,67] This is consistent with the fact that despite the presence of refluxing ureterointestinal anastomoses, many studies report upper tract stability in the majority of patients if there is no anastomotic or conduit obstruction.[60,68,69] On the other hand, the presence of conduit obstruction as well as ureteral reflux presents a very high risk for upper tract deterioration.[67,70] It is noteworthy that despite the lack of deliberate reflux prevention, Waldner et al, in a prospective study of renal function following ileal ureteral replacement as well as their review of the literature on ileal ureters, reported upper tract preservation in the majority of patients despite the documented presence of reflux to the kidneys in some.[53] They and others have noted generally that only in the presence of a neurogenic bladder or bladder outlet obstruction, both associated with elevated storage pressures, did upper tract deterioration occur.[53]

In an effort to better preserve renal function, the use of colon as a conduit became increasingly popular because it allowed for easier non-refluxing ureterointestinal anastomoses by tunneling the ureters submucosally.[71] While some studies did show improved renal preservation,[72,73] this was not reported by others. Elder et al, after a mean follow-up of 13 years, noted renal deterioration in approximately 50% of their patients with preoperatively normal kidneys and in 87% of patients with preoperatively abnormal kidneys following colon conduit diversion.[74] Twenty-two percent of renal units developed ureterointestinal strictures (a relatively high number) and reflux was noted in 58% despite antireflux anastomoses (combined nipple valve and submucosal tunnel). They did note that significantly more renal units not having reflux remained normal in follow-up compared to those renal units that did have reflux (73% vs. 21%) suggesting that the renal damage was possibly caused by the presence of reflux. However, they do not indicate how many of the patients with demonstrable reflux and renal deterioration also had evidence of conduit obstruction/dysfunction. It is noteworthy that 61.5% of their patients did require surgical correction of stomal stenosis. It is a reasonable hypothesis, therefore, that perhaps the reason that such a large proportion of patients did experience reflux and renal deterioration was related to the presence of conduit obstruction with resultant elevated conduit pressures which overcame the antirefluxing nature of the ureterointestinal anastomoses. Husmann et al similarly found an association between conduit obstruction and reflux.[36] They did tunneled ureterocolonic anastomoses and noted an 8% rate of postoperative reflux. However, 50% of these were in association with obvious stomal stenosis.

The ideal way to determine if antirefluxing ureterointestinal anastomoses are better than refluxing anastomoses in conduit diversion would be in a randomized study. This was done by Kristjansson et al who randomized patients into the type of conduit diversion (ileal or colon) and type of ureterointestinal anastomosis.[37] They performed both direct, refluxing anastomoses, as well as antirefluxing anastomoses using a split-cuff nipple technique in ileal conduits, and a submucosal tunnel technique in colon conduits. Thus patients had an antireflux anastomosis on one side and a direct anastomosis on the other side. They also compared their results to a group of patients undergoing continent diversion using a non-detubularized, catheterizable colon reservoir, all of whom had antirefluxing anastomoses using a submucosal tunnel technique (some were combined with a split-cuff nipple). Renal function was assessed using plasma clearance of ethylenediaminetetra-acetic acid (EDTA) as well as nuclear renal scans with a mean follow-up of 123 months. They found that while there was a moderate reduction in mean total GFR in all types of diversion that was larger than what would be expected with age-related decline, there were no significant intergroup differences. Furthermore, there was no significant difference in the decrease in mean separate GFR between refluxing and antirefluxing anastomoses in the two conduit groups. Unfortunately, they did not do imaging studies postoperatively to determine if reflux was present or absent, but these results do suggest that a deliberate effort to prevent reflux by performing antirefluxing anastomoses did not make any difference with respect to renal function in the long term, irrespective of the type of conduit performed. Patients with continent catheterizable colonic reservoirs and antirefluxing anastomoses had similar results. Interestingly, these were non-detubularized reservoirs which theoretically could achieve high pressures (although reservoir dynamics were not measured). Whether the similar results in the colonic reservoir group are because of the use of antirefluxing anastomoses is unknown because there was no control group with refluxing anastomoses and a colonic reservoir. Fifteen ureterointestinal anastomotic strictures developed in 12 patients (3/38 patients with an ileal conduit, 4/30 patients with a colonic conduit, and 5/26 patients with a colon reservoir). Ten of the 15 strictures involved the ureter that was tunneled beneath the sigmoid mesentery. There were 10 strictures occurring in patients with a conduit, of which 6 were on the antireflux side while 4 were on the refluxing side. In the second part of their study, the authors specifically addressed the issue of bacteriuria and renal scarring.[75] They noted evidence of more upper tract bacteriuria and renal scarring in renal units with direct ureterointestinal anastomoses to conduits compared to those with antireflux anastomoses (4/5 with direct anastomosis had the same organism grow in the renal pelvis as in the conduit vs. 1/4 with antireflux anastomosis; and 65% with direct anastomosis had renal scarring vs. 33% with antireflux anastomosis). However, 64% of renal units connected to a non-detubularized colonic reservoir in an antirefluxing fashion also had evidence of renal scarring, a proportion that is similar to the results in conduits with direct anastomoses. Since the presence of postoperative reflux was never determined, it still unclear if the actual prevention of reflux is what led to the difference in upper tract bacteriuria and renal scarring, although the suggestion was made that it did. However, the authors did identify that the presence of ureterointestinal obstruction was a definite risk factor for pyelonephritis and renal scarring. Others have found that antireflux anastomosis does not necessarily prevent bacterial colonization of the upper urinary tract. Gonzalez and Reinberg noted positive renal pelvic cultures by percutaneous aspiration in 6/8 patients with non-refluxing enterocystoplasties and one patient with a non-refluxing colon conduit.[76] Consistent with this is the fact that McDougal's review of the complications of conduit diversion noted a similar incidence of pyelonephritis in refluxing ileal and antirefluxing colon conduits (12% and 13%, respectively).[7]

It has become apparent that conduit diversion, while having improved upon the complications seen with ureterosigmoidostomy, is not without its own problems. In the long term, many patients do appear to sustain radiographic and functional deterioration of their upper tracts and the etiology appears to be multifactorial. While there is no question that obstruction to urine drainage either at the ureteral or conduit level is detrimental, what is still unclear is if the presence of ureteral reflux on its own is similarly harmful, and if the deliberate prevention of reflux is necessary. What is clear, however, is that long-term follow-up of patients with conduit diversions is necessary.

Results in continent diversions

The current trend in urinary diversion is that of continent diversion with an intestinal reservoir that is either drained by a continent catheterizable abdominal stoma or that is directly connected to the urethra. Reservoirs are fashioned using ileum, colon or both in a detubularized manner that serves to keep the intrareservoir pressures low. Whether or not an antireflux ureterointestinal anastomosis is necessary in these types of diversions is controversial.

Catheterizable reservoirs

In catheterizable intestinal reservoirs it is generally assumed that the urine in the reservoir is infected because the patient does not perform sterile catheterization and studies do confirm this.[77] The use of antirefluxing anastomoses has therefore been recommended.[78] In general, the literature on continent catheterizable reservoirs suggests preservation of renal function that is at least comparable to if not better than that of conduit diversions and usually antireflux anastomoses have been performed.[43] The issue is whether or not these are necessary. Recent reports have documented preservation of renal function in continent catheterizable diversions that have used simple, direct ureterointestinal anastomoses. Helal et al, frustrated by a significant rate of ureterointestinal obstruction after antireflux anastomosis (13.5%) in right colon pouches, began using direct anastomoses and saw a reduction in their rate of obstruction to 4.9%.[28] Interestingly, only 7% of these were found to reflux postoperatively compared with 3.3% of their antireflux anastomoses, and with a mean follow-up of 25 months, there was no renal deterioration on urography or renal scintigraphy. Hohenfellner et al had a similar experience with direct ureterointestinal anastomoses into catheterizable reservoirs.[29] They noted renal function to be preserved with no episodes of pyelonephritis and a low incidence of demonstrable reflux (5%) in patients with primary (median follow-up of 20 months) or secondary (median follow-up of 81 months) ureterointestinal anastomoses. It is clear that both of these reports are limited by short follow-up. As has been shown with conduit diversion, 15–20 years of follow-up is necessary to determine the true long-term effects of a diversion. However, they do legitimately question the need for antirefluxing anastomoses in low-pressure catheterizable reservoirs. It is interesting that despite direct ureterointestinal anastomoses, only 5–7% were shown to have reflux postoperatively. The authors hypothesize that there may be some inherent mechanism in the anastomosis itself, either by the backing created by the colonic wall or smooth kinking of the ureter as it traverses the colonic wall, that acts to prevent reflux.[28,29] This raises the question that perhaps the reason renal function was so well preserved is because reflux was unintentionally prevented by these anastomoses. Alternatively, these units may in fact have reflux that was simply missed due to technical reasons.

Orthotopic neobladders

Continent urinary diversion to an intestinal bladder substitute (orthotopic neobladder) is becoming increasingly popular and because these are generally low-pressure reservoirs, the need for antirefluxing ureterointestinal anastomoses has come into question. Some argue that because bacteriuria can be seen in up to 24% of patients,[79] and because voiding pressures can exceed 100 cmH_2O,[80] the prevention of reflux is crucial and every effort should be made to perform an antirefluxing anastomosis.[59] Others, however, believe that a deliberate antirefluxing anastomosis is not necessary, particularly if a Studer-type of neobladder is performed with an isoperistaltic afferent limb.[56] Using this technique, only 3% of patients develop ureterointestinal strictures and the upper tracts do appear to be well preserved.[34] However, the argument that reflux prevention is unnecessary in Studer-type neobladders because of their inherent low pressures cannot be made because in general, if a 20-cm isoperistaltic afferent limb is used, there is no demonstrable reflux to the kidneys as the isoperistaltic afferent limb is in fact a reflux prevention mechanism.[57] To say that antirefluxing anastomoses are not necessary in neobladders would require the ureters to be directly implanted into the neobladder proper, which has not been reported.

Conclusions

The literature is unclear about the need for antireflux ureterointestinal anastomoses in urinary diversion. While animal models do suggest that the prevention of reflux is important with respect to the development of pyelonephritis and renal scarring, clinical studies are far from conclusive. Issues related to the method of assessment and duration of follow-up continue to plague us and the lack of randomized prospective studies precludes definitive conclusions. It appears that conduit diversion has numerous problems in the long term regardless of the type of ureterointestinal anastomoses performed and it is difficult to separate the untoward effects of reflux, infection and obstruction in the reported studies. Conduit dysfunction and obstruction to conduit outflow can result in high-pressure storage and poor drainage which is detrimental to the upper tracts but whether antireflux ureterointestinal anastomoses can prevent these effects is still unknown. What can be concluded is that regardless of anastomotic type, careful long-term follow-up of patients is necessary.

As for continent urinary diversion using low-pressure reservoirs, there similarly is no conclusive evidence that antirefluxing are better than refluxing anastomoses. There is the suggestion that antirefluxing anastomoses are unnecessary because of the low-pressure nature of these reservoirs, and short- and medium-term follow-up studies do seem to confirm the lack of ill effects on the upper tracts in these diversions. Yet one cannot help to wonder whether in fact it is the lack of reflux that is contributing to these good results since the majority of patients in the studies that looked at the use of direct anastomoses in continent catheterizable reservoirs in fact did not have any demonstrable reflux. Similarly, patients with the Studer type of ileal neobladder with its afferent isoperistaltic limb generally do not have reflux despite direct refluxing ureterointestinal anastomoses. One could thus make the argument that perhaps it is truly the absence of reflux (whether deliberate or not) that is resulting in the preservation of the upper tracts.

Lastly, it does appear that deliberate attempts to perform antirefluxing anastomoses are associated, on average, with somewhat higher rates of anastomotic obstruction than simple, direct anastomoses and this risk must be considered when determining the necessity for antirefluxing anastomoses since there is no question as to the detrimental effects of ureterointestinal anastomotic obstruction. Until a randomized study using both truly refluxing and antirefluxing anastomoses in a standardized fashion with appropriate outcome assessment and long-term follow-up is performed, we will never have a definitive answer as to need for reflux prevention in urinary diversion.

References

1. Simon J. Ectopia vesicae; operation for directing the orifices of the ureters into the rectum; temporary success, autopsy. Lancet 1852; ii: 568.
2. Clarke BG, Leadbetter WF. Ureterosigmoidostomy: Collective review of results in 2897 reported cases. J Urol 1955; 73: 999–1008.
3. Williams DF, Burkholder GV, Goodwin WE. Ureterosigmoidostomy: a 15-year experience. J Urol 1969; 101: 168–70.
4. Wear JB Jr, Barquin OP. Ureterosigmoidostomy. Long-term results. Urology 1973; 1: 192–200.
5. Goodwin WE, Harris AP, Kaufman JJ, Beal JM. Open transcolonic ureterointestinal anastomosis: A new approach. Surg Gynecol Obstet 1953; 97: 295–300.
6. Bricker EM. Bladder substitution after pelvic evisceration. Surg Clin North Am 1950; 30: 1511–21.
7. McDougal WS. Use of intestinal segments and urinary diversion. In: Walsh PC, Retik AB, Vaughan ED, Wein AJ (eds). Campbell's Urology, 8th edn. Philadelphia: WB Saunders, 2002: 3745–88.
8. Winter AL, Hardy BE, Alton DJ et al. Acquired renal scars in children. J Urol 1983; 129: 1190–4.
9. Malek RS, Svensson JP, Torres VE. Vesicoureteral reflux in the adult. I. Factors in pathogenesis. J Urol 1983; 130: 37–40.
10. Ransley PG, Risdon RA. Renal papillary morphology and intrarenal reflux in the young pig. Urol Res 1975; 3: 105–9.
11. Ransley PG, Risdon RA. Reflux nephropathy: Effects of antimicrobial therapy on the evolution of the early pyelonephritic scar. Kidney Int 1981; 20: 733–42.
12. Edwards D, Normand ICS, Prescod N, Smellie JM. Disappearance of vesicoureteric reflux during long-term prophylaxis of urinary tract infection in children. BMJ 1977; 2: 285–8.
13. Malek RS, Svensson J, Neves RJ et al. Vesicoureteral reflux in the adult. III. Surgical correction: risks and benefits. J Urol 1983; 130: 882–6.
14. Guthman DA, Malek RS, Neves RJ et al. Vesicoureteral reflux in the adult. V. Unilateral disease. J Urol 1991; 146: 21–3.
15. Stefanovic KB, Bukurov NS, Marinkovic JM. Non-antireflux versus antireflux ureteroneocystostomy in adults. Br J Urol 1991; 67: 263–6.
16. Stamey TA. Pathogenesis and Treatment of Urinary Tract Infections. Baltimore: Williams & Wilkins, 1980: 122–209.
17. Ransley PG, Risdon RA. Reflux and renal scarring. Br J Radiol 1978; Suppl 14: 1–35.
18. Hodson CJ, Maling TMJ, Mcmanamon PJ, Lewis MG. The pathogenesis of reflux nephropathy. (Chronic atrophic pyelonephritis). Br J Radiol 1975; Suppl 13: 1–26.
19. Mendoza JM, Roberts JA. Effects of sterile high pressure vesicoureteral reflux on the monkey. J Urol 1983; 130: 602–6.
20. Roberts JA, Fischman NH, Thomas R. Vesicoureteral reflux in the primate IV: does reflux harm the kidney? J Urol 1982; 128: 650–2.
21. Danforth DN, Javadpour N, Bergman SM, Terrill R. Pressure effects of urinary reflux studies with renal autotransplantation and pyelocystostomy. Urology 1980; 25: 17–22.
22. Olbing H, Hirche H, Koskimies O et al. Renal growth in children with severe vesicoureteral reflux: 10-year prospective study of medical and surgical treatment: the International Reflux Study in Children (European branch). Radiology 2000; 216: 731–7.
23. Richie JP, Skinner DG. Urinary diversion: the physiological rationale for non-refluxing colonic conduits. Br J Urol 1975; 47: 269–75.
24. Kristjansson A, Abol-Enein H, Alm P et al. Long-term renal morphology and function following enterocystoplasty (refluxing or anti-reflux anastomosis): an experimental study. Br J Urol 1996; 78: 840–6.
25. Kristjansson A, Mansson W. Refluxing or nonrefluxing ureteric anastomosis. Br J Urol 1999; 76: 539–45.
26. Ekman H, Jacobsson B, Kock NG, Sundin T. High diuresis, a factor in preventing vesicoureteral reflux. J Urol 1966; 95: 511–15.
27. Mansson W, Colleen S, Forsberg L et al. Renal function after urinary diversion. A study of continent cecal reservoir, ileal conduit and colonic. Scand J Urol Nephrol 1984; 18: 307–15.

28. Helal M, Pow-Sang J, Sanford E, Figueroa E, Lockhart J. Direct (nontunneled) ureterocolonic reimplantation in association with continent reservoirs. J Urol 1993; 150: 835–7.
29. Hohenfellner R, Black P, Leissner J, Allhoff EP. Refluxing urteroointestinal anastomosis for continent cutaneous urinary diversion. J Urol 2002; 168: 1013–17.
30. St Clair SR, Hixson CJ, Ritchey ML. Enterocystoplasty and reflux nephropathy in the canine model. J Urol 1992; 148: 728–32.
31. Woodside JR, Borden TA, Dambon JR, Kiker JD. Isotope loopography, a new test: comparison with standard loopography and its relationship to renal function in patients with ileal conduit urinary diversion. J Urol 1978; 119: 31–4.
32. Lugagne PM, Herve JM, Lebret T et al. Ureteroileal implantation in orthotopic neobladder with the Le Duc–Camey mucosal-trough technique: risk of stenosis and long-term followup. J Urol 1997; 158: 765–7.
33. Chen K, Chang LS, Chen M, Yeh S. Prospective radionuclide renal function evaluation and its correlation with radiological findings in patients with Kock pouch urinary diversion. J Urol 1991; 145: 952–5.
34. Thoeny HC, Sonnenschein MJ, Madersbacher S, Vock P, Studer UE. Is ileal orthotopic bladder substitution with an afferent tubular segment detrimental to the upper urinary tract in the long term? J Urol 2002; 168: 2030–4.
35. Schwaibold H, Friedrich MG, Fernandez S, Conrad S, Huland H. Improvement of ureteroileal anastomosis in continent urinary diversion with modified Le Duc procedure. J Urol 1998; 160: 718–20.
36. Husmann DA, McLorie GA, Churchill BM. Non-refluxing colonic conduits: a long-term life-table analysis. J Urol 1989; 142: 1201–3.
37. Kristjansson A, Wallin L, Mansson W. Renal function up to 16 years after conduit (refluxing or anti-reflux anastomosis) or continent urinary diversion. 1. Glomerular filtration rate and patency of uretero-intestinal anastomosis. Br J Urol 1995; 76: 539–45.
38. Nesbit RM. Ureterosigmoid anastomosis by direct elliptical connection: a preliminary report. J Urol 1949; 61: 728–34.
39. Wallace DM. Uretero-ileostomy. Br J Urol 1970; 42: 529–34.
40. Coffey RC. Physiologic implantation of the severed ureter or common bile-duct into the intestine. JAMA 1911; 56: 397–403.
41. Le Duc A, Camey M, Teillac P. An original antireflux ureteroileal implantation technique: long-term follow-up. J Urol 1987; 137: 1156–8.
42. Kristjansson A, Engellau L, Willner J, Mansson W. Reflux, stricture and glomerular filtration rate after two antireflux techniques in continent urinary reconstruction using the right colon. Scand J Urol Nephrol 1997; 31: 425–9.
43. Rowland RG. Complications of continent cutaneous reservoirs and neobladders – series using contemporary techniques. AUA Update Series 1995; 14: 202–7.
44. Stein R, Fisch M, Beetz R et al. Urinary diversion in children and young adults using the Mainz pouch 1 technique. Br J Urol 1997; 79: 354–61.
45. Pantuck AJ, Han K, Perrotti M, Weiss RE, Cummings KB. Ureterointestinal implantation in continent urinary diversion: long term results and complications of refluxing versus non-refluxing techniques. J Urol 1999; 163: 450–5.
46. Roth S, van Ahlen H, Semjonow A, Oberpenning F, Hertle L. Does the success of ureterointestinal implantation in orthotopic bladder substitution depend more on surgeon level of experience or choice of technique? J Urol 1997; 157: 56–60.
47. Shaaban AA, Gaballah MA, El-Daisty TA, Ghoniem MA. Urethral controlled bladder substitution: a comparison between the intussuscepted nipple valve and the technique of Le Duc as antireflux procedures. J Urol 1992; 148: 1156–61.
48. Stone AR, MacDermott JPA. The split-cuff ureteral nipple reimplantation technique: reliable reflux prevention from bowel segments. J Urol 1989; 142: 707–9.
49. Sagalowsky AI. Further experience with split-cuff nipple ureteral reimplantation in urinary diversion. J Urol 1998; 159: 1843–4.
50. Kock NG, Nilson AE, Nilsson LO, Norlen LJ, Philipson BM. Urinary diversion via a continent ileal reservoir: clinical results in 12 patients. J Urol 1982; 128: 469–75.
51. Hinman Jr F, Oppenheimer R. Functional characteristics of the ileal segment as a valve. J Urol 1958; 80: 448–54.
52. Sarramon JP, Conte J, Bouisson SH. Ureteroileoplasty. Urologic and renal consequences. Experimental study in 13 dogs. J Urol Nephrol (Paris) 1971; 77: 579–93.
53. Waldner M, Hertle L, Roth S. Ileal ureteral substitution in reconstructive urological surgery: is an antireflux procedure necessary? J Urol 1999; 162: 323–6.
54. Studer UE, Danuser H, Merz VW, Springer JP, Zingg EJ. Experience in 100 patients with an ileal low pressure bladder substitute combined with an afferent tubular isoperistaltic segment. J Urol 1995; 154: 49–56.
55. Stein JP, Freeman JA, Esrig D et al. Complications of the afferent antireflux valve mechanism in the Kock ileal reservoir. J Urol 1996; 155: 1579–84.
56. Studer UE, Danuser H, Thalmann GN, Springer JP, Turner WH. Antireflux nipples or afferent tubular segments in 70 patients with ileal low pressure bladder substitutes: long-term results of a prospective randomized trial. J Urol 1996; 156: 1913–17.
57. Waidelich R, Rink F, Kriegmair M, Tatsch K, Schmeller N. A study of reflux in patients with an ileal orthotopic bladder. Br J Urol 1998; 81: 241–6.
58. Abol-Enein H, Ghoniem MA. A novel uretero-ileal reimplantation technique: the serous lined extramural tunnel. A preliminary report. J Urol 1994; 151: 1193–7.
59. Abol-Enein H, Ghoniem MA. Functional results of orthotopic ileal neobladder with serous-lined extramural ureteral reimplantation: experience with 450 patients. J Urol 2001; 165: 1427–32.
60. Pitts WR, Muecke EC. A 20-year experience with ileal conduits: the fate of the kidneys. J Urol 1979; 122: 154–7.
61. Madersbacher S, Schmidt J, Eberle JM et al. Long-term outcome of ileal conduit diversion. J Urol 2003; 169: 985–90.
62. Pernet FP, Jonas U. Ileal conduit urinary diversion: early and late results of 132 cases in a 25-year period. World J Urol 1985; 3: 140–4.
63. Orr JD, Shand JEG, Watters DAK, Kirkland IS. Ileal conduit urinary diversion in children. An assessment of long-term results. Br J Urol 1981; 53: 424–7.

64. Stern JM, Khan AU, Cass AS. Reversible upper tract dilatation with ileal conduit stomal ulceration or encrustation. Urology 1979; 13: 621–3.
65. Knapp PM. Konnak JW, McGuire EJ, Savastano JA. Urodynamic evaluation of ileal conduit function. J Urol 1987; 137: 929–32.
66. Neal DE, Hawkins T, Gallaugher AS, Essenhigh DM, Hall RR. The role of the ileal conduit in the development of upper tract dilatation. Br J Urol 1985; 57: 520–4.
67. Neal DE. Urodynamic investigation of the ileal conduit: upper tract dilatation and the effects of revision of the conduit. J Urol 1989; 142: 97–100.
68. Dunn M, Roberts JBM, Smith PJB, Slade N. The long-term results of ileal conduit urinary diversion in children. Br J Urol 1979; 51: 458–61.
69. Cass AS, Luxenberg M, Gleich P, Johnson CF. A 22-year followup of ileal conduits in children with a neurogenic bladder. J Urol 1984; 132: 529–31.
70. Magnus RV. Pressure studies and dynamics of ileal conduits in children. J Urol 1977; 118: 406–7.
71. Turner-Warwick RT. Colonic urinary conduits. Proc R Soc Med 1960; 53: 56–8.
72. Altwein JE, Jonas U, Hohenfellner R. Long-term follow-up of children with colon conduit urinary diversion and ureterosigmoidostomy. J Urol 1977; 118: 832–6.
73. Starr A, Rose DH, Copper JF. Antireflux ureteroileal anastomoses in humans. J Urol 1975; 113: 170–4.
74. Elder DD, Moisey CU, Rees RW. A long-term follow-up of the colonic conduit operation in children. Br J Urol 1979; 51: 462–5.
75. Kristjansson A, Bajc M, Wallin L, Willner J, Mansson W. Renal function up to 16 years after conduit (refluxing or anti-reflux anastomosis) or continent urinary diversion. 2. Renal scarring and location of bacteriuria. Br J Urol 1995; 76: 546–50.
76. Gonzalez R, Reinberg Y. Localization of bacteriuria in patients with enterocystoplasty and nonrefluxing conduits. J Urol 1987; 138: 1104–5.
77. Akerlund S, Campanello M, Kaijser B, Jonsson O. Bacteriuria in patients with a continent ileal reservoir for urinary diversion does not regularly require antibiotic treatment. Br J Urol 1994; 74: 177–81.
78. Stein JP, Skinner DG. Orthotopic urinary diversion. In: Walsh PC, Retik AB, Vaughan ED, Wein AJ (eds). Campbell's Urology. 8th edn. Philadelphia: WB Saunders, 2002: 3835–67.
79. Steven K, Poulsen AL. The orthotopic Kock ileal neobladder: functional results and urodynamic features, complications and survival in 166 men. J Urol 2000; 164: 288–95.
80. Gotoh M, Yoshikawa Y, Sahashi M et al. Urodynamic study of storage and evacuation of urine in patients with a urethral Kock pouch. J Urol 1995; 154: 1850–3.

32 Reflux prevention with intussuscepted nipple valves and tunnels

Arthur C Grabowski and Lesley K Carr

Introduction

The need for reflux prevention in adult urinary diversion is controversial. A detailed discussion of the evidence for it is presented in Chapter 31. The techniques for reflux prevention during ureteral reimplant into small bowel include the intussuscepted ileal nipple valve, the ureteric split-cuff nipple valve, the afferent tubular segment, various tunneled anastomoses and the Le Duc–Camey tunnel. Techniques for antireflux anastomosis into large bowel consist almost entirely of some type of a tunneled anastomosis. This chapter will cover the intussuscepted nipple valve and tunnel techniques for the prevention of reflux. The other techniques are outlined elsewhere in this book. Both of these have undergone significant modifications since their initial introduction and continue to be used in routine urologic practice.

General technical points

A few general principles are applicable to all ureterointestinal anastomoses. An anastomosis that opposes mucosa to mucosa for a watertight seal is essential. This is achieved by using a fine absorbable suture, preferably a 5-0. The ureters should be spatulated to create a wide anastomosis that is tension free and they need to be dissected with adequate periureteric tissue to avoid devascularization and consequent ischemic strictures. Anastomoses should be stented with soft silastic stents. Protection of the ureteric reimplant may be achieved by fixing the diversion to the retroperitoneum and by retroperitonealizing the anastomosis if possible. The path of the ureter should be free from kinks and severe angulation. Specifically, one must take care to avoid compression of the left ureter as it is tunneled under the bowel mesentery.

Tunneled anastomotic techniques

The attraction of the tunneled reimplant methods is that they are easy to perform and they mimic the natural antireflux mechanism. They have withstood the test of time and have known long-term results. The various tunneled anastomosis can be categorized based on whether they are performed intraluminally or extraluminally and whether they are performed on large or small bowel. The advantage of the extraluminal methods is the avoidance of opening of large bowel and consequent spillage of stool (i.e. ureterosigmoidostomy). However, modern reconstructive techniques almost always involve the opening, detubularization and refashioning of bowel, making this distinction less important.

Transluminal tunneled anastomosis: large bowel

The traditional transluminal ureterocolonic tunneled anastomosis was described by Goodwin in 1953.[1] The original description involves creating a 5-mm transverse incision in the mucosa and using a hemostat to create an oblique (medial to lateral) tunnel between the mucosa and muscularis for a distance of 1–1.5 cm after which the bowel muscularis and serosa are penetrated and the ureter is grasped and pulled through by a previously placed traction suture on the ureter (Figure 32.1a). Current descriptions advocate the creation of a 3–4-cm tunnel.[2] The spatulated ureteric mucosa is then anastomosed using interrupted sutures to the bowel mucosa under direct vision from the luminal side using a 5-0 absorbable suture (Figure 32.1b). Some bowel muscularis should be incorporated in the closure to firmly anchor the ureter. The ureter is also secured to the bowel seromuscular layer with interrupted stitches where it exits on the outside.

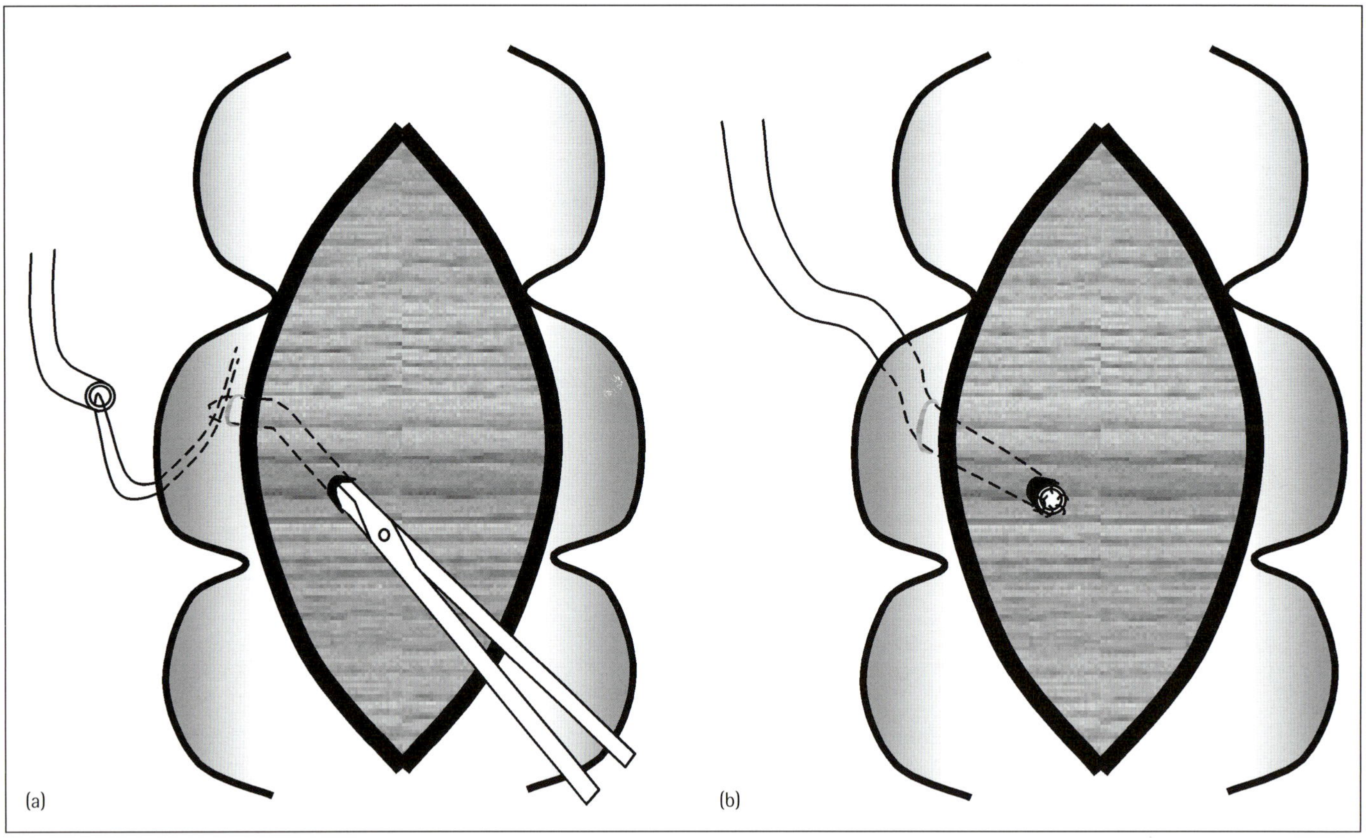

Figure 32.1 The Goodwin tunnel technique.[1] (a) The posterior wall of the colon is exposed. A curved instrument is used to tunnel underneath the mucosa of the large bowel for 1–1.5 cm and punch through the muscularis to the outside. (b) The ureter is brought into the bowel through the tunnel and anastomosed using interrupted sutures from within the bowel.

A modification of this technique involves injecting 2–3 ml of saline submucosally for 2 cm and then incising the mucosa and reflecting it from the muscularis, creating a trough for the ureter.[3] The ureter is brought in, spatulated and sutured to mucosa and muscularis of the bowel at the distal point of this trough. The reflected bowel mucosa of the trough is then closed over the ureter creating a tunnel. A small amount of periureteral tissue is incorporated in the closure to prevent tunnel shortening.

Shenfeld and Goldwasser described a further modification of the above technique which involves reflecting the mucosa from the muscularis on only the lateral aspect of the incision (Figure 32.2).[4] This avoids potential devascularization of the mucosa that lies between the two ureters if they are placed side by side.

Transluminal tunneled anastomosis: small bowel

Yang introduced a specialized needle that included a forceps to avoid incising of the bowel mucosa and allow for creation of submucosal tunnel in ileum.[5] (The Yang needle, although specialized, could be replaced by the needle passer used with the Carter–Thomason Closure system for laparoscopic port site closure.) The technique involves injecting 3–5 ml of normal saline submucosally to form a wheal. The needle is then used to pierce the mucosa at the margin of the wheal and tunnel submucosally for 1.5–2 cm before exiting through the bowel wall. The ureter is then grasped by the combined needle/forceps and brought out through the tunnel for a spatulated mucosa-to-mucosa anastomosis as previously described. Unfortunately, further reports on the success of this technique are lacking, therefore long-term results in a large number of patients are unknown.

Extraluminal tunneled anastomosis: large bowel

Leadbetter and Clarke[6] combined the direct spatulated anastomosis described by Nesbitt[7] with the tunneled anastomosis of Coffey to achieve good results with ureterocolonic implants. Their method involves incising the antimesenteric tenia for 2.5–3 cm slightly diagonally down to the colonic mucosa (Figure 32.3a). Flaps of muscle are created on either side of the mucosal trough by gently undermining the muscularis over the mucosa. The ureter is spatulated for 5–7 mm. A button of mucosa is then excised at the distal end of the trough and a mucosa-to-mucosa

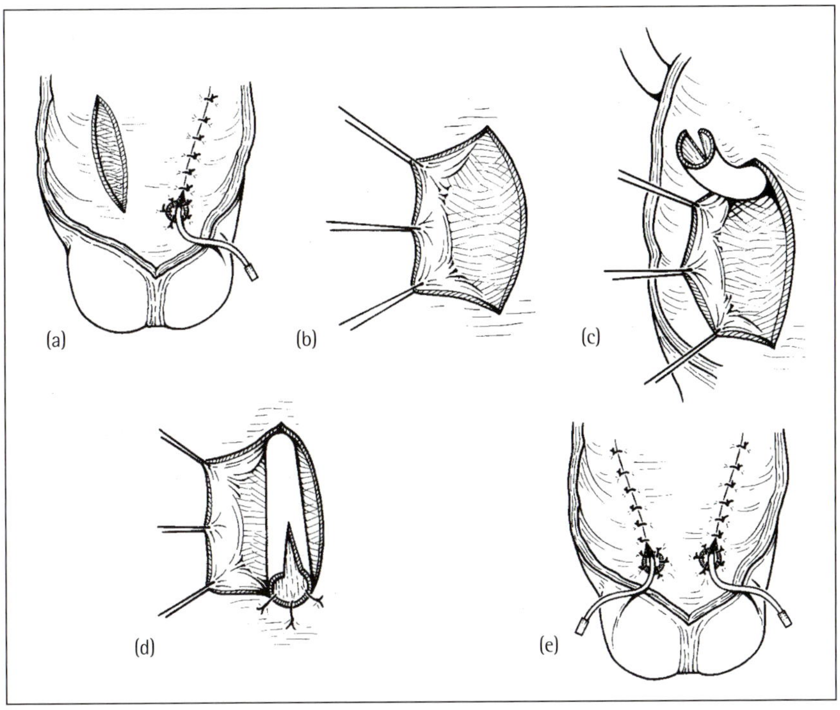

Figure 32.2 The Shenfeld and Goldwasser modification of the Goodwin tunnel.[4] (a) A 2–3-cm long trough is created in the mucosa of the posterior wall of the large bowel. (b) A mucosal flap is raised on the lateral side. (c) The ureter is brought in. (d) Three sutures are placed between the mucosa and muscularis and the spatulated end of the distal ureter. At the site of ureteral entry into bowel an anchoring suture is placed between the serosa of the ureter and the seromuscularis of the large bowel. (e) The mucosa is closed over the underlying ureter and a stent is left in place.

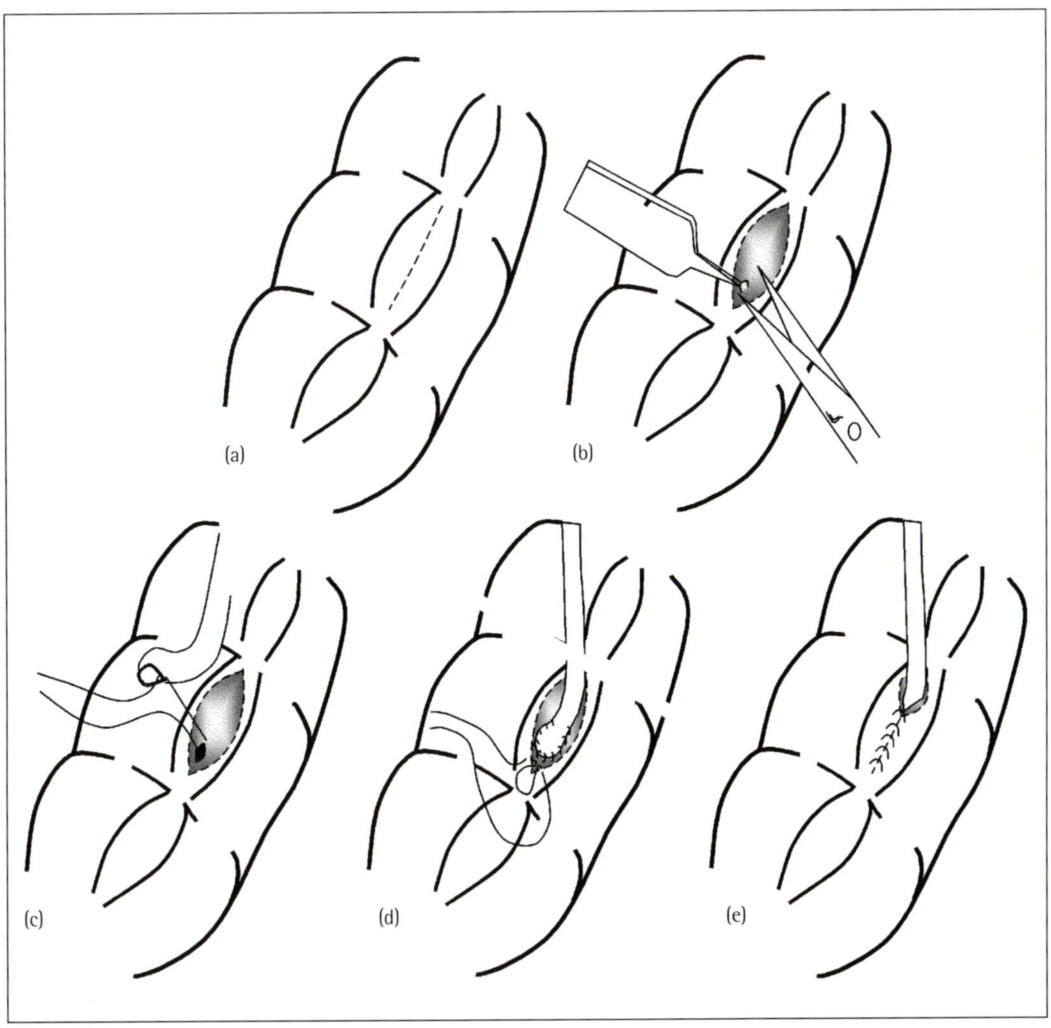

Figure 32.3 The Leadbetter and Clarke technique.[6] (a) The tenia is incised slightly obliquely and mucosa is separated from flaps of muscularis. (b) A small opening in the bowel is made. (c) Anastomosis is made between the full thickness of the ureteral wall and bowel mucosa using interrupted sutures starting at the apex of the spatulation. (d, e) A submucosal tunnel for the ureter is made by closing muscle flaps loosely over the ureter to avoid constriction.

anastomosis is made (Figure 32.3b, c). The muscularis flaps can then be loosely sutured over the ureter (Figure 32.3d, e). Care is taken to retroperitonealize the closure and to fix the bowel to the retroperitoneum to prevent future tension.

Strickler described an alternative method, which obviated the use of tenia, allowing for a less angulated, more natural course of the ureter.[8,9] Once the point of anastomosis is chosen, a 1–2 mm button of seromuscularis is excised down to intact mucosa (Figure 32.4a). Stay sutures are then placed on this seromuscular orifice and a submucosal tunnel is formed by blunt dissection with a mosquito hemostat for approximately 1.5 cm. The serosa is then penetrated, the ureter grasped and brought through the tunnel (Figure 32.4b). Care must be taken not to inadvertantly tent up the mucosa and enter it at this point. The colonic mucosa is incised at the distal orifice carefully to avoid an excessively large opening. The spatulated ureter is then anastomosed to the mucosa with interrupted 5-0 absorbable suture. The seromuscular opening is then closed perpendicular to the course of the ureter using interrupted 5-0 silk sutures (Figure 32.4c, d). The ureteric adventitial wall is secured to the proximal tunnel entrance using four quadrant sutures.

Pagano[10,11] published yet another modification of technique that is similar to Leadbetter and Clarke's, yet allows for a more natural path of the ureter. It involves infiltrating 0.5% procaine hydrochloride into the muscular layer of the anterior tenia which allows one to make a 5–6 cm midline incision in the tenia without entering the mucosa. The procaine diffusion also allows for easy dissection of the two seromuscular flaps away from the mucosa as far laterally as the lateral border of the colon (Figure 32.5). The ureters are then brought into this wide trough through separate stab incisions in the serosa at the proximal end of the trough. Two openings are then made at the

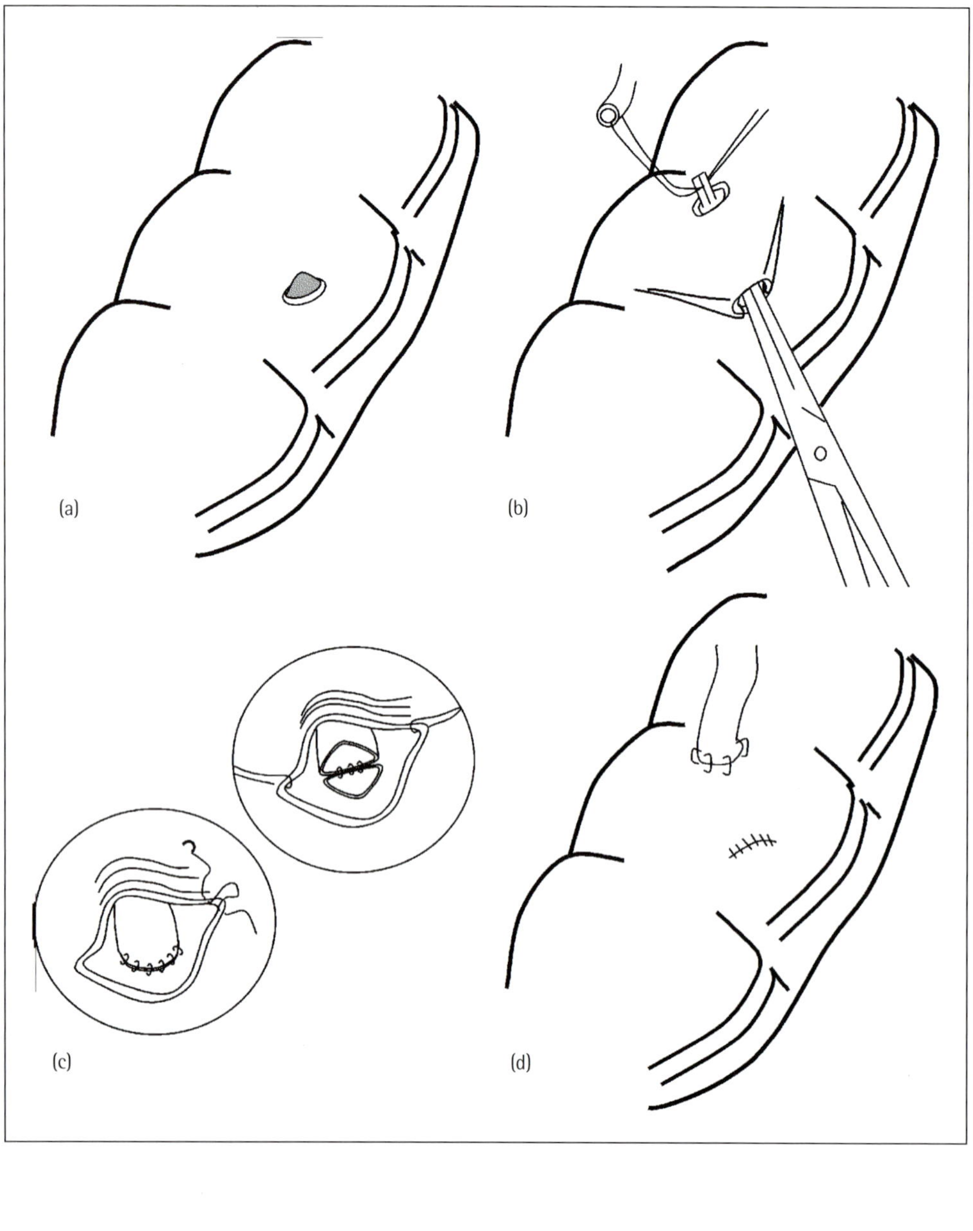

Figure 32.4 The Strickler technique.[8] (a) A button of seromuscular tissue is excised preserving intact mucosa. (b) A submucosal tunnel is created and the ureter is drawn through. (c) After incising the mucosa a mucosal anastomosis is made with interrupted fine sutures and the muscularis is closed over it. (d) Fixation sutures are placed where the ureter enters the tunnel.

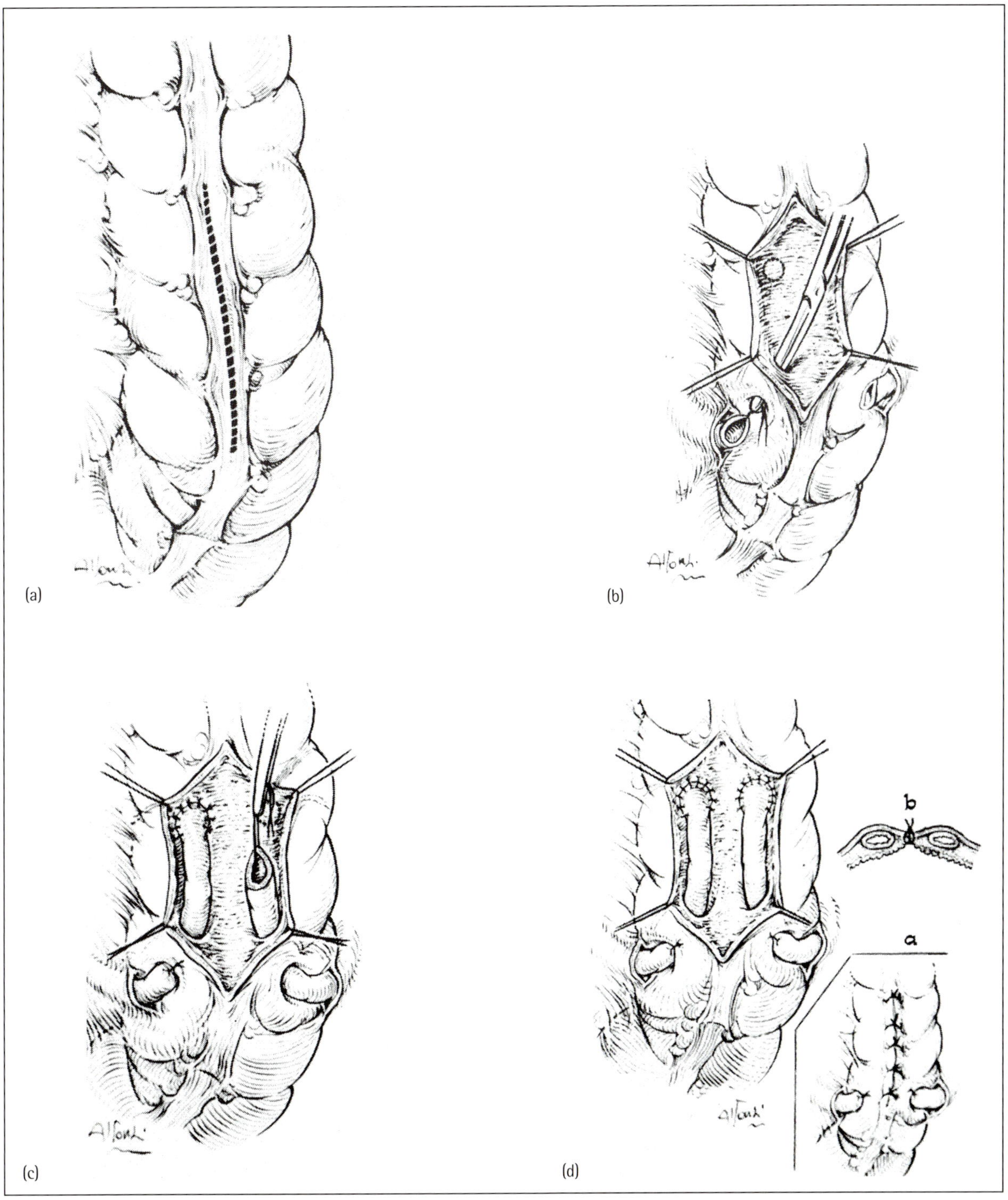

Figure 32.5 The Pagano technique. (a) After infiltration of 0.5% procaine hydrochloride into the muscularis layer of the anterior tenia a 5–6-cm midline incision is made through the seromuscular layer without entering mucosa. (b) Both edges are undermined separating mucosa from the muscularis and the ureters are brought in through a separate opening in the serosa at the proximal end of the dissected area. (c) A small opening in the mucosa is made at the distal end of the dissected area and the ureters are anastomosed as in the Leadbetter and Clarke technique. (d) The seromuscular layer is closed with interrupted sutures with each suture picking up the underlying dissected mucosa in the middle. (Reproduced from Pagano. J. Urol 1980; 123: 355–6[10] with permission from Lippincott Williams & Wilkins.)

distal end of the trough and the ureters are anastomosed as described by Leadbetter. The overlying seromuscular layer is then closed, incorporating the mucosa between the ureters in the interrupted sutures (Figure 32.5d). A stitch secures the ureteric adventitia to the bowel seromuscular layer at the proximal entry point into the bowel.

Extraluminal tunneled anastomosis: small bowel

Starr et al[12] described an extraluminal technique of ureterointestinal anastomosis that could be used on the ileum. The advantage of this method is that it can be used to anastomose ureters to ileal conduits without opening the bowel. It involves injecting normal saline with a 25-gauge needle under the serosa at the proximal end of the conduit. Then two 5-mm incisions are made approximately 2.5 cm apart (Figure 32.6). Mosquito hemostats are then used to develop the tunnel between serosa and muscularis. It is very important that the tunnel courses at right angles to the long axis of the conduit in order to avoid tearing the serosa. The ureter is then brought through the tunnel and a button of ileal muscularis and mucosa is the excised at the distal end. The spatulated ureter is then anastomosed to the bowel mucosa in the standard fashion. Since the original description there has been little use of this technique, so long-term results are unknown.

Serous-lined extramural tunnels in reservoirs

A novel approach to reflux prevention was described by Abol-Enein and Ghoneim.[13–15] They used opposing extramural serosa in the construction of a W-shaped ileal orthotopic neobladder to create a tunnel that would act as an antireflux mechanism. The advantage of this approach is that it is technically simple and does not necessitate submucosal or subserosal dissection. Furthermore, it does not require extra bowel to be used as is necessary for the intussuscepted valves. The neobladder is fashioned from 40 cm of distal ileum which is reconfigured into a 'W'. The two upper lateral limbs are joined to the central limb with seromuscular continuous 3-0 silk suture (Figure 32.7a). The antimesenteric border of the bowel is then opened in a fashion to leave a narrow strip of serosa on either side of this suture line as a trough for the ureters (Figure 32.7b). The two lower limbs of the 'W' are then closed using running through-and-through absorbable suture. The ureters are then placed into the previously created troughs and a spatulated anastomosis is made to the bowel mucosa present at the apex of each trough. The ureters are then covered by approximating the two edges of the bowel on either side of the trough with interrupted 4-0 polyglactin suture converting it into an extramural serous-lined tunnel. The anterior wall of the pouch is then closed. The suture line in the most dependent portion of the pouch is re-opened for 2 cm to perform the urethral anastomosis. This opening in the suture line is reinforced on either side with two interrupted sutures.

el-Mekresh et al reported using the same technique to anastomose ureters to an S-shaped rectosigmoid bladder.[16] The ureters were brought in between the three limbs of the 'S' and anastomosed in a manner similar to the W-pouch. It must be noted, however, that the results were not as good as with the W-pouch – 5% of the 57 patients evaluated developed strictures at the ureterosigmoid anastomosis and two patients developed signs of clinical pyelonephritis. De Filippo et al adapted the same technique to create a non-refluxing ileal bladder aug-

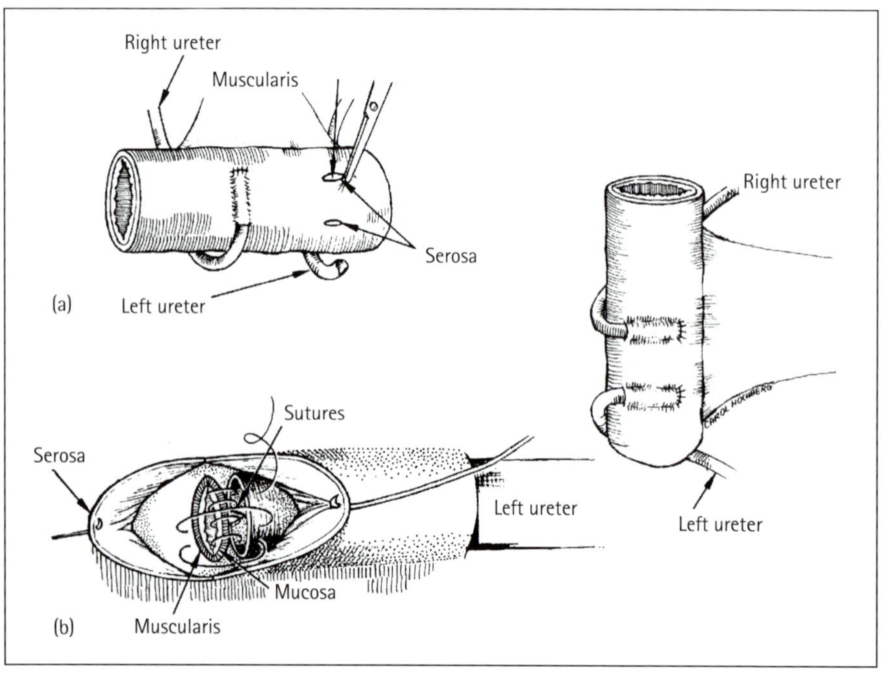

Figure 32.6 The Starr extraluminal small bowel tunnel technique. (a) Placement of initial serosal incisions and creation of the subserosal tunnel between serosa and muscularis. (b) Anastomosis of ureter to muscularis and mucosa. (Reproduced from Starr et al. J Urol 1975; 113: 170–4[12] with permission from Lippincott Williams & Wilkins.)

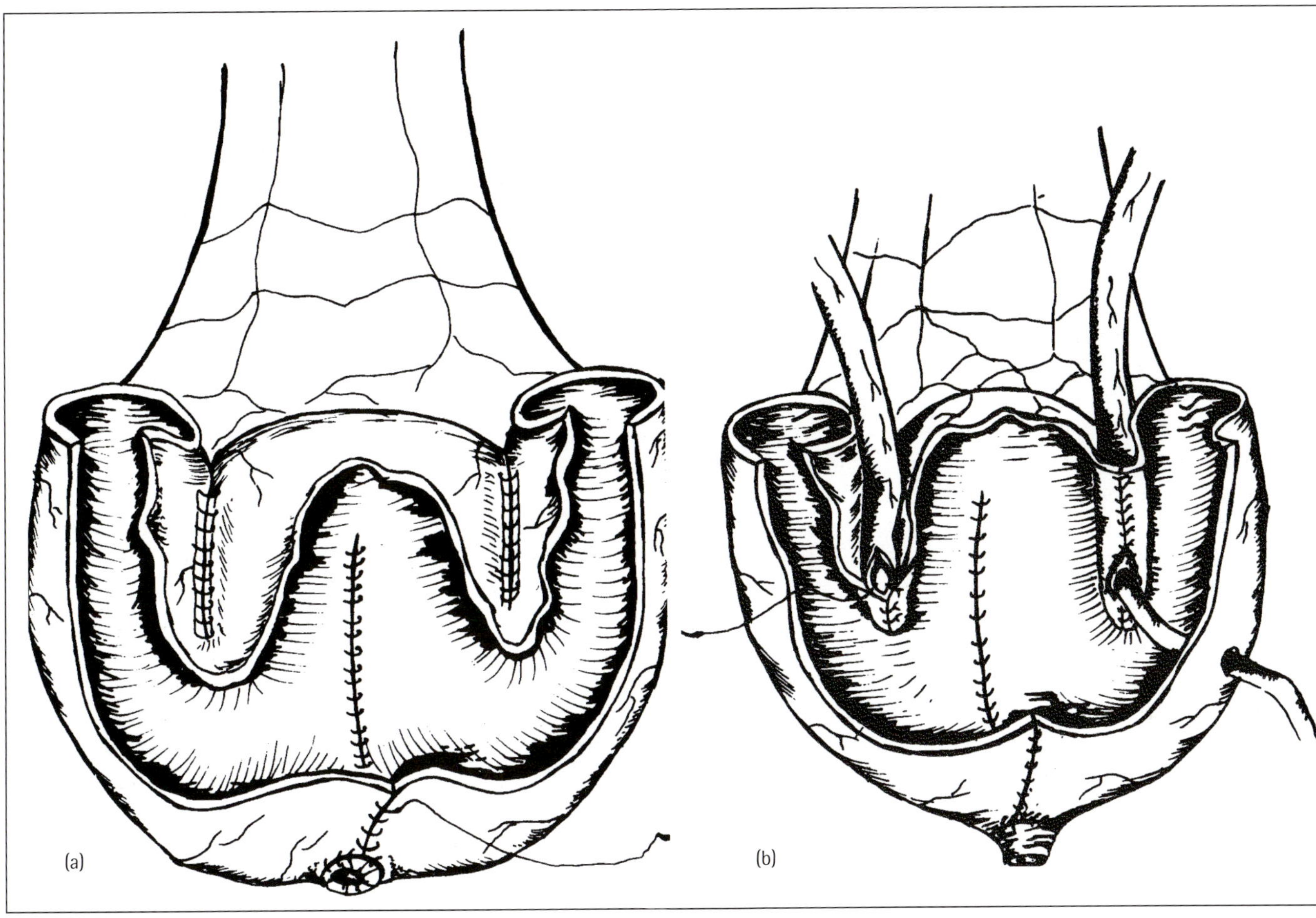

Figure 32.7 The extramural serous-lined tunnel. (a) Small bowel is refashioned into a 'W', detubularized and the lateral ileal limbs are joined together with seromuscular continuous suture to create two serous-lined intestinal troughs. (b) The ureters are brought into the troughs, anastomosed to the mucosa and the tunnel is closed over the implanted ureter. (Reproduced from Abol-Enein and Ghoneim. J Urol 1994; 151: 1193–7[13] with permission from Lippincott Williams & Wilkins.)

ment.[17] They used 30 cm of ileum reconfigured into a 'U'. The two arms of the 'U' were first opposed with a seromuscular stitch to create the serous trough. The ureters were then placed into the 3-cm trough side by side in a staggered fashion and then spatulated and anastomosed to the adjacent bowel. The trough was then closed by reapproximating the two edges in a running fashion. Although only one patient was reported on, it demonstrates the potential widespread applicability of this technique.

Results of antireflux procedures

The outcomes for the various antireflux procedures as reported by their innovators are summarized in Table 32.1. There are only a few studies comparing different tunneling methods. Kristjansson et al compared the Le Duc–Camey anastomosis to the Goodwin colonic tunnel using a retrospective cohort and found the Le Duc–Camey method superior with respect to stricture formation.[18] Five of 34 units using submucosal tunnel developed a stricture as opposed to none of the 35 performed using the Le Duc–Camey method. Overall, most of the tunneled methods demonstrate similar results. The Ahlering, Pagano and the extramural serous-lined tunnel appear somewhat better, however, confirmation of these initial results from other investigators is lacking. Each of the methods has its benefits and limitations, making it imperative for a surgeon to be familiar with many in order to apply them appropriately.

The intussuscepted ileal valve and intussuscepted ileocecal valve

History

There are two main types of intussuscepted nipple valve, the intussuscepted ileal valve and the intussuscepted ileocecal valve. The historical origins of the two are separate. The intussuscepted ileocecal valve can be traced back to the Nissen plication used to prevent gastroesophageal reflux, where the esophagus is wrapped in a collar of stomach.[19] Based on this,

Table 32.1 Success of various tunneled anti-reflux procedures

Antireflux method	Patients (n)	Stricture (%)	Reflux (%)	Leakage (%)
Intraluminal – large bowel				
Goodwin[18,37]	43	14	7	–
Ahlering[3]	70	7	–	0
Intraluminal – small bowel				
Yang[5]	7	0	14	14
Extraluminal – large bowel				
Leadbetter and Clarke[6,38–40]	127	14	4	3
Strickler[9]	28	14	–	–
Pagano[11]	63	7	6	3
Extraluminal – small bowel				
Starr[12]	10	10	0	0
Extramural serous-lined tunnel[15]	344	2	–	2.4

Zinman and Libertino intussuscepted terminal ileum into the cecum, forming a collar of cecum around the ileum as a means to prevent reflux in ileocecal conduits.[20] Hendren improved the stability of the intussusception by detaching the mesentery from a segment of terminal ileum, in effect forming an intussuscepted nipple valve to prevent reflux. Kock is responsible for devising the intussuscepted ileal valve, which was used in reservoirs of patients with permanent ileostomies to free them of an appliance by providing continence and preventing reflux.[21] The valve had obvious applicability to the urinary tract, where both continence and prevention of reflux were desirable.[22] However, the pouch required the use of staples in all four quadrants for stabilization of the intussusception and in the urinary tract these were lithogenic.[23] Additional problems were those of dessusception of the afferent valve and consequent upper tract damage, as well as problems with catheterization and incontinence stemming from the efferent valve.[23] Skinner et al described a number of modifications to the original description of the Kock pouch in order to address some of the above shortcomings.[24–27]

Mechanism of the intussuscepted valve

Hinman described a number of mechanisms through which antireflux or continent valves may function.[28] Applicable to both the ileocecal intussuscepted valve and the ileal intussuscepted valve is the concept of sphincteric compression. This mechanism relies on mucosal compression to increase intravalve pressure preventing reflux and providing continence. In the intussuscepted ileal valve, it is obtained by the compression of the inner sleeve by the outer sleeve created by the intussusception (Figure 32.8a). The ileocecal valve has an inherent sphincteric mechanism that is often reinforced by two rows of sutures to enhance inner channel compression.

Peristalsis is another mechanism that may be present in both the intussuscepted ileal and ileocecal valve. It is believed that the terminal ileum in the ileocecal valve may undergo reflex contractions that prevent reflux of contents in the antiperistaltic direction. Similarly, the intussuscepted ileal valve may have some peristaltic activity that prevents reflux, if it is oriented with the distal portion towards the reservoir.

The third proposed, but unproved mechanism of reflux prevention and continence is that of pressure equalization. The walls of the intussuscepted ileum by virtue of their presence within the reservoir are subject to intrareservoir pressures, which act to coapt the inner channel of the valve (Figure 32.8b). The short intussusception of the ileocecal valve may likewise be compressed by intracecal pressures.

The final mechanism preventing reflux and maintaining continence may be that of a flap valve which is the mechanism that normally functions to prevent ureteric reflux in the native bladder. Fixing the intussuscepted valve to the reservoir wall, one creates a flap valve allowing compression of the valve against the wall of the reservoir as the reservoir pressure increases (Figure 32.8c).

It is unknown to what degree these mechanisms contribute to continence, but it is likely that all of them play a role.

Construction

Details of the construction of the Kock pouch are given in Chapters 14 and 23. In this chapter we will focus on the construction of the afferent intussuscepted nipple and its modifications.

The afferent nipple valve as described by Kock consists of a segment of ileum that is intussuscepted onto itself to create a nipple that is 5 cm long and is stapled in four quadrants for stabilization (Figure 32.9a).[22] The intussuscepted portion protrudes into the reservoir and provides the antireflux mechanism. The non-intussuscepted portion is outside of the reservoir and it is to this portion that the ureters are implanted with a standard Bricker or Wallace type anastomosis. Skinner et al have made a number of modifications to the original description in order to address some of the previously mentioned problems.[24–27]

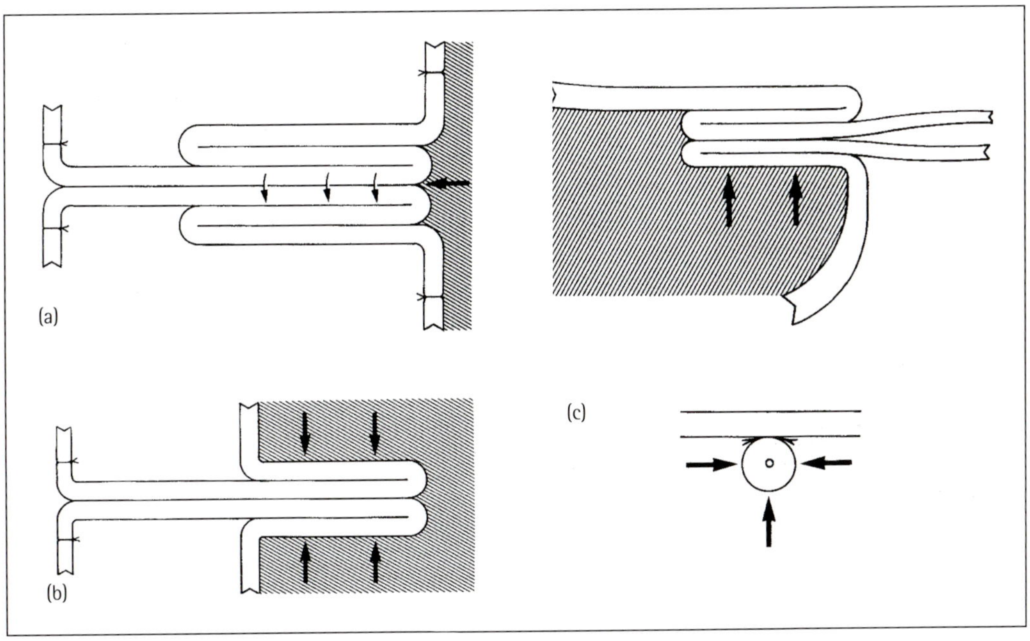

Figure 32.8 The mechanisms of the intussuscepted nipple valve. (a) Sphincteric compression principle: ileal intussusception generates sphincteric action (curved arrows) created by two additional layers within the ileal segment. (b) Pressure equilibration principle: reservoir pressure is delivered uniformly to the length of nipple equalizing the pressure in the lumen of the conduit. (c) Pressure equilibration with flap valve: fixing the nipple to the side of the reservoir has an added flap valve effect. (Reproduced from Hinman. J Urol 1990; 144: 27–30[28] with permission from Lippincott Williams & Wilkins.)

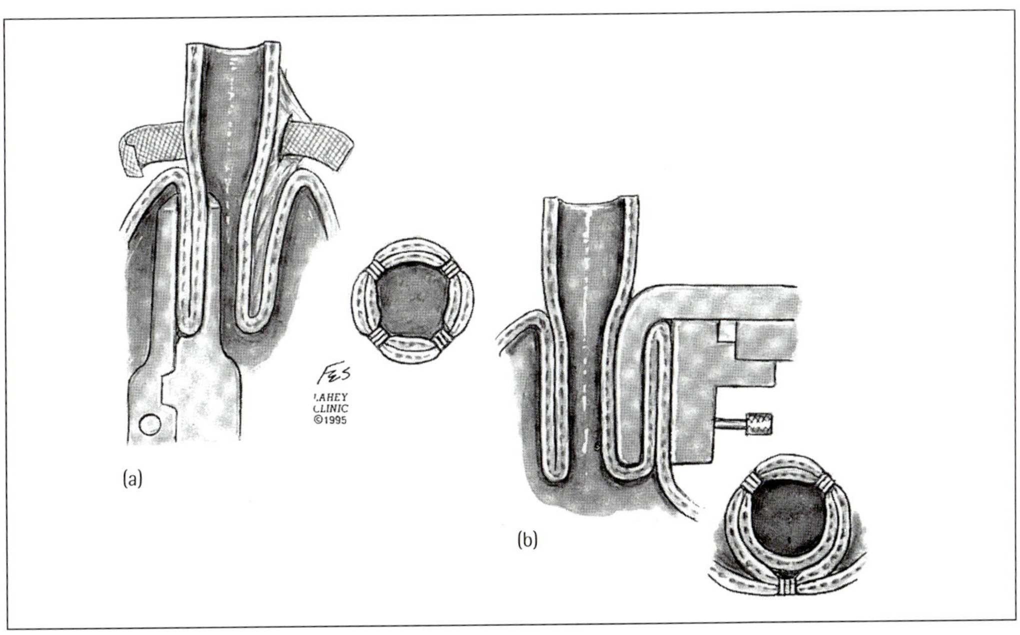

Figure 32.9 Construction of the intussuscepted ileal nipple valve. (a) Kock's initial description allowed for four staple lines as shown. (b) Skinner's modification uses three staple lines with one fixing the nipple valve to the pouch as shown. (Reproduced from Friedman et al. J Urol 1992; 147: 441–3[29] with permission from Elsevier.)

Some of the major modifications introduced by Skinner et al include the following:

- using 17 cm of bowel for the construction of the valve as opposed to 12–15 cm as originally described[24]
- stripping of 7–8 cm of mesentery off the intussuscepted portion of ileum to avoid future slippage and dessusception[24]
- replacing Marlex mesh collar with a 2-cm strip of polyglycolic acid mesh that is soaked in tetracycline solution (250 mg in 10 ml normal saline) before its application around the base of the nipple where it is fixed with interrupted 2-0 chromic catgut sutures to the reservoir in order to decrease the risk erosion[26]
- using a total of three rows of 4.8-mm stainless steel nonhemostatic staples to stabilize the intusussception (one to fix the nipple to the back wall of the reservoir and two equally spaced around the nipple) with the most proximal five staples removed to decrease the risk of stone formation[26] (Figure 32.9b)
- using the pin with the stapling device, but ensuring that the holes thus created are carefully closed to avoid fistula formation[26]
- the polyglycolic acid mesh is applied with a finger in the bowel to prevent overtightening which can lead to stenosis[24]

Other modifications to stomal stabilization have been proposed. King described a hand-sewn stabilization of the intussusception that avoided the use of staples in the urinary tract.[29,30]

A 2-cm longitudinal incision is made on the antimesenteric aspect through the mid-portion of the intussuscepted nipple. The incision is carried completely through the outer bowel segment and through the seromuscular layer of the inner leaf exposing the inner mucosa. Saline is used to raise a bleb on the pouch wall and a mirror incision is made through the mucosa of the pouch (Figure 32.10a). A 2-0 polyglycolic suture is used to oppose the muscularis of the pouch wall with the seromuscular cut edges of the outer leaf and the exposed seromuscular layer of the inner leaf of the nipple (Figure 32.10b, c). The cut mucosa of the outer leaf of the nipple is approximated to the cut mucosa of the pouch.

Atta proposed another technique of nipple stabilization, which avoided staples using an almost circumferential incision (excluding the mesentery) around the base of the nipple.[31] This incision was made through the outer leaf mucosal and seromuscular layer as well as the inner leaf seromuscular layer exposing the inner leaf mucosa (Figure 32.11a). The two inner seromuscular layers were then approximated using running 3-0 polyglycolic acid sutures (Figure 32.11b). The outer mucosa would then be closed over this incision (Figure 32.11c). A theoretical advantage of this method is the interruption of peristaltic contractions that produce dessusception. However, long-term follow-up and large series experience is lacking with this technique.

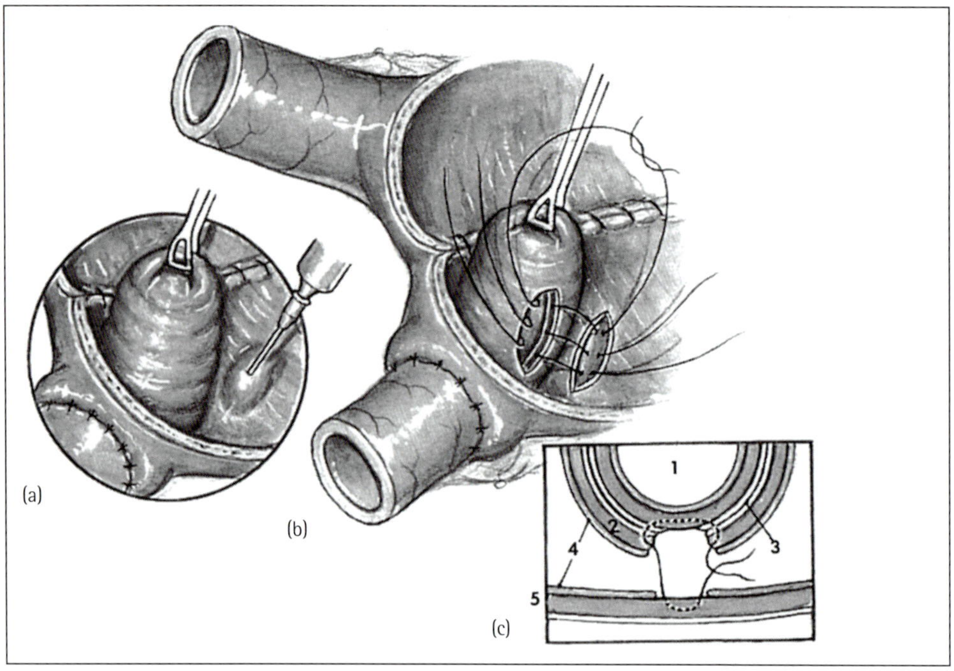

Figure 32.10 The King hand-sewn intussucepted nipple valve.[29,30] (a) Saline is used to raise a bleb facilitating the mucosal incision in the reservoir wall. (b) A corresponding incision is made through the full thickness of the outer bowel wall and through the seromuscular layer of the inner bowel wall. (c) Interrupted absorbable sutures are placed through the various layers as shown. (1, lumen of intussuscepted ileum; 2, outer bowel muscularis layer; 3, serosa of the two intussuscepted bowel segments; 4, mucosa of reservoir and outer bowel segment; 5, muscularis of reservoir).

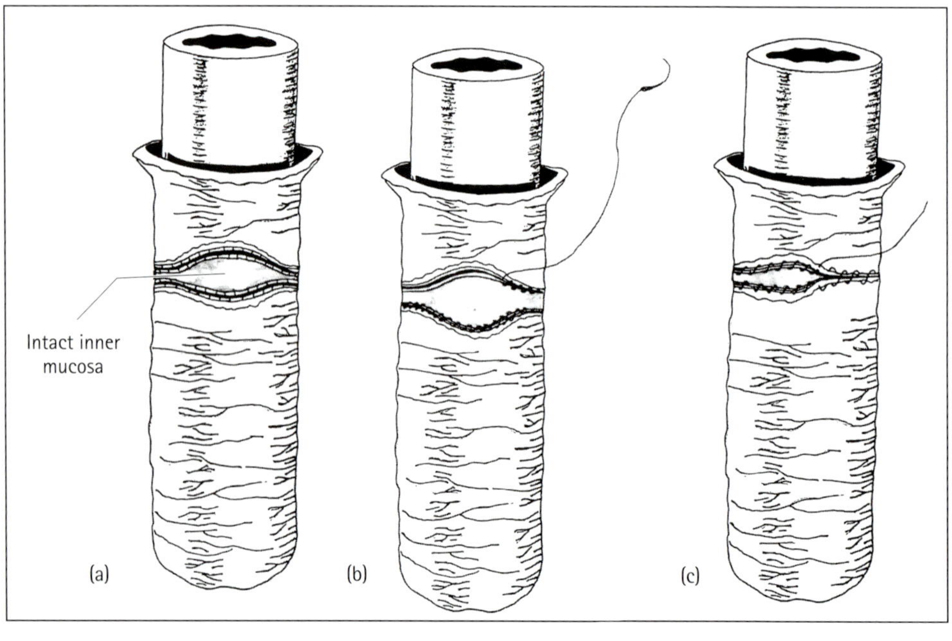

Figure 32.11 The Atta technique of nipple stabilization. (a) A full circumferential incision except for the mesenteric border is made through full thickness of outer ileum and seromuscular layer of inner ileum. (b) Muscularis of both ileal layers is sutured together on both the proximal and distal edges of the incision separately with continuous 3-0 polyglycolic acid suture. (c) The outer mucosa is closed. (Reproduced from Atta. J Urol 1990; 144: 1192–3[31] with permission from Lippincott Williams & Wilkins.)

The advent of absorbable staples has allowed for intussuscepted ileal valve construction that is fast and has a lower risk of stone formation. Arif et al conducted a prospective randomized study comparing absorbable and non-absorbable staples in constructing antireflux valves.[32] Although only 50 patients were randomized with a median follow-up of 3 years, there was a significant difference in stone formation rates and a non-significant difference in dessusception rates, both favoring the absorbable staples.

Results

Continual modifications made to the original technique of fashioning the intussuscepted ileal nipple have decreased the complication rates and improved results.[26] While early complications of the Kock pouch remain constant at about 16%, the incidence of late complications has decreased from 47% for the initial 150 patients operated on, to 22% for the last 239 patients.[26] When considered in isolation, the afferent antireflux nipple valve has an overall complication rate of 10.4% based on a large series of 802 patients.[33] Stone formation was reported in 5.2%, stenosis in 4.3% and valve prolapse in 0.9%.[33] Persistent reflux was seen in 6 of 292 (2%) men treated with a Kock ileal neobladder.[34] The rates of pyelonephritis were accordingly also low, occurring in 13 of 489 (2.6%) in Skinner's series.[26]

Comparisons with other methods of reflux prevention have been made. Shaaban et al reported a prospective randomized trial comparing the intussuscepted ileal nipple valve to the technique of Le Duc for reflux prevention.[35] Forty patients were randomized and the results were evaluated at 6 and 18 months postoperatively. The Le Duc method proved inferior, with 12 of 38 renal units showing evidence of radiographic dilatation while all of the nipple valves had normal postoperative studies. Of the 12 units 11 had stenotic ureters and one had reflux.

Another prospective randomized trial compared the intussuscepted ileal nipple valve (18 patients) or a ureteric split-cuff nipple valve (17 patients) to an 16–20 cm afferent tubular segment (35 patients). Follow-up varied from a median of 57 months for the antireflux nipples to 45 months for the afferent segments. The trial found significantly more upper tract dilatation in the nipple valve group compared to the afferent tubular segment group (13.5% vs. 3% $P<0.03$).[36] Unfortunately two different antireflux techniques, the intussuscepted ileal nipple and the ureteric split-cuff nipple, were analyzed together in this study preventing any conclusions about the intussuscepted ileal nipple valve. Furthermore, upper tract dilatation rates in this study are over twice as high as those reported in the large series by Skinner.[26, 33]

Summary

We have discussed a variety of tunneled anastomotic techniques for the prevention of ureteric reflux. Large scale outcome data using many of these techniques are lacking. Ultimately, the choice in technique will depend on the clinical situation and the surgeon's personal experience. However, it is useful for the reconstructive surgeon to have at his or her disposal many methods of reflux prevention – those presented in this chapter as well as others.

The use of the intussuscepted ileal nipple valve to prevent reflux has evolved over the years. However, it still remains a complex reconstructive technique that requires meticulous attention to detail. Its time-tested results must be examined with the knowledge that they come from high-volume centers and balanced against the results of other, less involved methods for which outcome data also appear initially favorable. Again, surgeon comfort and experience will likely dictate its continued use.

References

1. Goodwin WE, Harris AP, Kaufman JJ, Beal JM. Open, transcolonic ureterointestinal anastomosis. Surg Gynecol Obstet 1953; 97: 295–330.
2. McDougal WS. Use of intestinal segments and urinary diversion. In: Walsh PC, Retik AB, Vaughan ED, Wein AJ (eds). Campbell's Urolog, Vol. 4. Philadelphia: Saunders, 2002: 3763–7.
3. Ahlering TE, Weinberg AC, Razor B. Modified Indiana pouch. J Urol 1991; 145: 1156–8.
4. Shenfeld O, Goldwasser B. The tunneled, non-refluxing, uretero-enteric anastomosis in continent urinary reservoirs. In: Webster GD, Goldwasser B (eds). Urinary Diversion: Scientific Foundation and Clinical Practice. Oxford: Isis Medical Media Ltd, 1995: 310.
5. Yang WH. Yang needle tunneling technique in creating antireflux and continent mechanisms. J Urol 1993; 150: 830–4.
6. Leadbetter WF, Clarke BG. Five years' experience with ureteroenterostomy by the 'combined' technique. J Urol 1954; 73: 67–82.
7. Nesbit RM. Ureterosigmoid anastomosis by direct elliptical connection: a preliminary report. J Urol 1949; 61: 728–34.
8. Strickler WL. A modification of the combined uretero-sigmoidostomy. J Urol 1965; 93: 370–3.
9. Jacobs JA, Young JD Jr. The Strickler technique of ureterosigmoidostomy. J Urol 1980; 124: 451–4.
10. Pagano F. Ureterocolonic anastomosis: description of a technique. J Urol 1980; 123: 355–6.
11. Pagano F, Cosciani-Cunico S, Dal Bianco M, Zattoni F. Five years of experience with a modified technique of ureterocolonic anastomosis. J Urol 1984; 132: 17–18.
12. Starr A, Rose DH, Cooper F. Antireflux ureteroileal anastomoses in humans. J Urol 1975; 113: 170–4.
13. Abol-Enein H, Ghoneim MA. A novel uretero-ileal reimplantation technique: the serous lined extramural tunnel. A preliminary report. J Urol 1994; 151: 1193–7.
14. Abol-Enein H, Ghoneim MA. Further clinical experience with the ileal W-neobladder and a serous-lined extramural tunnel for orthotopic substitution. Br J Urol 1995; 76: 558–64.

15. Abol-Enein H, Ghoneim MA. Functional results of orthotopic ileal neobladder with serous-lined extramural ureteral reimplantation: experience with 450 patients. J Urol 2001; 165: 1427–32.
16. el Mekresh MM, Hafez AT, Abol-Enein H, Ghoneim MA. Double folded rectosigmoid bladder with a new ureterocolic antireflux technique. J Urol 1997; 157: 2085–9.
17. De Filippo RE, Bochner BH, Skinner DG. An alternative ureteroileal reimplantation used in augmentation cystoplasty for neurogenic bladder with bilateral vesicoureteral reflux. J Urol 1998; 160: 1416–17.
18. Kristjansson A, Engellau L, Willner J, Mansson W. Reflux, stricture and glomerular filtration rate after two antireflux techniques in continent urinary reconstruction using the right colon. Scand J Urol Nephrol 1997; 31: 425–9.
19. Nissen R. Eine einfache Operation zur Beeinflussung der Refluxesophagitis. Schweiz Med Wschr 1956; 86: 590.
20. Zinman L, Libertino JA. Ileocecal conduit for temporary and permanent urinary diversion. J Urol 1975; 113: 317–23.
21. Kock NG. Intra-abdominal 'reservoir' in patients with permanent ileostomy. Preliminary observations on a procedure resulting in fecal 'continence' in five ileostomy patients. Arch Surg 1969; 99: 223–31.
22. Kock NG, Nilson AE, Nilsson LO, Norlen LJ, Philipson BM. Urinary diversion via a continent ileal reservoir: clinical results in 12 patients. J Urol 1982; 128: 469–75.
23. Lieskovsky G, Skinner DG, Boyd SD. Complications of the Kock pouch. Urol Clin North Am 1988; 15: 195–205.
24. Skinner DG, Boyd SD, Lieskovsky G. Clinical experience with the Kock continent ileal reservoir for urinary diversion. J Urol 1984; 132: 1101–17.
25. Skinner DG, Lieskovsky G, Boyd SD. Continuing experience with the continent ileal reservoir (Kock pouch) as an alternative to cutaneous urinary diversion: an update after 250 cases. J Urol 1987; 137: 1140–5.
26. Skinner DG, Lieskovsky G, Boyd S. Continent urinary diversion. J Urol 1989; 141: 1323–7.
27. Nieh PT. The Kock pouch urinary reservoir. Urol Clin North Am 1997; 24: 755–72.
28. Hinman F Jr. Functional classification of conduits for continent diversion. J Urol 1990; 144: 27–30.
29. Friedman RM, Flashner SC, King LR. Effectiveness of a handsewn nipple valve for reflux prevention in bladder reconstruction. J Urol 1992; 147: 441–3.
30. Webster GD, King LR. Further commentary: cecal bladder. In: King LR, Stone AR, Webster GD (eds). Bladder Reconstruction and Continent Urinary Diversion. Chicago: Year Book Medical, 1987: 206–8.
31. Atta MA. A new technique for ileal nipple fixation: preliminary report. J Urol 1990; 144: 1192–3.
32. Arif H, Madbouly K, Mahran MR, Ashamallah A, Ghoneim MA. A prospective randomized study comparing absorbable and nonabsorbable staples in constructing antireflux valves of urethral hemi-Kock pouches. BJU Int 1999; 84: 440–3.
33. Stein JP, Freeman JA, Esrig D et al. Complications of the afferent antireflux valve mechanism in the Kock ileal reservoir. J Urol 1996; 155: 1579–84.
34. Elmajian DA, Stein JP, Esrig D et al. The Kock ileal neobladder: updated experience in 295 male patients. J Urol 1996; 156: 920–5.
35. Shaaban AA, Gaballah MA, el-Diasty TA, Ghoneim MA. Urethral controlled bladder substitution: a comparison between the intussuscepted nipple valve and the technique of Le Duc as antireflux procedures. J Urol 1992; 148: 1156–61.
36. Studer UE, Danuser H, Thalmann GN, Springer JP, Turner WH. Antireflux nipples or afferent tubular segments in 70 patients with ileal low pressure bladder substitutes: long-term results of a prospective randomized trial. J Urol 1996; 156: 1913–17.
37. Lockhart JL, Pow-Sang JM, Persky L, Sanford E, Helal M. Results, complications and surgical indications of the Florida pouch. Surg Gynecol Obstet 1991; 173: 289–96.
38. Hill JT, Ransley PG. The colonic conduit: a better method of urinary diversion? Br J Urol 1983; 55: 629–31.
39. King LR. Protection of the upper tracts in undiversion. In: King LR, Stone AF, Webster GD (eds). Bladder Reconstruction and Continent Urinary Diversion. Chicago: Year Book Medical, 1987: 127–53.
40. Hagen-Cook K, Althausen AF. Early observations on 31 adults with non-refluxing colon conduits. J Urol 1979; 121: 13–16.

33 The Le Duc–Camey method for reflux prevention

Alain Le Duc and Maurice Camey

Introduction

The earliest reported attempts at ureterointestinal implantation were by John Simon in 1852[1] and Thomas Smith in 1878. A number of implantation procedures were performed between 1880 and 1910, but most failed because of fistula formation. The first successes were achieved in 1920, with the arrival of ureteral stents. Ureteroileal antireflux implantations have always had more problems than ureterocolonic antireflux implantations[2] due to the structure of the submucosa of the small intestine, which is both more dense and more vascular than that of the colon. This renders the creation of a submucosal tunnel a more difficult procedure.

Four types of ureteroileal antireflux system are in current use:

- Implantation of the ureters proximal to an ileoileal invagination, which acts as an antireflux valve, as demonstrated by Kock's studies in 1982.[3]
- Partial replacement of the ureter by an isoperistaltic segment of small intestine which prevents reflux. The principle of this technique was described by Fenger in 1884[4] and then Shoemaker in 1906. More recently, Studer et al recommended this technique in 1989.[5]
- Eversion of the ends of the ureter to form a cuff, as described by Ricard at the beginning of the century, and popularized by Turner-Warwick in 1967.[6]
- Implantation of the ureters into a submucosal tunnel obtained by excision or incision of a strip of mucosa which is based on and improves upon the tube implantation described by Chalot in 1896. This technique is known by the name of Le Duc–Camey procedure.[7] Clinical experience with this type of implantation is primarily with reimplantation into small intestine, although it is easy to perform and sometimes used in the colon.[8]

Principle of the Le Duc–Camey technique

The principle is the creation of a mucosal tunnel by incision (Figure 33.1) or excision of a strip of mucosa (Figure 33.2). The ureter is drawn into the intestine through a hiatus made at the upper extremity of the tunnel and it is then laid in the base of the tunnel. The intra-ileal position is progressively covered with intestinal mucosa. The ureter is sometimes incompletely covered, leaving a segment of ureter exposed.

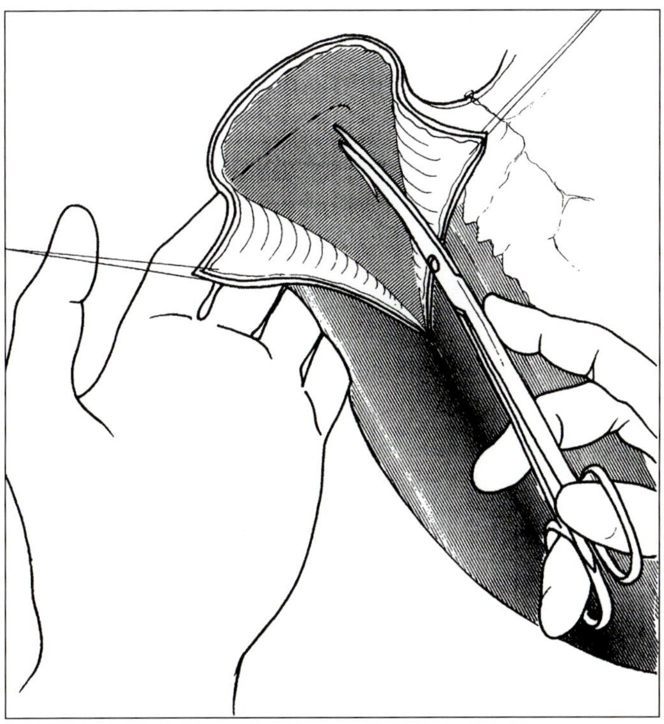

Figure 33.1 A 30-mm sulcus is created by incision of the ileal mucosa.

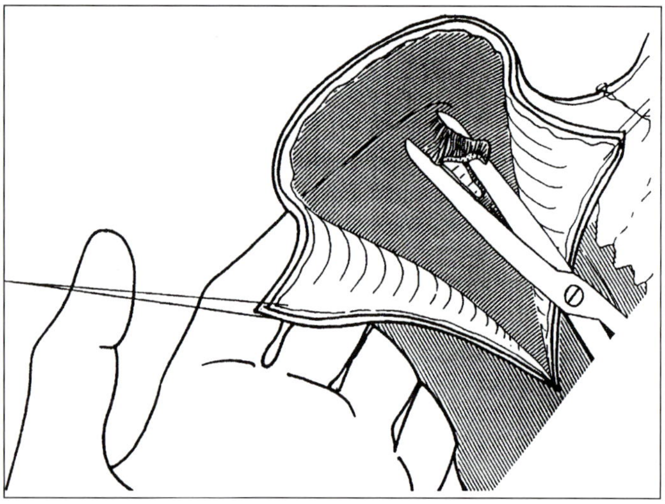

Figure 33.2 A 30-mm sulcus is created by excision of a strip of mucosa.

The technique is simple and has barely been modified since 1977, apart from the proposal by Hautmann of suturing the mucosal edges over the ureter.[9] However, a number of details should be emphasized:[10]

1. The ureter must be dissected widely to preserve its blood supply.
2. The ureter must be placed in contact with the implantation site without applying any traction, kinking or twisting.
3. The ureter enters the intestinal wall through an orifice sufficiently large to allow it to slide freely. The ureteral tract must be as straight as possible.
4. A length of 25–30 mm of ureter is introduced into the intestine.
5. The ureter is anchored solidly by two absorbable sutures, exterior to its intestinal orifice.
6. A 30-mm strip of mucosa is incised or excised superficially with scissors starting from the intestinal orifice of the ureter (see Figures 33.1 and 33.2).
7. The ureter is placed in the tunnel with the meso-ureter in contact with the base of the tunnel.
8. The ureter is spatulated on the anterior surface and solidly anchored to the end of the tunnel by a suture including the muscle coat in order to prevent retraction.
9. The muscosal edges are very carefully sutured by interrupted sutures to the ureteric adventitia without trying to cover the ureter if its caliber is too large (Figure 33.3). Alternatively, in the case of a narrow ureter, Hautmann's covering technique may be indicated.
10. A stent is inserted into the implanted ureter and is securely fixed at its entry (Figure 33.4).
11. The ureteral stents are removed after day 12 and the bladder catheter is removed after day 16.

The expected advantages of this procedure are:

- no hematoma at the operative site, as the zone of implantation remains open in the intestinal lumen

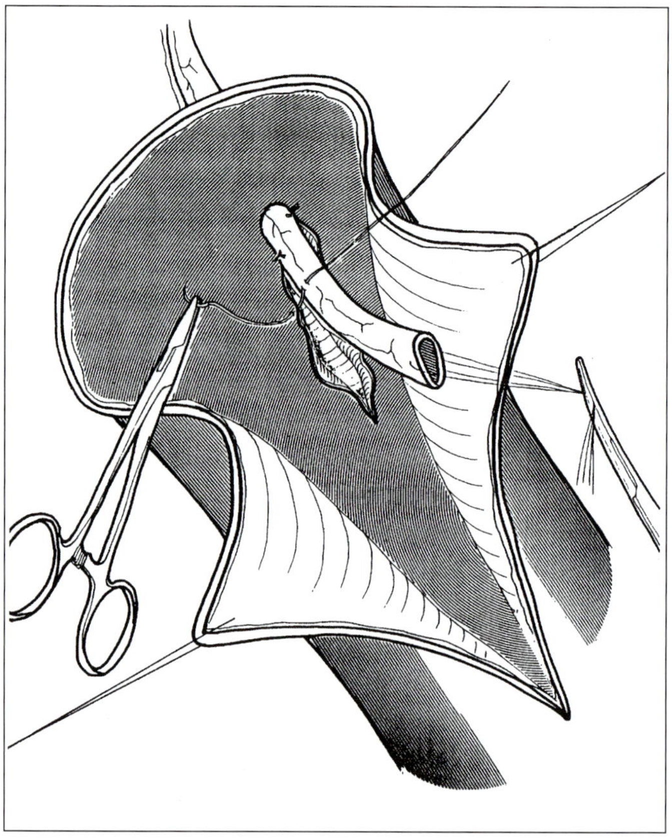

Figure 33.3 The ureter lies in the sulcus and is tacked to the ileal mucosa with interrupted sutures.

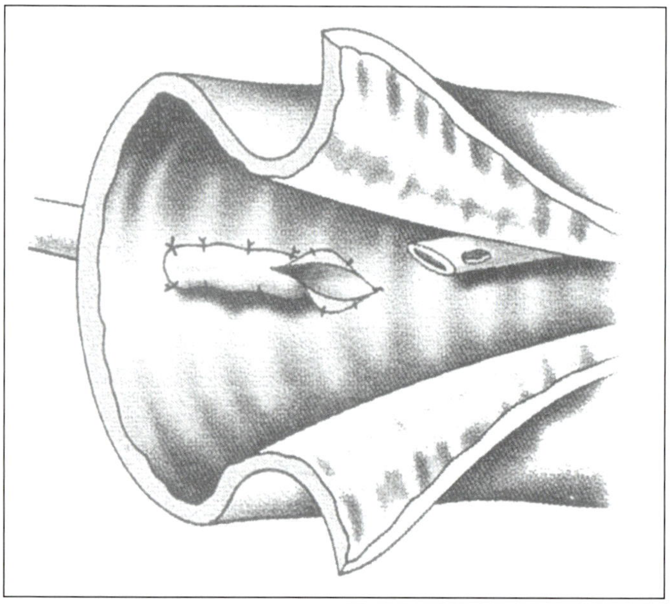

Figure 33.4 The ureter is firmly attached both at its entry in the ileal wall and at its end. The sulcus is sheltered from urine by the tacking sutures at the mucosal edges and by the ureteral stent. The ureter is widely spatulated on the anterior suface.

- no retractile cicatricial stenosis of the orifice, as there is no circumferential anastomosis between the ileal mucosa and the intestinal mucosa
- better blood supply to the distal ureter due to contact between the meso-ureter and the richly vascular ileal submucosa
- the possibility of retrograde catheterization of the ureters due to the anatomic position of this implantation.[8]

Clinical results

The results described here are based on a series of 796 reimplanted ureters, mostly in the context of Camey type I or II and Hautmann enterocystoplasties.[7–15]

Urine leaks

No urine leak or fistula was reported in this series, except for one case of Bricker diversion, in which urine leaked from the hiatus where the ureter enters the ileal wall, due to poor drainage of the intestinal segment causing accumulation of urine at this site.

Stenosis and impaired patency of the anastomosis

Three types of complication were observed:

- Immediate obstruction after removal of the ureteric stent on days 12–14 (4% of cases).
- Moderate unilateral or bilateral dilatation with no clinical signs (which generally resolves over several months: 15%).
- Tight secondary stenosis requiring reoperation (2.3% of cases) (Table 33.1).

Reflux

Reflux was detected in 10% of cases on routine follow-up by retrograde cystography (Table 33.2), and it may be as high as 15% in some series.[13]

Discussion

The absence of urinary fistulas at the site of ureteroileal reimplantation is directly related to the characteristics of this technique. The only precaution that must be taken is to ensure drainage of the plasty by a 22-Fr catheter for 2 weeks.

Stenosis of the ureteroileal implantation is certainly the most serious complication. Many factors can be responsible for stenosis. Some of them are not related to the implantation technique, such as extrinsic torsion, plication or compression of the ureter, while others are directly related to the technique iteslf. The frequency of stenotic complications is a subject of controversy, as many papers report a rate of about 5%, while others report a rate of more than 20% (see Table 33.1).

We have observed three types of situation in our practice.

- acute obstruction occurring after removal of the ureteric stent. This obstruction is due to odema in the tissues surrounding the suture. Treatment consists of administration of an anti-inflammatory drug, possibly combined with temporary nephrostomy drainage for 10–15 days.
- asymptomatic moderate obstructions that resolve spontaneously over several months.
- permanent stenoses due to ischemic fibrosis and chronic inflammation at the implantation site. These types of stenosis require surgical treatment, either by an endo-urologic procedure (30% success rate), or by surgical reimplantation, or by nephrectomy when the obstruction is detected too late.

Modified procedures have been proposed by Wenderoth et al,[9] Schwaibold et al[19] and Muraish et al[20] with stenosis rates

Table 33.1 Stenosis following ureteroileal implantation (mucosal sulcus) in reported series

Reference	No. of ureters	% stenosis
Lugagne et al[17]	246	5
Schwaibold et al[19]	117	5
Wenderoth et al[9]	169	2
Muraishi et al[20]	48	2
Le Duc et al[11]	120	4
Hautmann	933	3.6
Roth	142	20
Shaaban	38	29

Table 33.2 Reflux following ureteroileal implantation (mucosal sulcus) in reported series

Reference	Reno-ureteral units	Reflux
Camey	158	29
Pagano et al[14]	36	0
Hautmann	169	6
Le Duc	71	10
Nurmi and Puntala[13]	19	3
Sagalowsky et al[15]	28	3
Total	481	51

of less than 5%. All of these modifications retain the basic principle of the ureter lying in a mucosa groove. We have personally continued to use the same reimplantation technique but have modified the shape of the enterocystoplasty, by creating two horns for implantation of the ureters. This modification allows less extensive dissection of the ureters designed to preserve their distal blood supply (Figure 33.5). The antireflux mechanism is maintained by the segment of ureter buried in the mucosal groove. This mechanism is effective in 85% of cases (see Table 33.2).

Conclusion

The Le Duc–Camey reimplantation procedure is simple to perform. With a stenosis rate of 5% and antireflux protection in 85% of cases, this technique compares favorably with the other ureteroileal reimplantation procedures. Initially designed to protect the upper tract in high pressure neobladders (Camey I), this technique can also be recommended in low pressure detubularized bladders.[16]

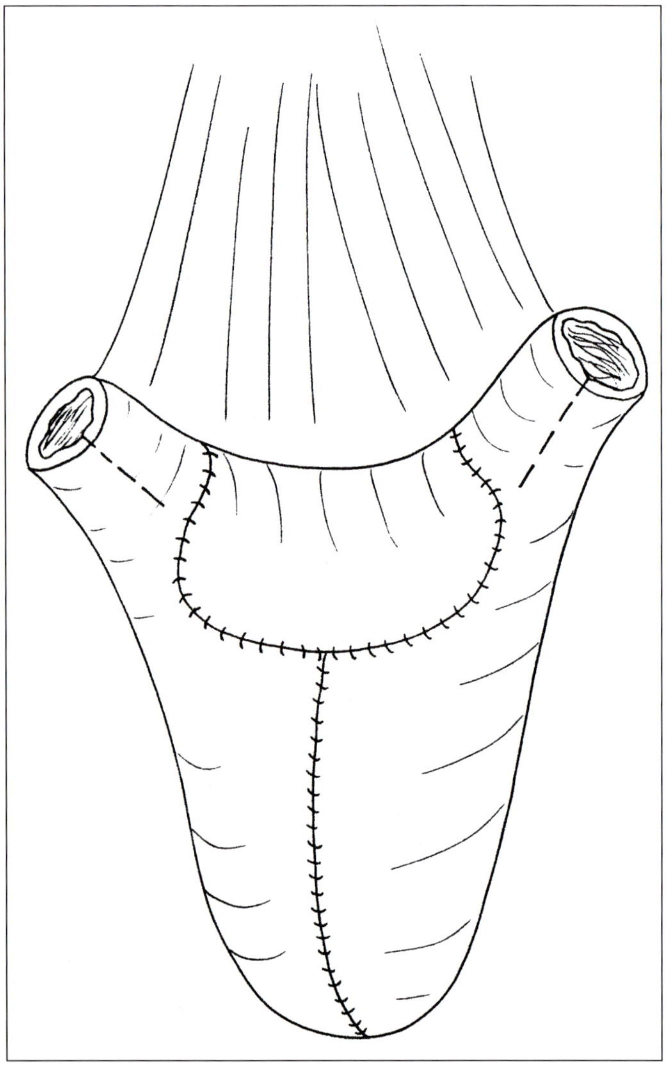

Figure 33.5 Technique of modified Hautmann ileal neobladder. Two horns are created in order to accept the ureterointestinal anastomoses. This modification allows less extensive dissection of the ureters.

References

1. Simon J. Ectopia vesica: operation for directing the orifices of the ureters into the rectum; temporary success; subsequent death; autopsy. Lancet 1852; ii: 568–70.
2. Coffey RC. Physiologic implantation of the severed ureter or common bile duct into the intestine. JAMA 1991; 56: 397–403.
3. Kock NG, Nilson AF, Nilson LO, Norlen LJ, Philipson BM. Urinary diversion via a continent ileum reservoir. Scand J Urol Nephrol 1982; 49: 23–31.
4. Fenger C. Surgery of the ureter. Ann Surg 1984; 20: 257–96.
5. Studer UE, Ackerman D, Casanova GA, Zingg EJ. 3 year experience with an ileal pressure bladder substitute. Br J Urol 1989; 63: 43.
6. Turner-Warwick RT, Ashken MA. The functional results of partial, subtotal and total cystoplasty with special reference to uretero-caeco-cystoplasty. Br J Urol 1967; 39: 3–12.
7. Le Duc A, Camey, M. Un précede d'implantation urétéro-iléale antireflux dans l'entérocystoplastie. J Urol Nephrol 1979; 85: 449–54.
8. Bejany DE, Politano V. Modified ileocolonic bladder: 5 years of experience. J Urol 1993; 149: 1441–4.
9. Wenderoth UK, Bachor R, Eggart G et al. The ileal neobladder experience and results of more than 100 consecutive cases. J Urol 1990; 143: 492–6.
10. Boccon-Gibod L, Leleu C, Peyret C, Conguy S. Entérocystoplastie de substitution continente par poche iléale détubularisée a basse pression après prostato-cystectomie radicale. Ann Urol 1998; 22: 16–20.
11. Le Duc A, Camey M, Teillac P. Original antireflux uretero-ileal implantation technique long term follow-up. J Urol 1987; 137: 1156–8.
12. Lilien OM, Camey M. 25 years experience with replacement of the human bladder (Camey procedure). J Urol 1984; 132: 886–91.
13. Nurmi M, Puntala P. Evaluation of upper and lower urinary tracts after Camey operation. Scand J Urol Nephrol 1989; 23: 275–7.
14. Pagano F, Artibani W, Ligato P et al. Vesica ileale padovana: a technique for total bladder replacement. Eur Urol 1990; 17: 149–54.
15. Sagalowsky AI. Experience with the ileal bladder (Camey procedure) and caeco-ileal resevoir for continent urinary diversion. Semin Urol 1987; 5: 28–45.
16. Keetch D, Klute CG, Catalona WJ. Late decompensation of neobladder. J Urol 1992; 148: 806–10.
17. Lugagne PM, Herve JM, Lebret T et al. Ureteroileal implantation in orthotopic neobladder with Le Duc–Camey mucosal through technique: risk of stenosis and long term follow up. J Urol 1997; 158; 765–7.

18. Minervini R, Morelli G, Fontana N et al. Functional evaluation of different ileal neobladder and ureteral reimplantation technique. Eur Urol 1998; 34: 198.
19. Schwaibold H, Friedrich MG, Fernandez S, Conrad S, Huland H. Improvement of ureteroileal anastomosis in continent urinary diversion with modified Le Duc procedure. J Urol 1998; 160: 718–20.
20. Muraishi O, Yamashita T, Ishikawa S, Yosuke H, Tokue A. Improvement of ureteroileal anastomosis in orthotopic ileal neobladder with modified Le Duc procedure: short submucosal tunnel technique. J Urol 2001; 165: 798–801.
21. Hautmann RE, Miller K, Steiner U, Wenderoth U. The ilea neobladder: 6 years of experience with more than 200 patients. J Urol 1993; 150: 40–45.
22. Roth S, Can Ahlen H, Semjonow A, Oberpenning F, Hertle L. Does the success of uterointestinal implantation in orthotopic bladder substitution depend more on surgeon level of experience or choice of technique? J Urol 1997; 157: 156–60.
23. Shaaban AA, Gaballah MA, El-Diasty TA, Ghonheim MA. Urethral controlled bladder substitution: a comparison between the intussuscepted nipple valve and the technique of Le Duc as antireflux procedures. J Urol 1992; 148; 1156–61.

34 Use of the split-cuff nipple technique for ureteral reimplantation

Regina Hovey, Anthony R Stone

Introduction

Creating a reliable antireflux mechanism from bowel segments has taxed reconstructive urologists for many years. Historically, this problem was first focused on during the development of ureterosigmoidostomy. The pioneering technical alterations developed first by Coffey in 1911[1] and later by Leadbetter in 1951[2] significantly improved the morbidity and mortality associated with this operation. These techniques require the formation of a submucosal tunnel similar to bladder reimplantation techniques. This is easily accomplished in large bowel segments, but cannot be used in reconstruction using small bowel. The attachment of the small bowel mucosa to the valvulae conniventes prevents the dissection of the mucosa through the submucosal layer.

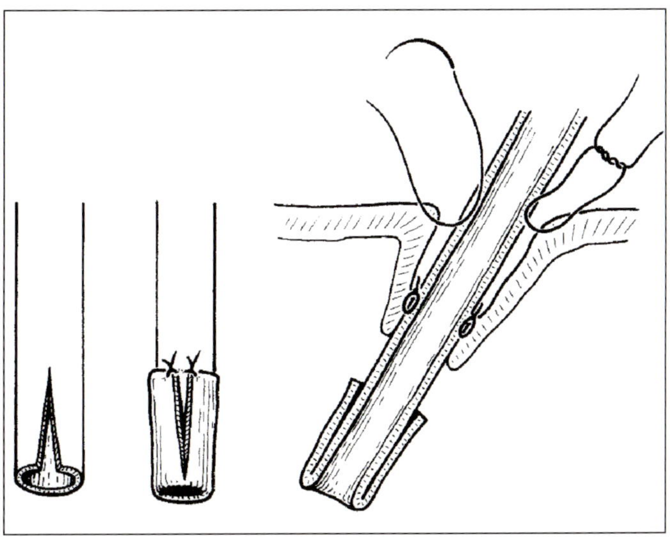

Figure 34.1 First description of 'split-cuff nipple' by Ricard in 1909 (From Heitz-Boyer M and Hovelacque A. J d'Urol Med Chir (Paris) 1912; 237.[9])

Techniques of ureteral reimplantation into small bowel, presently in use, are the intussuscepted ileal nipple technique,[3] the interpositioning of a non-detubularized isoperistaltic bowel segment,[4] the Le Duc–Camey technique[5] and the split-cuff nipple.[6] The first two techniques described above require additional bowel segments and there is experimental evidence that the Le Duc–Camey technique may have a relatively high stricture rate.[7]

The split-cuff nipple technique was popularized by Turner-Warwick and Ashken;[8] however, it was first described much earlier by Ricard in 1909[9] (Figure 34.1). It has the advantage of not requiring additional bowel for the reconstruction and complication rates are equivalent to other reliable reimplantation techniques. Similarly, antireflux function, in our hands, has been maintained in the long term.

This chapter will describe the surgical technique along with its applications and results.

Indications and contraindications

The split-cuff nipple ureteral reimplantation technique is applicable to reimplantation of ureters into any bowel segment used to reconstruct the lower urinary tract (cystoplasty, bladder replacement and continent diversion). It is not appropriate to use the technique if reimplantation into the native bladder is contemplated, as submucosal antireflux methods into the bladder are well established and reliable. The nipple may also be constructed from the ileal segment of a conduit in cases where undiversion from an ileal conduit is being carried out.

Contraindications to this technique are all relative. If the ureters are large and dilated, the nipples constructed may take up too much space in the reconstructed bladder and might also conceivably act as an obstructive ball valve. In cases where the ureters are deemed adynamic and acontractile, it is the author's opinion that any nipple or tunneled technique should not be used, in case the relative obstruction of these methods might further compromise renal function.

Surgical technique

The ureters are detached from the bladder as close to the native intravesical tunnels as possible, to leave the maximum ureteric length. It is not necessary to dissect the ureter out from within the bladder from the orifice, as in classic reimplantation techniques. This may often be difficult in the thickened, trabeculated, neurogenic bladder and may theoretically increase blood loss and the overall morbidity of the procedure. The small length of intramural refluxing ureter left behind is never of any significance.

The adipose tissue surrounding the distal ureter is carefully dissected off for 4–5 cm. This should be done sharply, aided by countertraction with non-toothed Gerald's forceps. The blood supply to the distal ureter is not compromised by this maneuver, as the adventitial vessels are always preserved. The vessels in the adipose tissue can be ligated or fulgurated at the proximal extent of this dissection.

The ureter is then spatulated away from any visible adventitial vessels for approximately 2 cm. The length of the spatulation should be four times the ureteral diameter, so that a nipple length of at least twice its diameter can be constructed (Figure 34.2). An 8-Fr infant feeding tube is placed in the ureter and passed up into the renal pelvis. If the ureter is very small, a 5-Fr catheter can be substituted. The catheter is secured to the apex of the spatulation with a 5-0 chromic catgut suture (Figure 34.3). This suture is passed from outside the ureter, then through the stent and back out of the ureter close to the initial suture pass. It is tied loosely to prevent necrosis of the ureter within the knot. The spatulation is then folded back to form the nipple. The catheter securing the suture should now be close to the apex of the nipple. The nipple is then stabilized with approximately four 4-0 polyglycolic acid (PGA) sutures. Three of these secure the spatulation to the underlying ureter passing through full thickness at the spatulation and into the seromuscular layer of the underlying ureter. These sutures should obviously avoid any adventitial vessels and be placed far enough down the ureter to stretch the spatulation proximally. The final suture of 4-0 PGA incorporates the two lateral edges of the spatulation and the ureteric adventitia between them. This suture is also tied loosely; it is not designed to draw the edges of the spatulation together, but to 'encourage' them to stay in the split-cuff nipple configuration (Figure 34.4).

Ureteroenteric anastomosis may be accomplished in two ways. In most cases, a small enterotomy is made at a suitable site in the bowel. This is readily done by passing a right-angle forcep out from the mucosal surface of the bowel and cutting down onto it from the adventitial side with cutting current Bovie. The right-angle forceps can then be used to stretch the enterotomy to the correct width. The ureteral stent is then grasped

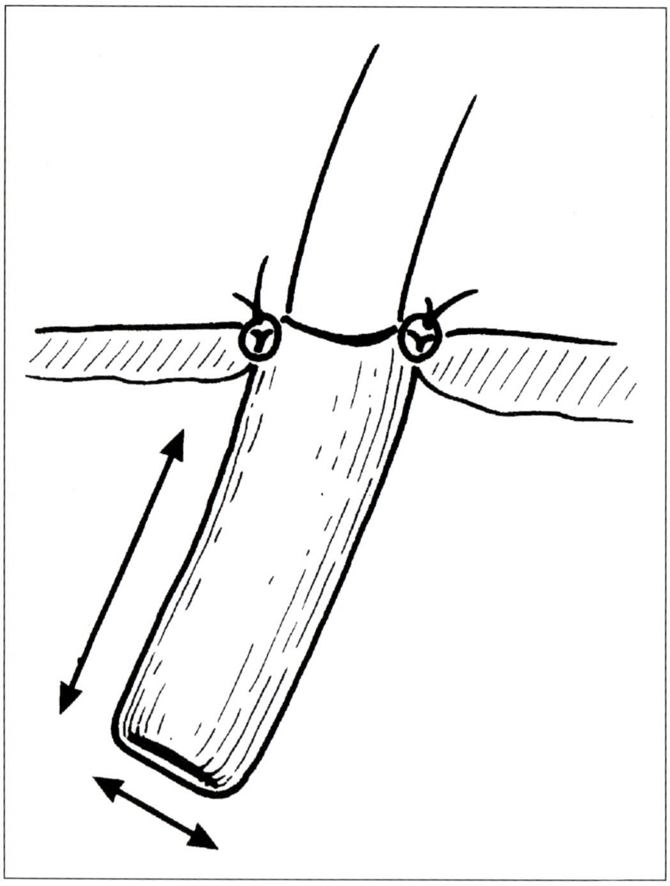

Figure 34.2 Diagrammatic representation of the nipple principle. The length should be at least twice the diameter for effective reflux prevention.

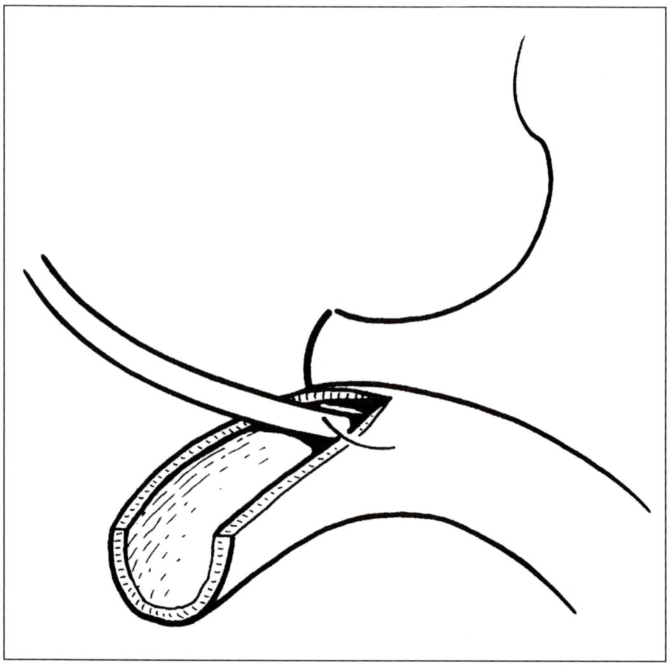

Figure 34.3 8-Fr feeding tube fixed to apex of spatulation with 5-0 chromic catgut suture.

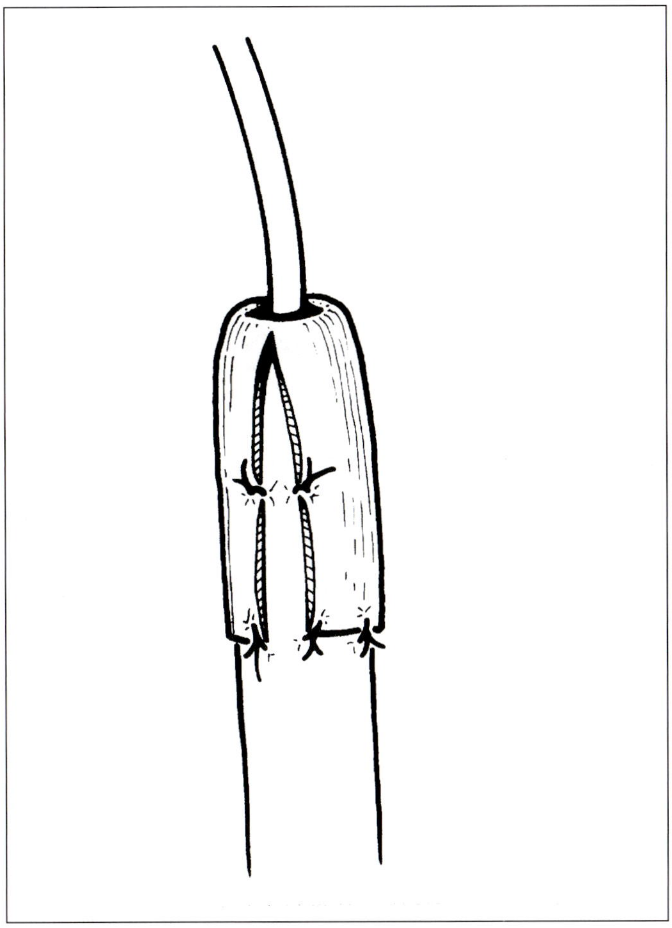

Figure 34.4 Construction of nipple using 4-0 PGA sutures.

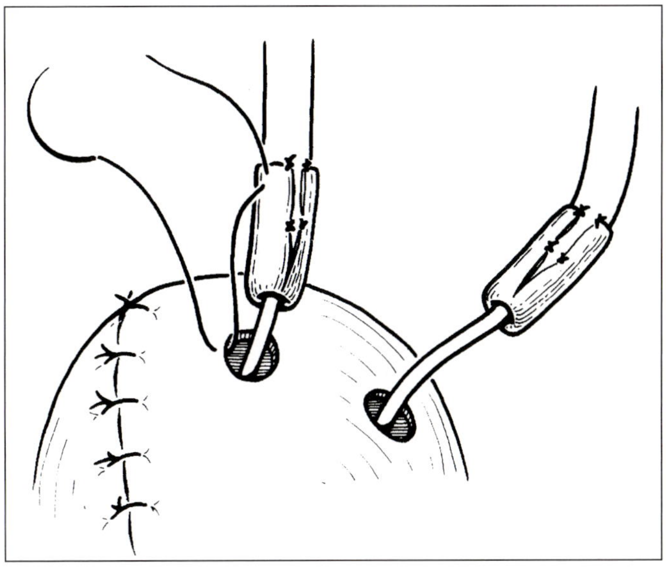

Figure 34.5 Attachment of nipple to bowel segment. Suture passes through seromuscular layer of ureter, spatulation and full thickness of edge of enterotomy.

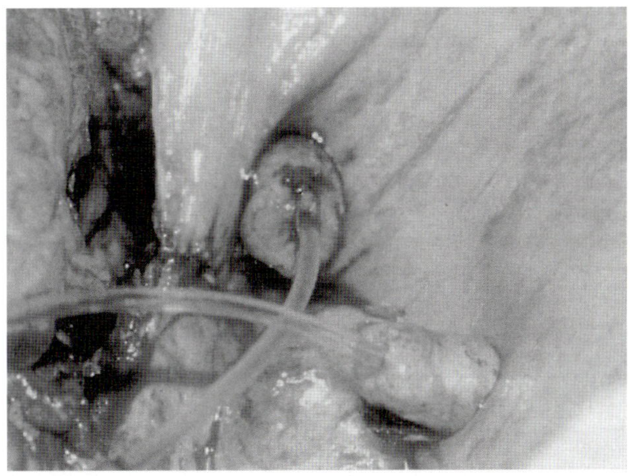

Figure 34.6 Two split-cuff nipple reimplants within lumen of augmentation cystoplasty.

and brought through into the lumen of the reconstructed lower urinary tract. The nipple is secured to the bowel with four or five 4-0 PGA sutures. These are placed seromuscularly through the ureter just below the spatulation, then through the spatulation, and then through full thickness of the edge of the enterotomy (Figure 34.5). Two or three of these sutures may be placed initially without trying to allow direct vision placement. When these are then tied down, the nipple will be pulled through the enterotomy and be seen protruding into the lumen of the bowel segment. Additional sutures can then be placed to support the nipple within the enterotomy (Figure 34.6).

Occasionally it may be suitable to place the nipples together through a corner of detubularized bowel. For instance, if this technique is used in an ileal orthotopic bladder replacement, both nipples may be placed within the left-hand corner of the open bowel segment. The nipples are then secured within the bowel by six or seven 4-0 Vicryl sutures, again placed into ureter, edge of spatulation and full thickness of bowel, to close the open bowel around both nipples.

Several additional steps will be outlined that may ensure a successful outcome of the procedure. We prefer to pass the stents through the bowel segment, usually alongside the Malecot catheter, and bring them directly out through the skin. This ensures control of the stent externally in the postoperative period. A pursestring suture is placed around the stent as they exit from the bowel segment and they are also secured to the skin. We have used this reimplantation technique in Kock pouch, in this case, bringing the stents through the stoma and securing them to the skin for extra stability.

If the ureters are reimplanted close together near the retroperitoneum, the peritoneum may be anchored to the bowel in front of the reimplants. This not only supports the bowel segment posteriorly, but places the reimplants in an anatomically correct retroperitoneal position. If the reimplants are not adjacent to the peritoneum, the omentum should be anchored close to the reimplantation, again ensuring healing without leakage.

All these reconstructions will need to be drained. We favor using a 10-Fr round Jackson-Pratt suction drain placed close to, but not absolutely adjacent to, the re-implantation sites.

Postoperative care

The stents are drained into separate bags (bile bags) in order to monitor output. Occasionally the stents will not drain. This usually means the urine is passing around the stent and should not be of immediate concern. The Jackson-Pratt drains are removed when they have stoppped draining (usually 3–5 days postoperatively). In general, in most reconstructions requiring split-cuff nipple reimplantation, the patient is sent home 1 week postoperatively with stents and Malecot in place. At about 2 ½–3 weeks, a cystogram is carried out to confirm healing and exclude any extravasation. This must be done under fluoroscopic control with the urologist present to prevent overzealous filling of the reconstructed lower urinary tract by the radiologist (Figure 34.7). If the cystogram is satisfactory, the stents are removed. The use of 5-0 chromic catgut to anchor the stents ensures that at about 17 days to 3 weeks they can be removed without difficulty.

At this point, spontaneous voiding or intermittent catheterization is commenced, as indicated.

Follow-up

Assuming no problems occur following removal of the stents, the patient's upper tracts will be restudied, initially, at around 3 months postoperatively. Routinely, a cystogram is carried out to confirm the lack of reflux and ultrasound to ensure stabilization or improvement of upper tracts. Occasionally mild upper tract dilatation is seen at this time, such that a repeat study is required at six months. In general, no further follow-up is required until 1 year postoperatively and yearly thereafter. Having established the reliability of this technique, we now follow these patients at 1 year with ultrasound only unless there have been extenuating problems such as recurrent upper tract infections and/or pain.

Complications

Early complications

Early complications have been very rare and are usually related to inadvertent migration of the stents into the bladder despite fixation. One case associated with edema at the reimplantation site following this migration necessitated nephrostomy drainage to resolve.

Late complications

Recurrent reflux has been seen in seven renal units (8%). In four of these units, the reimplantation was placed into the lumen of non-detubularized small bowel (two conduits, two Kock pouches). We believe that the small and narrow lumen of the native small bowel may not allow the normal compressive function of urine on the nipple, thus compromising its antireflux properties (Figure 34.8).

In three cases (three renal units), upper tract deterioration occurred (3%). In two of these cases, endoscopic manipulation was required with a successful long-term outcome. In the final case, the patient was asymptomatic and had metastatic disease, so treatment was not instigated.

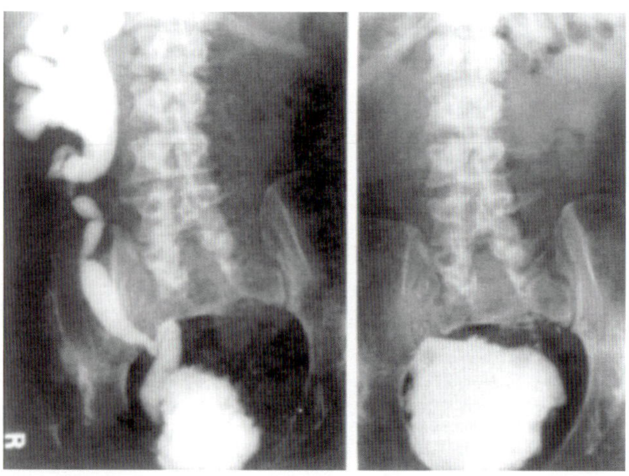

Figure 34.7 Pre- and postoperative cystograms. (Left) Grade IV reflux, (right) postoperative cystogram following ileal augmentation cystoplasty and split-cuff nipple reimplantation.

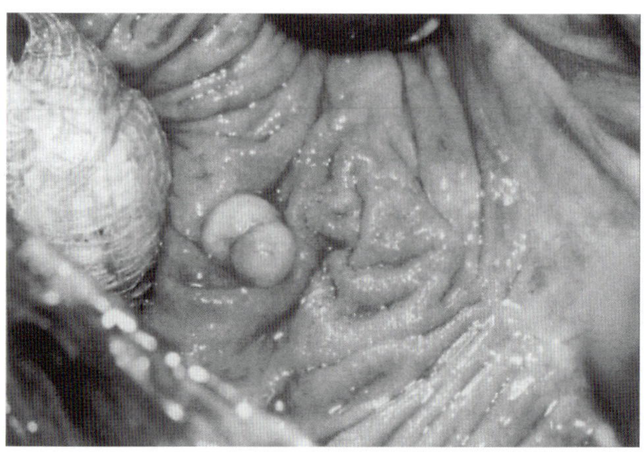

Figure 34.8 Split-cuff nipple within cystoplasty 4 years after construction.

Long-term follow-up

Split-cuff nipple ureteral reimplantation has been used in 52 cases comprising 92 renal units: 22 orthotopic bladder replacements (reconfigured ileal pouch), six Kock pouches, two ileal conduits and 23 augmentation cystoplasties. Apart from the specific complication described, no other problems occurred (follow-up 3 months to 8 years; average 4.5 years).

During this time, we have had an opportunity to endoscope or reoperate on several of these cases. In these circumstances, the nipple has always been seen to be maintained and discrete (see Figure 34.8).

Conclusions

Split-cuff nipple reimplantation technique is a useful and reliable adjunct for the reconstructive urologist. It is appropriate for reimplantation of the ureter into small bowel segments, but may be just as easily incorporated into gastrocystoplasty or colocystoplasty. It also has a distinct place in undiversion from ileal conduit.

The technique has been shown in our hands to be safe and reliable and has the theoretical advantage of decreased stenosis rate compared to submucosal tunnel techniques or the Le Duc–Camey technique. It also allows reimplantation without the need for an extra bowel segment, bowel nipple or ureteral staples.

References

1. Coffey RC. Physiologic implantation of the severed ureter or common bile-duct into the intestine. JAMA 1911; 56: 397.
2. Leadbetter WF. Consideration of problems incident to performance of uretero-enterostomy: report of a technique. J Urol 1951; 65: 818.
3. Skinner DG, Boyd SD, Lieskovsky G. Clinical experience with the Kock continent ileal reservoir for urinary diversion. J Urol 1984; 132: 1101.
4. Studer UE, Ackermann D, Casanova GA, Zingg EJ. Three years' experience with an ileal low pressure bladder substitute. Br J Urol 1989; 63: 43–52.
5. Le Duc A, Camey M. Un procédé d'implantation uréteroiléale anti-reflux dans l'entéro-cystoplastie. J Urol Nephrol 1979; 85: 449.
6. Stone AR and MacDermott JPA. The split-cuff ureteral nipple reimplantation technique: reliable reflux prevention from bowel segments. J Urol 1989; 142: 707–9.
7. Abol-Enein H, El-Baz M, Ghoneim MA. (1993) Optimization of uretero-intestinal anastomosis in urinary diversion: an experimental study in dogs. Urol Res 1993; 21: 125–9.
8. Turner-Warwick RT, Ashken MH. The functional results of partial, subtotal and total cystoplasty, with special reference to ureterocaecocystoplasty, selective sphincterotomy and cystocystoplasty. Br J Urol 1967; 39: 3.
9. Heitz-Boyer M, Hovelacque A. Création d'une nouvelle vessie et d'un nouvel urètre. J d'Urol Méd Chir (Paris) 1912; 237.

35 Ileal conduit urinary diversion

Christophe E Iselin

Introduction

When Eugen Bricker more than 50 years ago popularized urinary diversion by an ileal conduit,[1] he probably had not foreseen that this type of diversion would still be the one most frequently performed in the world at the beginning of the twenty-first century. Reasons for its popularity have, however, evolved over the years, and partly depend on the technical versatility of the surgeon to perform the two basic dry diversions now validated: orthotopic and continent cutaneous bladder replacement. In the 1950s and 1960s, the ileal conduit was favored because it overcame four main problems of urinary diversion. It markedly decreased the problems of electrolyte imbalance and pyelonephritis following ureterosigmoidostomy,[2] and provided the patient with a unique single stoma whose appliance was much simpler and more reliable than that of bilateral uretero-, nephro- or pyelostomies. Nowadays, the ileal conduit remains very much appreciated throughout the world owing to its technical simplicity and long-term effectiveness.[3,4] Indeed, although not devoid of late complications,[3–6] the procedure has undoubtedly stood the test of time. Except after pelvic irradiation, ileum is the best small bowel segment to be used for conduit construction, and it remains superior to the jejunum which carries a 40–65% risk of electrolyte imbalance.[7–8] Moreover, although conduit diversion has long carried the reputation of poor self body image associated with a low quality of life, studies have shown that a large proportion of patients are well satisfied with this type of diversion.[9–11] Interestingly, the underlying cause for the diversion appears more likely to affect subsequent quality of life issues, and cancer patients seem more prone to curtail social activities compared with those undergoing diversion for a benign pathology, such as incontinence or bladder dysfunction.[12] This chapter reviews the indications, complications of and quality of life after one of the classical urologic operations. It does not cover the laparoscopic aspect, which is dealt with in Chapter 38.

Indications

Ureteroileal conduit urinary diversion is a valid option for any pathology which renders the bladder non-functional or requires its removal. However, as discussed elsewhere in this text, the indications for orthotopic or cutaneous continent diversions are now well defined (see Chapter 13), and have increased over the past 10 years. Besides the fact that surgeons may choose urinary ileostomy for matters of technical simplicity, there are distinct indications for conduit diversion: poor renal function, decreased bowel availability, lack of motivation because of cosmetic aspects, insufficient dexterity for self-catheterization and poor compliance for forming a habit of regular micturition or self-catheterrization. Practically, it is often an array of arguments which lead to preference for ileal conduit in up to 45–50% of diversion candidates.[5,13]

In patients with malignant pathology risk of local recurrence, especially in the urethra, may preclude orthotopic bladder replacement, although the issue remains debated.[14,15] A continent stoma is then the next option, followed finally by urinary ileostomy, as often chosen when a salvage cystectomy is performed. Building a continent neobladder requires twice to three times as much bowel as an ileal conduit and may employ the ileocecal valve. Prior intestinal resection, radiation therapy or intestinal disease such as ulcerative colitis or Crohn's disease often decrease significantly bowel availability, which may preclude elaborate bladder reconstruction. In such situations, the limited length of ileum needed for a standard loop is a safe way out. Poor dexterity and foreseeable poor compliance with the mandatory discipline of continent neobladders are relative contraindications for these diversions, since patients either do not benefit from their reservoirs or may ruin neobladder function by excessive voiding intervals. In such instances, a simple urostoma is the best solution. Due to their large surface area, intestinal urinary reservoirs have a significantly higher resorption capacity than conduits. This may lead to electrolyte disturbances in patients with poor renal function.[16,17] Therefore, a conduit is a better option than a neobladder when serum creatinine exceeds 2.5 mg/dl or 225/umol/L. Finally, cosmetic motivation may be lacking even in relatively young patients, and has been found to significantly decrease in older patients, who are often very satisfied with a urostoma.[10]

Following these selection criteria is the requirement of course, that the patient has been fully informed of the benefits and disadvantages offered by conduit, cutaneous continent and orthotopic reconstruction of the lower urinary tract.

Preparation of the patient for ileal conduit

Patient counseling

Counseling is a determinant step in providing the patient with the type of urinary diversion, that will meet his needs and expectancies. Adjustment problems should be addressed in a positive fashion. Helping the patient to understand the functional characteristics of urinary conduit and dry diversions requires a close partnership between the surgeon and enterostomal therapist. Illustration of the practical and simple anatomic aspects of the various diversions by videos helps to illustrate postoperative life in a more realistic fashion[18] and increase the chances of making the correct choice. Ultimately, communicating with urinary diversion patients may help to convince the diversion candidate which a particular form of bladder replacement will be best for them.

Once the initial selection procedure described above is accomplished, patient counseling continues by the physician who provides information about the perioperative period, essentially the milestones of recovery from the surgery. Simple outcome facts in terms of bowel function resumption, removal of the various drains, management of the stoma appliance are also given to the patient and the importance of undergoing regular follow-up evaluation is stressed. The stoma therapist further explains the practical characteristics of the various appliances available. In this respect, a video is most helpful since an accurate picture can be given with the possibility to review the sequence of stoma care.

Stoma siting

The success of urostomy surgery is predominantly determined by the optimal selection of the stoma position. The surgeon and/or stoma therapist will examine the patient supine, sitting and standing to select a site in the superior part of the iliac fossa. This site must provide a good surface for optimal adherence of the appliance plate and ideally resides equidistant from the umbilicus and the anterior superior iliac spine (Figure 35.1). To prevent herniation, stoma position should ensure that the conduit passes *through* the rectus muscle, usually just medial to its lateral border (see Figure 35.1). To ensure waterproof adherence of the appliance, the stoma should also be sufficiently far from the umbilicus and from major abdominal scars or creases. Finally, an appliance filled with 100–200 ml of saline is fixed on the selected site, and the patient is asked to dress and walk around to ensure correct leakproof positioning. Once located, the site should be indelibly marked with a needle as a cruciate scratch, which ensures that it will be easily located peroperative.

Bowel preparation

The customary policy is to start a low residue diet 24–48 hours before surgery, and to mechanically prepare the bowel with an oral gastrointestinal lavage solution the afternoon before surgery, to reduce as far as possible the microbiological load of the intestinal contents. At the author's institution, the patient drinks 3 l of an electrolyte solution (Fordtran) rendered reasonably tasty by adding citric acid, saccharin and aspartame. This usually leads to clear rectal efflux the same evening. Since oral antibiotics such as neomycin or erythromycin reduce normal intestinal flora with the potential resultant emergence of resistant strains,[20] and have not been shown to significantly improve postoperative outcome, there appears to be no rationale to prescribe them.

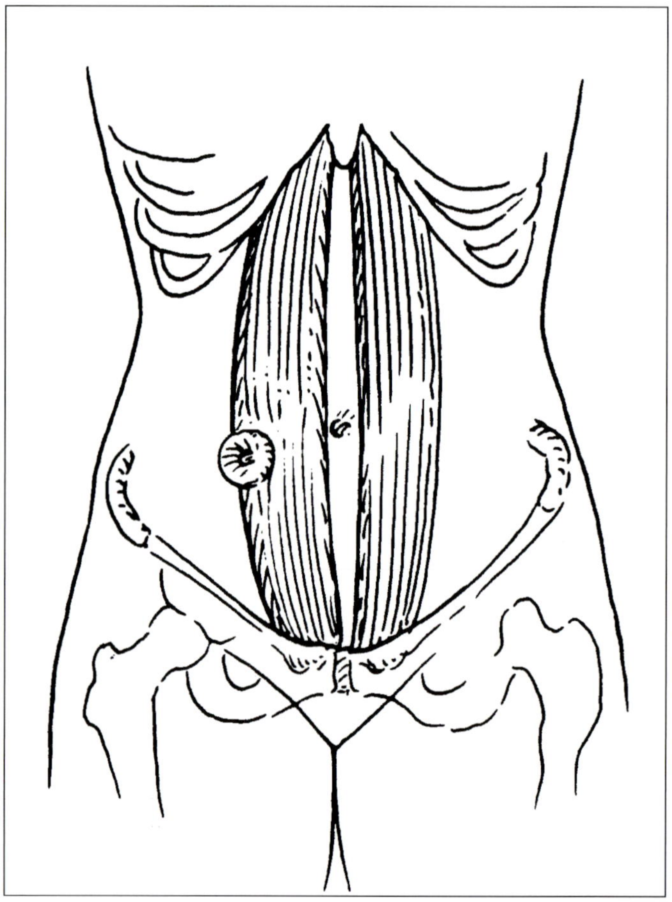

Figure 35.1 Stoma location. The ideal stoma site is to the right of the midline just medial to the border of the rectus and between the umbilicus and the anterior superior iliac spine. (Reproduced with permission from Vickers MA et al. In: Mastery of Surgery: Urologic Surgery. Chicago: Little Brown and Co, 1992[19].)

The surgeon must also be aware that the necessity of preoperative mechanical bowel preparation has been questioned over the past 15 years, even for left colonic surgery.[21,22] Arguments include fluid overload by reabsorption of 20% of saline used in whole-gut lavage,[23] metabolic complications[24,25] and significant prolongation of postoperative ileus as recently described in a radical cystectomy and ileal conduit series.[26] Nevertheless, until more evidence-based arguments are available, the policy remains in a majority of institutions to proceed with preoperative mechanical bowel preparation.

Surgical technique

Incision and preparation of the field

The abdominal midline is incised from the superior rim of the pubic bone to approximately 3–6 cm above the umbilicus. An abdominal ring retractor (Bookwalter type) facilitates the exposure. The ureters are identified where they cross the iliac vessels, and are circumferentially dissected distally close to the ureterovesical junction, where they are transected. In case of bladder cancer, a frozen section of each ureteral end is obtained. Left ureteral mobilization should be sufficient to allow it to pass without kinking and strangulation through the base of the sigmoid mesocolon, so that it rejoins the right ureter over the sacral promontory.

Isolation of the ileum segment

The terminal ileum remains a particularly well adapted bowel segment for urinary conduit construction because it is easily accessed and isolated. However, prior radiation therapy, bowel resection or Crohn's disease may preclude its use. Only seldom does a short or abnormally inserted mesentery leads the surgeon to select another bowel segment.

To tailor the ileal segment to an adequate length, four principles should be kept in mind. First, the distal 15–20 cm of the ileum must not be used to preserve bile salts and vitamin B_{12} reabsorption. Secondly, one should use a segment as short as possible to reduce the nutritional and metabolic effects of its removal and the electrolyte effects of its inclusion in the urinary tract. Usually a patient of standard habitus needs a 15–20-cm length. However, construction of a short loop must avoid excessive ureteral mobilization which carries risk of ischemia which may lead to ureteroileal anastomotic stricture. Too short a loop may also compromise correct stoma construction, which may lead to retraction with potential major appliance-fitting problems. Thirdly, at least four vascular arcades should supply the segment to avoid ischemia. Lastly, one must incise the distal mesentery in the avascular space between the ileocolic and the right colic arteries (Figure 35.2), since this avascular space allows a particularly long incision which is necessary to permit an easy tension-free transfer of the distal end of the segment through the abdominal wall.

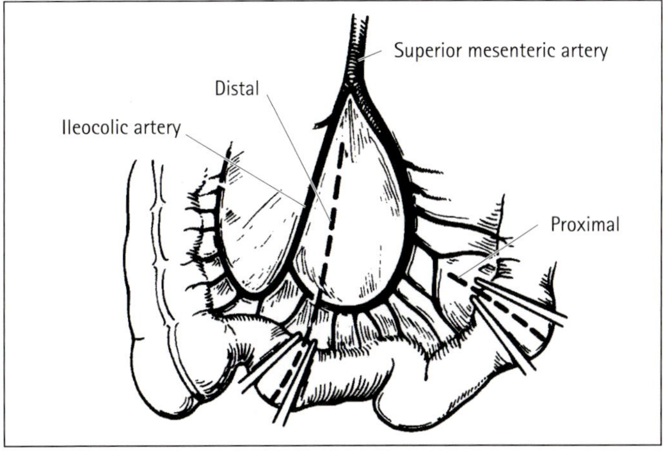

Figure 35.2 Isolation of the ileal conduit. Note the sufficient number of vascular arcades and the extended distal mesenteric incision in the avascular plane between the ileocolic and superior mesenteric artery. (Reproduced from Loughlin KR et al. In: Surgical Management of Urologic Disease: An Anatomic Approach. St Louis: Mosby Year Book, 1992[27] with permission from Elsevier.)

Ileoileal anastomosis is then performed cephalad to the conduit using a single layer of an absorbable 3-0 or 4-0 running suture or a stapling device according to the surgeon's preference, and the mesenteric hiatus is closed to avoid intestinal hernia.

Ureteroileal anastomosis

This step of ileal conduit construction is of paramount importance, since a significant number of early and late complications arise here, such as urinary leak and stricture, respectively. Several precautions, if followed, lead to efficient prevention of these complications. First, ureteral vascularization of the ureters must be kept intact. The ureteral vascular system is divided in two layers which anastomose, the peripheral one being just under the adventitia. Hence, respecting ureteral vasculature means strictly avoiding any breach of the ureteral adventitia, leaving periureteral fat whenever possible and avoiding excessive ureteral length. Secondly, atraumatic ureteral handling and careful suture technique using 5-0 absorbable sutures are mandatory. The indications, necessity and usefulness of performing an antireflux technique, is discussed in the 'Tunneled anastomosis' section of this chapter.

The two classic techniques of ureteroileal anastomosis are the Nesbit end-to-side anastomosis[28] and the Wallace anastomosis which has two variants: end-to-end or side-by-side.[29] Seldom, Le Duc[30] or Leadbetter[31] non-refluxing reimplantations are performed.

Nesbit end-to-side anastomosis

The proximal end of the ileal loop is closed with a one- or two-layer inverting suture. The ileal wall is incised over 1 cm close to the proximal end of the loop, and the redundant mucosa is excised. The ureter is spatulated for a short distance and anastomosed with 5-0 absorbable interrupted sutures, which encompass the full thickness of the ureteral wall and include a large bite of the serosa of the ileum and a smaller bite of the mucosa (Figure 35.3). After long-term follow-up, anastomotic stricture rates range between 3 and 8% of renal units.[5,32–36]

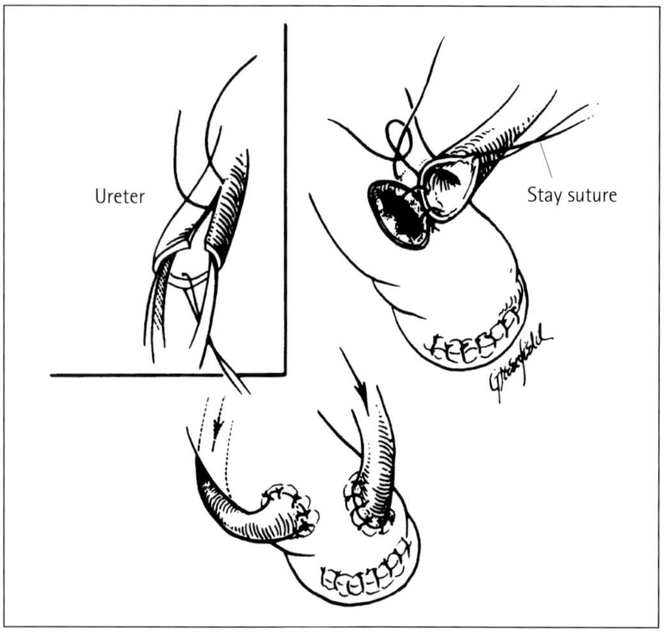

Figure 35.3 Nesbit anastomosis. The ureter is spatulated for a short distance and anastomosed with 5-0 absorbable interrupted sutures, which encompass the full thickness of the ureteral wall and include a large bite of the serosa of the ileum and a smaller bite of the mucosa. (Reproduced from Richie JB. In Genitourinary Cancer Surgery. Philadelphia: Lea and Febiger, 1982[2] with permission from Lippincott Williams & Wilkins.)

Wallace anastomosis

The principle of this type of anastomosis is to construct a plate by uniting both spatulated ureters, which is then anastomosed to the proximal open end of the ileal loop, thereby closing it.

The Wallace 1 anastomosis unites the ureters in a parallel side-by-side fashion (Figure 35.4), while the Wallace 2 suture the ureters end-to-end (Figure 35.5). Both techniques are simple, require a spatulation length of approximately 2 cm, and are performed with running 5-0 absorbable sutures, or eventually 4-0 when anastomosing the ureteral plate to the ileum. There are many advantages of both variants. These include (i) a single large anastomosis of ureters to ileum, (ii) direct visualization of the ureteral lumen throughout closure, (iii) avoidance of separate closure of the proximal end of the conduit, (iv) easy entire retroperitonealization of the anastomosis, (v) elimination of proximal end dead space leading to a possibly shorter conduit, and (vi) a shorter operating time.[32] A suggested disadvantage in cases in whom diversion is being performed following cystectomy for transitional cell cancer is the possibility of ureteral recurrence causing bilateral ureteral obstruction, however this is unreported as yet. After long-term follow-up, anastomotic stricture rates range between 0 and 11% of renal units.[6,32,36,37]

Tunneled anastomosis

The principle to reimplant a ureter with an antireflux mechanism has always challenged urologists in conceptual and technical matters, and led to elaborate non-refluxing anastomotic techniques. The incentive was reinforced by the concept of putative high-pressure reflux through ureteroileal anastomoses.[40]

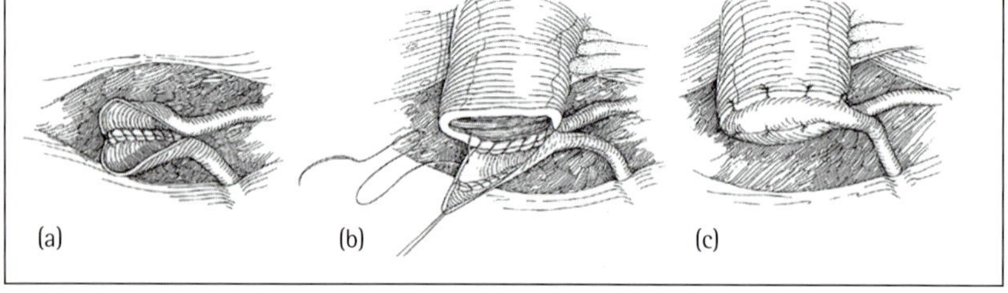

Figure 35.4 Wallace side-by-side anastomosis. This anastomosis unites the ureters in a parallel fashion (a,b). It requires a spatulation length of approximately 2 cm. Eventually, a second layer of interrupted sutures may reinforce the anastomosis (c). (Reproduced from Kelalis PP. In: Atlas of Urologic Surgery, 2nd edn. Philadelphia: WB Saunders, 1998: 661[38] with permission from Elsevier.)

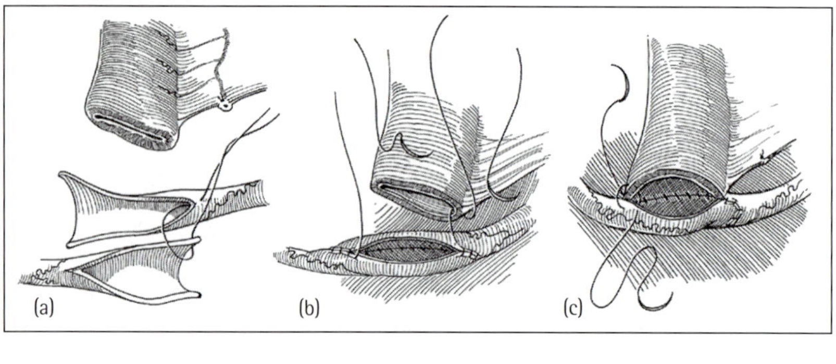

Figure 35.5 Wallace end-to-end anastomosis. This anastomosis unites the ureters end-to-end sites (a–c). The spatulation length is approximately 2 cm. (Reproduced from Kelalis PP. In: Atlas of Urologic Surgery, 2nd edn. Philadelphia: WB Saunders, 1998: 661[38] with permission from Elsevier.)

An antireflux tunnel can be created by placing the ureter in a mucosal trough either by an intraluminal (Le Duc or Goodwin variants; for illustrations, see Chapters 32 and 33) or extraluminal (Leadbetter variant; see Chapter 32) technique. The initial long-term follow-up series by Le Duc reports an 85% antireflux effectiveness associated with a 2% stricture rate.[41] However, further cohort studies of dry diversions using this technique have reported a significantly higher stricture rate ranging between 13 and 29%.[41–43] Hence, it appears at this time that the higher stricture rate of non-refluxing anastomosis outweighs any theoretical benefit of preventing pyelonephritis, stones or azotemia.

Ureteroileal anastomosis drainage

Once completed, ureteroileal anastomoses are retroperitonized by delicately suturing the proximal end of the loop to the posterior peritoneum. Drainage of the anastomoses may be performed externally, and internally by ureteral stents. Although the anastomoses are retroperitonealized, suction drainage of the area is customary, for instance by a Jackson-Pratt drain. Ureteral stenting is the rule nowadays, although it has not been for years.[39] Stents may prevent delayed urine output due to anastomotic edema, and may also favor healing of a leaking anastomosis. Many surgeons use a 8-Fr single J-stent draining through the conduit to the exterior. Single J-stents obviate the need to suture them in position, as was the case with straight catheters. If stents are not used, drainage of the ileal conduit should be favored by placement of a 22–24-Fr fenestrated catheter, which may be removed between the seventh and tenth day. Ureteral stents are left longer, and removed between the tenth and twentieth day under broad spectrum antibiotic coverage, once anastomotic patency and absence of leakage has been assessed by contrast study.

Stoma construction

A small skin disk of approximately 2.5-cm diameter is excised, and the subcutaneous fat separated or removed as a plug according to the body habitus, The rectus fascia is incised in a cruciate fashion, the underlying muscle split and the peritoneum incised. This creates a hiatus that should accommodate two fingers, which is usually large enough to allow passage of the distal end of the conduit without compressing its blood supply. Two to three centimeters of conduit should be brought above skin level without tension, the redundant length being excised. Once the distal end of the loop is passed through the abdominal wall hiatus created at the end of the procedure, the loop is sutured posteriorly and laterally to prevent any bowel hernia between the abdominal wall and the conduit.[1]

The ileum may be fixed to the anterior rectus fascia by seromuscular stitches, although some surgeons find this unnecessary, and often deleterious to sufficient stoma eversion. This most important step of stoma construction is achieved by cardinal 3-point absorbable 3-0 sutures picking up skin edge, the seromuscular layer of the ileum 2 cm under its distal edge and the edge itself (Figure 35.6). Further sutures inbetween the previous four cardinal sutures finally approximate the edge of the stoma to the skin (Figure 35.6, inset). Patency of the stoma should be tested by passing one finger through it deep enough so that its tip easily reaches inside the abdominal wall with a straight axis.

When the ileum has insufficient mobility to allow for a tension-free protrusion 2–3 cm above its distal end, a Turnbull loop stoma can be performed,[45] some recommend it routinely in obese patients. The distal end of the ileal loop is closed in two layers and a knuckle of the terminal end of the loop is then drawn through a larger abdominal wall hiatus. The antimesenteric edge of the ileal knuckle is incised and matured to the skin as described above after the two bowel segments have been fixed to the rectal fascia. This technique boasts a better arterial blood supply and venous drainage, and leaves a larger stomal hiatus with one small blind opening cephalad (Figure 35.7). However, controversy remains regarding the benefit of this technique.[46]

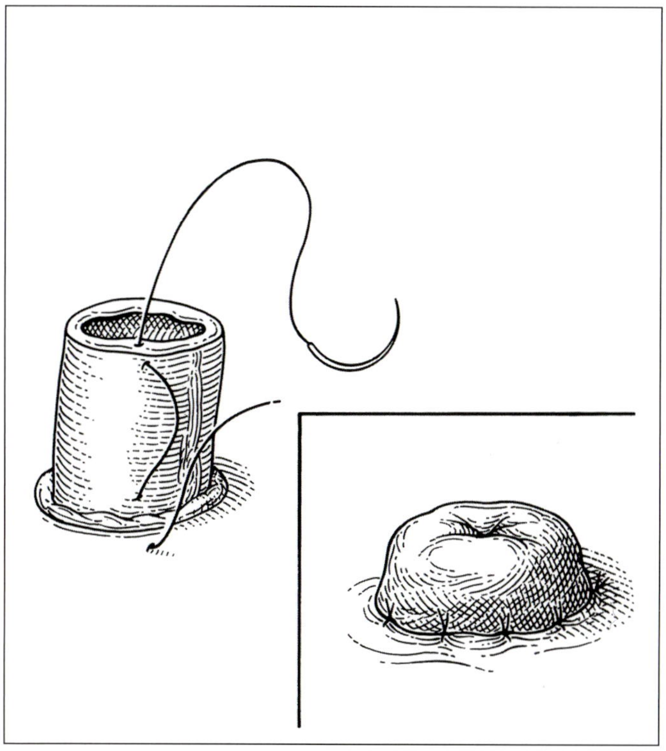

Figure 35.6 Stoma eversion. Cardinal 3-point absorbable 3-0 sutures picking up skin edge, the seromuscular layer of the ileum 2 cm under its distal edge and the edge itself. Further sutures inbetween the previous four cardinal sutures finally approximate the edge of the stoma to the skin (inset). (Reproduced with permission from Persky L. In Urologic Surgery. 4th edn. Philadelphia: JB Lippincott Company, 1991: 1004–12.[44])

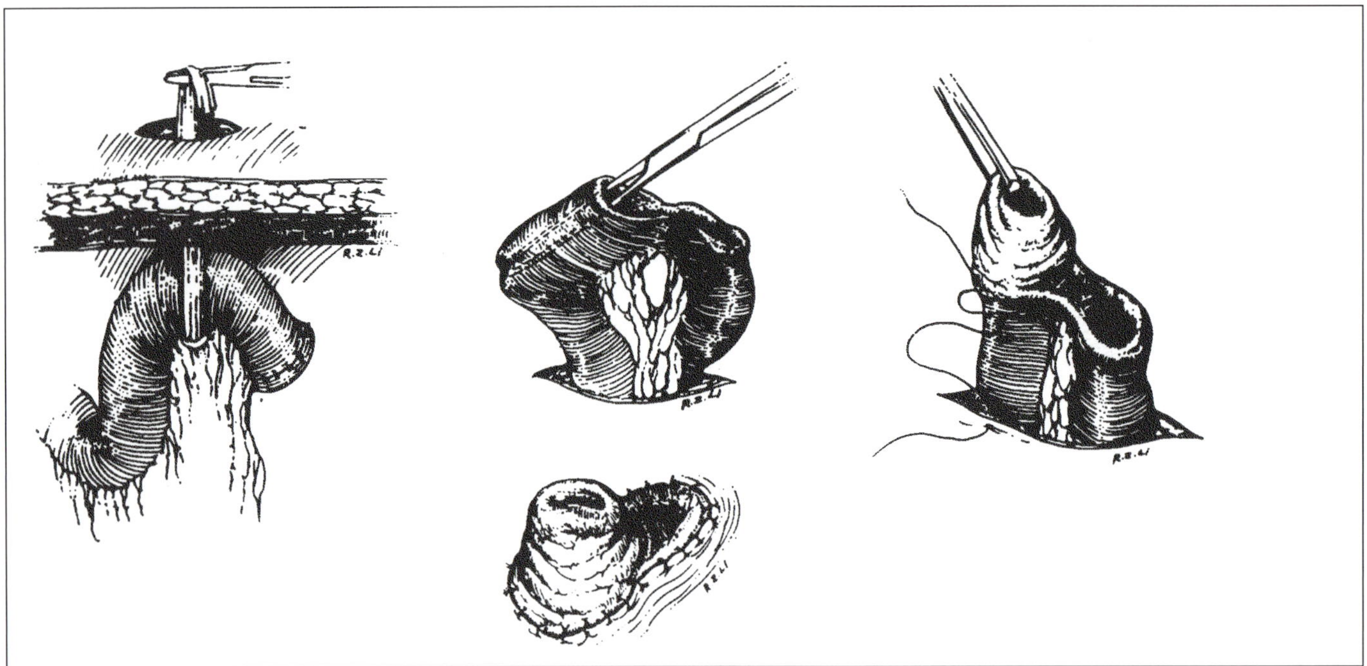

Figure 35.7 Modified Turnbull loop stoma. (Reproduced with permission from Vickers MA et al. In: Mastery of Surgery : Urologic Surgery Chicago: Little Brown and Co., 1992.[19])

Postoperative care

Usually, 8–15 days of hospitalization are needed, length of stay depending mainly on the occurrence of an extirpative procedure, its anatomic magnitude and patient age. Thromboembolic prophylaxis may be achieved by daily subcutaneous low-weight heparin and/or alternatively compressive boots. Broad spectrum antibiotic coverage is provided for 24–48 hours. The surgeon may then decide to pursue antibiotic prophylaxis because of the indwelling ureteral stents. For this purpose, a limited spectrum antibiotic may be prescribed at a prophylactic dosage (for instance amoxicillin 375 mg once daily, or trimethoprim-sulfamethoxazole 480 mg once daily). Intravenous hydration is continued until bowel activity returns, which triggers progressive oral diet resumption. Stents and stomal catheters have been previously discussed, and suction drains are removed once there is no more fluid production. If drainage persist, one should assess the creatinine content of the fluid to make sure if it is serum or lymph. If creatinine approximates that of urine levels, a contrast study should be performed to disclose an eventual urinoma, which may eventually be drained percutaneously. Gastrointestinal decompression is routinely done following urinary diversion, customarily by nasogastric aspiration, although some surgeons favor placement of a percutaneous gastrostomy tube peroperatively, which appears to significantly reduce postoperative patient discomfort.[47]

Upon completion of the diversion, the stoma is immediately fitted with an adequate appliance, whose adaptation will be checked closely on a regular basis during the early postoperative days by the stomatherapist.

Before bilateral antegrade ureteropyelography and stent removal, a broad spectrum antibiotic should be administered, and a kidney ultrasound performed to easily follow upper tracts in further sonograms, the initial one 3–4 weeks after stent removal. If there has been an extirpative oncologic procedure, at 3 months an abdominopelvic computed tomography (CT) scan with intravenous contrast is done followed by a KUB (kidney-ureter-bladder radiography). In benign instances, kidney ultrasound may suffice, and be performed at 6, 12 and 24 months. Serum electrolytes should be periodically checked because of the risk of impairment of renal function and metabolic acidosis. Vitamin B_{12} and folates need also to be assessed on a long-term basis, since their absorption occurs in the distal parts of the ileum.

Complications of ileal conduit urinary diversion

As in any major surgery, complications of ileal conduit can be prevented by careful preoperative strategy, meticulous peroperative technique, safe anesthesia and attentive postoperative care. By following these principles, one may markedly decrease the complication rate in the early postoperative period, and hence limit the occurrence of a 'cascade effect', in that one initial complication increases the risk for others. Late complications are frequent, occurring in up to two-thirds of patients, 40% requiring reintervention.[5] The occurrence of secondary malignancy is rare, and is discussed in Chapter 9.

Early complications

Mortality

Between 1950 and 1970, ileal conduit associated with cystectomy had an operative mortality ranging from 7 to 14%,[48–50] two-fifths of the deaths being attributable to ileal conduit.[50] Half of the patients die from those urinary or intestinal leaks that evolve unfavorably to sepsis, the other half from myocardial infarction, pneumonia associated with respiratory failure and thromboembolic complications.[4,51,52] Since the 1970s, death rates from radical cystectomy and ileal conduit have decreased from initially to approximately 3–4%,[4,53] and is presently down to 0–2% when the operative team is familiar with the operation.[54,55]

Ureteroileal leak

A urine leak was reported in 2–8% of patients in the pre-stent era,[49–51,53] and as exemplified above, is one of the most dreaded complications of conduit diversion, carrying a 50% risk of death in early series.[51,56] While it may heal spontaneously with drainage improvement, a urinary leak exposes the patient to ileus, respiratory problems secondary to difficulty in fluid management, thromboembolic events secondary to an increased inflammatory response in the abdomen, infections and nutritional problems. A 50% early reoperative rate is reported in series before the 1980s.[50,51] In this context, and with the improvement in stent material, endoureteral drainage was progressively introduced 25 years ago. Stent advantage has never been demonstrated in a randomized fashion. However, abolition of ureteroileal leaks has been reported in a stented group of 126 patients, whereas the rate was 3% in the control group including 236 patients.[57] On the other hand, stents may become obstructed if not rinsed when necessary, and lead to potentially severe infections.[58] However, modification of stent design to prevent obstruction has markedly improved their function.[59] Actually, wide stent usage and adequately indicated percutaneous abdominal or nephrostomy drainage account for the significant decrease rate of lethal urinary leaks, as demonstrated by the continent neobladder literature (see Sections 3 and 4).

Intestinal complications

Ileus may occur in 2–24% of patients, but responds most often to nasogastric tube aspiration. Mechanical obstruction may signify the presence of an anastomotic urinary and/or bowel leak, in which case appropriate drainage or judicious early re-exploration is indicated.

Leakage at the ileoileal anastomosis is rare, however with potentially lethal consequences[52] as described above, and if serious requires prompt reintervention. Abdominal revision is best performed within the first 15 postoperative days, since bowel distension, edema and adhesions may result later in a very tricky operative field.

Thrombosis of the ileal loop is exceedingly rare in the immediate postoperative period, and rather has been reported to occur years later in association with conduit volvulus.[60,61]

Wound infection

The incidence of wound infection is high, ranging from 10 to 30% of patients,[50,51,62] its association with fascial dehiscence being fortunately low. The former requires drainage and subsequent daily local wound healing care, while the latter prompts immediate surgical revision.

Late complications

Ureteroileal obstruction

Since it is most often asymptomatic, obstruction may lead to significant renal deterioration, patients at risk being those not followed routinely. Obstruction most often occurs at the ureteroileal anastomosis, but also where the left ureter crosses under the sigmoid mesentery. Mild pyelocalyceal dilation is not uncommon in the initial weeks postoperatively, but require precise radiologic work-up if it persists after 3 months.

Ureteroileal stricture occurs in up to 11% of renal units after refluxing anastomosis,[5,6,32–37] and ranges from 2 to 29% with the more seldom performed non-refluxing techniques.[40,42,43] Several investigators have reported an increased incidence of left versus right strictures,[50,63,64] most probably related to the additional mobilization required for the left ureter when it is brought under the sigmoid mesentery, which may jeopardize its distal vascularization. Open surgery remains the gold standard treatment of these strictures, especially when their length exceeds 2 cm. A midline or retroperitoneal Gibson incision is used to perform either a pyloroplasty type repair (Figure 35.8), a side-to-side bypass or an end to side reimplantation.[66] Parallel with the minimally invasive trend of surgery, endoscopy has been extensively used over the past 15 years to treat short strictures with various success rates. High-pressure balloon dilation was the first method used endourologically, but long-term follow-up has proved its minor efficiency in significant series, with success rates at 3 years of 5–15%,[67,68] whereas the 3-year success rate of open surgery was 76–80%.[68,69] Balloon dilation associated with electrocautery cutting wire (Acucise) appears somewhat more effective in series mixing various types of diversions, however the 3-year success rate does not go beyond 40%.[70,71] Cold-knife endoureterotomy approaches open surgery showed a 74% success rate at 2 years in a cohort including over two-thirds of ileal conduit patients, however, decreasing down to 61% a year later.[72,73] Holmium:Yag laser performs no better, with 1-year efficiency rates of 75–85%[74,75] decreasing to 56% at 3 years.[75] At a mean follow-up of 2 years, the latter series also reports 90% success for strictures equal or less than 1 cm. In conclusion, although open surgery remains the gold standard, endourology may manage a significant number of ureteroileal strictures when their length is less than 2 cm,[73,75] the optimal cutting modalities appearing to be the cold-knife or the Holmium:Yag laser. Permanent self-expandable metallic stents have been recently tried with an encouraging success at mid-term follow-up, however with a risk of stone formation, and a longer evaluation period.[76,77]

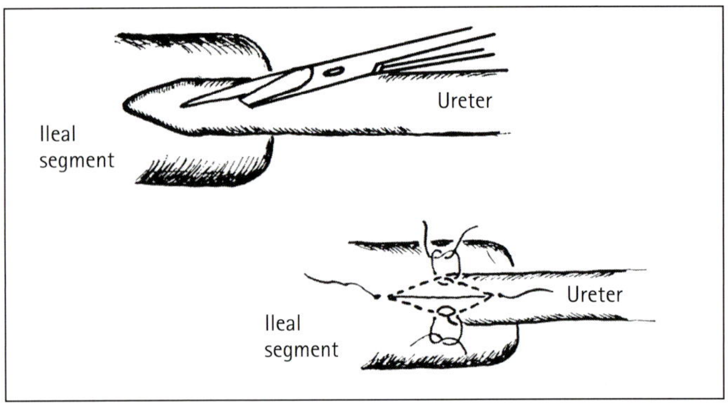

Figure 35.8 Pyloroplasty type repair of a ureteroileal stenosis. The strictured area is incised along the ureteral axis, and sutured in the perpendicular axis. (Reproduced from Bowles et al. J Urol 1964; 92: 630[65] with permission from Lippincott Williams & Wilkins.)

Strictures under the sigmoid mesentery usually belong to a long stenotic disease of the anastomosis and require open surgery as discussed above.

Stoma problems

Some problems usually occur late, and have fortunately been markedly reduced by the regularly increasing expertise of enterostomal therapists, but may affect a quarter of the patients.[5] A residual urine of 10 ml, free passage of a 12-Fr catheter and normal upper tracts characterize a healthy stoma.[78] Stenosis is the most serious stomal complication and has been reported in 5–10% of adults,[33,53,79] but is higher in children. In some instances, it may be due to an insufficiently protruding stoma which finally retracts and allows chronic irritation of the skin by urine, leading to hyperkeratosis and scarring which ends up in stomal stricture. Using irradiated ileum may also place the patient at risk for stomal stenosis (reference 79; Figure 35.9). The skin at the stoma site has also often been irradiated, and this may lead in conjunction with stoma retraction to marked deterioration (see Figure 35.9) with peristomal skin unsuitable for correct fitting of an appliance. A stenosed stoma initially causes dilation of the conduit, residual urine and infection, and may end up on the long run with upper tract damage. The stenosis may be at the muscle, fascial or skin level. The length of residual healthy conduit, the site and length of obstruction and the quality of adjacent skin will determine whether simple peristomal revision is possible, or whether laparotomy is needed with eventual addition of a bowel segment. When performing a local stoma revision, one incises circumferentially around the stenosed stoma and through the fascia and muscle, and the intra-abdominal portion of the ileal loop is mobilized so that its stenotic end can be resected and a new budded stoma fashioned (Figure 35.10). Obstruction at the fascial level may result from a shuttering effect due to the loss of alignment between the anterior and posterior fascia, which can be prevented by pulling to the midline the skin and fascial edges with clamps of similar lengths while creating the transparietal orifice for the loop. An inadequately sized fascial incision may also be the culprit, and requires surgery to revise the fascial incision circumferentially.[66]

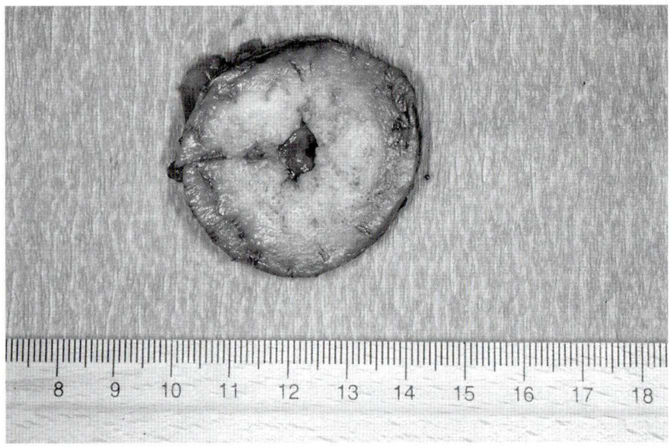

Figure 35.9 Excised strictured and inverted postactinic ileal stoma, with peristomal dermatitis (scale in cm). Ileal conduit performed for neurogenic postactinic bladder 34 years after radical hysterectomy with subsequent external beam and brachytherapy for invasive carcinoma of the uterine cervix. Reconstruction with distal amputation was needed after 6 months. This revision failed, and a further 15 months later, replacement of the distal part of the ileal loop was performed with a segment of transverse colon.

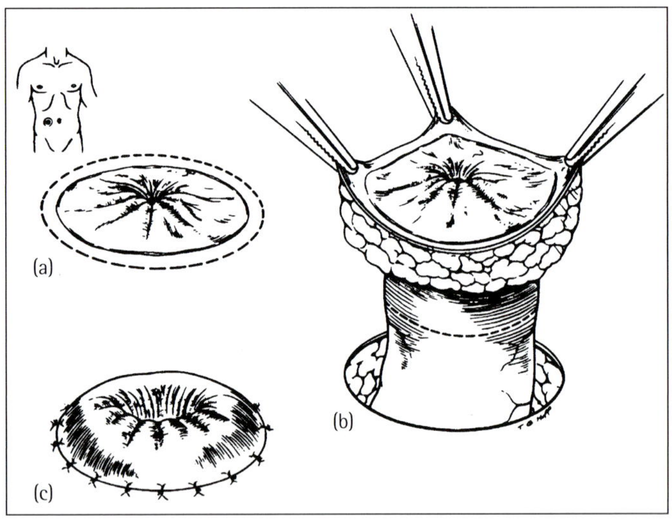

Figure 35.10 Reconstruction with distal amputation. (a) A circumferential incision is made around stoma; (b) mobilization of stoma and distal conduit and amputation of distal segment are performed, and (c) a new stoma is fashioned. (Reproduced from Bloom DA et al. In: Complications of Urologic Surgery. Philadelphia: WB Saunders, 1990[78] with permission from Elsevier.)

Other stomal problems include peristomal hernia (4–14%), stomal retraction (1–2%) and stomal prolapse (1–2%), each requiring surgical management in most cases.[78,80]

Kidney complications

Upper urinary tract stones occur in approximately 5–10% of conduit diversion patients usually more than 5 years later.[5,81,82] Pathogenesis is related to obstruction, increased chloride-bicarbonate exchange, acidosis, buffering by calcium absorption from bone and precipitation of calcium in the acid urine.[83] As for the rest of stone disease in urology, extracorporeal shockwave lithotripsy and endourology are now the two basic therapeutic lines used with a high success rate.[74,84–86]

Pyelonephritis was reported to occur in 6% of 500 patients undergoing ileal diversion for benign disease,[82] but in another series of 131 long-term survivors in 12%.[5] Also, chronic asymptomatic bacteriuria is a very common phenomenon in ileal conduit patients,[78] because of bacterial colonization of the distal 2–3 cm of the conduit,[66] its proximal part usually remaining sterile possibly because of secretory IgA produced by intestinal mucosa.[87] To detect a true urinary infection of the loop, catheterization is performed with a double catheter technique which bypasses the distal segment, a pediatric feeding tube being inserted through a 14-Fr Robinson catheter.[88] Treatment of pyelonephritis requires a targeted antibiotic and sufficient hydration. Obstruction has been noted in up to 87% of pyelonephritis cases in ileal conduit patients,[5] and must hence be ruled out by an emergency ultrasound, and eventually drained with a nephrostomy tube. In case of an obstacle, subsequent contrast studies are indicated to identify it and plan a therapeutic strategy once acute pyelonephritis has resolved.

In the long run, renal function deterioration is a common problem in urinary conduit patients, occurring in between 16 and 27% of patients,[5,89] and is due in half of the cases to hydronephrosis and in a quarter to nephroangiosclerosis.[5] This decrease in renal function appears to be identical to that of continent neobladders, as shown by a series with a mean 10-year follow-up after ileal loop, colonic conduit or continent cecal reservoir which found a similar fall in glomerular filtration rate in all three groups of about 15–20%. However, there is no anatomic obstructive explanation in conduit diversion for two-thirds of patients with bilateral upper tract dilation on long term follow-up,[35] which seems to be attributed rather to high-pressure reflux, unrelated to patient position.[89,90] Hence, regular long-term renal function follow-up is warranted in ileal conduit patients to prevent renal deterioration by prompt detection of obstruction, and adequate monitoring of blood electrolyte balance in those patients with preoperative damaged upper tracts.

Quality of life following ileal conduit

Interestingly, in over three-quarters of patients, ileal conduit does not reduce activity levels[91,92] which parallels the general satisfaction reported above. This emphasizes the astonishingly user-friendly aspect of this type of appliance-dependent diversion, and the high capacity of humans to react positively to significant body changes. However, subpopulations do not adapt as easily, such as patients receiving chemotherapy,[91] those treated for cancer[12] and females,[91] who also commonly report the negative aspect of an altered body image.[12] Several investigators have compared quality of life in conduit and continent neobladder patients. Surprisingly, there is no unanimity concerning the benefits of the latter[93–95] which, however, tends to report a better outcome in some series.[96–99] This dilemma appears to be related to the absence of prospective longitudinal studies, the lack of appropriate assessment instruments, and to confounding variables such as age, which is often different in the two populations and renders them inept to comparison.[11] Moreover, it is partly the upfront decision by the patient and the surgeon that minimizes differences in quality of life after surgery: once a type of diversion has been selected and performed, there is a strong tendency for the patient to want to believe that they made the right choice.[100] Nevertheless, continent diversion patients report less reduction in physical contact with partners,[96] less urinary leakage problems,[99] less decrease in mental health quality of life,[98] and less stoma-related problems.[97] Integrating these aspects would mean that patients with an active life benefit from continent diversions.[97]

Conclusions

During the early 1990s, it appeared that ileal conduit would be increasingly superseded by continent neobladders. However, distinct indications, its technical simplicity and the fairly recent significant reduction of its early complication rate still place ileal conduit as a major actor in urology at the beginning of the twenty-first century. Nevertheless, continent diversions will continue to challenge ileal conduit diversion over the next 10 years because of the evolving surgical education. Time will also tell whether the significant long-term rate of complications of ileal conduit will stand the comparison with the upcoming long-term follow-up reports of continent diversion series.

References

1. Bricker EM. Bladder substitution after pelvic evisceration. Surg Clin North Am 1950; 30: 1511–21 .
2. Ferris DO Hodel HM. Electrolyte pattern of the blood after bilateral ureterosigmoidostomy. JAMA 1950; 142: 634–41.
3. Pernet FPPM, Jonas U. Ileal conduit urinary diversion: early and late results of 132 cases in a 25-year period. World J Urol 1985; 3: 140–4.
4. Frazier HA, Robertson JE, Paulson DF. Complications of radical cystectomy and urinary diversion: a retrospective review of 675 cases in 2 decades. J Urol 1992; 148: 1401–5.
5. Madersbacher S, Schmidt J, Eberle JM et al. Long-term outcome of ileal conduit diversion. J Urol 2003; 169: 985–90.
6. Singh G, Wilkinson JM, Thomas DG. Supravesical diversion for incontinence: a long-term follow-up. Br J Urol 1997; 79: 348–53.
7. Golimbu M, Morales PA. Electrolyte disturbances in jejunal urinary diversion. Urology 1973; 1: 432–8.
8. Mansson W, Lindstedt E. Electrolyte disturbances after jejunal conduit diversion. Scand J Urol Nephrol 1978; 12: 17–21.
9. Hart S, Skinner EC, Meyerowitz BE et al. Quality of life after radical cystectomy for bladder cancer in patients with an ileal conduit, or cutaneous or urethral Kock pouch. J Urol 1999; 162: 77–81.

10. Mansson A, Mansson W. When the bladder is gone: quality of life following different types of urinary diversion: World J Urol 1999; 17: 211–18.
11. Dutta SC, Chang SS, Coffey CS et al. Health related quality of life assessment after radical cystectomy: comparison of ileal conduit with continent orthotopic neobladder. J Urol 2002; 168: 164–7.
12. Nordström G, Nyman CR, Theorell T. Psychological adjustment and general state of health in patients with ileal conduit urinary diversion. Scand J Urol Nephrol 1992; 26: 139–47.
13. Montie JE. Ileal conduit diversion after cystectomy. Urology 1997; 49: 659–62.
14. Iselin CE, Robertson CN, Webster GD, Vieweg J, Paulson DF. Does prostate transitional cell carcinoma preclude orthotopic bladder reconstruction after radical cystoprostatectomy for bladder cancer? J Urol 1997; 158: 2123–6.
15. Tefilli MV, Gheiler EL, Tiguert R et al. Urinary diversion-related outcome in patients with pelvic recurrence after radical cystectomy for bladder cancer. Urology 1999; 53: 999–1004.
16. Koch MO, McDougal WS. The pathophysiology of hyperchloremic metabolic acidosis after urinary diversion through intestinal segments. Surgery 1985; 98: 561–70.
17. Koch MO, McDougal WS, Reddy PK, Lange PH. Metabolic alteration following continent urinary diversion through colonic segments. J Urol 1991; 145: 270–3.
18. Mayer F, Lataillade L, Beyeler S, Iselin CE. La dérivation continente cutanée cathéterisable. Video presented at the Annual Meeting of the Swiss Urological Society, Lausanne, June 2002.
19. Vickers MA, Richie JP. Ileal and colon urinary diversions .In: Fowler JA (ed). Mastery of Surgery: Urologic Surgery. Chicago: Little Brown and Co., 1992.
20. Hewitt J, Reeve J, Rigby J et al. Whole-gut irrigation in preparation for large bowel surgery. Lancet 1973; ii: 337–40.
21. Irving AD, Scrimgeour D. Mechanical bowel preparation for colonic resection and anastomosis. Br J Surg 1987; 74: 580–1.
22. Santos JCM, Batista J, Sirimarco MT et al. Prospective randomized trial of mechanical bowel preparation in patients undergoing elective colorectal surgery. Br J Surg 1994; 81: 1673–6.
23. Kujat R, Creutzig H, Gams E et al. Metabolic changes after whole gut washout with an electrolyte solution. Dtsch Med Wochenschr 1982; 107: 537–40.
24. Kim HJ, Yoon YM, Park KN. The change in electrolyte and acid base balance after artificially induced acute diarrhoea by laxatives. J Korean Med Sci 1994; 9: 388–93.
25. Takada H, Ambrose NS, Galbraith K et al. Quantitative appraisal of picolax in the preparartion of the large bowel for elective surgery. Dis Colon Rectum 1990 ; 33: 679–83.
26. Shafil M, Murphy DM, Donovan MG, Hickey DP. Is mechanical bowel preparation necessary in patients undergoing cystectomy and urinary diversion ? BJU Int 2002; 89: 879–81.
27. Loughlin KR, Richie JP. Approaches in urinary tract replacement. In: Droller MJ (ed). Surgical Management of Urologic Disease: An Anatomical Approach. St Louis: Mosby Year Book, 1992.
28. Nesbit RM. Ureterosigmoid anastomosis by direct elliptical connection: a preliminary report. J Urol 1949; 61: 728–34.
29. Wallace DM. Ureteric diversion using a conduit: a simplified technique. Br J Urol 1966; 38: 522–7.
30. Le Duc A, Camey M. Un procédé d'implantation urétéro-iléale anti-reflux dans l'entérocystoplastie. J Urol (Paris) 1979; 85: 449–54.
31. Leadbetter WF, Clarke BG. Five years experience with ureteroenterostomy by the 'combined' technique. J Urol 1955; 73: 67–82.
32. Esho JO, Vitko RJ, Ireland GW, Cass AS. Comparison of Bricker and Wallace methods of uretero-ileal anastomosis in urinary diversions. J Urol 1974; 111: 600–2.
33. Pitts WR, Muecke EC. A 20-year experience with ileal conduits: the fate of the kidneys. J Urol 1979; 122: 154–7.
34. Svare J, Walter S, Kristensen JK, Lunf F. Ileal conduit urinary diversion – early and late complications. Eur Urol 1985; 11: 83–6.
35. Neal DE. Complications of ileal conduit diversion in adults with cancer followed up at least five years. BMJ 1985; 290: 1695–7.
36. Wiederhorn AR, Roberts M. Ureteroileal anastomosis. Comparison of Wallace and Bricker techniques. Urology 1974; 3: 168–70.
37. Morgan PR, Murdoch JB, Lopes A, Piura B, Monaghan JM. The Wallace technique of uretero-ileal anastomosis and its use in gynaecologic oncology: a study of 81 cases. Obstet Gynecol 1993; 82: 594–7.
38. Kelalis, PP. Ileal conduit. In: Hinman F Jr (ed). Atlas of Urologic Surgery. 2nd edn. Philadelphia: WB Saunders, 1998: 661.
39. Bricker EM. Current status of urinary diversion. Cancer 1980; 45: 2986–91.
40. Le Duc A, Camey M, Teillac P. An original antireflux ureteroileal implantation technique: long-term follow-up. J Urol 1987; 137: 1156–8.
41. Pantuck AJ, Han K-R, Perrotti M, Weiss RE, Cummings KB. Ureteroenteric anastomosis in continent urinary diversion: long-term results and complications of direct versus nonrefluxing techniques. J Urol 2000; 163: 450–5.
42. Shaaban AA, Gaballah MA, El-Diasty TA et al. Urethral controlled bladder substitute: a comparison between the intussuscepted nipple valve and the technique of Leduc as antireflux procedures. J Urol 1992; 148: 1156–61.
43. Roth S, van Ahlen H, Semjonow A, et al. Does the success of ureterointestinal implantation in orthotopic bladder substitution depend more on surgeon level of experience or choice of technique? J Urol 1997; 157: 56–60.
44. Persky L. Large and small bowel urinary conduits. In: Glenn JF (ed). Urologic Surgery. 4th edn. Philadelphia: JB Lippincott, 1991: 1004–12.
45. Turnbull RB, Fazio V. Advances in the surgical technique in ulcerative colitis surgery. In Nyhus L (ed). Surgery Annual Appleton-Century-Crofts, New York, 1975: 315.
46. Chechile G, Klein EA, Bauer L, Novick AC, Montie JE. Functional equivalence of end and loop ileal conduit stomas. J Urol 1992; 147: 582–6.
47. Van Poppel H, Baert L. The percutaneous operative gastrostomy for gastric decompression in major urological surgery. J Urol 1991; 145: 100–2.
48. Jaffe BM, Bricker EM, Butcher HR Jr, Surgical complications of ileal segment urinary diversion. Ann Surg 1968; 167: 367–76.

49. Daughtry JD, Susan LP, Stewart BH et al. Ileal conduit and cystectomy: a 10 year retrospective study of ileal conduits performed in conjunction with cystectomy and with a minimum five years follow up. J Urol 1977; 118: 556–7.
50. Sullivan JW, Grabstald H, Whitmore WF. Complications of ureteroileal conduit with radical cystectomy: a review of 336 cases. J Urol 1980; 124: 797–801.
51. Richie JP, Skinner DG, Kaufmann J. Radical cystectomy for carcinoma of the bladder: 16 years of experience. J Urol 1975; 113: 186–9.
52. Chahal R, Sundaram SK, Iddenden R et al. A study of the morbidity, mortality and long-term survival following radical cystectomy and radical radiotherapy in the treatment of invasive bladder cancer in Yorkshire. Eur Urol 2003; 43: 246–57.
53. Johnson DE, Lamy SM. Complications of a single stage radical cystectomy and ileal conduit diversion: a review of 214 cases. J Urol 1977; 117: 171–3.
54. Montie JE, Wood DP Jr. The risk of radical cystectomy. Br J Urol 1989; 63: 483–6.
55. Rosario DJ, Becker M, Anderson JB. The changing pattern of mortality and morbidity from radical cystectomy. BJU Int 2000; 85: 427–30.
56. Nichols WK, Krause AH, Donegan WL. Urinary fistulas after ureteral diversion. Am J Surg 1972; 124: 311–16.
57. Regan JB, Barrett DM. Stented versus nonstented ureteroileal anastomoses: is there a difference with regard to leak and strictures? J Urol 1985; 134: 1101–3.
58. Walther PJ, Robertson CN, Paulson DF. Lethal complications of standard self-retaining ureteral stents in patients with ileal conduit urinary diversion. J Urol 1985; 133: 851–3.
59. Gittes RF. Editorial: to stent or not to stent. J Urol 1985; 134: 1179.
60. Gardner TA, Poppas DP, Wei JT, Blaivas JG. Volvulus of the ileal conduit: a late complication. J Urol 1994; 152: 948–50.
61. Coxon JP, Jones CR. Two cases of patients with renal transplants presenting with anuria due to an infarcted ileal conduit. Transplant Int 2002; 15: 515–16.
62. Benson MC, Slawin KM, Wechsler MH, Olsson CA. Analysis of continent versus standard urinary diversion. Br J Urol 1992; 69: 156–62.
63. Skinner DG, Crawford DE, Kaufmann JJ. Complications of radical cystectomy for carcinoma of the bladder. J Urol 1980; 123: 640–3.
64. Vandenbroucke F, Van Poppel H, Vandeursen H, Oyen R, Baert L. Surgical versus endoscopic treatment of non-malignant uretero-ileal anastomotic strictures. Br J Urol 1993; 71: 408–12.
65. Bowles WT, Cordonnier JJ, Parsons RP. et al. Treatment of late ureteroileal stenosis following ileal segment urinary diversion. J Urol 1964; 92: 630.
66. Loughlin KR, Richie JP. Complications of urinary conduit diversion. Smith RB, Ehrlich RM (eds). Complications of Urologic Surgery – Prevention and Management, 2nd edn. 1990: 301–18.
67. Shapiro AW, Banner MP, Amendola MA et al. Balloon catheter dilation of ureteroenteric strictures: long-term results. Radiology 1988; 168: 385–7.
68. DiMarco DS, LeRoy AJ, Thieling S, Bergstrahl EJ, Segura JW. Long-term results of treatment for ureteroenteric strictures. Urology 2001; 58: 909–13.
69. Laven BA, O'Connor RC, Gerber GS, Steinberg GD. Long-term results of endoureterotomy and open surgical revision for the management of ureteroenteric strictures after urinary diversion. J Urol 2003; 170: 1226–30.
70. Wolf JS Jr, Elashry OM, Clayman RV. Long-term results of endoureterotomy for benign ureteral and ureteroenteric strictures. J Urol 1997; 158: 759.
71. Lin DW, Bush WH, Mayo ME. Endourological treatment of ureteroenteric strictures: efficacy of acucise endoureterotomy. J Urol 1999; 162: 696–8.
72. Poulakis V, Witzsch U, de Vries R, Becht E. Antegrade percutaneous endoluminal treatment of non-malignant ureterointestinal anastomotic strictures following urinary diversion. Eur Urol 2001; 39: 308–15.
73. Poulakis V, Witzsch U, de Vries R, Becht E. Cold-knife endoureterotomy for non-malignant ureterointestinal anastomotic strictures. Urology 2003; 61: 512–17.
74. DelVecchio FC, Kuo RL, Iselin CE, Webster GD, Preminger GM. Combined antegrade and retrograde endoscopic approach for the management of urinary diversion-associated pathology. J Endourol 2000; 14: 251–6.
75. Watterson JD, Sofer M, Wollin TA, Nott L, Denstedt JD. Holmium:Yag laser endoureterotomy for ureterointestinal strictures. J Urol 2002; 167: 1692–5.
76. Barbalias GA, Liatsikos EN, Karnabatidis D, Yarmenitis S, Siablis D. Ureteroileal anastomotic strictures: an innovative approach with metallic stents. J Urol 1998; 160: 1270–3.
77. Palascak P, Bouchareb M, Zachoval R et al. Treatment of benign ureterointestinal anastomotic strictures with permanent ureteral wallstent after Camey and Wallace urinary diversion: long-term follow-up. J Endourol 2001; 15: 575–80.
78. Bloom DA, McGuire EJ. Complications of urinary stomas. Smith Ehrlich (eds). Complications of Urologic Surgery – Prevention and Management, 2nd edn. 1990: 319–28.
79. Malgieri JJ, Persky L. Ileal loop in the treatment of radiation-treated pelvic malignancies: a comparative review. J Urol 1978; 120: 32–4.
80. Webster GD. Conduit urinary diversion. Webster GD, Goldwasser B (eds). Urinary Diversion – Scientific Foundation and Practice, 1st edn. Oxford: Isis Medical Media, 1995: 318–28.
81. Richie JP. Intestinal loop urinary diversion in children. J Urol 1974; 111: 687–9.
82. Koehler PR, Bowles WT, McAlister WH. Roentgenographic evaluation of late results of ileal loop urinary diversion in infants and children. Am J Roentgenol Radium Ther Nucl Med 1967; 100: 177–85.
83. Dretler S., Urinary tract calculi and ileal conduit diversion. Am J Surg 1972; 123: 480–3.
84. Wolf JS, Stoller ML. Management of upper tract calculi in patients with tubularized urinary diversions. J Urol 1991; 145: 266–9.
85. Cohen TD, Streem SB, Lammert GK. Selective minimally invasive management of calculi in patients with urinary diversions. J Urol 1994; 152: 1091–4.

86. Deliveliotis C, Varkarakis J, Argiropoulos V et al. Shockwave lithotripsy for urinary stones in patients with urinary diversion after radical cystectomy. J Endourol 2002; 16: 717–19.
87. Mansson W, Colleen S, Low K, Mardh PA, Lundblad A. Immunoglobulins in urine from patients with ileal and colonic conduits and reservoirs. J Urol 1985; 133: 713–16.
88. Smith ED. Followup studies on 150 ileal conduits in children. J Pediatr Surg 1972; 7: 1–10.
89. Neal DE, Hawkins T, Gallaugher AS, Essenhigh DM, Hall RR. The role of the ileal conduit in the development of upper tract dilatation. Br J Urol 1985; 57: 520–4.
90. Baltaci S, Bozlu M, Kosucu P, Beduk Y, Gogus O. Does the position of the patient affect the presence and/or degree of reflux in an ileal conduit urinary diversion? BJU Int 1999; 84: 433–5.
91. Babaian JR, Smith DB. Effect of ileal conduit on patients activities following radical cystectomy. Urology 1991; 37: 33–5.
92. Fossa SD, Reitan JB, Ous S, Kaalhus O. Life with an ileal conduit in cystectomized bladder cancer patients: expectations and experience. Scand J Urol Nephrol 1987; 21: 97.
93. Kitamura H, Miyao N, Yanase M et al. Quality of life in patients having an ileal conduit, continent reservoir or orthotopic neobladder after cystectomy for bladder carcinoma. Int J Urol 1999; 6: 393–9.
94. Fujisawa M, Isotani S, Gotoh A et al. Health-related quality of life with orthotopic neobladder versus ileal conduit according to the SF-36 survey. Urology 2000; 55: 862–5.
95. Hara I, Miyake S, Hara A et al. Health-related quality of life after radical cystectomy for bladder cancer: a comparison of ileal conduit and orthotopic bladder replacement. BJU Int 2002; 89: 10–13.
96. Bjerre BD, Johansen C, Steven K. Health-related quality of life after urinary diversion: continent diversion with the Kock pouch compared with ileal conduit – a questionnaire study. Scand J Urol Nephrol 1994; Suppl 157: 113–18.
97. Gerharz EW, Weingärtner K, Dopatka T et al. Quality of life after cystectomy and urinary diversion: results of a retrospective interdisciplinary study. J Urol 1997; 158: 778–5.
98. McGuire MS, Grimaldi G, Grotas J, Russo P. The type of urinary diversion after radical cystectomy significantly impacts on the patient's quality of life. Ann Surg Oncol 2000; 7: 4–8.
99. Hobisch A, Tosun K, Kinzl J et al. Quality of life after cystectomy and orthotopic neobladder versus ileal conduit urinary diversion. World J Urol 2000; 18: 338–44.
100. Smith AJ. Urological survey of urinary diversion. J Urol 2003; 170: 331.

36 Colon conduit diversion and special considerations in radiated patients

Joseph A Costa

Introduction

The colon possesses unique physiologic qualities which can be used to the surgeon's advantage: it consists of true serosal and mucosal layers which are easily separated for creation of non-refluxing ureteral anastomoses; it has a larger lumen than small bowel segments which reduces risk of stenosis; it has a much more mobile vascular pedicle which allows greater flexibility for stoma location; and it has multiple segments useable for diversion depending on specific patient needs.

The colon is a reasonable option in most patients requiring urinary diversion. Specific contraindications to the use of large bowel segments are listed in Box 36.1. The small bowel has been the preferred segment of choice for diversion for the majority of urologists since its population by Bricker in the 1950s.[1] Large bowel is an ideal option in patients who have been previously exposed to radiation therapy for treatment of pelvic neoplasia, who have had prior or are scheduled for fecal diversion, and in those who are best treated with a non-refluxing anastomosis.

BOX 36.1 CONTRAINDICATIONS OF USE OF COLON FOR URINARY DIVERSION

- Inflammatory diseases of the colon
- Active neoplastic processes
- Prior radiation exposure to segment
- Extensive polyp disease
- Extensive diverticular disease

Historically, anterior, posterior, or total pelvic exenteration has been associated with a high complication rate relative to other urologic procedures. Morbidity and mortality are certainly higher in patients who have received radiation therapy prior to major pelvic surgery. Survival rates of only 40% have been reported in the radiated patient requiring re-operation or salvage pelvic exenteration secondary to complications of primary therapy for pelvic malignancy.[2] With modification of technique and the advancement of technology more contemporary large series reports have a lower but still significant re-operation and mortality rate.[3] The most predictive factor of postoperative complications in the patient who has received radiotherapy is total dose.[4]

Experience with large groups who have undergone urinary diversion after prior exposure to or due to complications of radiation therapy support the use of transverse colon as a superior bowel segment of choice. In a study of 119 patients undergoing pelvic exenteration (98.3% receiving prior radiotherapy) secondary to gynecologic malignancy, Orr et al reported a 10.3% conduit/ureteral leak rate and a 3.4% stomal complication rate. Of their series of 119 patients, 97 were diverted with ileal bowel segments and 18 were diverted with transverse colon, the remaining four were not described. Three of four conduit and stomal complications were in ileal segments and the fourth experienced distal stenosis of a ureterocutaneous stoma.[5] Similar outcomes and recommendations of the use of transverse colon in radiation exposed patients have been reported.[6,7]

An additional 'subpopulation' of patients ideal for colon conduit diversion are those who have had prior or are scheduled for planned permanent fecal diversion. No large series for patients with this specific condition exists; however, several smaller series of patients have been reported.[8–10] This population allows for the prior defunctionalized limb or the existing or planned fecal conduit to be used for urinary diversion and for the surgeon to avoid the potential complications of an additional bowel-to-bowel anastomosis.

Preoperative evaluation

It is recommended that patients aged 50 years or more have a colonoscopy prior to pelvic exenteration and/or urinary diversion.[11] In centers where colonoscopy is not available, or if the patient age is less than 50 years, air contrast barium enema is a reasonable alternative. If contraindications to the use of colon segments are diagnosed on preoperative evaluation it becomes the surgeon's task to weigh the risks and benefits of using an isolated non-diseased portion of colon or operatively locate 'viable non-irradiated', ileum or jejunum at the time of diversion.

Standard oral and intravenous prophylactic antibiotics are used in addition to a mechanical bowel preparation. Preoperative discussion with the patient should include the possibility of placing the colon conduit stoma on either the right or left side of the abdominal wall. Contractile properties of colon when compared with ileum allow for placement of the colonic limb in either an oral to anal or an anal to oral orientation with satisfactory urine drainage[12–14] Therefore, bilateral abdominal wall marking for stoma location is recommended preoperatively in order to maximize operative options. Patient evaluation for stoma site marking should include the standing, sitting and supine position. Additionally, it is useful to have the patient wear trousers that best represent their usual attire including belt and height of waistband. When in doubt the patient may be allowed to wear an appliance for a period of time preoperatively to best decide where it is the least obtrusive during daily activities.

The radiation-exposed patient

Radiotherapy applications have undergone great change over the past 30 years. Improved treatment in the form of conformal, three- and four-field arc technique, and brachytherapy have allowed delivery of higher total dose and greater local recurrence-free survival. With the escalation of total dose delivered the recipient remains at risk for potentially devastating post-treatment complications (Figure 36.1). It cannot be understated how important it is to know the total dose of radiation previously delivered, width of fields treated, and whether or not additional brachytherapy or 'boost' doses were given to any fields of interest. Generally speaking, those receiving radiotherapy for rectal cancer undergo pelvic doses in the range of 45–55 Gy and those being treated for cervical cancer 60–80 Gy.[15,16] However, many protocols exist which call for much higher than standard dose delivery. Therefore, it is prudent to inquire as to whether or not the individual patient received boost doses to regions of unusually large tumor burden, a wider lymph region

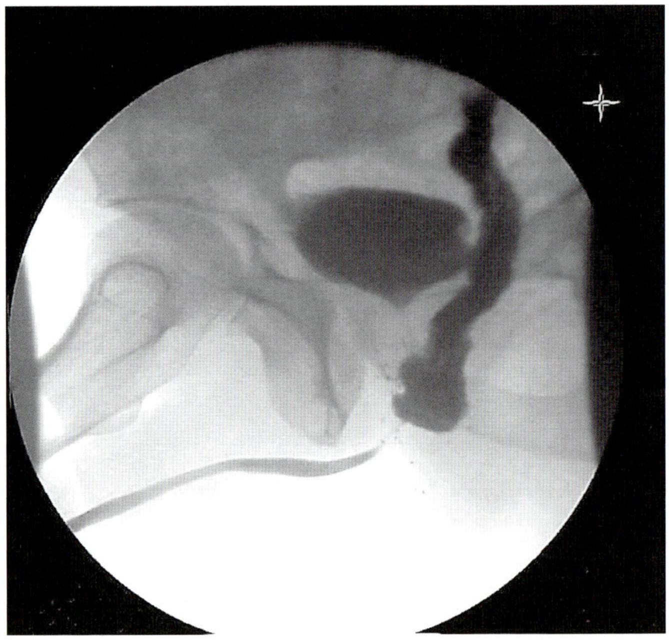

Figure 36.1 Example of a prostatorectal fistula secondary to interstitial seed therapy for prostate cancer.

secondary to positive nodes, or any other 'special' factors that involved the specific case. For example, a patient in the RTOG 97–07 (Radiation Therapy Oncology Group) locally advanced cervical cancer protocol may receive a 9.6 Gy boost dose over an 8 × 12 × 16 cm area over the cervix, mass, or involved parametrium in addition to the 85 Gy combined external beam and interstitial radiation.[17] This is a very high dose protocol, therefore future diversion complications should be anticipated and the operative procedure modified to minimize their likelihood. Time from radiation dose is another very important variable. The effect of radiation therapy on tissue viability can take years to develop.[18] Therefore, in the relatively recent post-radiation therapy patient, the surgeon may only have the known therapeutic field as a guide to determine how much or little ureter to excise and which specific colonic segment is the 'best choice' for use. Prior oral and intravenous contrast-enhanced computed tomography (CT) scans are extremely useful studies to review. In addition to thorough evaluation of the urinary system, they are helpful in predicting the likelihood of aberrant vascular supply to the colon, diagnosing aortic abnormalities, and helping to anticipate redundancy or other unusual characteristics in the bowel segment anticipated for use in diversion.

The patient with prior or planned fecal diversion

The patient who has a planned or a prior permanent fecal diversion presents a unique opportunity to the reconstructive surgeon. The stoma for fecal diversion can be converted to use for urinary diversion. In a retrospective review of 12 patients requiring combined urinary and fecal diversion, Costa and

Kreder found no difficulty with appliance continence or increased infection rate in patients who had prior fecal colostomies converted to urinary conduits.[8] If a large defunctionalized sigmoid limb was left after fecal diversion, and there is no history of pelvic radiation, it is reasonable to consider use of this limb for urinary diversion. Preoperative imaging with barium is very useful in evaluating the length of the intraperitoneal portion of the segment as well as evaluates it for disease, which would contraindicate its use. If the defunctionalized limb is not available for further use (i.e. prior pelvic radiation) or the patient has not yet undergone fecal diversion then the distal-most 20 cm of the segment of colon intended for diversion can be isolated for the urinary diversion.

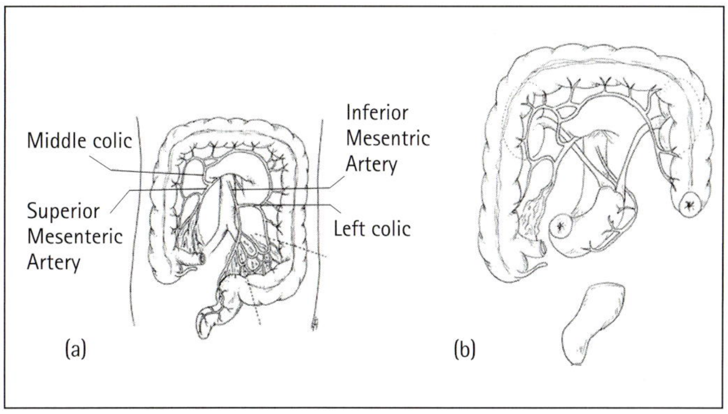

Figure 36.2 Combined urinary diversion in a patient without previous intestinal surgery. (a) Segment of sigmoid colon supplied by inferior mesenteric artery and its sigmoid branch is selected. (b) Urinary conduit fashioned from sigmoid colon and brought out in right lower quadrant in isoperistaltic fashion. End descending colonic colostomy brought out through left lower quadrant. (Reprinted from Costa JA et al. J Urol 2002; 167: 2063–5.[7] Copyright © 2002 American Urological Association, Inc. ®. All rights reserved. With permission from Lippincott Williams & Wilkins.)

Surgical technique

The patient is supine and dorsally flexed. The break is positioned at the level of the umbilicus to allow for the greatest increase in distance between the umbilicus and pubic symphysis. An infraumbilical incision is often all that is necessary for colon harvest, however, it is sometimes necessary to extend the incision a few centimeters cephalad in order to safely take down the hepatic, splenic or both ligaments for mobilization. Complete mobilization of the antimesenteric colon and removal of the greater omentum at the distal-most ends is recommended in preparation of the colon segment for harvest. Often, at least one of the colonic flexures needs mobilization for diversion and tension-free realignment of bowel continuity. The transverse colon conduit requires mobilization of the hepatic and splenic flexures, and transverse colon to allow for a tension free restoration of bowel continuity as well as good mobilization of the segment for urinary diversion. In the case of prior fecal diversion multiple options are available. The three most readily available options are: use of the prior sigmoid stump (not recommended in the case of prior pelvic irradiation); conversion of the current fecal diversion into a dual 'double-barreled wet' anastomosis;[19] and conversion of the fecal stoma into the urinary conduit and mobilization of the proximal colon to the contralateral lower quadrant with creation of a new permanent stoma. Examples of these options are demonstrated in Figures 36.2–36.4. Conversion of the fecal conduit for urinary diversion is relatively simple. At a point 20 cm proximal to the stoma the colon can be transected and is available for ureteral anastomosis. The remaining proximal limb is mobilized (usually requiring release of the splenic flexure) to the contralateral lower abdominal quadrant and a second stoma is created.

The transverse colon conduit is based off the middle colic artery. It is the most ideal segment for use in patients who have undergone prior radiation exposure because of its hepatic and splenic attachments 'hanging' this segment out of the pelvic therapeutic fields. Due to its mobile mesentery, vascular pedicles for colon segments do not need to be isolated as aggressively as with ileum. As previously stated, it is not absolutely imperative the transverse colon be aligned in an isoperistaltic manner. The colon's properties of 'mass contraction', as opposed to the primarily peristaltic waves of ileum allow for efficient emptying regardless of orientation. This physiologic property of colon allows for much greater intraoperative flexibility when determining stoma location or when which ureter to preferentially direct the proximal end of the conduit ureteral length is a concern. The colon is brought out through a cruciate incision in the fascia that will easily allow the passage of two fingers and a straight course for the colon to pass to the skin of the abdomen. The conduit is fixed at three points to the fascia. A fourth fixation point to the fascia can be avoided if concerns of accidental injury to the mesentery exist. The stoma is then matured in a standard 'rose bud', fashion with at least a 3-cm prominence from the skin to assure good appliance fit with a low likelihood of incontinence.

The most ideal form of ureteral anastomosis remains somewhat controversial. There are advantages and disadvantages of all forms. The benefits of a non-refluxing anastomosis and the more popular techniques are reviewed in Chapters 31–34 of this text. Whether a refluxing or non-refluxing anastomosis is desired, the colon is suitable for each. Surgeon preference may dictate the type of ureteral anastomosis; it is our preference to perform a modified Wallace 'end-to-end', anastomosis. The length of ureter used should be dictated by the field of radiation exposure, visual inspection of the ureter for viability, frozen section evidence of freedom of urothelial disease if applicable, and proper length depending which side of the body the stoma is going to be placed. For the surgeon planning a non-refluxing anastomosis, the possibility of aborting this technique should be anticipated due to inadequate 'viable' ureteral length. Stenting the ureteral anastomosis is much less controversial in the patient undergoing urinary diversion. In the case of the patient who has received prior radiation there is compelling evidence that the incidence of ureteral enteric anastomotic leaks are

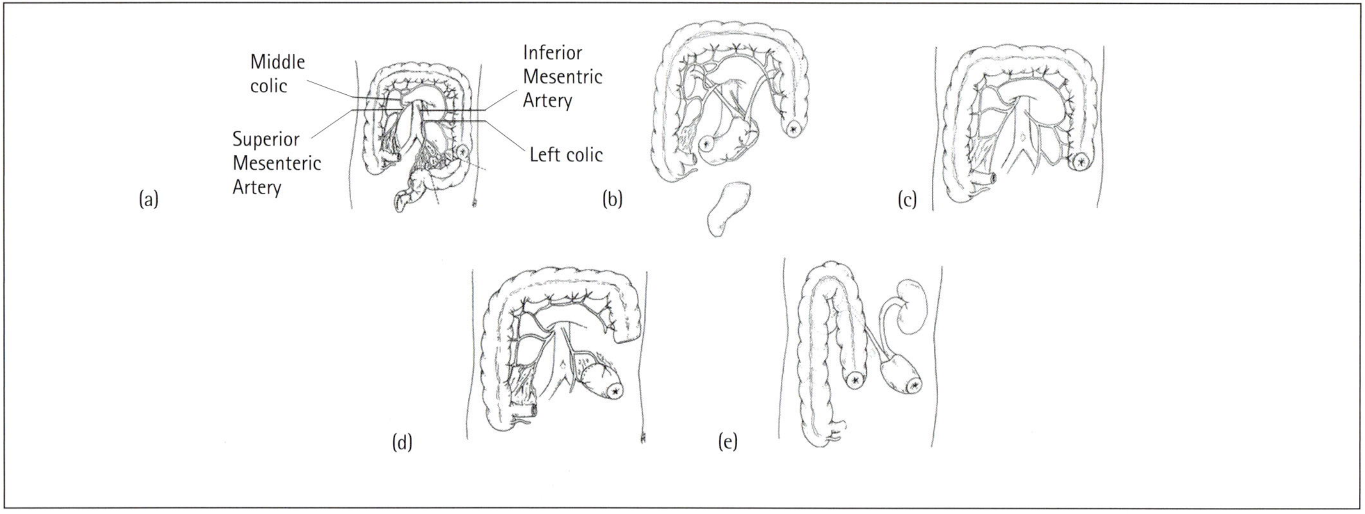

Figure 36.3 Combined urinary diversion in patient with colostomy. (a, b) Loop colostomy. (a) Distal sigmoid is transected (dotted lines) and colostomy remains in situ. (b) Sigmoid is then rotated in isoperistaltic fashion, ureters are anastomosed and ostomy is formed in right lower quadrant. Distal colon remains in place as Hartmann pouch. (c–e) End colostomy. (d) Distal 20 cm of colon are isolated, colostomy remains in situ and ureters are attached to isolated segment. (e) Colon is then mobilized to splenic flexure and brought to the patient's right lower quadrant. (Reprinted from Costa JA et al. J Urol 2002; 167: 2063–5.[7] Copyright © 2002 American Urological Association, Inc. ®. All rights reserved. With permission from Lippincott Williams & Wilkins.)

decreased when stents are placed at the time of surgery. Beddoe et al reported on a series of 75 women who underwent pelvic exenteration for gynecologic malignancy.[18] All 75 were diverted to transverse colon conduits and 74 of the 75 had prior radiotherapy. Thirty-seven women had stented ureterocolonic anastomoses and 38 did not have stents placed intraoperatively; other than stent placement, the technique of ureteral anastomosis was the same in both groups. Stents were removed on postoperative days 14–21. In the stented group

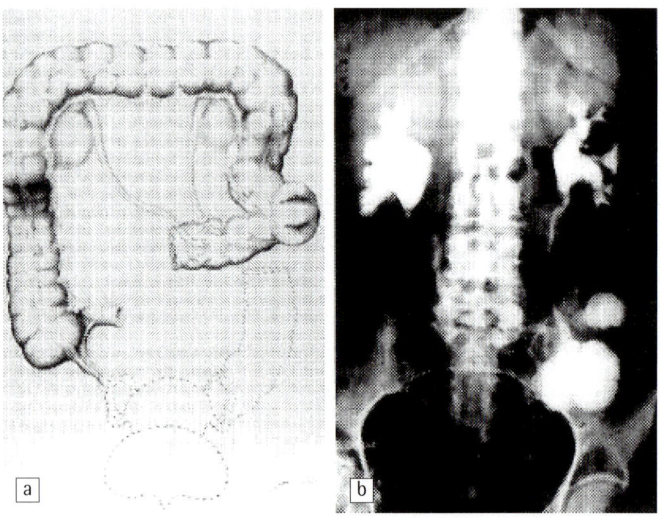

Figure 36.4 An example of the 'double-barreled wet colostomy'. (a) Double-barreled colostomy: surgical technique. (b) Intravenous pyeolography performed 6 months after surgery, showing good evacuation to the colonic conduit. (Reprinted from Osorio Gullan A et al. Int J Colorectal Dis 1997; 12: 37–41[9] with permission from Springer.)

there was a single ureteral unit that had an anastomotic leak (3%) while seven patients in the non-stented group experienced leaks at eight anastomotic sites (18% patients, 11% renal units). Among the stented patients three (8%) developed ureteral strictures and among the non-stented seven (18%) developed strictures.[18]

At least two closed suction drains are recommended after exenteration and diversion. One is left dependently in the pelvis and one approximates the area near the ureteral colonic anastomosis. Stents are typically removed on postoperative day 10 unless prior radiation is a factor (postoperative days 14–28) or the closed drain output near the anastomosis remains elevated. In the case of prolonged drain output a loopogram or intravenous pyelogram (IVP) are performed prior to stent removal to assure the conduit has no leak.

Postoperative concerns

Nasogastric tube suction is typically removed after the patient has active bowel sounds and tube output is lower then physiologic expectations. Perioperative antibiotics are continued for 24 hours. Daily, low-dose oral prophylactic antibiotics are started in the case of colon segment diversion until the stents are removed. It is not our practice to image the patient routinely at the time of stent removal unless the integrity of the anastomosis is in question. At 6 weeks postoperatively an IVP is performed as a useful baseline study of function and drainage. Additionally, basic serum chemistries are followed to assure the absence of metabolic disturbances from the diverted urine in contact with the colonic lumen.

References

1. Bricker EM. Bladder substitution after pelvic exenteration. Surg Clin North Am 1950; 30: 1511.
2. Symmonds RE, Pratt JH, Webb MJ. Extenterative operations: Experience with 198 patients. Am J Obstet Gynecol 1975; 121: 907.
3. Orr JW, Shingleton HM, Hatch KD et al. Urinary diversion in patients undergoing pelvic exenteration. Am J Obstet Gynecol 1982; 142: 883–9.
4. Swan RW, Rutledge FN. Urinary conduit in pelvic cancer patients, a report of 16 years' experience. Am J Obstet Gynecol 1974; 119: 6–13.
5. Bladou F, Houvenaeghel G, Delpero JR, Guerinel G. Incidence and management of major urinary complications after pelvic exenteration for gynecological malignancies. J Surg Oncol 1995; 58: 91–6.
6. Schmidt JD, Buschbaum HJ, Nachtsheim DA. Long-term follow-up, further experience with and modifications of the transverse colon conduit in urinary tract diversion. Br J Urol 1985; 57: 284–8.
7. Beckley S, Wajsman Z, Pontes JE, Murphy G. Transverse colon conduit: a method of urinary diversion after pelvic irradiation. J Urol 1982; 128: 464–8.
8. Costa JA, Kreder KJ. Combined urinary and fecal diversion using a no bowel anastamosis technique. J Urol 2002; 167: 2063–5.
9. Davis BE, Noble MJ. Simplified urinary diversion in patients with pre-existing or eminent colostomy. J Urol 1992; 147: 1245–7.
10. Osorio Gullon A, de Oca J, Lopez Costea MA et al. Double-barreled wet colostomy: a safe and simple method after pelvic exenteration. Int J Colorectal Dis 1997; 12: 37–41.
11. Mitka M. Colon cancer screening guidelines stress initial test's importance. JAMA 2003; 289: 1089–90.
12. Hinman F Jr. Volume and pressure in intestinal segments. Pediatr Urol Corresp Club Letter, 1987.
13. Kock NG, Hulten L, Leandoer L. A Study of the motility in different parts of the human colon. Resting activity, response to feeding and to prostigmin. 1968; 3: 163–9.
14. Schmidt JD, Buchsbaum HJ. Transverse colon conduit diversion. Urol Clin North Am 1986; 13: 233–9.
15. Gerard JP, Xie C, Carrie C et al. Curative external beam radiotherapy for prostate carcinoma: results in 231 patients treated in Lyon. Aust N Z J Surg 1999; 69: 707–11.
16. Perez CA, Lee HK, Georgiou A, Lockett MA. Technical factors affecting morbidity in definitive irradiation for localized carcinoma of the prostate. Int J Radiat Oncol Biol Phys 1994; 28: 811–19.
17. Clifford Chao KS, Grigsby PW, Stevens R. Phase I/II Study of concomitant parametrial boost radiation therapy for locally advanced cervical cancer. Radiation Therapy Oncology Group 97–07. Closure date December 1998.
18. Wammack R, Hohenfellner R. Reconstructive surgery in females with pelvic malignancy and radiation Injury. AUA Update Series 2000; 19.
19. Beddoe AM, Boyce JG, Remy JC, Fruchter RG, Nelson JH. Stented versus nonstented transverse colon conduits: a comparative report. Gynecol Oncol 1987; 27: 305–13.

37 Special considerations in neurogenic bladder patients

Thiagarajan Nambirajan and Ian K Walsh

Introduction

Since the major publications by Bors,[1] Comarr,[2] Guttmann[3] and others in the 1950s our understanding of and approach to managment of patients with neurogenic voiding dysfunction have evolved significantly. The management goals for these patients involve low-pressure storage, near complete bladder emptying at low voiding pressure, avoiding incontinence and protecting the upper urinary tract to preserve renal function. Since all these goals can be achieved by conservative treatment, this has become the mainstay of urologic management. Urologic complications accounted for the death of 30–50% of patients who sustained spinal cord injury during the Second World War.[4] In patients who could not be managed with indwelling catheterization, urinary diversion with ileal conduit was proposed and popularized by Bricker in 1952.[5] However, the long-term follow-up of ileal conduit diversion shows upper tract deterioration in 30–48% of patients and the need for reoperation in 32–60% of patients.[6–8] The introduction of clean intermittent self-catheterization (CISC) by Lapides and associates in 1972 revolutionized the management of neurogenic bladder.[9] By the end of the 1970s, there were very few indications for urinary diversion.[10] Urinary diversion is a viable option for patients who cannot be maintained on an effective conservative management program. A number of urinary diversion procedures are currently available and they continue to evolve. All options should be discussed with the patient and tailored to each individual patient's neuro-urologic status.

Initial management

In spinal cord injury patients during the initial shock period (4–6 weeks), the bladder is usually managed with an indwelling urethral catheter or intermittent catheterization. After the spinal shock resolves, reflexes return and the neurological state of the lower urinary tract changes according to the level and degree of injury. Clinical examination and urodynamic evaluation provide useful information regarding the storage and voiding function and coordination between detrusor muscle and sphincter complex. The conservative management program depends on the following: level of spinal injury; degree of neurological recovery; detrusor pressure – storage and voiding phases; sphincteric competence; manual dexterity and mobility; patient's wishes and expectations; and desire to maintain sexual function.

Conservative management

Madersbacher et al[11] have standardized the various types of neurogenic lower urinary tract dysfunction. The innervation to detrusor or sphincter is affected and both can become either hyperreflexic or areflexic. Clinically, four combinations are usually seen: (i) hyperreflexic detrusor and hyperreflexic sphincter, i.e. detrusor sphincter dyssynergia (DSD); (ii) hyperreflexic detrusor and hypo/areflexic sphincter; (iii) hypo/areflexic detrusor and hyperreflexic sphincter; and (iv) hypo/areflexic detrusor and hypo/areflexic sphincter.

CISC with or without antimuscarinic agents is suitable for motivated patients with good manual dexterity. Techniques such as triggered voiding and bladder expression have a minimal role in present day management. Indwelling urethral catheterization is usually offered as a temporary measure and the occasional patient especially someone with quadriplegia may tolerate urethral catheterization in the long term. A suprapubic catheter (SPC) might be necessary if patients cannot self-catheterize. SPC may not alleviate urethral leakage completely, especially in females. Any indwelling catheter carries the risk of repeated blockage, infection, stone formation, and bladder contraction, and the risk of neoplasia in the long term due to chronic irritation and infection. In the presence of the devastated urethra (urethral incompetence due to sphincteric weakness or pressure from longstanding indwelling urethral catheterization), it may be necessary to close the urethra or bladder neck surgically.[12] Condom catheterization has been used in male patients with urodynamically safe, low storage and voiding intravesical pressures. It can be combined with external sphincterotomy in patients with DSD. The major drawbacks are difficulty in retaining the condom catheter, penile skin erosion and bacteriuria.

Indications for urinary diversion

The majority of patients are initially managed with conservative treatment. There are a few patients who are unable or unwilling to perform self-catheterization. Complications include urethral erosion, bladder neck dilatation, devastated urethra, vesicoureteric reflux, recurrent pyelonephritis, persisting incontinence (urethral or pericatheteric). Decubitus skin ulcers associated with ammoniacal dermatitis, impaired quality of life and renal function deterioration can also occur in these patients. For most patients some form of urinary diversion is still the final solution to provide continence and protect renal function.

Bladder augmentation

High-pressure, non-compliant bladders can damage the upper urinary tract and result in incontinence if the detrusor pressure exceeds resting urethral closure pressure. If CISC and antimuscarinic agents fail to keep the detrusor pressure low, bladder augmentation can be considered to increase the bladder capacity and to keep vesical pressures low, thereby controlling incontinence and protecting the upper tracts. The patient should have good hand–eye coordination and be willing to carry out CISC. It is vital to establish that the urethra is competent for adequate storage. If not, a procedure to increase the outlet resistance such as placement of a sling or artificial urinary sphincter may be necessary.[13] If vesicoureteric reflux is present preoperatively, it is often due to high intravesical pressure from detrusor overactivity. As the augmentation lowers the intravesical pressure, the reflux disappears or is of a lesser grade. Rarely ureteric reimplantation is required to prevent recurrent pyelonephritis. Either small or large bowel can be used for augmentation, provided renal function is normal. In the presence of impaired renal function, stomach is preferred as this minimizes reabsorption and acidosis.

To date 30 tumors have been reported in enterocystoplasties and hence it is essential to follow these patients with cystoscopy or cytology, but the optimal method of surveillance is yet to be determined.[14]

Bladder augmentation with continent diversion

Bladder augmentation with continent diversion is suitable for the patient with a small hyperreflexic bladder and a devastated urethra requiring urethral closure or patients who cannot catheterize urethrally. The continence mechanism of such a conduit is based on the principle of an intussuscepted valve, e.g. intussuscepted ileocaecal valve or flap valve, or Mitrafanoff's principle using appendix, fallopian tube, ureter or small bowel reconfigured as a Monti tube.

Continent diversion

In severely contracted, fibrotic bladders not suitable for reconstruction, if the patient is willing to perform catheterization, continent diversion is a viable option. The continent reservoir is constructed based on small or large bowel or combination of both (see Section IV). The choice of the continent reservoir depends upon the availability of bowel and preference of the surgeon.

BOX 37.1 INDICATIONS FOR URINARY DIVERSION IN PATIENTS WITH NEUROGENIC BLADDERS

Bladder augmentation
High-pressure, small capacity, non-compliant bladder
Ability to perform CISC
Failed conservative management

Bladder augmentation with continent diversion
High-pressure, small capacity, non-compliant bladder
Incompetent urethral sphincter
Ability to perform CISC
Failed conservative management

Continent diversion
Catheter and condom drainage not suitable
Bladder not suitable for reconstruction
Ability to perform CISC

Ileal/colon conduit diversion
Catheter or external device unsuitable
Bladder not suitable for reconstruction
Inability to perform CISC

Incontinent ileovesicostomy
Catheter or external device unsuitable
High-pressure, small capacity, non-compliant bladder
Inability to perform CISC

CISC, clean intermittent self-catheterization.

Ileal/colon conduit diversion

The techniques for conduit diversions have been already discussed in Chapters 35 and 36. The main issue in these forms of diversion is long-term renal function. Long-term follow-up of ileal and colonic conduit diversions has shown renal function deterioration in 30–48% of patients and the need for reoperation in 32–60% of patients.[6–8] Early reports suggested a lower incidence of renal deterioration with colonic conduits but recent studies suggest that the incidence is the same. However, Stein et al showed 78% preservation of upper tracts with colonic conduits and continue to advocate colonic conduit over ileal conduit diversion.[15] Despite the drawbacks of these forms of diversion, the conduit has been shown to be a reasonable option in selected patients unsuitable for other forms of diversion. Bennett et al showed that the ileal conduit remained an effective option for female spinal cord injury patients.[16] Chartier-Kastler et al recently reviewed their experience with ileal conduits.[17] All patients achieved perineal dryness and all problems related to catheters and incontinence had resolved. Conduit urinary diversion has also been proposed in children as a temporizing procedure to either maximize renal function or to allow the child to grow older and become capable of coping with the responsibilities associated with orthotopic or continent diversion.

The issue of whether cystectomy should be performed at the same time as urinary diversion is still controversial. The estimated risk of need for subsequent extra peritoneal cystectomy is around 30% and the risk is higher in males.

Incontinent ileovesicostomy

Because of the complications associated with ileal conduits and retained bladders, investigators began to conceive a form of diversion incorporating the native bladder. In 1955, Smith and Hinmann described a series of canine experiments in which the animal's native bladder was left in situ and connected to the skin surface by an intestinal conduit.[18] The intent was to create a continent reservoir which would allow storage and drainage of urine. They theorized that by leaving the bladder essentially intact, the animals could void by normal detrusor contraction, and the urine would flow preferentially to the outside through the ileal conduit rather than the urethra. Incontinent ileovesicostomy or 'bladder chimney' in humans was initially described by Cordonnier.[19] He described a procedure where a tubularized portion of ileum was anastomosed end on to the bladder dome with a limited transverse cystotomy. Cordonnier's technique did not gain popularity because of failure of adequate bladder drainage in these patients. This was probably because of high outlet resistance across the tubularized ileum. The technique was later modified and perfected by Schwartz et al.[20]

Patients with neurogenic voiding dysfunction who cannot self-catheterize because of impaired manual dexterity (typically quadriplegics or patients with progressive multiple sclerosis) and patients developing complications because of indwelling catheters may be candidates for this form of urinary diversion.

Preoperative evaluation involves videourodynamic examination, renal function estimation, urine culture and ultrasonography to evaluate the upper tracts. Cystoscopy is warranted in patients with previous long-term indwelling catheters to exclude premalignant and malignant lesions. Preoperative preparation includes mechanical bowel preparation. Prophylactic intravenous broad-spectrum antibiotics are administered at the time of surgery. A 15-cm segment of ileum is mobilized about 30–45 cm proximal to the ileocecal junction. Longer ileal segments are selected in obese individuals. It is essential to keep the length to the necessary minimum as redundancy will impair the flow of urine and potentially contribute to electrolyte reabsorption. The native bladder is mobilized from the lateral pelvic sidewalls and opened by a transverse cystotomy. The proximal portion of the ileal tube is detubularized and anastomosed to the bladder in single layer. The distal end is brought out through the rectus muscle and fascia in the standard fashion for an ileal stoma. Both urethral and suprapubic catheters are left in situ (indwelling) to ensure adequate postoperative urinary drainage. We employ nasogastric tube drainage in the immediate postoperative period since these patients have neurogenic bowel dysfunction as well. Cystography is carried out at the end of 3 weeks and the catheters are removed if there is no extravasation of contrast (Figures 37.1 and 37.2).

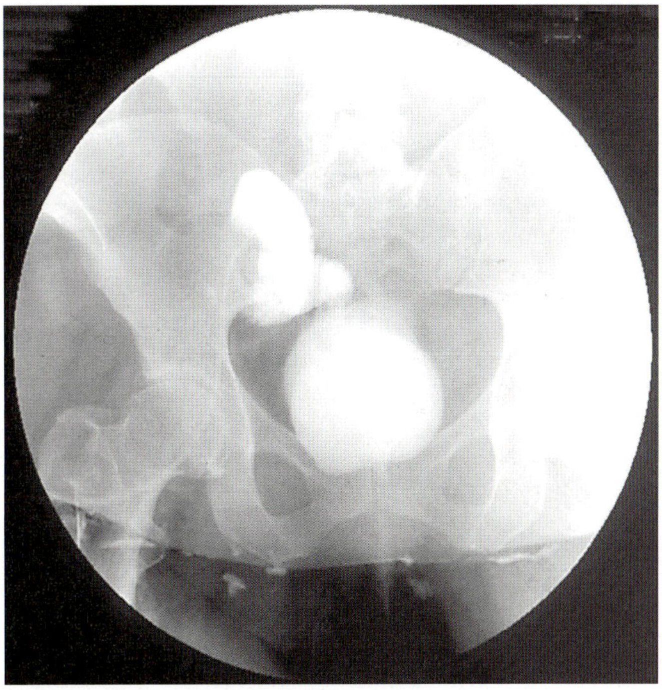

Figure 37.1 Incontinent ileovesicostomy – cystogram showing bladder chimney.

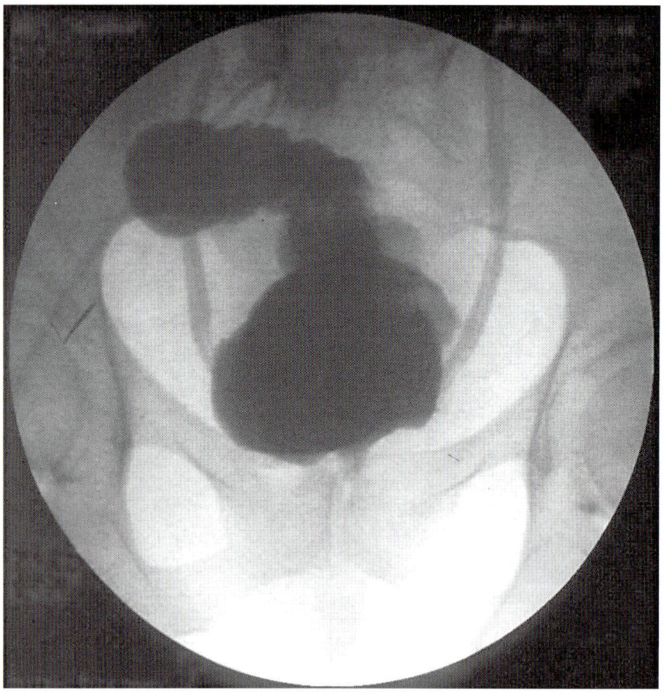

Figure 37.2 Incontinent ileovesicostomy – cystogram showing mild vesicoureteric reflux.

Results of various series of urinary diversion in neurogenic bladder patients

The first experience was reported by Schwartz et al.[20] A total of 23 patients underwent diversion and were followed-up for a mean of 43 months. Of 23 patients 22 achieved low-pressure storage and drainage. Upper tract function improved or remained stable in all patients. Complications included stomal stenosis in three patients and poor drainage across the ileovesical junction requiring revision in two patients.

Mutchink et al[21] reported their experience in six patients with no perioperative complications. Postoperatively, urodynamic examination demonstrated subjects to have a mean stomal leak point pressure of 7.7 cmH_2O (range 5–10). Radiographically, patients carried low urinary residuals (less than 100 ml) and did not exhibit vesicoureteric reflux. In the follow-up of 12–15 months, no patient demonstrated calculus formation, hydronephrosis, autonomic dysreflexia, or worsening renal function.

Atan et al[22] reported following up 15 patients for a mean of 23.2 months after ileovesicostomy. Fourteen patients had low-pressure drainage. Four women had persistent urge incontinence, which was managed with oral antimuscarinic therapy. One woman required cystectomy and ileal conduit for refractory urge incontinence. Renal function was preserved in all patients. Long-term complications included stomal stenosis in two patients, bladder and kidney stone formation in five patients and symptomatic urinary tract infections in three patients. The authors concluded that ileovesicostomy could be safely performed in both male and female patients with neurogenic bladders.

Routine surveillance for infection and stones is mandatory. It is a versatile procedure, as it can be converted to a conventional ileal conduit if necessary. In cases of neural recovery, the ileal 'chimney' can be excised and the patient's original lower urinary tract preserved.

Gudiazk et al reported their experience in 13 patients followed-up for a mean period of 23 months (6–57 months).[23] There were no intraoperative complications and no need for blood transfusion. The mean leak point pressure through the stoma was 8.2 cmH_2O. One patient underwent reoperation for stomal stenosis. One patient had a ureteric stone 2 years after surgery and one patient continued to have urinary tract infections.

Long-term follow-up (mean 52 months) of 38 patients (25 men and 13 women) was reported by Leng et al.[24] Before ileovesicostomy, the incidence of serious complications associated with an indwelling catheter was significant, including poor bladder compliance in 50% of cases, urosepsis in 45%, hydronephrosis in 21%, renal calculi in 18%, urethrocutaneous fistula in 18%, autonomic dysreflexia in 13% and bladder calculi in 2%. After conversion to ileovesicostomy, the results showed that 83–91% of this high-risk population maintained a normal upper urinary tract and normal bladder storage compliance. They concluded that ileovesicostomy is an excellent long-term management option for severe lower urinary dysfunction in patients who are unable to perform CISC.

Advantages of incontinent ileovesicostomy

- Technically simple with low intraoperative morbidity.
- Retains native bladder and avoids pyocystis and need for subsequent cystectomy.
- Achieves low-pressure drainage and protects upper tracts.
- Avoids complications associated with catheters.
- Avoids the complications of ureterointestinal anastomosis such as reflux and stenosis while maintaining native antireflux mechanism at the urethrovesical junction.
- Such reconstruction is reversible if the patient's bladder function is regained spontaneously or restored by neural stimulation techniques.
- Can be combined with ancillary procedures like slings or bladder neck closure for the incompetent bladder neck or devastated urethra.
- Its inherent design allows simultaneous bladder augmentation.
- Can be converted to ileal conduit easily, if needed.

Complications

Apart from complications associated with the stoma (stenosis) and bowel resection (stenosis, dehiscence), the specific complication related to ileovesicostomy is narrowing at the ileovesical junction. This hourglass contracture is avoided by taking care to construct a wide anastomosis between the ileum and bladder. Recurrent urosepsis is rare, but if seen would warrant videourodynamic examination. Other potential mechanical problems include kinking of the redundant ileal limb during bladder filling or stenosis at the abdominal fascial level.

In contrast to ileal conduit formation, there is a larger surface area of ileum exposed to urine with a longer contact time and hence the potential risk of electrolyte reabsorption is higher in patients who have undergone ileovesicostomy. This procedure is, therefore, best avoided in patients with compromised renal function. Patients with large capacity, atonic bladders tend to have higher residual urine volumes and are not ideal candidates for this form of diversion.

Summary

While the majority of patients with neurogenic lower urinary tract dysfunction are now managed with drugs and CISC, there is a subset of patients who need some form of urinary diversion. After the various options of urinary diversion have been discussed, the procedure can be tailored to the individual patient's needs, expectations, manual dexterity and the status of bladder reservoir and outlet.

References

1. Bors E. Urologic aspects of rehabilitation in spinal cord injuries. JAMA 1951; 146: 225.
2. Comarr AE. The practical urological management of the patients with spinal cord injury. Br J Urol 1959; 31: 1–46.
3. Guttmann L. Discussion on the treatment and prognosis of traumatic paraplegia. Proc R Soc Med 1947; 40: 219–25.
4. Graham SD. Present urological treatment of spinal cord injury patients. J Urol 1982; 126: 1–4.
5. Bricker EM. Bladder substitution after pelvic eviceration. Surg Clin North Am 1950; 30: 1511.
6. Dunn M, Roberts JBM, Smith PJB et al. The long-term results of ileal conduit urinary diversion in children. Br J Urol 1979; 51: 158.
7. Pernet F, Jonas U. Ileal conduit urinary diversion: early and late results of 132 cases in 25-year period. World J Urol 1985; 3: 140.
8. Svare J, Walter S, Kirstensin JK et al. Ileal conduit urinary diversion – early and late complications. Eur Urol 1985; 11: 83.
9. Lapides J, Diokno AC, Silber SJ et al. Clean intermittent self-catheterisation in the treatment of urinary tract disease. J Urol 1972; 107: 458.
10. Hackler RH. When is an ileal conduit indicated in spinal cord injured patients. Paraplegia 1979; 8: 135.
11. Madersbacher H, Wyndaelle JJ, Igawa Y et al. Conservative management in the neuropathic patient. In: Abrams P, Khoury S, Wein A (eds). Incontinence. Health publications, 1999: 775–812.
12. Hollander JB, Diokno AC. Urol Clin North Am 1993; 20: 465–74.
13. Strawbridge LR, Dramer SA, Castillo OA et al. Augmentation cystoplasty and artificial genitourinary sphincter. J Urol 1989; 142: 297.
14. Kälbe T, Austen M. Sekundäre Malignome nach Harnableitungen unter Verwendung von Darm. Akt Urol 2002; 33: 120–3.
15. Stein R, Fisch M, Stockle M et al. Colonic conduit in children: protection of the upper urinary tract 16 years later? J Urol 1996; 156: 1146–50.
16. Bennett C, Young MN, Atkins RH, Diaz F. Comparison of bladder management complication outcomes in female spinal cord injury patients. J Urol 1995; 153: 1458–60.
17. Chartier-Kastler EJ, Mozer P, Denys P et al. Neurogenic bladder management and cutaneous non-continent ileal conduit. Spinal Cord 2002; 40: 443–8.
18. Smith GI, Hinmann F. The intussuscepted ileal cystostomy. J Urol 1955; 73: 261–9.
19. Cordonnier JJ. Ileocystostomy for neurogenic bladder. J Urol 1957; 78: 605–10.
20. Schwartz SL, Kenneky MJ, McGuire EJ, Faerber GJ. Incontinent ileo-vesicostomy urinary diversion in the treatment of lower urinary tract dysfunction. J Urol 1994; 152: 99–102.
21. Mutchnik SE, Hinson JL, Nickell KG, Boone TB. Ileovesicostomy as an alternative form of bladder management in tetraplegic patients. Urology 1997; 49: 353–7.
22. Atan A, Konety BR, Nangia A, Chancellor MB. Advantages and risks of ileovesiocostomy for the management of neurogenic bladder. Urology 1999; 54: 636–40.
23. Gudziak MR, Tiguert R, Puri K, et al. Management of neurogenic bladder dysfunction with incontinent ileovesicostomy. Urology 1999; 54: 1008–11.
24. Leng WW, Faeberer G, Terzo MD, McGuire EJ. Long-term outcome of incontinent ileovesicostomy management of severe lower urinary tract dysfunction. J Urol 1999; 161: 1803–6.

38 Troubleshooting the problematic patient after conduit urinary diversion

Vincent Tse

Introduction

Urinary diversion – in the non-continent or continent form – has featured prominently in lower urinary tract reconstruction over the past few decades, with non-continent urinary diversion beginning in 1950 when Eugene Bricker[1] first reported the use of the ileal conduit, and continent diversion, especially the orthotopic neobladder in its various forms, featuring more prominently in the past two or so decades. Urinary diversions are performed for many different indications the most common following cystectomy for bladder malignancies.

There are many different types of urinary diversion, using various intestinal segments including jejunum, ileum and colon, and with respect to continent diversion, the segments can be made into a myriad of configurations. Since the advent of the ileal conduit, ureterosigmoidostomy is now almost of historical interest, mainly because of its many disadvantages, among which are diarrhea, fecal incontinence and the high incidence of malignant change at the ureterointestinal anastomosis.[2]

Although urinary diversion has been successful in offering patients a satisfactory quality of life,[3] it is not without complications. It is therefore of utmost importance that multiple disciplines, both medical and paramedical, are involved in order to offer the best preoperative, intraoperative and postoperative management if a successful, durable outcome is to be achieved. This chapter highlights specific aspects of pre-, peri- and postoperative care of the patient undergoing urinary diversion so that the risks of complications can be minimized. Metabolic sequelae, as well as voiding dysfunction after orthotopic bladder replacement, are covered elsewhere in this book.

Non-continent urinary diversion: the ileal conduit

Although many types of urinary conduit have been described, the most commonly used is the ileal conduit, which forms the focus on this section, with specific mention of other types of conduit where appropriate.

Complications of ileal conduit diversion

In order to troubleshoot complications associated with the ileal conduit, the reconstructive urologist needs to have a good working knowledge of its complication profile. Complications can be classified into general or specific. General complications are similar to those associated with any major intra-abdominal surgery, such as anesthetic, cardiac, pulmonary and thromboembolic events, as well as complications relating to the surgical wound. Box 38.1 gives a list of some common specific complications which may be encountered during the care of a patient undergoing an ileal conduit diversion.

Troubleshooting problems associated with the ileal conduit

In a large retrospective review (between 1971 and 1995) of the long-term outcome of ileal conduit diversion with a mean follow-up of 98 months (range 60–354), Madersbacher et al identified a total of 131 long-term survivors and an overall conduit-related complication rate of 66%.[4] The most common

BOX 38.1 COMMON SPECIFIC COMPLICATIONS ASSOCIATED WITH ILEAL CONDUIT DIVERSION

Intra operative complications
Short ileal conduit
Short ureter(s)
Ischemic conduit or stoma
Irradiated bowel
Abnormal intestinal position (e.g. in spina bifida)
Presence of Meckel's diverticulum

Postoperative short-term complications
Anastomotic leaks
  Enteroenteric
  Ureteroileal
Enterocutaneous fistula
Ischemic/necrotic stoma
Paralytic ileus
Metabolic derangements
Urosepsis

Postoperative long-term complications
Ureteroileal anastomotic stricture
Stomal stenosis
Stoma retraction
Parastomal hernia
Stomal prolapse
Peristomal skin disorders
Urinary tract infection
Calculi
Metabolic derangements
Malignancy
Pyocystis
Renal failure

complications were related to renal function and morphology (27%), stoma (24%), bowel (24%), symptomatic urinary sepsis (23%), ureteroileal anastomosis (14%) and urolithiasis (9%). At 5 years, 45% of patients experienced a complication. This figure increased to 50%, 54% and 94% when follow-up was extended to 10, 15 and longer than 15 years, respectively. Some 40% of patients in the series required surgical re-intervention. This study underpins the importance of meticulous attention to detail in the total care of these patients and that vigorous long-term follow-up is crucial in identifying potential problems as some complications do not surface until late in follow-up.

Troubleshooting preoperatively

Preoperative assessment

Effective troubleshooting starts with a comprehensive clinical assessment of the patient, because patient selection is a major factor in determining long-term success.

The patient's general medical condition, mental state, manual dexterity, body habitus and social support are important considerations. Death from anesthesia is uncommon, whereas the risk of acute myocardial infarction is reported to be 0.1–0.7% within 5 days of surgery, and increases to 6% in patients with a previous myocardial infarct.[5] In patients with an impaired sensorium such as dementia, a conduit may not be ideal as they may dislodge stomal appliances during periods of confusion, causing skin excoriations and undesirable nursing difficulty for the carer. Impaired manual dexterity will be an issue in patients who wish to care for their own stoma. Obese patients always pose a challenge but preoperative assessment will allow for more careful stoma siting to avoid urine leakage, thought given to troubleshoot by using a longer conduit length or a Turnbull's loop. If the diversion is not medically urgent, assessment by a dietitian and a weight loss program may also be beneficial. Patients with spina bifida often have very little abdominal wall on which to place the stoma, and careful stomal siting is paramount. Patients who live in remote areas may have limited access to stomal appliances and specialist urological care, so they should be given adequate contact information and warned to send for supplies well in advance and to attend regular urological follow-up so problems can be minimized, or tackled expeditiously if encountered.

A detailed medical history needs to be elicited. A history of inflammatory bowel disease, diverticular disease, previous bowel resection and pelvic irradiation may alter the selection of bowel segments and length used. Crohn's disease has been reported to develop in ileal conduits causing diffuse conduit inflammation and subsequent stenosis.[6,7] Consistency and frequency of bowel motions may worsen in patients who have had previous bowel resections. Both ileum and colon results in similar functional and metabolic outcomes. Hyperchloremic metabolic acidosis is expected secondary to luminal bicarbonate loss and active hydrogen ion and ammonium reabsorption. Severity of the acidosis is dependent on renal function, contact time of urine with the conduit mucosa, and the effectiveness of conduit drainage. The patient should give informed consent and needs to understand the potential need for long-term oral bicarbonate supplementation, and the long-term risks of the untreated acidosis such as bone demineralization, neuromuscular dysfunction from hypomagnesemia, encephalopathy, and malabsorption.[8] Patients with chronically raised intra-abdominal pressure (e.g.

chronic cough from chronic obstructive airways disease) may have increased incidence of incisional hernia and stomal prolapse.[9] Poor nutritional status, diabetes mellitus and post-pelvic radiotherapy patients may be associated with poorer and prolonged wound healing, wound infection and dehiscence.

Selection of bowel segments

Jejunal conduits have largely fallen out of favor due to the high incidence of metabolic complications secondary to salt and water loss. Ileal and colonic conduits have stood the test of time and continued to be used. Although there are no randomized trials, in terms of complications related to the stoma and uretero–conduit anastomosis, as well as to long-term renal function, the ileal and colonic conduits appear to have similar outcomes.[10–12] Due to the relative ease of performing an ileal conduit, this remains the bowel segment of choice. Colonic segments are limited to selected scenarios, such as short ureters, irradiated small bowel, and loss of terminal ileum from other causes such as inflammatory bowel disease.

Troubleshooting intraoperatively

'Short' ileal conduit

Generally, a length of 12–15 cm of bowel is measured and then harvested for conduit formation. In an ileal conduit, the distal 61 cm of terminal ileum is spared to reduce the incidence of vitamin B_{12} and bile salt malabsorption. A conduit often shrinks immediately after it is harvested due to smooth muscle spasm. This should not be mistaken for a short conduit. In obese patients, a longer conduit should be judiciously planned preoperatively to traverse the thick abdominal wall. If the conduit does appear too short to be able to reach the skin without tension, several maneuvers have been described to lengthen the mobility of the distal conduit.

Aggressive division of the mesentery, taking care not to damage the proximal ileocolic artery, may provide more length. A series of short horizontal slits in the avascular portions of the small bowel mesentery may allow the mesentery to lengthen to a small degree when the conduit is brought towards the skin. Daniel's technique of discarding a segment of bowel immediately distal to the conduit will reduce the incidence of conduit ischemia as it traverses through a thick abdominal wall.[13] However, this needs to be planned preoperatively since a longer segment of ileum needs to be harvested because the distal end will be discarded. Another technique based on a similar rationale of reducing mesenteric tension is the Turnbull's loop stoma. A knuckle of the distal conduit is brought through the rectus sheath. The antimesenteric border is longitudinally incised, forming a short loop urostomy, allowing circumferential stomal maturation without tension on mesenteric blood supply.

It is not common practice to add another bowel segment to the already short conduit because an additional two bowel anastomoses need to be created and increase the incidence of anastomotic complications. Bringing the short conduit out to the skin via the shortest possible route is also ill-advised as the patient may experience urine leakage when the stoma is not sited where it should be.

'Short' ureters

The ureters should be left as long as possible. They may have to be shortened because of the need to resect tumor or carcinoma in situ on intraoperative frozen section, poor condition (e.g. ischemia or pelvic irradiation), or poor surgical technique (ureters transected too high). The mesenteric window of the sigmoid needs to be generous so that the left ureter can be brought into the right hemiabdomen without tension or kinking. If the left ureter needs to be mobilized, care must be taken to preserve the subadventitial vascular plexus to prevent ischemia. If both ureters are short, a transverse colon conduit should be contemplated. If one ureter is short, options include an ileal interposition, transureteroureterostomy, ipsilateral renal autotransplant, and nephrectomy.

Intraoperative conduit or stomal ischemia

This situation is best avoided by careful assessment of the mesenteric vasculature before its division. The mesentery must not be stretched or pulled with force. This can lead to intimal tears in the arteries and subsequent thrombosis. All vessels should be carefully dissected out and ligated to prevent mesenteric hematomas. Attention should also be paid to the anatomical lie of the conduit. There should be no twisting or kinking as both vasculature and urinary drainage may be compromised. During closure of the mesenteric defect, care should be exercised to avoid laceration of mesenteric vessels. In the intraoperative or early postoperative period, it is not unusual for the stoma to appear a little dusky from edema and associated venous congestion. This often settles after a few days.

Irradiated bowel

The reconstructive urologist should be familiar with the distinct features of irradiated bowel. The bowel wall is often thickened and indurated to palpation and appears edematous compared with normal segments. The bowel may look pale with telangiectasia on its serosa. Its wall may even be friable on suturing. Segments with these features should be avoided to minimize postoperative complications, such as anastomotic leakage, fistula, stricture and conduit necrosis or stenosis. If no suitable ileum is identified, consideration should be given for a transverse colon conduit in the upper abdomen.

Other intraoperative problems

Patients with spina bifida may have unusual intra-abdominal anatomy. Their cecum and ascending colon may assume an abnormally high position towards the right upper quadrant. Hence the ileocecal junction and terminal ileum may not be where they normally rest. The surgeon should watch out for a Meckel's diverticulum. Although there are reports of using Meckel's diverticulum during Mitrofanoff procedures,[14] attention should be paid not to inadvertently incorporate a Meckel's diverticulum into the ileal conduit lest it becomes inflamed and causes an acute abdomen.

Troubleshooting early postoperative problems

Anastomotic leaks

Leaks may occur at two sites, the enteroenteric and the ureteroileal anastomoses. They occur usually due to two major causes – poor quality tissues and suboptimal surgical technique.

Enteroenteric anastomotic leak

Leakage in this area is a major postoperative morbidity. There are several issues which the surgeon needs to bear in mind intraoperatively to prevent its occurrence. Healthy bowel needs to be used. Irradiated segments must be avoided. Any ischemic or dusky ends should be resected before anastomosis. Meticulous attention is paramount when performing the anastomosis. If a stapler gun is used, one must ensure the segments are approximated at the antimesenteric border to avoid compromising intestinal blood supply. The anastomosis should be checked to ensure correct firing of the stapler. A 'safety' absorbable suture at the mesenteric end of the stapled anastomosis is preferred by many surgeons. In cases where there had been pelvic irradiation and extensive division of adhesions, the entire intestinal tract should be inspected at the end of the operation to exclude any inadvertent perforation of the bowel.

An extensive retrospective review with a mean follow-up of 8 years reported that bowel fistula occurred when a double-layer small bowel anastomosis with interrupted silk and chromic catgut was used. Bowel fistulas were not seen after the technique was changed to a single-layer seromuscular end-to-end anastomosis.[4] Unless the leak is small, most patients are managed by total parenteral nutrition or a low residual diet until the leak or fistula heals. Prompt surgical revision of the anastomosis is necessary in major leaks.

Ureteroileal anastomotic leak

A basic surgical principle in any good anastomosis is that it should be well vascularized, tension-free, mucosa-to-mucosa, water-tight and without distal obstruction. This is especially true of the ureteroileal anastomosis which is unforgiving to a deficit in any of the above.

Utmost care must be taken during mobilization of the ureter to preserve the subadventitial ureteric arterial plexus which run longitudinally along the entire length of the ureter.[15] This is especially important in the irradiated patient because blood supply is already tenuous from the effects of endarteritis obliterans. An adequate mesenteric window is crucial in preventing kinking of the ureter when brought under the sigmoid mesocolon. This also prevent excessive tension on the anastomosis. When preparing the distal ureteric ends, the author prefers to leave a tongue of ureteric sheath (adventitia) distal to the spatulated end which can be used to cover up the anastomosis. This tissue is supple and well vascularized and may aid in preventing leaks and providing blood supply toward a healthy anastomosis.

The two common types of anastomosis used nowadays are the Bricker[1] and Wallace anastomoses.[16] Favorable results have been seen with both techniques: the risk of stricture is slightly greater with the Bricker technique, and the risk of leakage is possibly greater with the Wallace anastomosis.[17] The Bricker anastomosis is preferred in conduits performed for urothelial malignancies. It may be easier to catheterize the ureters retrogradely with the Wallace anastomosis and hence may be a better option in patients who may require retrograde instrumentation, e.g. in those with recurrent urolithiasis. The author prefers using 4-0 Vicryl interrupted sutures with particular attention paid to the apical suture. A variety of ureterocolic anastomoses have been described, with the most commonly used being the antireflux subtenial anastomosis, although the issue of whether an antireflux mechanism is beneficial remains controversial.

Although not evidence based, most surgeons prefer the use of a stent across the anastomosis in the early postoperative period. There are many types of stent used, including single and double J stents, and 5-Fr infant feeding tubes. Stents may reduce leakage by channeling urine away from the anastomosis during the healing phase. They ensure patency of the anastomosis during the first few postoperative days when edema may narrow the anastomosis. They also provide access to the pelvicalyceal system if imaging studies are required to check for healing of the anastomoses.

Conservative management of the leak include ensuring conduit patency and maximizing drainage with a catheter without inflating the balloon, removing suction from the surgical drains, percutaneous nephrostomies and prophylactic antibiotics. If leakage is profuse despite the above, surgical revision may be indicated. In delayed leakage more than 7–10 days postoperatively, ischemic ureteric necrosis is likely. Surgical revision is usually required either early for a major leak, or after a 2–3-month period if leakage is reduced but persists as a fistula after percutaneous nephrostomies. Due to the suboptimal state of the distal ureteric ends and the surrounding friable tissues, revision reimplantation of the ureter often require meticulous attention. A new site on the conduit should be made and the old defect closed. Surgical diathermy should be kept to a minimum during preparation of the anastomosis to prevent ischemia and necrosis. Bipolar diathermy should be sparingly used if required. Interrupted sutures should be used. A stent should be left across the new anastomosis. The patient's nutritional status should also be maximized, possibly with the assistance of a hospital dietitian, to effect optimal wound healing.

Stomal ischemia and necrosis

Most conduit-related long-term morbidity centers around the stoma, affecting between 25 and 63% of cases.[4,18–20] Meticulous attention needs to be paid to the preparation of the stoma as it may lead to long-term complications and it is the component with which the patient has direct contact and ultimately influences quality of life.

Several technical points are important in preventing stomal ischemia or necrosis. Sufficient abdominal opening is needed to avoid strangulation of the conduit as it traverses through the abdominal wall. As mentioned earlier, the conduit mesentery must not be under excessive tension when the conduit is carried through to the skin. A dusky looking stoma in the early postoperative period may not always signify an impending disaster as early edema may impair venous drainage and gives rise to the dusky discoloration which often settle after 2–3 days. However, if there is progressive deterioration of the viability of the stoma or if frank necrosis occurs, urgent surgical revision is required to prevent subsequent urine extravasation and sepsis. Vascular insufficiency and scarring caused by chronic infection may contribute to the reported 'pipe stem' deformity of the conduit.[21]

Paralytic ileus

It is not unusual to see paralytic ileus in the early postoperative period. It often resolves spontaneously with patient recovery and mobility. It is important to ensure plasma electrolytes are within normal limits and replenish as necessary as low potassium, magnesium and calcium states may retard gut motility. More sinister causes of ileus include anastomotic leaks, fistulaes, bowel ischemia and infarction.

Urosepsis

The occurrence of early pyelonephritis is reported to be between 1.8 and 3.1%.[17] This incidence is low perhaps due to the common use of prophylactic antibiotics in the early postoperative period, especially when ureteric stents are still in place. It is important to give the patient prophylactic antibiotics if a retrograde study is to be performed through the stents to reduce the risk of bacteremia and possible septic shock, as the stents are often colonized with bacteria. Patients at risk of postoperative urosepsis are those with poorly controlled diabetes, chronic corticosteroid ingestion and other immunosuppressed conditions.

Troubleshooting long-term postoperative problems

Ureteroileal anastomotic stricture

Ureteroileal strictures following urinary diversion have an incidence of 2–18%.[22,23] Causes include previous urinary extravasation, tension at the anastomosis, vascular compromise, prior pelvic irradiation and tumour recurrence in cases of previous urothelial malignancies. These patients may be totally asymptomatic, or present with impaired renal function, hydronephrosis, flank pain or urosepsis.

The principles of management include determining the nature of the anastomotic stricture, whether the kidney is obstructed and exacting the best possible therapeutic maneuver from the least to the more invasive approaches. It is important in the initial assessment to perform a conduitogram and a computed tomography (CT) scan in conjunction with a conduitoscopy. With this investigative triad, one can assess free reflux to rule out obstruction; renal function can be assessed; recurrent cancer may be excluded, and if seen, may be biopsied simultaneously; and the stricture can be better localized and its length defined. In patients with impaired renal function, magnetic resonance urography may be indicated in place of the CT scan. It should be noted that although reflux on a conduitogram excludes significant stenosis, its absence does not always mean obstruction.[17] De novo carcinomas at the anastomotic site have been reported and must be excluded in stricture cases.[24]

The stricture may be treated either endoscopically or through open surgical reconstruction. Many endoscopic approaches have been described, including balloon dilation, cold-knife incision, diathermy incision, holmium:YAG laser stricturotomy, and ureteral endoluminal stenting.[23,25–28] These can be performed either retrogradely or antegradely. With antegrade laser stricturotomy, a success rate of 71% was reported after a mean follow-up of 22 months. However, its success dropped to 56% at 3 years. Although the majority of studies are small and non-randomized, it seems that for an uncomplicated stricture of short length (<1 cm) endoscopic treatment should be initially attempted in most patients.[17] Endoluminal ultrasound should be used if available to identify adjacent bowel or vascular structures. Blind incisions are not encouraged. The antegrade approach is preferred by most surgeons as the patient is left with a nephrostomy as a safety port. Longer complicated strictures should be approached initially by an open approach. Care must be taken during the dissection not to damage the conduit and the contralateral ureteroileal anastomosis.

Shortened conduit

Repeated stomal revisions due to stomal stenosis can give rise to a short conduit. Complete conduit reconstruction is often necessary. However, recent reports of augmentation of the conduit with a new isolated bowel loop, leaving the well functioning ureteroenteric anastomoses intact, have been published, in both ileal as well as colonic conduits.[29,30]

Stoma-related complications (stomal stenosis, retraction, prolapse and parastomal hernias)

Stomal-related complications may occur in 25–60% of patients, with an average time to stomal complications of 54 months.[17,20] The most common are parastomal hernias, stenosis, and recurring bleeding and skin excoriation.

Parastomal hernia

The incidence of parastomal hernia ranges from 4.5 to 15% for ileal conduit surgery.[4,17] Risk factors may include obesity, chronic raised intra-abdominal pressure, wound infection, malnourished states and suboptimal surgical technique. In patients with the above, meticulous attention is needed when constructing the stoma. The occurrence of parastomal hernia can be minimized by placing the stoma through the rectus muscle, and anchoring the conduit segment to the anterior and posterior rectus sheath. Care must be taken to ensure that all fascial layers are aligned when making the stoma and that the entire fascial opening is within the rectus sheath. The portion of the conduit that traverses the rectus muscle should be anchored to the cruciated fascial edge by a generous four-point fixation. It is the author's preference not to remove the core of subcutaneous fat together with the skin when creating the stomal opening.

Surgery for parastomal hernia is often complicated and is associated with significant morbidity such as recurrent hernia. However, parastomal hernias often enlarge if not treated, hence earlier surgical treatment should be considered in the symptomatic patient if it is interfering with quality of life. Surgical repair may be performed via an open, or more recently, laparoscopic approach. The reconstruction may involve relocating the stoma to a new site via an open approach, or taking down the herniated contents, then repairing the fascial defect with or without mesh, which can be performed open or laparoscopically. As parastomal hernia is often associated with incisional hernia, the laparoscopic approach may offer the advantage of correcting two conditions simultaneously (SB Chew, personal communication, 2004).

Stomal stenosis and retraction

Stomal stenosis is reported to occur in 3–20% of patients undergoing a conduit diversion.[17,31] Possible causes include vascular insufficiency, constriction at the rectus sheath, stomal retraction, alkaline urine, poor-fitting stomal appliance with repeated leakage causing skin excoriations and hyperkeratosis, and rarely secondary to recurrent inflammation from inflammatory bowel disease. The stenosis may be clinically obvious with a narrow stomal meatus. It can be as small as a pinhead in severe cases. More subtle cases may be diagnosed by attempting to calibrate it by passing a catheter. Conduitography may demonstrate proximal conduit dilatation, tortuosity, or hydroureteronephrosis. Patients may present with reduced urine output, flank pain, urosepsis or renal failure.

Prophylaxis against stomal stenosis include careful harvesting of the conduit, especially its blood supply, obtaining an adequate fascial opening by making a cruciate incision on the rectus sheath (the author prefers not to excise part of the sheath or the subcutaneous fat to minimize the risk of parastomal hernia), and ensuring a spouting and generously everted mucosal nipple so that urine is directly emitted into the bag rather than trickling into it via skin contact. The opening on the bag should just exceed the diameter of the stoma to minimize urine–skin contact. Persistent alkaline urine may cause stomal encrustation and epithelialization with subsequent stomal stenosis.[32] Management consists of vitamin C 500 mg four times daily or 0.25% acetic acid washes twice daily. If there is significant stomal stenosis with retraction, early revision with excision of the hyperkeratotic skin is recommended.[17]

Stomal retraction is a nuisance to the patient, the urologist, as well as the stomal therapist. It may be avoided by anchoring the conduit onto the rectus fascial opening by interrupted absorbable sutures, and by generously everting the distal end so it protrudes approximately 2 cm from the skin.

Although a single revision may suffice, some require multiple revisions.[33] There are several techniques for reconstructing a stenosed or retracted stoma. The simplest approach is distal stomal amputation. The distal conduit end needs to be carefully mobilized, avoiding the mesenteric vessels. Then the end is resected together with the surrounding indurated skin, and a new stoma is fashioned. Another approach, more suitable for a longer stenotic segment, is the skin inlay reconstruction. The stenotic ring is longitudinally incised and spatulated, and an adjacent inverted triangular skin flap is harvested and sutured onto the spatulated stoma with interrupted absorbable sutures. A 14-Fr or 16-Fr catheter is then placed across the new stomal meatus for maturation to take place. For severe cases of stomal stenosis involving significant length of the conduit, complete reconstruction of a new conduit may be required. The very proximal healthy segment harboring the ureteroileal anastomoses may be spared and the stenosed distal segment excised. This shortened segment can then be augmented by a new loop of ileum and brought out as a stoma.[30]

Calculi, malignancy and miscellaneous issues

The incidence of calculi in ileal conduits ranges from 8 to 20%.[17,22,34] Both calcium as well as struvite lithiasis can occur. The stones may be in the upper tracts or in the conduit itself. Upper tract calculi are usually managed in a similar way as in patients without conduit, except that extracorporeal shockwave lithotripsy (ESWL) is preferred over ureteroscopy as retrograde instrumentation may be difficult and tedious, and at times impossible. Stone clearance up to 95% has been reported with ESWL.[35] Percutaneous nephrolithotomy combined with ESWL is preferred for larger stones and has stone clearance rates of up to 100%. Open ureterolithotomy may be indicated for a selected few patients with large impacted ureteric calculi. Any underlying metabolic abnormality should be looked for and treated to prevent further stone episodes. Intraoperatively, attention should be paid to exclude or remove any metallic staples that are exposed at the mucosal surface as calculus has a predilection to form on these foreign niduses.

Presently, data regarding the incidence of malignancies in urinary conduits are lacking. Adenocarcinomas have been reported to occur in ileal and colonic conduits and transitional cell carcinomas in ileal conduits.[36–38] The etiology of carcinogenesis is unclear, but may include chronic urine infection, nitrosamines, prolonged contact of carcinogens with intestinal mucosa, and oxygen-free radicals. Due to lack of solid data, close monitoring during follow-up is suggested with intravenous pylogram, cytology and conduitoscopy.

Of those patients in whom the bladder is left in place, a significant number experience morbidities: pyocystis (67%), hemorrahge (23%), chronic pelvic pain (13%) and sensation of incomplete emptying and spasm (17%).[39] These complications resulting in emergency hospital admission amount to almost 45%, and 13% required cystectomy for symptom control. Hence, specific consideration should be given to primary cystectomy at time of supravesical diversion, particularly in the presence of outflow obstruction. In situations where the bladder is spared, monthly irrigation with normal saline or neomycin solution may be indicated to reduce the incidence of pyocystis.

Conclusion

Overall, provided patients are given adequate information before obtaining informed consent and counseled appropriately both pre- and postoperatively, up to 80% do not experience a reduction in their preoperative activity following ileal conduit diversion.[40–42] Nordstrom and colleagues found that almost 80% of employed patients returned to work after surgery.[43] The ileal conduit had stood the test of time and is the current gold standard urinary diversion with which new diversion approaches need to be compared. However, the reconstructive urologist needs to be familiar with its complications and can develop proficiency by close surveillance and management of these problems when they arise.

References

1. Bricker E. Bladder substitution after pelvic evisceration. Surg Clin North Am. 1950; 30: 151.
2. Husmann DA, Spence HM. Current status of tumor of the bowel following ureterosigmoidostomy: a review. J Urol 1990; 144: 607–10.
3. Turner WH, Bitton A, Studer UE. Reconstruction of the urinary tract after radical cystectomy: the case for continent urinary diversion [Editorial]. Urology 1997; 49: 663–7.
4. Madersbacher S, Schmidt J, Eberle JM et al. Long-term outcome of ileal conduit diversion. J Urol 2003; 169: 985–90.
5. Tarhan S, Moffitt EA, Taylor WF et al. Myocardial infarction after general anaesthesia. Anesth Analg 1977; 56: 455–61.
6. Walser EM, Kopecky KK, Rowland R. Diffuse ileal conduit stenosis from Crohn's Disease. Urol Radiol 1990; 12: 160–2.
7. McLaughlin TC. Crohn's disease developing in an ileal conduit. J Urol 1981; 125: 420–1.
8. McDougal WS. Metabolic complications of urinary intestinal diversion. J Urol 1992; 147: 1199–208.
9. Fontaine E, Barthelemy Y, Houlgatte A et al. Twenty-year experience with jejunal conduits. Urology 1997; 50: 207–13.
10. Jahnson S, Pedersen J. Cystectomy and urinary diversion during twenty years – complications and metabolic complications. Eur Urol 1993; 24: 343–9.
11. Singh G, Wilkinson JM, Thomas DG. Supravesical diversion for incontinence: a long-term follow-up. Br J Urol 1997; 79: 348–53.
12. Morales P, Golimbu M. Colonic urinary diversion: 10 years of experience. J Urol 1975; 113: 302–7.
13. Ehrlich R. Ileal conduit. J Urol 1973; 109: 994.
14. Boemers TM. Mitrofanoff procedure using Meckel's diverticulum. BJU Int 2001; 88: 799–800.
15. Hinman F Jr. Kidney, ureter and adrenal gland. In: Atlas of Urosurgical Anatomy. 1st edn. Philadelphia: WB Saunders, 1993: 287.
16. Wallace D. Ureteroileostomy. Br J Urol 1970; 42: 529–34.
17. Gitlin J, Taneja SS. Complications of conduit urinary diversion. In: Taneja SS, Smith RB, Ehrlich RM (eds). Complications of Urologic Surgery – Prevention and Management. 3rd edn. Philadelphia: WB Saunders, 2001: 437–53.
18. Bricker EM. The evolution of the ileal segment bladder substitution operation. Am J Surg 1978; 135: 834–41.
19. Klein EA, Montie JE, Montague DK et al. Stomal complications of intestinal conduit urinary diversion. Cleve Clin J Med 1989; 56: 48–52.
20. Cheung MT. Complications of an abdominal stoma: an analysis of 322 stomas. Aust N Z J Surg 1995; 65: 808–11.
21. Williams O, Vereb MJ, Libertino JA. Noncontinent urinary diversion. Urol Clin North Am 1997; 24: 735.
22. Sullivan JW, Grabstald H, Whitmore WF Jr. Complications of ureteroileal conduit with radical cystectomy: review of 336 cases. J Urol 1980; 124: 797–801.
23. Palascak P, Bouchareb M, Zachoval R et al. Treatment of benign ureterointestinal anastomotic strictures with permanent ureteral wallstent after Camey and Wallace urinary diversion: long-term follow-up. J Endourol 2001; 15: 575–80.
24. Filmer RB, Spencer JR. Malignancies in bladder augmentations and intestinal conduits. J Urol 1990; 143: 671–8.
25. Kramolowsky EV, Clayman RV. Advances in endosurgery. Treatment of ureteral-enteric anastomotic strictures. Urol Clin North Am. 1988; 15: 413–18.
26. Shapiro MJ, Banner MP, Amendola MA et al. Balloon dilation of uretroenteric strictures: long-term results. Radiology 1988; 168: 385–7.
27. Wolf JS Jr, Elashry OM, Clayman RV. Long-term results of

endoureterotomy for benign ureteral and ureteroenteric strictures. J Urol 1997; 158: 759–64.

28. Watterson JD, Sofer M, Wollin TA et al. Holmium: YAG laser endoureterotomy for ureterointestinal strictures. J Urol 2003; 167: 1692–5.
29. Kirby RS, Baltitude MI, Lloyd-Davies RW. Isolated ileal loop augmentation of existing ileal conduit. Br J Urol 1983; 55: 183–4.
30. Ramon J, Goldwasser B, Nativ O et al. Augmentation of existing ileal and colonic conduits and stomal revision. Isr J Med Sci 1990; 26: 395–8.
31. Frazier HA, Robertson JE, Paulson DF. Complications of radical cystectomy and urinary diversion: a retrospective review of 675 cases in 2 decades. J Urol 1992; 148: 1401–5.
32. Wood DP Jr, Spencer M, Hocevar BJ et al. Office management of urinary stomas. Urol Clin North Am 1988; 15: 753–67.
33. Redman JF. Techniques to enhance the ileal conduit. Urol Clin North Am 1990; 17: 125–9.
34. Engel EM. Complications of bilateral uretero-ileal cutaneous diversion: a review of 208 cases. J Urol 1969; 101: 508–12.
35. Cohen TD, Streem SB. Minimally invasive endourologic management of calculi in continent urinary resovoirs. Urology. 1994; 43: 865–8.
36. Sakano S, Yoghihiro S, Joko K et al. Adenocarcinoma developing in an ileal conduit. J Urol 1995; 153: 146–8.
37. Ng FC, Woodhouse CR, Parkinson MC. Adenocarcinoma in an ileal conduit. Br J Urol 1996; 77: 321–2.
38. Mulholland C, McCallion WA, Biggart JD et al. Transitional cell carcinoma in an ileal conduit. Br J Urol 1993; 71: 618–19.
39. Lynch TH, Fitzpatrick JM. Non-continent urinary diversion. In: Colleen S, Mansson W (eds). Reconstructive Surgery of the Lower Genito-urinary Tract in Adults. 1st edn. Oxford: Isis Medical Media, 1995: 73–91.
40. Babaian RJ, Smith DB. Effect of ileal conduit on patients' activities following radical cystectomy. Urology. 1991; 37: 33–5.
41. Fossa SD, Reitan JB, Ous S et al. Life with an ileal conduit in cystectomised bladder patients: expectations and experience. Scand J Urol Nephrol 1987; 21: 97–102.
42. Hautmann RE. Trouble shooting. In: Hohenfellner R, Wammack R (eds). Societe Internationale D'urologie (SIU) Reports – Continent Urinary Diversion. 1st edn. New York: Churchill Livingstone, 1992: 279–83.
43. Nordstrom GM, Nyman CR, Theorell T. The impact on work ability of ileal conduit urinary diversion. Scand J Soc Med 1990; 18: 115–24.

39 Laparoscopic bladder augmentation and urinary diversion

Raymond R Rackley, Joseph B Abdelmalak, Ahmed S El-Azab, Sandip P Vasavada and Inderbir S Gill

Laparoscopic augmentation

Augmentation cystoplasty remains the most widely accepted reconstructive technique for creating a compliant, large capacity bladder that protects the upper urinary tract and provides urinary continence in people with bladder dysfunction secondary to non-compliance or reduced functional capacity.[1–4] This form of bladder reconstruction may even be combined with a continent catheterizable stoma for use as an accessible port for bladder emptying. In 1888, Tizzoni and Poggi demonstrated the feasibility of performing ileocystoplasty in a canine model. Ten years later, Mickulicz performed the first clinical ileocystoplasty.[5] Since that time, the standard enterocystoplasty has classically evolved as a procedure performed through an open laparotomy incision utilizing various segments of well-vascularized segments of the gastrointestinal system that are reconfigured before anastomosis with the urinary bladder.[6] One hundred years have passed since the original open approach for this procedure has become an established reconstructive technique performed laparoscopically. No matter what approach is chosen, the use of any bowel segment for augmentation is associated with advantages and disadvantages, but the versatility of choosing a particular bowel segment, for both open and laparoscopic approaches, provides a variety of clinical options based on an individualized set of objectives for the person requiring this form of bladder reconstruction.

Enterocystoplasty is effective in providing a durable increase in bladder capacity and compliance; however, the morbidity and postoperative discomfort associated with the open laparotomy incision are a major deterrent. For patients with pre-existing debilitating neurologic and other comorbid conditions, the open procedure may significantly prolong the hospital stay, increase the metabolic needs for wound healing, and delay postoperative recovery. Laparoscopy has distinct advantages when compared with open surgical procedures with regard to postoperative pain and morbidity, improved cosmetics, and a shorter hospital stay and decreased convalescence period. Recent studies have indicated that postoperative intra-abdominal adhesions are significantly reduced after laparoscopic surgery when compared with open surgery.[7]

Despite the established role of laparoscopy in diagnostic and ablative urologic surgery, the use of laparoscopic techniques in reconstruction has been limited because of the technical complexity of the procedures involved. The technical steps in performing a laparoscopic bladder augmentation are designed to emulate the open surgical counterpart in every aspect, thereby producing similar functional results with improved recovery.

Indications and patient selection

The goal of augmentation cystoplasty is to restore the compliant storage properties of the urinary bladder. Non-compliant, small capacity bladders that typically do not respond to more conservative forms of treatment can be surgically augmented. Interruption of the bladder musculature and the use of bowel to patch the resultant defect may decrease efficiency of the spontaneous voiding mechanism. People with neurological causes of bladder dysfunction will require clean intermittent catheterization for prolonged or indefinite periods postoperatively to empty the bladder effectively. People with physical disabilities or limitations due to neurologic conditions may be unable to catheterize themselves via the urethra and a continent catheterizable abdominal stoma should be considered in addition to bladder augmentation. A relative contraindication specific to laparoscopic bladder augmentation is the presence of extensive intra-abdominal and pelvic adhesions that would preclude laparoscopic bowel dissection. Our experience in open and laparoscopic approaches for this procedure suggests that people with ventriculoperitoneal shunts typically have increased abdominal adhesions that may preclude a successful laparoscopic approach.

Routine laboratory studies include renal function and serum electrolytes, whole blood cell count, urinalysis, and when appropriate, a urine culture. Upper and lower urinary tract studies are important baseline evaluations. A urodynamic study and cystoscopy will provide additional useful information about the competence of the urinary sphincter.

Preparation of the patient

Mechanical and antibiotic bowel preparation includes a clear liquid diet for 2 days before the operation, a bowel preparation the day before the operation, preoperative antibiotics for bowel and urinary tract surgical prophylaxis, and antifungal medication when indicated. Many patients with neurological diseases have chronic constipation and may need more time for an adequate bowel preparation.

The patient is placed in the supine position and pneumatic compression stockings are applied to both legs. After induction with general anesthesia and endotracheal intubation, an oral gastric tube is inserted, and the patient is placed in the low-lithotomy position for the remainder of the operation. Both arms are tucked and protected along the sides so that the surgical team may direct their operative movements deep into the pelvis. In our early experience, we performed cystoscopy and inserted internal-external ureteral stents (70Fr, 90 cm, Circon Surgitek, Santa Barbara, CA) into the renal pelvis for intraoperative and postoperative drainage. The straight ends of the stents remained outside the external urethral meatus and were secured to a urethral catheter in order to provide maximal drainage of urine from the operative field during the procedure. Currently, we do not use ureteral stents and can acheive effective intraoperative urine and pelvic fluid drainage by intermittently opening the urethral catheter to preserve the pneumoperitoneum. The internal-external ureteral stents that pass through the urethra and subsequently into the urethral catheter also prevent effective bladder irrigation of potential blood clots and bowel mucus in the intraoperative and postoperative period by precluding an adequate seal of the bladder neck and urethra around the urethral catheter.

Surgical technique

For laparoscopic or open approaches the surgical technique of enterocystoplasty is based on the following fundamentals: (i) selection of an optimal segment of bowel based on a broad, well-vascularized mesenteric pedicle, (ii) isolation of the bowel segment, (iii) re-establishment of bowel continuity and closure of the mesenteric defect, (iv) detubularization and reconfiguration of the bowel segment without peritoneal soiling of bowel contents, (v) bladder mobilization with formation of an adequate sized cystotomy, (vi) creation of a tension-free, watertight, full-thickness, circumferential anastomosis of the bowel to the bladder, and (vii) confirmation of adequate postoperative urinary drainage.

An incision is made at the inferior umbilical crease and a disposable 10-mm port with occluding balloon and cuff is introduced under direct vision into the peritoneal cavity at the superior umbilical crease. A 10-mm 0-degree laparoscope is introduced and the subsequent reusable ports are introduced under visual guidance. The 10- and 5-mm ports are inserted bilaterally at the lateral borders of the rectus muscle at the level of the umbilicus (Figure 39.1). Most of the operative suturing takes place via the two paraumbilical ports. The 10-mm port not only facilitates the introduction of sutures on large needles, but also may be useful for extracorporeal knot tying. An additional 5-mm port is inserted at the level of the anterior superior iliac spines. Other ports may be placed depending on the bowel mobilization required and surgeon's preference.

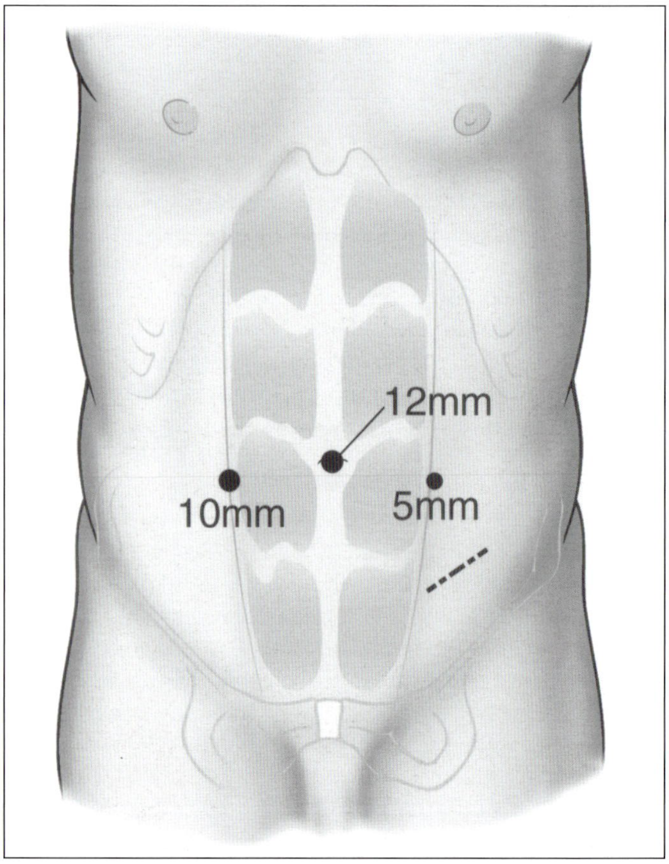

Figure 39.1 Selection of port sizes and location for laparoscopic enterocystoplasty procedures. (Reprinted with the permission of The Cleveland Clinic Foundation.)

Selection and mobilization of the bowel segment

As is true in open enterocystoplasty, various segments of the gastrointestinal system may be used for the procedure depending on the clinical requirements of the patient. A length of 20 cm of bowel is usually desirable to attain an adequate augmented bladder capacity. An appropriate segment of bowel is identified based on the following criteria: (i) the bowel segment will reach the area of the bladder neck without tension, and (ii) a well-defined arterial arcade should be present in the bowel mesentery.

In laparoscopic ileocystoplasty, the initial step is identification of the ileocecal junction. With the use of 5-mm laparoscopic small bowel clamps, a 20-cm segment of ileum at least 15 cm proximal to the ileocecal junction is identified. A 5-mm laparoscope may be introduced through the lower left port to transilluminate the mesentery and identify its vascular pedicle. The mesentery adjacent to the proximal and distal ends of the selected bowel loop is scored with laparoscopic electrosurgical scissors for subsequent extracorporeal identification.

In laparoscopic sigmoidocystoplasty, a loop of sigmoid colon is selected using similar techniques. Many patients with neurogenic bladder dysfunction also have defecating dysfunction resulting in a redundant sigmoid colon. In patients who can easily perform intermittent catheterization via the urethra, the sigmoid colon may be the preferred segment of bowel for harvesting if a continent catheterizable stoma formation is not required. Extracorporeal manipulation of the sigmoid is achieved via extension of the left lower abdominal port defect (Figure 39.2).

The right colon and terminal ileum are selected in patients who in addition to bladder augmentation require a continent catheterizable abdominal stoma in addition to bladder augmentation. The cecum and ascending colon are used for the bladder augmentation, and 10 cm of terminal ileum is used to create the catheterizable conduit and stoma at the umbilicus. The peritoneum lateral to the cecum and ascending colon and the peritoneum of the terminal aspect of the Z line are incised and the entire right colon and terminal ileum are mobilized for extracorporeal manipulation via the extended incision of the umbilical port. Ensuring a low position of the patient's thighs via the low-lithotomy position enables proper manipulation of the laparoscopic instruments through the lower abdominal ports for mobilization of the right colonic flexure.

Exclusion and reanastomosis of the bowel

Following mobilization of the bowel for extracorporeal manipulation, the pneumoperitoneum is desufflated and the umbilical port removed. The umbilical incision is enlarged circumumbilically and extended inferiorly in obese patients for an additional 2 cm. The preselected loop of bowel is

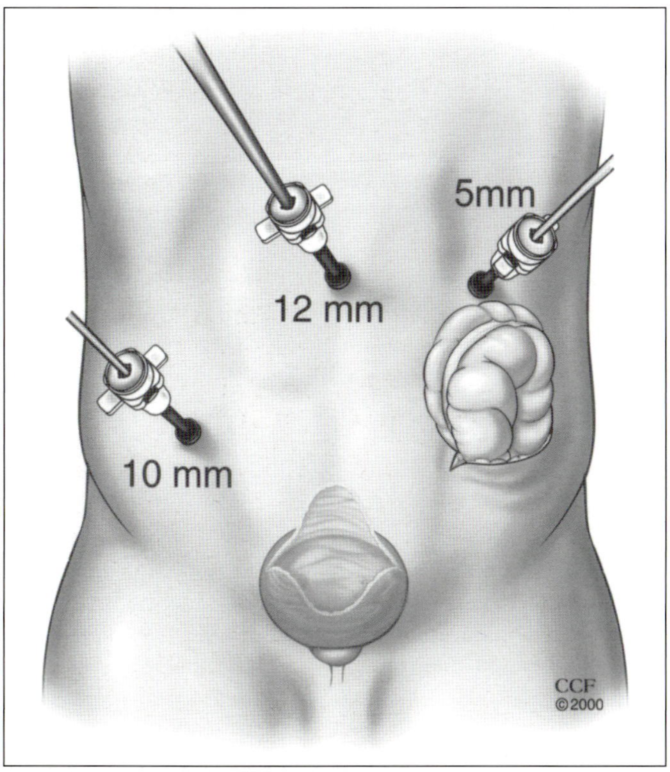

Figure 39.2 Selection of port sizes and location for laparoscopic sigmoidocystoplasty. (Reprinted with the permission of The Cleveland Clinic Foundation.)

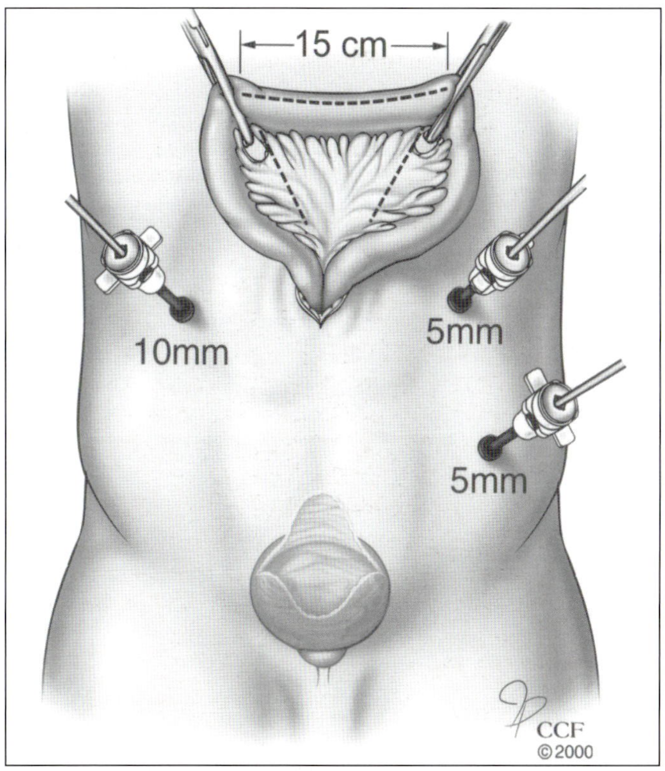

Figure 39.3 Extracorporeal isolation and manipulation of the small bowel via the umbilical port site. (Reprinted with the permission of The Cleveland Clinic Foundation.)

delivered outside the abdomen through this incision. Care is taken to prevent any twisting of the mesenteric pedicle and to ensure proper proximal–distal orientation of the loop. Using traditional open surgical techniques, the 20-cm bowel segment with its pedicle is divided between bowel clamps and isolated as in ileocystoplasty (Figure 39.3). Bowel continuity is re-established using traditional open techniques and the mesenteric window is closed. The bowel anastomosis is performed cephalad to the excluded segment of bowel and the reanastomosed bowel is returned to the abdominal cavity before any further manipulation. This step reduces the potential need to enlarge the circumumbilical incision for reintroduction of an edematous combination of both the bowel reanastomosis and the reconfigured bowel segment for augmentation.

Refashioning of the isolated bowel segment

The excluded bowel segment is draped in moist warm sponges and then irrigated thoroughly with normal saline until the returning irrigation is clear. The antimesenteric border of the bowel is incised using electrocautery. For the small bowel or sigmoid, a U-shaped plate is created by a side-to-side anastomosis with a 2-0 absorbable suture (Figure 39.4). After the isolated bowel segment for augmentation is reintroduced into the peritoneal cavity, the ports are replaced to re-establish the pneumoperitoneum. In ileocystoplasty, reintroducing a disposable

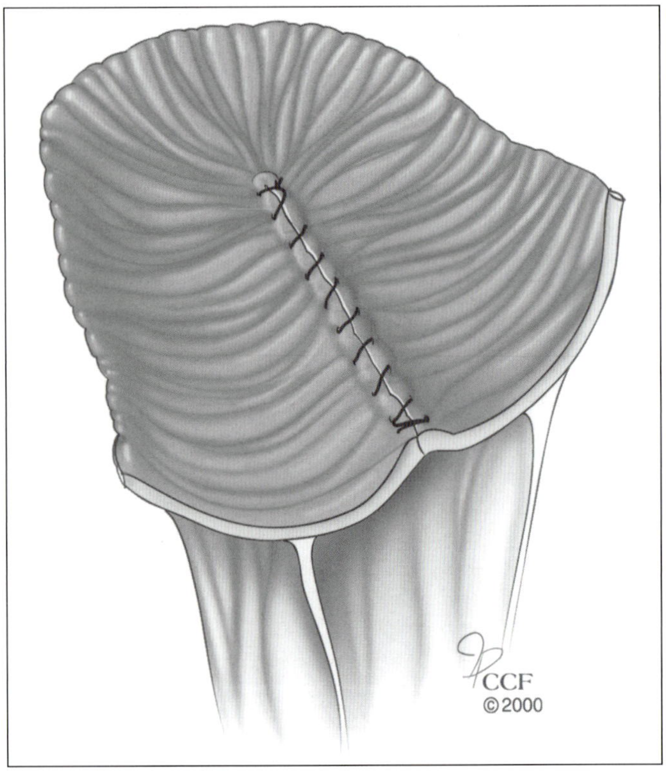

Figure 39.4 Detubularization and reconfiguration of the isolated bowel segment. (Reprinted with the permission of The Cleveland Clinic Foundation.)

10-mm blunt-tip port with a fascial retention balloon and foam cuff to minimize gas leakage is appreciated. In sigmoidocystoplasty, the extended left lower abdominal port incision is reduced to accommodate a 5-mm port. The pneumoperitoneum is then re-established and the laparoscope inserted. The isolated bowel segment is oriented appropriately and inspected to exclude torsion of the pedicle.

For patients requiring a catheterizable stoma, the right colon and terminal ileum are utilized. Following detubularization of the cecum and proximal colon, an appendectomy is performed. The terminal ileum is narrowed over a a 16-Fr red rubber catheter using a gastrointestinal anastomosis stapling device (GIA stapler), and the ileocecal junction is imbricated and intussuscepted to augment the continence mechanism of the ileocecal valve using 2-0 permanent sutures (Figure 39.5). Orientation sutures are placed at the cephalic ends of the bowel patch to facilitate intracorporeal laparoscopic identification and manipulation. The 16-Fr red rubber catheter is secured to the terminal end of the catheterizable segment of ileum with a suture for atraumatic intracorporeal manipulation and for delivering this terminal segment to the umbilicus for stoma maturation at the end of the procedure. The isolated bowel patch is then returned to the abdominal cavity and the infraumbilical incision is closed over a 10-mm blunt-tip port with a fascial retention balloon and foam cuff to minimize gas leakage for the remainder of the operation. After the pneumoperitoneum is re-established and the laparoscope inserted, the isolated bowel segment is oriented appropriately and inspected to rule out torsion of the pedicle.

Exclusion of the bowel segment and subsequent restoration of bowel continuity can be performed intracorporeally using Endo-GIA staplers and is thought to reduce any theoretical complications from undue tension placed on the bowel mesentery during the extracorporeal manipulation of the bowel in obese patients. We have not experienced any complications related to this proposed concern during our use of this maneuver in obese patients. We prefer to perform these manipulations extracorporeally by delivering the bowel outside the abdomen through the umbilical or lower abdominal port site respectively for the following reasons: (i) the bowel segment can be measured precisely and the mesentery incised after ensuring good vascularity, (ii) the bowel may be reanastomosed meticulously using open surgical techniques with increased confidence; (iii) the excluded loop may be irrigated without any peritoneal spillage, thereby eliminating the potential for subsequent pelvic abscess formation; (iv) the detubularization and desired modification of the isolated loop can be performed expeditiously by traditional open suturing; (v) if the mesenteric length allows the segment to be delivered outside the anterior abdominal wall comfortably without evidence of bowel ischemia, it is also likely to reach the bladder without tension; and (vi) the extracorporeal approach allows considerable savings in overall operative time and cost.

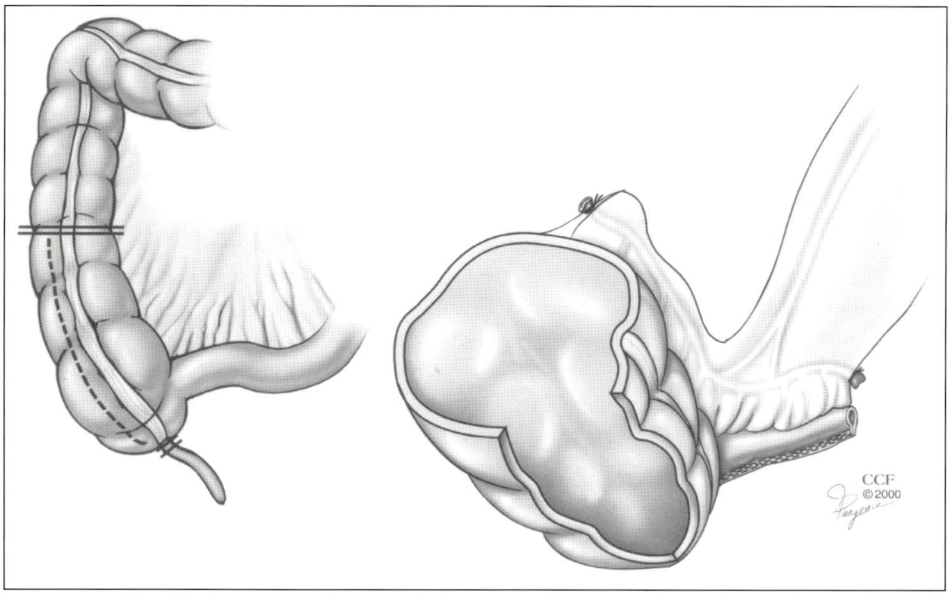

Figure 39.5 Detubularization and reconfiguration of the right colon and ileum for cecocolocystoplasty in preparation for formation of a catheterizable stoma. (Reprinted with the permission of The Cleveland Clinic Foundation.)

Bladder mobilization and cystotomy

Placing the patient in the Trendelenberg position aids in displacement of the bowel loops from the pelvic cavity and facilitates the subsequent steps of the procedure. The bladder is distended with saline through the urethral catheter. The peritoneum overlying the bladder is incised at the medial border of the left medial umbilical ligament and extended to the right in a linear fashion to the right medial umbilical ligament. The median umbilical ligament is taken down during the procedure using electrosurgical scissors. If needed, the lateral peritoneum incisions are extended down along the medial umbilical ligaments to increase exposure. The loose areolar tissue surrounding the bladder is bluntly dissected to expose the anterior bladder neck and perivesical spaces. A large cystostomy is created by making an anterior bladder wall flap through a curvilinear incision that positions the apex at the dome of the bladder and the base extending to the level approaching the trigone (see Figures 39.2 and 39.3). This type of cystostomy ensures a large dysfunctional disruption of the bladder musculature for increasing the linear length of bladder wall for bowel anastomosis. It is most useful in cases where the uterus is present and potentially prevents an adequate cystostomy incision. Furthermore, adequate exposure for enterovesical anastomosis in all of the procedures described previously is preserved by avoiding a closure of the deep posterior bladder wall incision in the pelvis that will be obscured by bowel and the isolated bowel segment to be used for the augmentation.

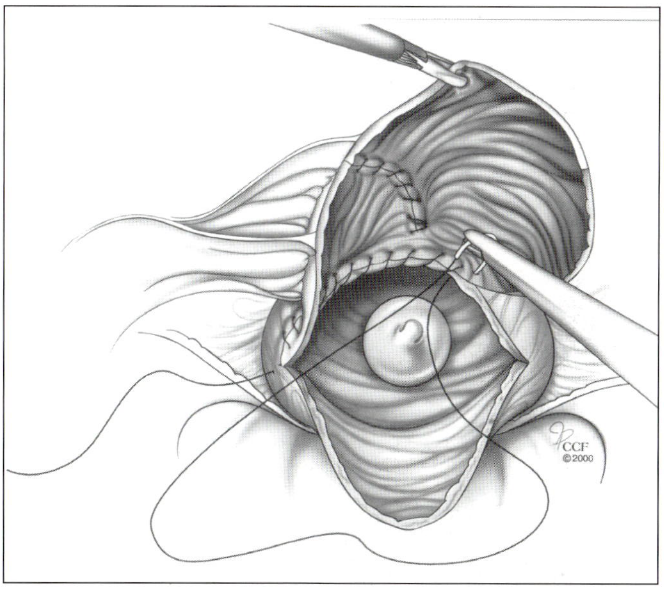

Figure 39.6 Intracorporeal suturing of the isolated bowel segment to the bladder. Point A is at the apical aspect of the newly formed bladder flap that was derived from the anterior aspect of the bladder wall near the bladder neck. (Reprinted with the permission of The Cleveland Clinic Foundation.)

Enterovesical anastomosis

Although different approaches can be used for intracorporeal suturing of the bowel segment to the bladder as shown in Figure 39.6, we prefer to begin by running the pre-placed suture on the 'posterior' wall of the reconfigured bowel patch to the apical aspect of the bladder flap in a medial to lateral direction on each side. Completion of the 'posterior' wall of the reconfigured bowel segment from an intravesical approach beginning medially (point A) and finishing laterally (points B and C, respectively) facilitates the best exposure to ensure a watertight anastamosis. If one attempts to complete the 'anterior' wall of the reconfigured bowel patch to the bladder first as shown in Figure 39.6, it may be difficult to visualize the suturing of the 'posterior'

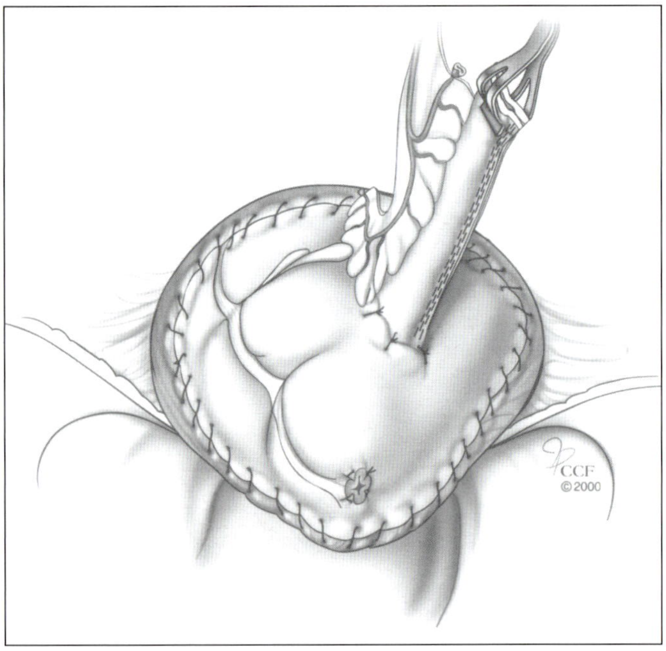

Figure 39.7 View of the completed bowel-to-bladder anastomosis in preparation for maturation of the catheterizable stoma to the umbilicus. (Reprinted with the permission of The Cleveland Clinic Foundation.)

wall anastomosis to the bladder owing to the constraints of the pelvic anatomy.

To complete a circumferential, continuous, full-thickness, single-layer anastomosis of the bowel to the bladder, we finish by running the pre-placed sutures of the 'anterior' wall of the reconfigured bowel patch and additional sutures as required (Figure 39.7). Free hand laparoscopic suturing and intracorporeal knot tying techniques are used exclusively for the entire suturing. Exposure of the operative field for intracorporeal suturing can be improved by temporarily fixing the anterior bladder flap to the rectus fascia. This not only opens the operative suturing field for easier identification of the bladder and bowel mucosal edges, but also stabilizes the tissues for rapid suture placement. At the completion of the anastomosis, the bladder is distended to confirm a watertight anastomosis. A Jackson-Pratt drain is inserted into the pelvic cavity through one of the lower lateral 5-mm port sites. Postoperative bladder drainage is maintained with a 22- or 24-Fr urethral catheter. Because a smaller urethral catheter may be preferred for postoperative drainage in males, a suprapubic tube may be placed through the bladder wall and externalized via the remaining lower port site. The umbilical and remaining 10-mm ports are closed in layers.

In patients who require a catheterizable stoma, the previously refashioned ileal segment is located and the attached red rubber catheter is grasped with an endoscopic clamp via the umbilical port site. After the pneumoperitoneum is decompressed, the terminal end of the ileal segment is delivered to the umbilicus and secured to the anterior rectus fascia and skin at the level of the umbilicus. A Y-V flap maturation of the stoma to the skin of the umbilicus is performed using 4-0 chromic sutures. In obese patients, use of the umbilicus as the site of stoma formation decreases the amount of ileum needed to mature the stoma to the skin. A 16-Fr catheter is placed through the stoma and into the bladder to optimize bladder drainage and healing of the newly created catheterizable segment in the early postoperative period.

Postoperative management

The oral-gastric decompression tube is removed before extubation. The Jackson-Pratt drain is removed when the drainage is less than 25 ml or fluid chemistries suggest peritoneal fluid. The patient can be discharged when they are afebrile and able to complete three consecutive meals without abdominal distension; the first meal is usually started on the first postoperative day. Patients are discharged with the indwelling urethral catheter used for bladder drainage and daily bladder irrigation with 100 ml of sterile saline. Low dose prophylactic antibiotics are continued during the first 3 postoperative weeks. At that time, the urinary catheter is removed and intermittent catheterization is initiated. For patients who have an indwelling catheter via the umbilical stoma, the catheter is usually capped at the time of hospital discharge, but may be used to flush the augmented bladder at the time of daily bladder irrigation.

Results

From 1999 to 2001, we performed laparoscopic enterocystoplasty in 18 patients with functionally reduced bladder capacities owing to neurogenic causes (Table 39.1). The procedures included: ileocystoplasty (n=5), sigmoidocystoplasty (n=3), colocystoplasty (n=1) and cecocolocystoplasty with a continent catheterizable ileal stoma (n=9). Total surgical time (including cystoscopy, stent placement, and extracorporeal bowel anastomosis and refashioning of the isolated loop, and laparoscopic dissection and suturing) ranged from 5.3 to 8 hours (average 7.0 hours). The time for laparoscopic suturing ranged from 1.7 to 3.1 hours (average 2.4 hours). Blood loss was minimal and did not exceed 250 ml in any of the cases (average 175 ml). The only intraoperative complication was a trocar-induced rectus sheath hematoma during the course of the sigmoidocystoplasty that was controlled laparoscopically. Oral feeding was resumed by 24 hours in 17 of 18 patients. Our first patient had a self-limited paralytic ileus that responded to conservative treatment. Although most of the study group had moderate to severe forms of neurological dysfunction owing to multiple sclerosis, the average hospital stay until the patient was discharged home was 5.7 days and ranged from 3 to 7 days. Most notable was the absence of long-term or extended care needs for the patients with multiple sclerosis because of demands of wound healing or functional neurological loss that typically occur with an open procedure in this subset of patients.

All patients gave consent to participate in a long-term outcome study using preoperative and postoperative validated